# Embryonic Development in Days

| | | | |
|---|---|---|---|
| **Day 5** Late blastocyst | **Day 6-7** Events during first week: Fertilization to implantation | 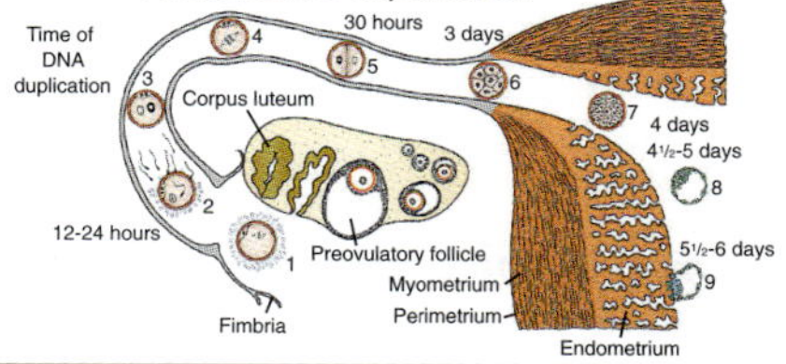 | **Development Week 1** |
| **Day 12** Extraembryonic mesoderm develops | **Day 13** Uteroplacental circulation begins | **Day 14** Embryonic disc: dorsal view | **Development Week 2** |
| **Day 19** CNS induction | **Day 20** Neurulation: Neural folds elevate | **Day 21** Transverse section through somite region | **Development Week 3** |
| **Day 26** Pharyngeal arches present | **Day 27** | **Day 28** Neurulation complete | **Development Week 4** |
| **Day 33** Umbilical ring | **Day 34** Optic cup and lens placode | **Day 35** Branchial arches and clefts | **Development Week 5** |
| **Day 40** Auricular hillocks | **Day 41** Atrial septum formed | **Day 42** Digit formation | **Development Week 6** |
| **Day 47** External genitalia | **Day 48** Facial prominences fused | **Day 49** Digits present, eyelids forming | **Development Week 7** |

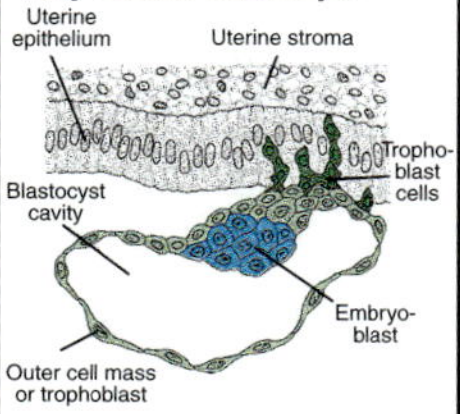

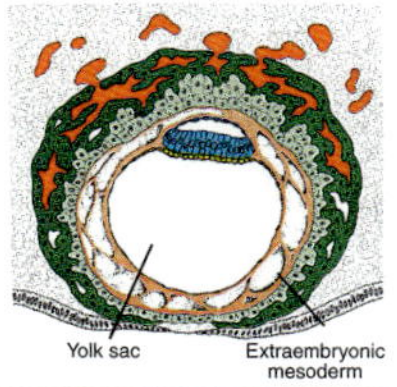

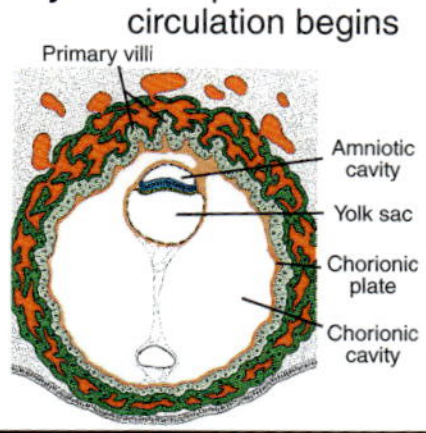

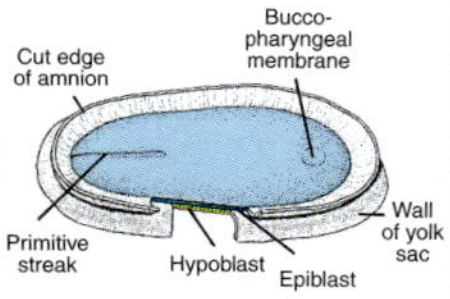

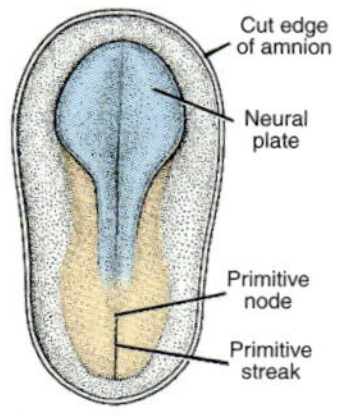

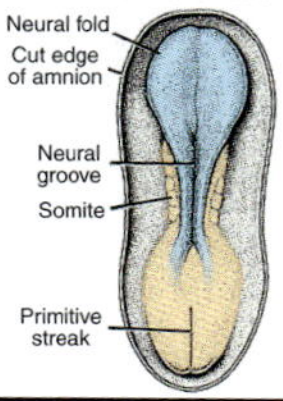

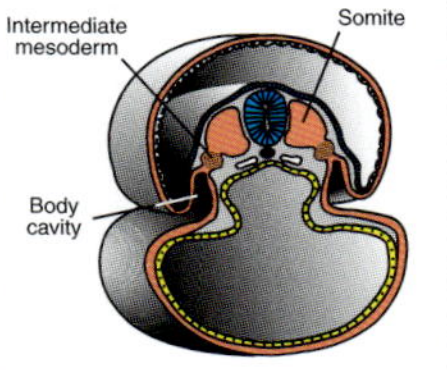

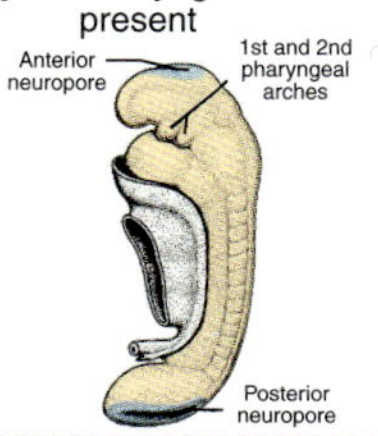

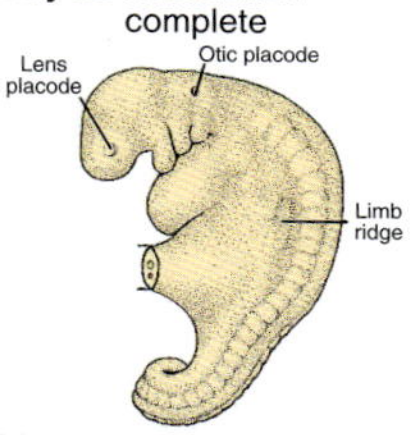

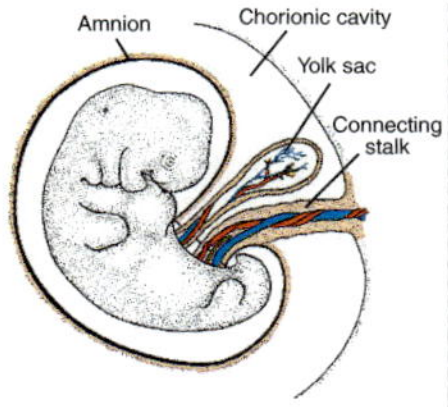

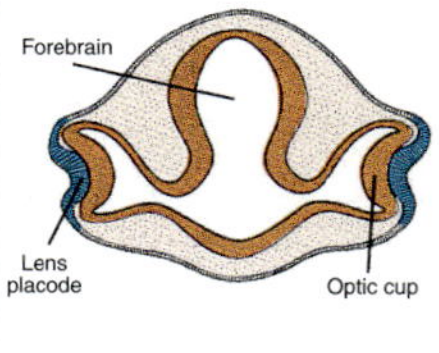

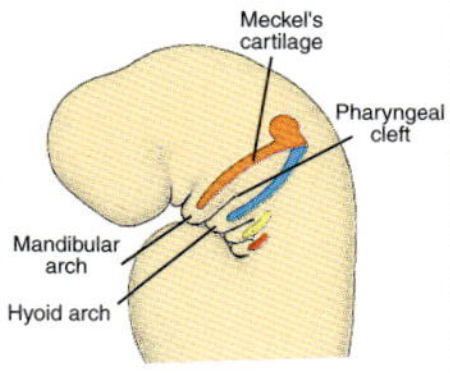

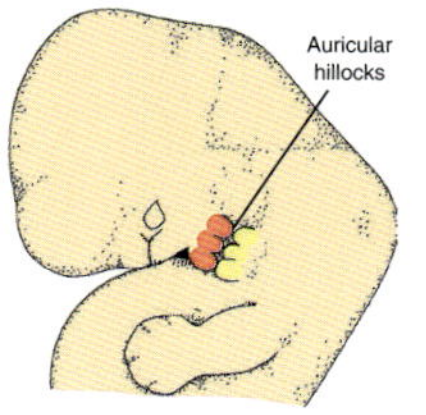

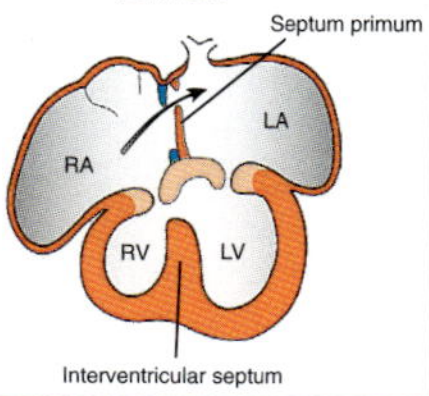

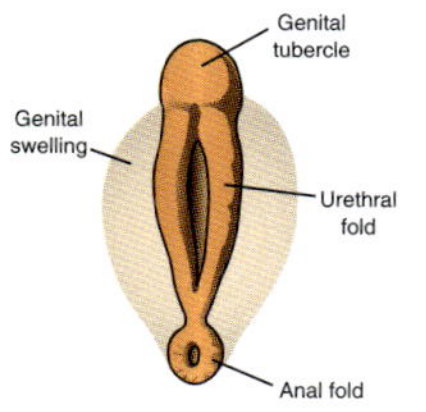

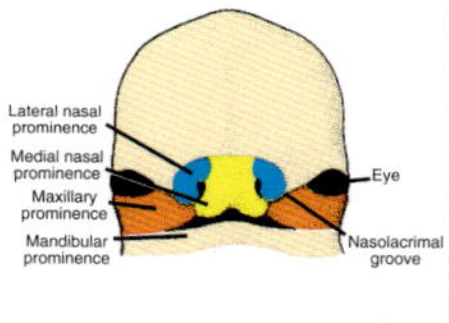

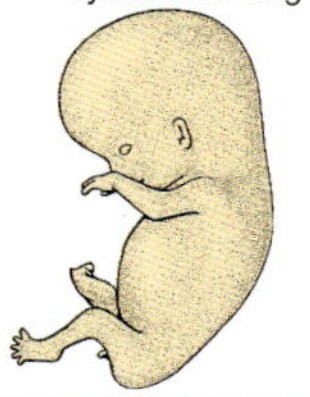

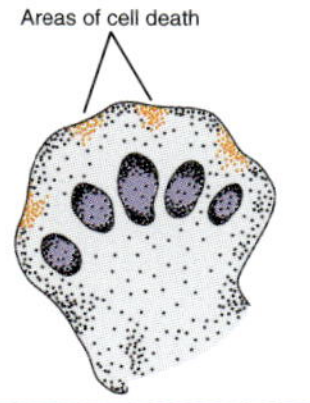

**Day 27**

| Approx. Age (Days) | No. of Somites |
|---|---|
| 20 | 1-4 |
| 21 | 4-7 |
| 22 | 7-10 |
| 23 | 10-13 |
| 24 | 13-17 |
| 25 | 17-20 |
| 26 | 20-23 |
| 27 | 23-26 |
| 28 | 26-29 |
| 30 | 34-35 |

**Placode:** **A local thickening in the embryonic ectoderm layer that develops into a sensory organ or ganglion.**

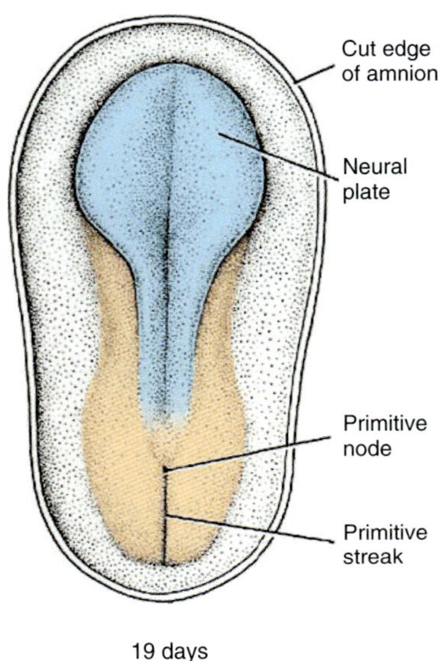

19 days

## ODE TO A PLACODE

There once was a flat sheet of cells
That were stumpy and ugly as hell;
But one day they arose, stood tall on their toes,
and declared they were the best cells of all.

Presumptuously they cried that their lineage was high
and right proudly they bragged of their codes;
But soon it was clear, they weren't like the ear
and they were nixed in their dreams as placodes.

Semantics, they screamed, please maintain our dreams,
but their pleas were unheeded and late;
And now to this day in repast they must lay
as a misconstrued, flat neural plate!

**T.W. Sadler**
*Sheridan, MT*

LANGMAN'S

# Medical Embryology

Second South Asian Edition

As per the Indian Competency-Based Medical Curriculum

# LANGMAN'S

# Medical Embryology

## Second South Asian Edition

**As per the Indian Competency-Based Medical Curriculum**

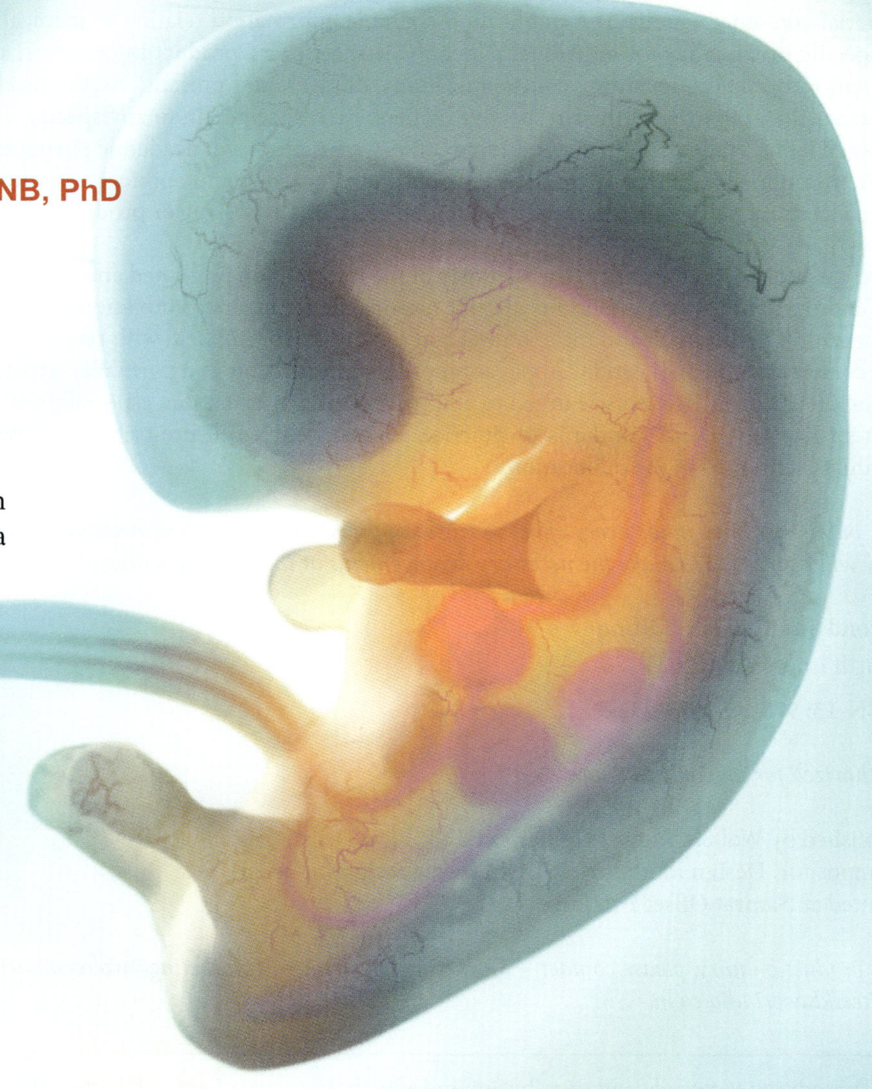

***SAE Editor***

**Sabita Mishra** MBBS, DNB, PhD
Director Professor *and* Head
Department of Anatomy
Maulana Azad Medical College
Delhi

***International Editor***

**T. W. Sadler** PhD
Consultant, Birth Defects Prevention
Sheridan, Madison County, Montana
Adjunct Professor of Pediatrics
University of Utah
Visiting Professor of Embryology
East Tennessee State University
Quillen School of Medicine
Senior Scholar
Greenwood Genetics Center
Greenwood, South Carolina

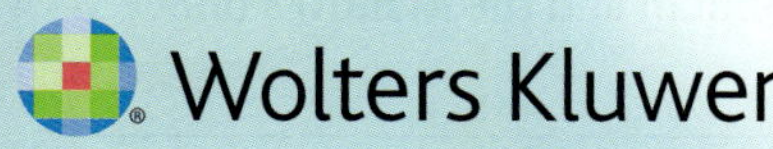

*Publishing Manager:* Ravi Vishwakarma
*Development Editor:* Dr. Satheesh Kumar
*Production Editor:* Pooja Chauhan
*Asstt Manager Manufacturing:* Sumit Johry

Copyright © 2023 by Wolters Kluwer (India) Pvt Ltd

3rd Floor, Tower B, Building No. 10, Phase II, DLF Cyber City, Gurgaon, Haryana - 122002

All rights reserved. This product, consisting of the printed book, is protected by copyright. No part of this book may be reproduced in any form or by any means, including photocopying, or utilized by any information storage and retrieval system without written permission from the copyright owner.

The publisher is not responsible (as a matter of product liability, negligence, or otherwise) for any injury resulting from any material contained herein. This publication contains information relating to medical embryology that should not be construed as specific instructions for individual patients. Manufacturers' product information and package inserts should be reviewed for current information, including contraindications, dosages, and precautions. All products/brands/names/processes cited in this book are the properties of their respective owners. Reference herein to any specific commercial products, processes, or services by trade name, trademark, manufacturer, or otherwise is purely for academic purposes and does not constitute or imply endorsement, recommendation, or favoring by the publisher. The views and opinions of authors expressed herein do not necessarily state or reflect those of the publisher, and shall not be used for advertising or product endorsement purposes.

Care has been taken to confirm the accuracy of the information presented and to describe generally accepted practices. However, the authors, editors, and publishers are not responsible for errors or omissions or for any consequences from application of the information in this book and make no warranty, expressed or implied, with respect to the currency, completeness, or accuracy of the contents of the publication. Application of this information in a particular situation remains the professional responsibility of the practitioner. Readers are urged to confirm that the information, especially with regard to drug dose/usage, complies with current legislation and standards of practice. Please consult full prescribing information before issuing prescription for any product mentioned in the publication.

*The publishers have made every effort to trace copyright holders for borrowed material. If they have inadvertently overlooked any, they will be pleased to make the necessary arrangements at the first opportunity.*

**Second South Asian Edition**
Fourth Impression, 2025
**ISBN-13:** 978-93-95736-36-7

*Authorized for sale only in South Asia*

Published by Wolters Kluwer (India) Pvt. Ltd., New Delhi
Compositor: Design Modus, New Delhi (www.designmodus.in)
Printed at: Samrat Offset Pvt. Ltd.

*For product enquiry, please contact – Marketing Department (marketing@wolterskluwerindia.co.in) or log on to our website www.wolterskluwerindia.co.in.*

This edition is for sale and distribution in India, Pakistan, Sri Lanka, Bangladesh, Nepal, Bhutan and the Maldives only. It is prohibited and illegal to distribute this edition outside of these territories.

# Preface

*Langman's Medical Embryology* has been one of the most preferred books for understanding the developmental processes of human embryo. The concepts are clearly explained and amply supported by numerous well-labeled line diagrams and enriching clinical pictures.

I have thoroughly evaluated the book vis-à-vis the new competency-based curriculum and have made modifications and additions, wherever necessary, to make the book fully meet the new standards set by the NMC. The Specific Learning Objectives given at the beginning of each chapter state the subtopics around which the newly developed embryology course is built. Competencies recommended by NMC are given at the beginning of respective chapters for better correlation of the content. The Clinical Correlates have been revisited and updated. New tables have been added in some chapters to make exam-relevant information easy to learn. In addition, the clinical aspect has been further strengthened by adding more questions and answers to "Problem Solving Questions" section at the end of each chapter to enhance the analytical ability of the students. Also, comprehensive questions and multiple-choice questions have been added in this edition to help students understand their level of preparation for the MBBS as well as NExT and other competitive PG examinations.

Eminent anatomists from all over India have contributed by making suggestions and recommendations which have been incorporated as far as possible.

## Features of the Book

To accomplish its goal of providing a basic understanding of embryology and its clinical relevance, the second South Asian edition of *Langman's Medical Embryology* retains its unique approach of combining an economy of text with excellent diagrams and clinical images. The following pedagogic features help facilitate student learning.

**Organization of Material:** This edition is organized into three parts. The first provides an overview of early development from gametogenesis through the embryonic period. Also included in this section are chapters on placental and fetal development as well as prenatal diagnosis and birth defects. The second part of the text provides a description of the fundamental processes of embryogenesis for each organ system. The third part provides an idea of molecular regulation and signaling pathways.

**Clinical Correlates:** In addition to describing normal events, each chapter contains clinical correlates that appear in highlighted boxes. This material is designed to demonstrate the clinical relevance of embryology and the importance of understanding key developmental events as a first step to improving birth outcomes and having healthier babies. Clinical pictures and case descriptions are used to provide this information, and this material has been increased and updated in this edition.

**Genetics:** Because of the increasingly important role of genetics and molecular biology in embryology and the study of birth defects, basic genetic and molecular principles are discussed. The last chapter provides an introduction to molecular processes, defines terms commonly used in genetics and molecular biology, and describes key pathways used in embryonic development. Throughout the text, major signaling pathways and genes that regulate embryological development are identified and discussed.

**Extensive Art Program:** The artwork has always been designed to enhance understanding of the text and includes four-color line drawings, scanning electron micrographs, and clinical pictures.

**Summary:** At the end of each chapter is a summary in which the key points are listed for easy recap. Key terms are highlighted and defined in these summaries.

**Self-Assessment:** Problems related to the key elements of each chapter are provided to assist the students in assessing their understanding of the material. Detailed answers are provided in an appendix at the end of the book. Multiple choice and comprehensive questions have also been added to enhance the analytical skills of the readers and help them understand their level of preparation for the MBBS as well as NExT and other competitive examinations.

**Assessing Learning Outcomes:** These are a list of frequently asked medical exam questions to help students assess the knowledge gained.

**Glossary:** A glossary of key terms is listed at the end of the book.

Besides undergraduates, this book would also benefit postgraduate students as it describes the molecular regulation of each developmental process extensively. Online content includes lecture videos, lecture ppts, question bank, and image bank.

I wish all students happy learning!

**Sabita Mishra**

# Acknowledgments

At the outset, I gratefully acknowledge my teachers, especially Dr T.S. Roy, Dr Shashi Wadhwa, Dr J.M. Kaul, Dr Anita Tuli, and Dr Neelam Vasudeva, for imparting their knowledge and for always being there for me.

I would also like to sincerely thank my friends and colleagues, Dr Rima Dada, Dr Surbhi Wadhwa, Dr Babita Pangtey, Dr Anita Mahajan, and Dr Swati Tiwari for helping out in the editing process.

I wish to express my gratitude to my residents and students for giving me the opportunity to follow my passion in teaching embryology.

I acknowledge my husband Dr Pradeep Misra for his support in all my endeavors. My daughter Sunayana and son-in-law Vikrant and daughter Shivani and son-in-law Sebastian and grandson Vinayak have given me their unconditional love and support.

I express my gratitude to Wolters Kluwer (India) for providing me the opportunity to associate with such an acclaimed embryology book. My sincere thanks to Mr Ravi Vishwakarma, Senior Content & Publishing Analyst, for his perseverance, support, and valuable inputs in timely completion of the book. I have no words to express my thanks to Dr Satheesh, Senior Technical Writer, for going through the contents thoroughly and diligently editing the book. His skillful editing has brought about the changes effectively. I would also thank Ms. Pooja Chauhan, Content Management Analyst, for her editorial inputs.

**Sabita Mishra**

# Publisher's Acknowledgments

The publisher would like to thank the following reviewers for providing their valuable suggestions:

## Faculty

**Adithya Krishnadas**
Professor and Head
Department of Anatomy
Sree Narayana Institute of Medical Sciences
Ernakulam, Kerala

**Alok Tripathi**
Professor
Department of Anatomy
Subharti Medical College
Meerut, Uttar Pradesh

**A. Anupriya**
Assistant Professor
Sri Ramachandra Medical College and Research Institute
Chennai, Tamil Nadu

**Avanish Kumar**
Professor and Head
Indira Gandhi Institute of Medical Sciences
Patna, Bihar

**Farah Ghaus**
Professor
Department of Anatomy
Jawaharlal Nehru Medical College
Aligarh Muslim University
Aligarh, Uttar Pradesh

**Hitendra LOH**
Director Professor
Department of Anatomy
VMMC and Safdarjung Hospital
New Delhi

**Kalpana Sharma**
Assistant Professor
Department of Anatomy
Pacific Institute of Medical Sciences
Udaipur, Rajasthan

**P. Kanagavalli**
Head
Department of Anatomy
Government Medical College
Tiruvallur, Tamil Nadu

**Kanchan Wankhede**
Associate Professor
Department of Anatomy
Government Medical College
Nagpur, Maharashtra

**Kumar Satish Ravi**
Professor and Head
Department of Anatomy
AIIMS
Gorakhpur, Uttar Pradesh

**Lathikumari K**
Professor and Head
Department of Anatomy
Government Medical College
Thiruvananthapuram, Kerala

**Leena Raichandani**
Senior Professor
Department of Anatomy
Dr S N Medical College
Jodhpur, Rajasthan

**D. Malar**
Professor and Head
Sri Venkateswaraa Medical College Hospital and Research Centre

**Mamata Chimmalgi**
Department of Anatomy
Sree Gokulam Medical College
Thiruvananthapuram, Kerala

**Md. Jawed Akhtar**
Associate Professor
Department of Anatomy
Indira Gandhi Institute of Medical Sciences
Patna, Bihar

**A. Meharunnisa**
Professor and Head
Department of Anatomy
SUT Academy of Medical Science
Thiruvananthapuram, Kerala

**Minnie Pillay**
Professor and Head
Department of Anatomy
School of Medicine
Amrita Vishwa Vidyapeetham
Kochi, Kerala

**Nikha Bhardwaj**
Associate Professor
Department of Anatomy
AIIMS
Jodhpur, Rajasthan

**Nirupma Gupta**
Dean and Professor
Department of Anatomy
SMSR Sharda University
Greater Noida, Uttar Pradesh

**Parveen Ojha**
Professor and Head
Department of Anatomy
RNT Medical College
Udaipur, Rajasthan

**G. Prabavathy**
Professor
Department of Anatomy
Mahatma Gandhi Medical College and Research Institute
Puducherry

**Priyanka Katara**
Associate Professor
Department of Anatomy
SMS Medical College
Jaipur, Rajasthan

**Rajiv Ranjan**
Assistant Professor
Department of Anatomy
Rajendra Institute of Medical Sciences (RIMS)
Ranchi, Jharkhand

**Ranjana Verma**
Professor and Head
Department of Anatomy
Government Institute of Medical Sciences (GIMS)
Greater Noida, Uttar Pradesh

**Rema Devi**
Professor and Head
Division of Human Genetics
Department of Anatomy
Pondicherry Institute of Medical Sciences
Puducherry

**Rima Dada**
Professor
Department of Anatomy
AIIMS
New Delhi

**Sajan Skaria**
Assistant Professor
Department of Anatomy
American International Institute of Medical Sciences
Udaipur, Rajasthan

**S. Saravana Kumar**
Assistant Professor
Department of Anatomy
Meenakshi Medical College
Kanchipuram, Tamil Nadu

**K. Santhini Arulselvi**
Professor and Head
Department of Anatomy
Vinayaka Missions Medical College
Karaikal, Puducherry

**Satyam Khare**
Professor and Head
Department of Anatomy
Subharti Medical College
Meerut, Uttar Pradesh

**Shobha Rawalani**
Professor
Department of Anatomy
JNMC - Datta Meghe Institute of Medical Sciences (Deemed to be University)
Sawangi (Meghe), Wardha, Maharashtra

**Shruthy K M**
Associate Professor
Department of Anatomy
ACS Medical College and Hospital
Chennai, Tamil Nadu

**Shweta Asthana**
Associate Professor
Department of Anatomy
RNT Medical College
Udaipur, Rajasthan

**Simmi Mehra**
Professor and Head
Department of Anatomy
AIIMS
Rajkot, Gujarat

**Smruti Rekha Mohanty**
Professor and Head
Department of Anatomy
Kalinga Institute of Medical Sciences
Bhubaneshwar, Odisha

**Sudipa Biswas**
Professor and Head
Department of Anatomy
ESI-PGIMSR
Joka, Kolkata

**Suma HY**
Professor and Head
Department of Anatomy
Jawaharlal Institute of Postgraduate Medical Education and Research
Puducherry

**Suriyakumari K V P**
Professor and Head
Department of Anatomy
Sri Manakula Vinayagar Medical College and Hospital
Madagadipet, Puducherry

**Susan Varghese**
Professor and Head
Department of Anatomy
Government Medical College
Kollam, Kerala

**Sushant Swaroop Das**
Assistant Professor
Department of Anatomy
AIIMS
Bilaspur, Himachal Pradesh

**Vahini**
Senior Assistant Professor
Department of Anatomy
Madras Medical College
Chennai, Tamil Nadu

**Vaibhav P. Anjankar**
Professor
Department of Anatomy
JNMC - Datta Meghe Institute of Medical Sciences (Deemed to be University)
Sawangi (Meghe), Wardha, Maharashtra

**Vandana Mehta**
Director Professor and Head
Department of Anatomy
VMMC and Safdarjung Hospital
New Delhi

**R. Vijaya**
Associate Professor
Department of Anatomy
AIIMS
Madurai, Tamil Nadu

**Vinay Sharma**
Professor
Department of Anatomy
Muzaffarnagar Medical College
Muzaffarnagar, Uttar Pradesh

**Vipin Kumar**
Professor and Head
Department of Anatomy
ESIC Medical College and Hospital
Bihta, Patna

## Student

**Pranjal Prasoon**
Intern
VMMC and Safdarjung Hospital
New Delhi

# Contents

# Figure Credits

**FIGURE 2.2** Courtesy of Dr. Roger Stevenson, Greenwood Genetic Center, Greenwood, SC.

**FIGURE 2.16A,B** Reprinted with permission from Gelehrter TD, Collins FS, Ginsburg D. *Principles of Medical Genetics*. 2nd ed. Baltimore, MD: Williams & Wilkins; 1998:166.

**FIGURE 2.17** Courtesy of Dr. Barbara DuPont, Greenwood Genetic Center, Greenwood, SC.

**FIGURE 2.18A,B** Courtesy of Dr. Roger Stevenson, Greenwood Genetic Center, Greenwood, SC.

**FIGURE 2.19** Courtesy of Dr. Roger Stevenson, Greenwood Genetic Center, Greenwood, SC.

**FIGURE 2.20** Courtesy of Dr. Roger Stevenson, Greenwood Genetic Center, Greenwood, SC.

**FIGURE 2.21A–D** Courtesy of Dr. David Weaver, Department of Medical and Molecular Genetics, Indiana University School of Medicine.

**FIGURE 2.22** Courtesy of Dr. David Weaver, Department of Medical and Molecular Genetics, Indiana University School of Medicine.

**FIGURE 2.23** Courtesy of Dr. R. J. Gorlin, Department of Oral Pathology and Genetics, University of Minnesota.

**FIGURE 2.24A,B** Courtesy of Dr. Barbara DuPont, Greenwood Genetic Center, Greenwood, SC.

**FIGURE 3.8A** Courtesy of Dr. P. Motta, Department of Anatomy, University of Rome.

**FIGURE 3.10A,B** Courtesy of the Carnegie Collection, National Museum of Health and Medicine, Washington, DC.

**FIGURE 3.12A,B** Courtesy of Dr. Caroline Ziomeck, Genzyme Transgenics Corporation, Framingham, MA.

**FIGURE 3.13A** Courtesy of the Carnegie Collection, National Museum of Health and Medicine, Washington, DC.

**FIGURE 4.2** Courtesy of the Virtual Human Embryo Project (http://virtualhumanembryo.lsuhsc.edu). Provided by John Cork.

**FIGURE 4.5** Courtesy of the Virtual Human Embryo Project (http://virtualhumanembryo.lsuhsc.edu). Provided by John Cork.

**FIGURE 4.7** Courtesy of the Virtual Human Embryo Project (http://virtualhumanembryo.lsuhsc.edu). Provided by John Cork.

**FIGURE 4.8** Modified from Hamilton WJ, Mossman HW. *Human Embryology*. Baltimore, MD: Lippincott Williams & Wilkins; 1972.

**FIGURE 5.2C** Courtesy of Dr. K. W. Tosney, Molecular, Cellular, and Developmental Biology Department, University of Michigan.

**FIGURE 5.5** Courtesy of Dr. Roger Stevenson, Greenwood Genetic Center, Greenwood, SC.

**FIGURE 5.8A,B** Courtesy of Dr. Roger Stevenson, Greenwood Genetic Center, Greenwood, SC.

**FIGURE 5.9** Courtesy of Dr. David D. Weaver, Department of Medical and Molecular Genetics, Indiana University School of Medicine.

**FIGURE 6.1C** Courtesy of the Carnegie Collection, National Museum of Health and Medicine, Washington, DC.

**FIGURE 6.2B,D** Courtesy of Dr. Kohei Shiota, Department of Anatomy and Developmental Biology, Kyoto, Japan.

**FIGURE 6.3B,D** Courtesy of Dr. Kohei Shiota, Department of Anatomy and Developmental Biology, Kyoto, Japan.

**FIGURE 6.5D** Courtesy of Dr. K. W. Tosney, Molecular, Cellular, and Developmental Biology Department, University of Michigan.

**FIGURE 6.7A,C** Courtesy of Dr. Roger Stevenson, Greenwood Genetic Center, Greenwood, SC.

**FIGURE 6.7B** Courtesy of Dr. David D. Weaver, Department of Medical and Molecular Genetics, Indiana University School of Medicine.

**FIGURE 6.9** Courtesy of Dr. K. W. Tosney, Molecular, Cellular, and Developmental Biology Department, University of Michigan.

**FIGURE 6.10** Courtesy of Dr. K. W. Tosney, Molecular, Cellular, and Developmental Biology Department, University of Michigan.

**FIGURE 6.16A,B** Courtesy of Dr. Roger Stevenson, Greenwood Genetic Center, Greenwood, SC.

**FIGURE 6.25** Reprinted with permission from Coletta PL, Shimeld SM, Sharpe PT. The molecular anatomy of Hox gene expression. *J Anat*. 1994;184:15–22.

**FIGURE 6.20A,B** Courtesy of the Carnegie Collection, National Museum of Health and Medicine, Washington, DC.

**FIGURE 6.21** Courtesy of Dr. E. Blechschmidt, Department of Anatomy, University of Gottingen.

**FIGURE 6.22** Courtesy of Dr. E. Blechschmidt, Department of Anatomy, University of Gottingen.

**FIGURE 6.23** Reprinted with permission from Hamilton WJ, Mossman HW. *Human Embryology*. Baltimore, MD: Lippincott Williams & Wilkins; 1972.

**FIGURE 7.3A–C** Courtesy of Dr. Roger Stevenson, Greenwood Genetic Center, Greenwood, SC.

**FIGURE 7.3D** Courtesy of Dr. David D. Weaver, Department of Medical and Molecular Genetics, Indiana University School of Medicine.

**FIGURE 7.4B** Courtesy of Dr. Roger Stevenson, Greenwood Genetic Center, Greenwood, SC.

**FIGURE 7.8C** Courtesy of Dr. Don Nakayama, Department of Surgery, University of North Carolina.

**FIGURE 8.4** Courtesy of Dr. E. Blechschmidt, Department of Anatomy, University of Gottingen.

**FIGURE 8.15A–D** Reprinted from Reeder, Martin, Koniak, Griffin. Maternity Nursing. Family, Newborn and Women's Health Care, 19th edn. Wolters Kluwer India: New Delhi; 2014.)

**FIGURE 8.17** Courtesy of Dr. Roger Stevenson, Greenwood Genetic Center, Greenwood, SC.

**FIGURE 8.18B–E** Reprinted from Reeder, Martin, Koniak, Griffin. Maternity Nursing. Family, Newborn and Women's Health Care, 19th edn. Wolters Kluwer India: New Delhi; 2014.)

**FIGURE 8.20A,B** Courtesy of Dr. Roger Stevenson, Greenwood Genetic Center, Greenwood, SC.

**FIGURE 8.23** Courtesy of Dr. Roger Stevenson, Greenwood Genetic Center, Greenwood, SC.

**FIGURE 8.24** Courtesy of Dr. Roger Stevenson, Greenwood Genetic Center, Greenwood, SC.

**FIGURE 8.26A,B** Courtesy of Dr. Roger Stevenson, Greenwood Genetic Center, Greenwood, SC.

**FIGURE 9.3** Courtesy of Dr. Roger Stevenson, Greenwood Genetic Center, Greenwood, SC.

**FIGURE 9.4** Courtesy of Dr. David D. Weaver, Department of Medical and Molecular Genetics, Indiana University School of Medicine.

**FIGURE 9.5A,B** Courtesy of Dr. Roger Stevenson, Greenwood Genetic Center, Greenwood, SC.

**FIGURE 9.6** Courtesy of Dr. Andre Luiz Santos Pessoa, Professor of Medicine at State University of Ceara-UECE, Brazil.

**FIGURE 9.7** Courtesy of Dr. Roger Stevenson, Greenwood Genetic Center, Greenwood, SC.

**FIGURE 9.8A–D** Courtesy of Dr. Hytham Imseis, Department of Obstetrics and Gynecology, Mountain Area Health Education Center, Asheville, NC.

**FIGURE 9.9A,B** Courtesy of Dr. Hytham Imseis, Department of Obstetrics and Gynecology, Mountain Area Health Education Center, Asheville, NC.

**FIGURE 9.10A–D** Courtesy of Dr. Jan Byrne, Department of Obstetrics and Gynecology, University of Utah Health Sciences Center.

**FIGURE 9.11** Reprinted with permission from Dr. Hanmin Lee, MD, UCSF Benioff Children's Hospital and University of California, San Francisco, School of Medicine, published by Medscape Drugs and Diseases (http://emedicine.medscape.com) 2011, available at: http://reference.medscape.com/features/slideshow/fetal-surg.

**FIGURE 10.3** Modified from Gilbert SF. *Developmental Biology*. 9th ed. Sunderland, MA: Sinauer Associates, Inc.; 2010.

**FIGURE 10.8A,B** Courtesy of Dr. Roger Stevenson, Greenwood Genetic Center, Greenwood, SC.

**FIGURE 10.9A** Courtesy of Dr. Roger Stevenson, Greenwood Genetic Center, Greenwood, SC.

**FIGURE 10.9B,C** Courtesy of Dr. Michael L. Cunningham, Division of Craniofacial Medicine, Children's Craniofacial Center, University of Washington.

**FIGURE 10.10A** Courtesy of Dr. Roger Stevenson, Greenwood Genetic Center, Greenwood, SC.

**FIGURE 10.10B** Courtesy of Dr. J. Jane, Department of Neurosurgery, University of Virginia.

**FIGURE 10.10C** Courtesy of Dr. Michael L. Cunningham, Division of Craniofacial Medicine, Children's Craniofacial Center, University of Washington.

**FIGURE 10.11A,B** Courtesy of Dr. David D. Weaver, Department of Medical and Molecular Genetics, Indiana University School of Medicine.

**FIGURE 10.12** Courtesy of Dr. Roger Stevenson, Greenwood Genetic Center, Greenwood, SC.

**FIGURE 10.13** Courtesy of Dr. David D. Weaver, Department of Medical and Molecular Genetics, Indiana University School of Medicine.

**FIGURE 10.14** Courtesy of Dr. David D. Weaver, Department of Medical and Molecular Genetics, Indiana University School of Medicine.

**FIGURE 10.15B** Reprinted with permission from Moore KL, Dalley AF. *Clinically Oriented Anatomy*. 5th ed. Philadelphia, PA: Lippincott Williams & Wilkins; 2006.

**FIGURE 10.17** Courtesy of Mr Ravi Kumar (artist), Maulana Azad Medical College, New Delhi.

**FIGURE 10.18A,B** Courtesy of Dr. Jan Byrne, Department of Obstetrics and Gynecology, University of Utah Health Sciences Center.

**FIGURE 11.5** Courtesy of Dr. Roger Stevenson, Greenwood Genetic Center, Greenwood, SC.

**FIGURE 11.6** Courtesy of Dr. Roger Stevenson, Greenwood Genetic Center, Greenwood, SC.

**FIGURE 12.2A,B** Courtesy of Dr. K. W. Tosney, Molecular, Cellular, and Developmental Biology Department, University of Michigan.

**FIGURE 12.5** Modified from Gilbert SF. *Developmental Biology*. 9th ed. Sunderland, MA: Sinauer Associates, Inc.; 2010.

**FIGURE 12.8** Reprinted with permission from Moore KL, Dalley AF. *Clinically Oriented Anatomy*. 5th ed. Philadelphia, PA: Lippincott Williams & Wilkins; 2006.

**FIGURE 12.11** Courtesy of Dr. Roger Stevenson, Greenwood Genetic Center, Greenwood, SC.

**FIGURE 12.12A** Courtesy of Dr. David D. Weaver, Department of Medical and Molecular Genetics, Indiana University School of Medicine.

**FIGURE 12.12B** Courtesy of Dr. Roger Stevenson, Greenwood Genetic Center, Greenwood, SC.

**FIGURE 12.13A–D** Courtesy of Dr. Roger Stevenson, Greenwood Genetic Center, Greenwood, SC.

**FIGURE 12.14** Courtesy of Dr. David D. Weaver, Department of Medical and Molecular Genetics, Indiana University School of Medicine.

**FIGURE 12.15** Courtesy of Dr. David D. Weaver, Department of Medical and Molecular Genetics, Indiana University School of Medicine.

**FIGURE 12.16** Courtesy of Dr. David D. Weaver, Department of Medical and Molecular Genetics, Indiana University School of Medicine.

**FIGURE 12.17** Courtesy of Dr. Roger Stevenson, Greenwood Genetic Center, Greenwood, SC.

**FIGURE 15.16** Reprinted with permission from Agur AMR, Dalley AF. *Grant's Atlas of Anatomy*. 14th ed. Philadelphia, PA: Wolters Kluwer; 2017.

**FIGURE 15.21** Modified from Gilbert SF. *Developmental Biology*. 8th ed. Sunderland, MA: Sinauer Associates, Inc.; 2006.

**FIGURE 15.23** Courtesy of Dr. Swati Tiwari, Maulana Azad Medical College, New Delhi.

**FIGURE 15.31B,C** Courtesy of Dr. Roger Stevenson, Greenwood Genetic Center, Greenwood, SC.

**FIGURE 15.31D,E** Courtesy of Dr. Jan Byrne, Department of Obstetrics and Gynecology, University of Utah Health Sciences Center.

**FIGURE 15.35** Courtesy of Dr. D. Nakayama, Department of Surgery, University of North Carolina.

**FIGURE 16.9** Courtesy of Dr. Roger Stevenson, Greenwood Genetic Center, Greenwood, SC.

**FIGURE 16.10D,E** Reprinted with permission from Stevenson RE, Hall JG, Goodman RM, eds. *Human Malformations and Related Anomalies*. New York, NY: Oxford University Press; 1993.

**FIGURE 16.11A–C** Courtesy of Dr. Roger Stevenson, Greenwood Genetic Center, Greenwood, SC.

**FIGURE 16.16A** Courtesy of Dr. Roger Stevenson, Greenwood Genetic Center, Greenwood, SC.

**FIGURE 16.16B** Courtesy of Dr. David D. Weaver, Department of Medical and Molecular Genetics, Indiana University School of Medicine.

**FIGURE 16.34B,C** Courtesy of Dr. Roger Stevenson, Greenwood Genetic Center, Greenwood, SC.

**FIGURE 16.36** Courtesy of Dr. David D. Weaver, Department of Medical and Molecular Genetics, Indiana University School of Medicine.

**FIGURE 17.5C** Courtesy of Prof. Shigehito Yamada, MD, PhD, Congenital Anomaly Research Center, Kyoto University Graduate School of Medicine, Japan.

**FIGURE 17.13** Courtesy of Dr. A. Shaw, Department of Surgery, University of Virginia.

**FIGURE 17.16A–D** Courtesy of Dr. David D. Weaver, Department of Medical and Molecular Genetics, Indiana University School of Medicine.

**FIGURE 17.20** Courtesy of Dr. A. Shaw, Department of Surgery, University of Virginia.

**FIGURE 17.21C** Courtesy of Prof. Shigehito Yamada, MD, PhD, Congenital Anomaly Research Center, Kyoto University Graduate School of Medicine, Japan.

**FIGURE 17.22C,D** Courtesy of Prof. Shigehito Yamada, MD, PhD, Congenital Anomaly Research Center, Kyoto University Graduate School of Medicine, Japan.

**FIGURE 17.23C** Courtesy of Prof. Shigehito Yamada, MD, PhD, Congenital Anomaly Research Center, Kyoto University Graduate School of Medicine, Japan.

**FIGURE 17.30A,D** Courtesy of Dr. David D. Weaver, Department of Medical and Molecular Genetics, Indiana University School of Medicine.

**FIGURE 17.31A** Courtesy of Prof. Shigehito Yamada, MD, PhD, Congenital Anomaly Research Center, Kyoto University Graduate School of Medicine, Japan.

**FIGURE 17.31B,C** Courtesy of Dr. Roger Stevenson, Greenwood Genetic Center, Greenwood, SC.

**FIGURE 17.34** Reprinted with permission from Moore KL, Dalley AF. *Clinically Oriented Anatomy*. 5th ed. Philadelphia, PA: Lippincott Williams & Wilkins; 2006.

**FIGURE 18.2D** Courtesy of Dr. K. W. Tosney, Molecular, Cellular, and Developmental Biology Department, University of Michigan.

**FIGURE 18.6B** Courtesy of Dr. K. W. Tosney, Molecular, Cellular, and Developmental Biology Department, University of Michigan.

**FIGURE 18.16** Courtesy of Dr. Roger Stevenson, Greenwood Genetic Center, Greenwood, SC.

**FIGURE 18.32A,B** Redrawn from Rubenstein JLR, Beachy PA. Patterning of the embryonic forebrain. *Curr Opin Neurobiol.* 1998;8:18–26.

**FIGURE 18.34** Courtesy of Dr. Roger Stevenson, Greenwood Genetic Center, Greenwood, SC.

**FIGURE 18.36** Courtesy of Dr. Roger Stevenson, Greenwood Genetic Center, Greenwood, SC.

**FIGURE 18.37A,B** Courtesy of Dr. Roger Stevenson, Greenwood Genetic Center, Greenwood, SC.

**FIGURE 18.38** Courtesy of Dr. J. Warkany. Reprinted with permission from Warkany J. *Congenital Malformations: Notes and Comments*. Chicago, IL: Year Book Medical Publishers; 1971.

**FIGURE 18.39** Courtesy of Dr. David D. Weaver, Department of Medical and Molecular Genetics, Indiana University School of Medicine.

**FIGURE 19.8** Reprinted with permission from Moore KL, Dalley AF. *Clinically Oriented Anatomy*. 5th ed. Philadelphia, PA: Lippincott Williams & Wilkins; 2006.

**FIGURE 19.3F** Courtesy of Dr. Sabita Mishra, Department of Anatomy, Maulana Azad Medical College, Delhi.

**FIGURE 19.11A–D** Courtesy of Dr. David D. Weaver, Department of Medical and Molecular Genetics, Indiana University School of Medicine.

**FIGURE 20.2D,E** Courtesy of Dr. K. W. Tosney, Molecular, Cellular, and Developmental Biology Department, University of Michigan.

**FIGURE 20.12** Courtesy of Dr. David D. Weaver, Department of Medical and Molecular Genetics, Indiana University School of Medicine.

**FIGURE 20.13** Courtesy of Dr. David D. Weaver, Department of Medical and Molecular Genetics, Indiana University School of Medicine.

**FIGURE 21.2** Courtesy of Dr. Roger Stevenson, Greenwood Genetic Center, Greenwood, SC.

**FIGURE 21.4** Courtesy of Dr. Roger Stevenson, Greenwood Genetic Center, Greenwood, SC.

**FIGURE 21.6** Courtesy of Dr. Roger Stevenson, Greenwood Genetic Center, Greenwood, SC.

# CBME Topics*

## Competency-Based Undergraduate Curriculum Topics: Chapter-Wise Coverage

| Code | Competency | Chapter/s | Page/s |
|---|---|---|---|
| AN9.3 | Describe the development of the breast. | 21 | 302–304 |
| AN13.8 | Describe the development of the upper limb. | 12 | 138–144 |
| AN20.10 | Describe the basic concept of the development of the lower limb. | 12 | 138–144 |
| AN25.2 | Describe the development of the heart. | 13 | 148–160 |
| AN25.2 | Describe about the development of the pleura and lung. | 14 | 183–188 |
| AN25.3 | Describe fetal circulation and changes occurring at birth. | 13 | 177, 178 |
| AN25.4 | Describe embryological basis of the following: (1) atrial septal defect, (2) ventricular septal defect, and (3) Fallot's tetralogy. | 13 | 166–168 |
| AN25.4 | Describe the embryological basis of tracheoesophageal fistula. | 14 | 184 |
| AN25.5 | Describe the developmental basis of congenital anomalies, transposition of great vessels, dextrocardia, patent ductus arteriosus, and coarctation of the aorta. | 13 | 171–173 |
| AN25.6 | Mention the development of aortic arch arteries, SVC, IVC, and coronary sinus. | 13 | 169–176 |
| AN26.1 | Explain the concept of bone ossification. | 10 | 121–124 |
| AN39.1 | Describe the embryological basis of nerve supply, blood supply, lymphatic drainage, and actions of extrinsic and intrinsic muscles of the tongue. | 17 | 244–245 |
| AN43.4 | Describe the development and developmental basis of congenital anomalies of the face, palate, tongue, branchial apparatus, pituitary gland, thyroid gland, and eye. | 17, 18 | 236–251, 269 |
| AN43.4 | Describe the development of the face and branchial apparatus (Development of Year). | 17, 19 | 236–251, 284–289 |
| AN43.4 | Describe the development and developmental basis of congenital anomalies of the eye. | 20 | 292–298 |
| AN52.4 | Describe the development of the anterior abdominal wall. | 7 | 8, 80, 81 |
| AN52.5 | Describe the development and congenital anomalies of the diaphragm. | 7 | 83–85 |
| AN52.6 | Describe the development and congenital anomalies of the foregut, midgut, and hindgut. | 15 | 190–209 |
| AN52.7 | Describe the development of the urinary system. | 16 | 212–220 |
| AN52.8 | Describe the development of the male and female reproductive system. | 16 | 220–232 |
| AN64.2 | Describe the development of neural tube, spinal cord, medulla oblongata, pons, midbrain, cerebral hemisphere, and cerebellum. | 18 | 255–274 |
| AN64.3 | Describe the various types of open neural tube defects with their embryological bases. | 18 | 274–276 |
| AN74.3 | Describe multifactorial inheritance with examples. | 2, 9 | 17–22, 105–114 |
| AN75.1 | Describe the structural and numerical chromosomal aberrations. | 2 | 17–22 |
| AN75.2 | Explain the terms mosaic and chimera with examples. | 2 | 22 |
| AN75.3 | Describe the genetic basis and clinical features of Prader-Willi syndrome, Edward syndrome, and Patau syndrome. | 2 | 19–21 |
| AN75.4 | Describe the genetic basis of variation: polymorphism and mutation. | 2 | 21 |
| AN75.5 | Describe the principles of genetic counseling. | 2 | 17 |
| AN76.1 | Describe the stages of human life. | 1 | 5 |

*Reference: National Medical Commission. Competency Based Undergraduate Curriculum for the Indian Medical Graduate. Vol. 1 (2018), pages 40 to 90. Available at https://www.nmc.org.in/wp-content/uploads/2020/01/UG-Curriculum-Vol-I.pdf

| Code | Competency | Chapter/s | Page/s |
|---|---|---|---|
| AN76.2 | Explain the terms ontogeny and phylogeny. | 1 | 5 |
| AN77.1 | Describe the uterine changes occurring during the menstrual cycle. | 3 | 26–30 |
| AN77.2 | Describe the synchrony between the ovarian and menstrual cycles. | 3 | 26–30 |
| AN77.3 | Describe spermatogenesis and oogenesis along with diagrams. | 2 | 10–15 |
| AN77.4 | Describe the stages and consequences of fertilization. | 3 | 31–34 |
| AN77.5 | Enumerate and describe the anatomical principles underlying contraception. | 3 | 33 |
| AN77.6 | Describe fertility and sterility and surrogate motherhood. | 3 | 33 |
| AN77.6 | Describe teratogenic influences. | 9 | 105, 111–113 |
| AN78.1 | Describe cleavage and formation of a blastocyst. | 3 | 34–36 |
| AN78.2 | Describe the development of trophoblast. | 4 | 40–44, 53, 55–57 |
| AN78.3 | Describe the process of implantation and common abnormal sites of implantation. | 4 | 44, 45 |
| AN78.4 | Describe the formation of extraembryonic mesoderm and coelom, bilaminar disc, and prochordal plate. | 4 | 42, 43 |
| AN78.5 | Describe in brief abortion, decidual reaction, and pregnancy test. | 4 | 44–46 |
| AN79.1 | Describe the formation and fate of the primitive streak. | 5 | 48–51 |
| AN79.2 | Describe the formation and fate of the notochord. | 5 | 53 |
| AN79.3 | Describe the process of neurulation. | 6 | 59–63 |
| AN79.4 | Describe the development of somites and intraembryonic coelom. | 6 | 66 |
| AN79.4 | Describe the development of somites. | 6, 11 | 66–68 |
| AN79.5 | Explain the embryological basis of congenital malformations, nucleus pulposus, sacrococcygeal teratomas, and neural tube defects. | 6 | 54, 65 |
| AN79.5 | Explain the embryological basis of nucleus pulposus and the embryological basis of vertebral defects. | 10 | 128, 129 |
| AN80.1 | Describe the formation, functions, and fate of chorion: amnion, yolk sac, allantois, and decidua. | 8 | 90, 91 |
| AN80.2 | Describe the formation and structure of the umbilical cord. | 8 | 96, 97 |
| AN80.3 | Describe the formation of placenta, its physiological functions, fetomaternal circulation, and placental barrier. | 8 | 90, 91, 93–95 |
| AN80.4 | Describe the embryological basis of twinning in monozygotic and dizygotic twins. | 8 | 99–101 |
| AN80.5 | Describe the role of placental hormones in uterine growth and parturition. | 8 | 96, 99, 100 |
| AN80.6 | Explain the embryological basis of estimation of the fetal age. | 8 | 87–89 |
| AN80.7 | Describe the various types of umbilical cord attachments. | 8 | 94, 96, 97 |
| AN81.1 | Describe various methods of prenatal diagnosis. | 9 | 114–116 |
| AN81.2 | Describe indications, process, and disadvantages of amniocentesis. | 9 | 115 |
| AN81.3 | Describe indications, process, and disadvantages of chorion villus biopsy. | 9 | 116 |
| BI7.1 | Describe the structure and functions of DNA and RNA and outline the cell cycle. | 22 | 307–310 |
| BI7.2 | Describe the processes involved in replication and repair of DNA and the transcription and translation mechanisms. | 22 | 309 |
| BI7.3 | Describe gene mutations and the basic mechanism of regulation of gene expression. | 22 | 310–314 |

# Part 1

# General Embryology

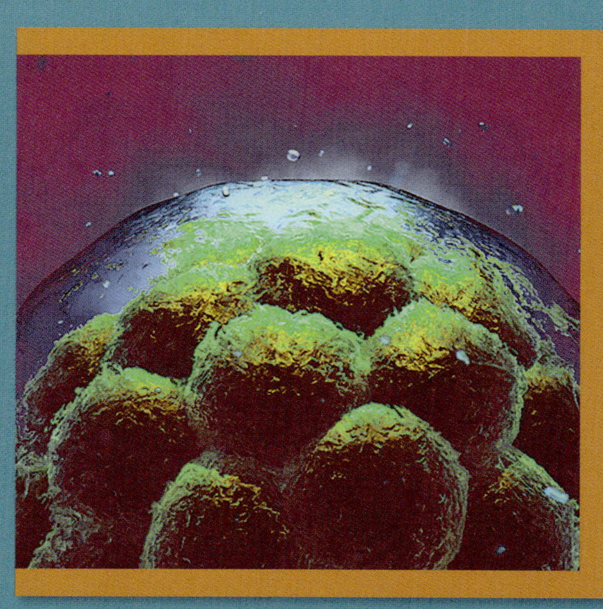

CHAPTER

# 1 Embryology: Clinical Relevance, Historical Perspective, and Phases of Human Development

Part 1

**Specific Learning Objectives**

- Introduction to embryology
- Clinical relevance
- Historical perspective
- Phases of human development
- Ontogeny and phylogeny
- Life cycle of humans
- Important phases of development
- Important terms used in development

**Competencies Covered**

AN76.1 Describe the stages of human life.
AN76.2 Explain the terms ontogeny and phylogeny.

"The one who sees things from the beginning will have the finest view of them."

Aristotle, 322 to 384 BC

## CLINICAL RELEVANCE

From a single cell to a baby in 9 months—a developmental process that represents an amazing integration of increasingly complex phenomena. The study of these phenomena is called **embryology**, and the field includes investigations of the molecular, cellular, and structural factors contributing to the formation of an organism. These studies are important because they provide knowledge essential for creating health care strategies for better reproductive outcomes. Thus, our increasingly greater understanding of embryology has resulted in new techniques for prenatal diagnoses and treatments; therapeutic procedures to circumvent problems with infertility; and mechanisms to prevent birth defects, the leading cause of infant mortality. These improvements in prenatal and reproductive health care are significant not only for their contributions to improved birth outcomes but also for their long-term effects postnatally. For example, both our cognitive capacity and our behavioral characteristics are affected by our prenatal experiences, and factors such as maternal smoking, nutrition, stress, diabetes, etc., play a role in our postnatal health. Furthermore, prenatal experiences, in combination with molecular and cellular factors, determine our potential to develop certain adult diseases, such as cancer and cardiovascular disease. Thus, our prenatal development produces many ramifications affecting our health for both the short and long term, making the study of embryology and fetal development an important topic for all health care professionals. Also, with the exception of a few specialties, most physicians and health care workers will have an opportunity to interact with women of childbearing age, creating the potential for these providers to have a major impact on the outcome of developmental processes and their sequelae.

## A BRIEF HISTORY OF EMBRYOLOGY

The process of progressing from a single cell through the period of establishing organ primordia (the first 8 weeks of human development) is called the period of **embryogenesis** (sometimes called the period of **organogenesis**); the period from that point on until birth is called the **fetal period**, a time when differentiation continues while the fetus grows and gains weight. It is interesting to note that the ancient Ayurvedic teachings described the growth of the fetus in utero as the "Garbha Upanishad." The Greek and the Egyptians also have evidence of embryology documented in paintings and scriptures. Scientific approaches to study embryology have progressed over hundreds of years. Not surprisingly, anatomical approaches dominated early investigations. Observations were made, and these became more sophisticated with advances in optical equipment and dissection techniques. Comparative and evolutionary studies were part of this equation as scientists made comparisons among species and so began to understand the progression of developmental phenomena. Also investigated were offspring with birth defects, and these examples were compared to organisms with normal developmental patterns. The study of the embryological origins and causes for these birth defects was called **teratology**.

In the 20th century, the field of experimental embryology blossomed. Numerous experiments were devised to trace cells during development to determine their cell lineages. These approaches included observations of transparent embryos from tunicates that contained pigmented cells which could be visualized through a microscope. Later, vital dyes were used to stain living cells to follow their fates. Still later in the

1960s, radioactive labels and autoradiographic techniques were employed. One of the first genetic markers also arose about this time with the creation of chick-quail chimeras. In this approach, quail cells, which have a unique pattern to their heterochromatin distribution around the nucleolus, were grafted into chick embryos at early stages of development. Later, host embryos were examined histologically, and the fates of the quail cells were determined. Permutations of this approach included development of antibodies specific to quail cell antigens that greatly assisted in the identification of these cells. Monitoring cell fates with these and other techniques provides valuable information about the origins of different organs and tissues.

Grafting experiments also provided the first insights into signaling between tissues. Examples of such experiments included grafting the primitive node from its normal position on the body axis to another and showing that this structure could induce a second germ disc. In another example, employing developing limb buds, it was shown that if a piece of tissue from the posterior axial border of one limb was grafted to the anterior border of a second limb, then digits on the host limb would be duplicated as the mirror image of each other. This posterior signaling region was called the **zone of polarizing activity (ZPA)**, and it is now known that the signaling molecule is **SONIC HEDGEHOG (SHH)**.

In 1961, the science of teratology became prominent because of the drug **thalidomide** that was given as an antinauseant and sedative to pregnant women. Unfortunately, the drug caused birth defects, including unique abnormalities of the limbs in which one or more limbs was absent (amelia) or was lacking the long bones such that only a hand or foot was attached to the torso (phocomelia). The association between the drug and birth defects was recognized independently by two clinicians, W. Lenz and W. McBride, and showed that the conceptus was vulnerable to maternal factors that crossed the placenta. Soon, numerous animal models demonstrating an association between environmental factors, drugs, and genes provided further insights between developmental events and the origin of birth defects.

Today, molecular approaches have been added to the list of experimental paradigms used to study normal and abnormal development. Numerous means of identifying cells using reporter genes, fluorescent probes, and other marking techniques have improved our ability to map cell fates. Using other techniques to alter gene expression, such as knockout, knock-in, and antisense technologies, has created new ways to produce abnormal development and allowed the study of a single gene's function in specific tissues. Thus, the advent of molecular biology has advanced the field of embryology to the next level, and as we decipher the roles of individual genes and their interplay with environmental factors, our understanding of normal and abnormal developmental processes progresses.

## PHASES OF HUMAN DEVELOPMENT

Human development starts from conception; the product of conceptus is the zygote which divides and differentiates to form a full-term fetus.

Human development can be categorized into the prenatal, neonatal, and postnatal periods.

The prenatal period consists of the embryonic period from conception to 8 weeks and the fetal period starts after 8 weeks to birth (Fig. 1.1).

The prenatal period is divided into three trimesters as the first trimester, the second trimester, and the third trimester.

The neonatal period is the first 4 weeks after birth. The neonate is at a vulnerable stage during this period as it needs to adjust to the external environment. The respiratory system and the cardiovascular system have to develop and function efficiently.

The phases of the postnatal period have been depicted in Figure 1.2 as infancy, childhood, puberty, adolescence, young adults, middle-aged adults, and old age.

## TRIMESTERS

The entire pregnancy has been divided into three stages which are known as trimesters, as they each are of 3-month duration.

The first trimester is the critical period as organogenesis takes place during this period. This is when the expectant mothers have to be very careful with their diet and activities.

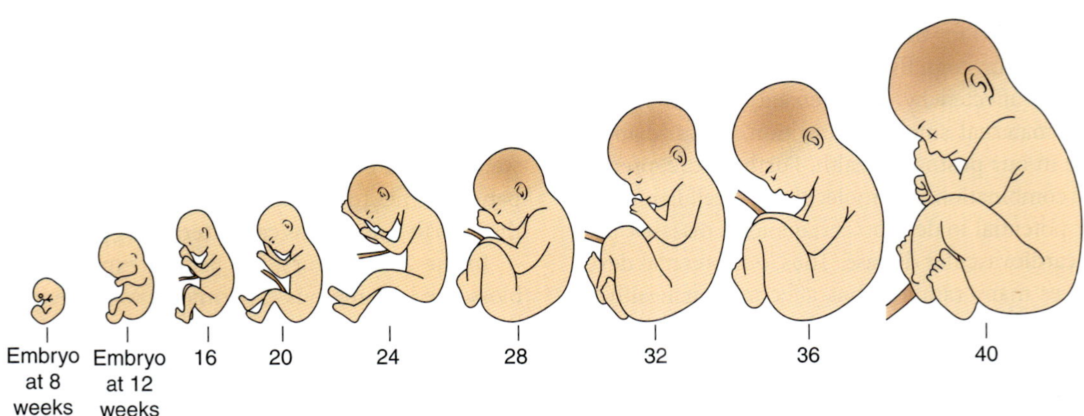


**FIGURE 1.1** Fetal growth from 8 to 40 weeks.

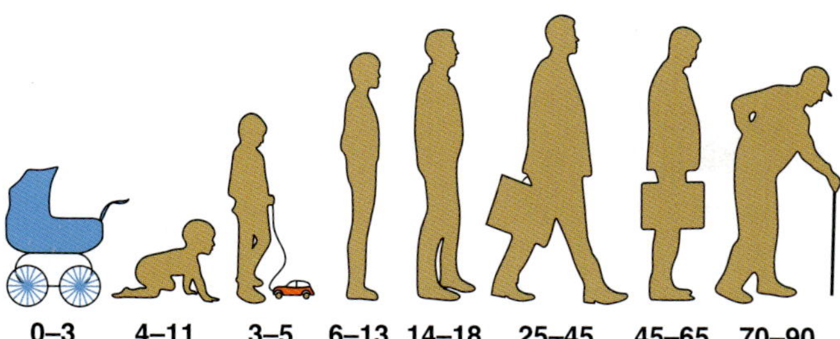


**FIGURE 1.2** Postnatal development: stages of life from birth to old age.

A viable pregnancy is when the fetus is growing as expected. When it is not viable, the fetus is expelled spontaneously leading to an abortion. Medical termination of pregnancy (MTP) is conducted when congenital defects are detected on the prenatal ultrasound examination. In India, MTP is legal under the MTP Act of 1971 for pregnancy less than 20 weeks. It has been amended recently in 2021 till 24 weeks under special circumstances. The baby born before 20 weeks is not viable.

Embryology is like a story which unfolds the mystery of formation of human life.

## ONTOGENY AND PHYLOGENY

Haeckel formulated his theory as "ontogeny recapitulates phylogeny." The notion later became simply known as the recapitulation theory. Ontogeny is the growth (size change) and development (structure change) of an individual organism; phylogeny is the evolutionary history of a species. Haeckel claimed that the development of advanced species passes through stages represented by adult organisms of more primitive species. As explained, each successive stage in the development of an individual represents one of the adult forms that appeared in its evolutionary history.

For example, Haeckel proposed that the pharyngeal grooves between the pharyngeal arches in the neck of the human embryo not only roughly resembled gill slits of fish but also directly represented an adult "fish-like" developmental stage, signifying a fish-like ancestor. Embryonic pharyngeal slits, which form in many animals when the thin branchial plates separating pharyngeal pouches and pharyngeal grooves perforate, open the pharynx to the outside. Pharyngeal arches appear in all tetrapod embryos: in mammals, the first pharyngeal arch develops into the lower jaw, the Meckel's cartilage.

## LIFE CYCLE OF HUMANS (FIG. 1.2)

The following are the different stages of development in the human life cycle:

1. **Fetus:** The sperm from the adult male human and the egg from the adult female human fuse and form a zygote inside the uterus of the female. Over time, the zygote develops and forms an embryo. Initially, the embryo looks like a cluster of cells, but after 8 weeks, the embryo resembles the human body and is called a fetus. During this stage, the fetus is entirely dependent on the mother for respiration, nutrition, and growth.
2. **Infancy:** After around 9 months, the fetus is fully developed to be born. This stage in human development marks the period from birth to age 1. Infancy is the earliest part of childhood, in which the infant undergoes increase in height and weight. During this stage, infants require a lot of attention as they are completely dependent on their mothers. Infants develop their behavior, physiology, and cognition. Gradually, they learn to suck, swallow, and cry if they are in an uncomfortable situation. Since infants are unable to speak, crying is their way of communicating. The mother tends to breastfeed her infant during this stage.
3. **Toddler years:** The term "to toddle" means to walk unsteadily and the child has a clumsy walk during this period. During the toddler years, a child is crawling for mobility and eventually gains the unsteady gait. This stage marks the end of early childhood. This stage lasts till the child is 2 to 3 years old. This stage in a child's life is where he or she undergoes immense cognitive, emotional, and social development.
4. **Childhood:** In this stage, the child eventually learns to walk, run, jump, talk, and eat independently, and becomes more aware of his or her surroundings. The child is more social and active during this period and intrigued to learn new things. This stage lasts till the child is 3 to 8 years old.
5. **Adolescence:** The beginning of adolescence is from age 9-19 years. In this stage, the child grows into an adolescent, through a period called puberty. Puberty occurs during the initial stages of the child's teenage years, and that is why adolescents are also called teenagers. In this stage, the teenager grows rapidly and physical changes begin to appear. These changes include hair growth, structural changes in body shape, voice cracking in adolescent males, and breast growth and menarche (starting of the menstrual cycle) in adolescent females. There are certain behavioral changes also which take place in the adolescents.
6. **Adulthood:** Human beings who are between the age of 20 and 50 years are known as adults. During this stage, human beings are sexually mature and capable of reproducing. The body is fully developed at this stage of life. Adults have full mental and social development by this stage. The time period of adulthood is between the age of 30 and 50 years (middle age).
7. **Old age:** This period starts from 60 years of age, until the end of their lives. During this stage, the intestine absorbs fewer nutrients from food sources. The physical capabilities of doing tasks are also reduced and the individuals again depend on external support to do things.

The behavior of old people in this stage varies depending on the immunity and lifestyle of the person. The average life expectancy of human beings varies from 70 to 85 years. But this also changes depending on their lifestyle.

## IMPORTANT PERIODS IN EMBRYOLOGY

The important periods in embryology are shown in Figure 1.3.

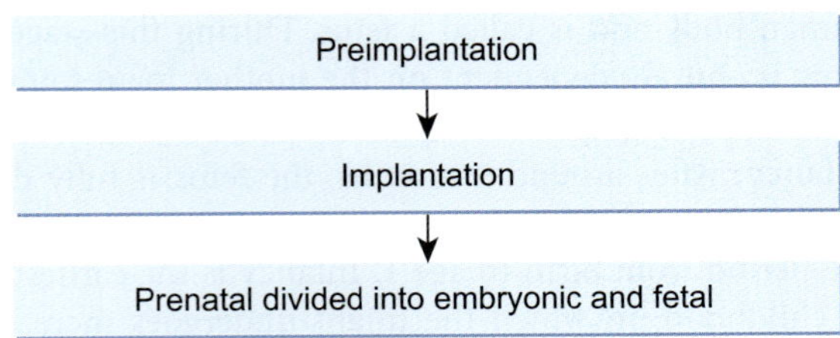


**FIGURE 1.3** Important periods in embryology.

## IMPORTANT TERMS USED IN DEVELOPMENT

- In utero
- Conceptus
- Primordium
- Abortus
- Trimester
- Congenital anomalies—birth defects
- Teratology
- Applied embryology (IVF, surgical interventions)



## SUMMARY

- Evolution of a single cell to a baby in 9 months is a developmental process that represents an amazing integration of increasingly complex phenomena; the study of these phenomena is called **embryology**.
- Embryology includes investigations of the molecular, cellular, and structural factors contributing to the formation of an organism.
- Studies on the molecular, cellular, and structural factors are important because they provide knowledge essential for creating healthcare strategies for better reproductive outcomes.
- Understanding of embryology has resulted in new techniques for prenatal diagnoses and treatments; therapeutic procedures to circumvent problems with infertility; and mechanisms to prevent birth defects, the leading cause of infant mortality.
- The process of progressing from a single cell through the period of establishing organ primordia (the first 8 weeks of human development) is called the period of **embryogenesis** (sometimes called the period of **organogenesis**); the period from that point on until birth is called the **fetal period**.
- **History:** Ancient Ayurvedic teachings described the growth of the fetus in utero as the "Garbha Upanishad." The Greek and the Egyptians also have evidence of embryology documented in paintings and scriptures.
- Scientific approaches to study embryology have progressed over hundreds of years while anatomical approaches dominated early investigations.
- The study of the embryological origins and causes for birth defects is called **teratology**.
- Molecular biology has revolutionized the study of embryology.
- Numerous experiments were conducted to trace cells during development to determine their cell lineages.
- Human development starts from the product of conceptus—a zygote to a full-term baby.
- **Viable pregnancy** is when a fetus is growing as expected. In case of any abnormality, the fetus is expelled spontaneously.
- Haeckel formulated his theory as "Ontogeny recapitulates phylogeny." The development of advanced species passes through stages represented by adult organisms of more primitive species. Each successive stage in the development of an individual represents one of the adult forms that appeared in its evolutionary history.
- Phases of human development are categorized into
  - Prenatal: divided into 3 trimesters
  - Neonatal: first 4 weeks after birth
  - Postnatal: infancy, childhood, puberty, adolescence, young adults, middle age adults, and old age.

## Self-Assessment

### Comprehensive Question

1. What is phylogeny and ontogeny?

### Multiple Choice Questions

1. Which is the most critical period of development?
   (a) First trimester
   (b) Second trimester
   (c) Third trimester
   (d) Neonatal period
2. At what week of gestation can a preterm baby survive?
   (a) 20
   (b) 22
   (c) 24
   (d) 28
3. At what age would one be referred to as an old person?
   (a) 50
   (b) 55
   (c) 60
   (d) 70
4. MTP Act (1971) allows termination of pregnancy before
   (a) 20 weeks
   (b) 24 weeks
   (c) 26 weeks
   (d) 30 weeks

### Answers

1. (a) 2. (d) 3. (d) 4. (a)

CHAPTER 2

# Gametogenesis: Conversion of Germ Cells into Male and Female Gametes



### Specific Learning Objectives

- Primordial germ cells
- Mitosis and meiosis
- Spermatogenesis and oogenesis
- Chromosomal theories of inheritance
- Birth defects: Genetic factors responsible
- Diagnostic techniques to identify genetic abnormalities

### Competencies Covered

AN77.3 Describe spermatogenesis and oogenesis along with diagrams.
AN74.3 Describe multifactorial inheritance with examples.
AN75.1 Describe the structural and numerical chromosomal aberrations.
AN75.2 Explain the terms mosaic and chimera with examples.
AN75.3 Describe the genetic basis and clinical features of Prader-Willi syndrome, Edward syndrome, and Patau syndrome.
AN75.4 Describe the genetic basis of variation: polymorphism and mutation.
AN75.5 Describe the principles of genetic counseling.

## PRIMORDIAL GERM CELLS

Development begins with fertilization, the process by which the male gamete, the **sperm**, and the female gamete, the **oocyte**, unite to give rise to a **zygote**. Gametes are derived from **primordial germ cells (PGCs)** (Fig. 2.1).

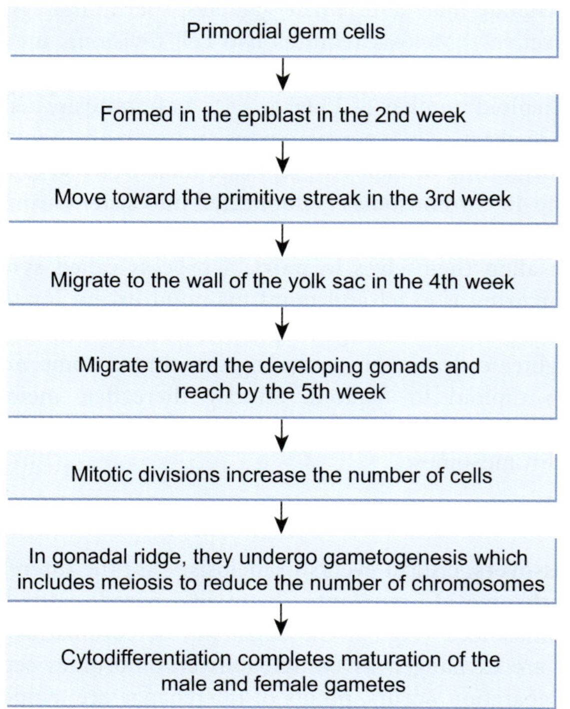


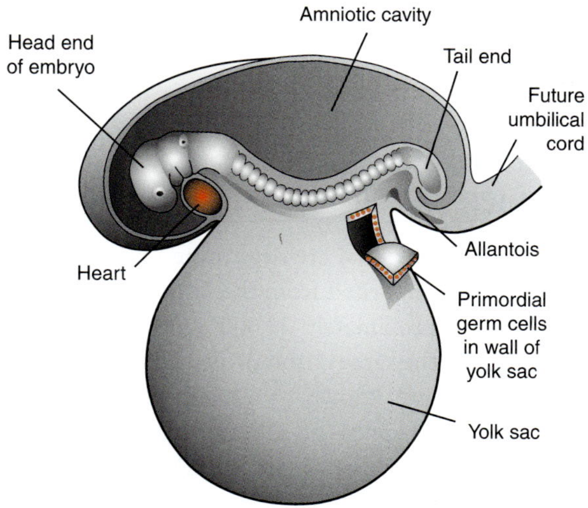


**FIGURE 2.1** An embryo at the end of the third week, showing the position of primordial germ cells (PGCs) in the wall of the yolk sac, close to the attachment of the future umbilical cord. From this location, these cells migrate to the developing gonad.

## Clinical Correlates

### Primordial Germ Cells and Teratomas

**Teratomas** are tumors of disputed origin that often contain a variety of tissues, such as bone, hair, muscle, gut epithelia, and others. It is thought that these tumors arise from pluripotent stem cells that can differentiate into any of the three germ layers or their derivatives. Some evidence suggests that PGCs that have strayed from their normal migratory paths could be responsible for some of these tumors (Fig. 2.2). Another source may be epiblast cells that give rise to all three germ layers during gastrulation (see Fig. 5.9, p. 54).

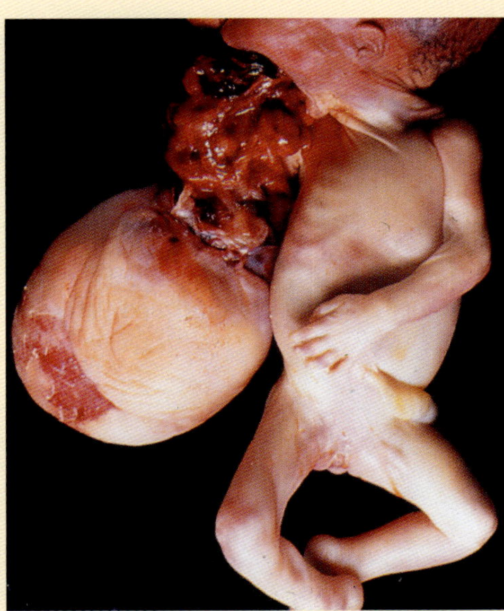

**FIGURE 2.2** Oropharyngeal teratoma. These tumors may arise from PGCs or from epiblast cells (see Chapter 5), both of which are pluripotent. Tissues within the tumors include derivatives of all three germ layers and may include gut, bone, skin, teeth, and so forth.

## THE CHROMOSOME THEORY OF INHERITANCE

Traits of a new individual are determined by specific genes on chromosomes inherited from the father and the mother. Humans have approximately 23,000 genes on 46 chromosomes. Genes on the same chromosome tend to be inherited together and so are known as **linked genes**. In somatic cells, chromosomes appear as 23 **homologous** pairs to form the **diploid** number of 46. There are 22 pairs of matching chromosomes, the **autosomes**, and one pair of **sex chromosomes**. If the sex pair is XX, the individual is genetically female; if the pair is XY, the individual is genetically male. One chromosome of each pair is derived from the maternal gamete, the **oocyte**, and one from the paternal gamete, the **sperm**. Thus, each gamete contains a **haploid** number of 23 chromosomes, and the union of the gametes at **fertilization** restores the diploid number of 46.

### Mitosis

**Mitosis** is the process whereby one cell divides, giving rise to two daughter cells that are genetically identical to the parent cell (Fig. 2.3). Each daughter cell receives the complete complement of 46 chromosomes. Before a cell enters mitosis, each chromosome replicates its **DNA**. During this replication phase, chromosomes are extremely long, they are spread diffusely through the nucleus, and they cannot be recognized with the light microscope. With the onset of mitosis, the chromosomes begin to coil, contract, and condense; these events mark the beginning of **prophase**. Each chromosome now consists of two parallel subunits, **chromatids**, that are joined at a narrow region common to both called the **centromere**. Throughout prophase, the chromosomes continue to condense, shorten, and thicken (Fig. 2.3*A*), but only at prometaphase do the chromatids become distinguishable (Fig. 2.3*B*). During metaphase, the chromosomes line up in the equatorial plane, and their doubled structure is clearly visible (Fig. 2.3*C*). Each is attached by **microtubules** extending from the centromere to the centriole, forming the **mitotic spindle**. Soon, the centromere of each chromosome divides, marking the beginning of anaphase, followed by migration of chromatids to opposite poles of the spindle. Finally, during telophase, chromosomes uncoil and lengthen, the nuclear envelope reforms, and the cytoplasm divides (Fig. 2.3*D–F*). Each daughter cell receives half of all doubled chromosome material and thus maintains the same number of chromosomes as the mother cell.

### Meiosis

**Meiosis** is the cell division that takes place in the **germ cells** to generate male and female gametes, sperm and egg cells, respectively. Meiosis requires two cell divisions, **meiosis I** and **meiosis II**, to reduce the number of chromosomes to the haploid number of 23 (Fig. 2.4). As in mitosis, male and female germ cells (**spermatocytes** and **primary oocytes**) at the beginning of meiosis I replicate their DNA so that each of the 46 chromosomes is duplicated into sister chromatids. In contrast to mitosis, however, **homologous chromosomes** then align themselves in **pairs**, a process called **synapsis**. The pairing is exact and point for point except for the XY combination. Homologous pairs then separate into two daughter cells, thereby reducing the chromosome number from diploid to haploid. Shortly thereafter, meiosis II separates sister chromatids. Each gamete then contains 23 chromosomes.

#### *Crossover*

**Crossovers**, critical events in meiosis I, are the **interchange of chromatid segments** between paired homologous chromosomes (Fig. 2.4*C*). Segments of chromatids break and are exchanged as homologous chromosomes separate. As separation occurs, points of interchange are temporarily united and form an X-like structure, a **chiasma** (Fig. 2.4*C*). The approximately 30 to 40 crossovers (one or two per

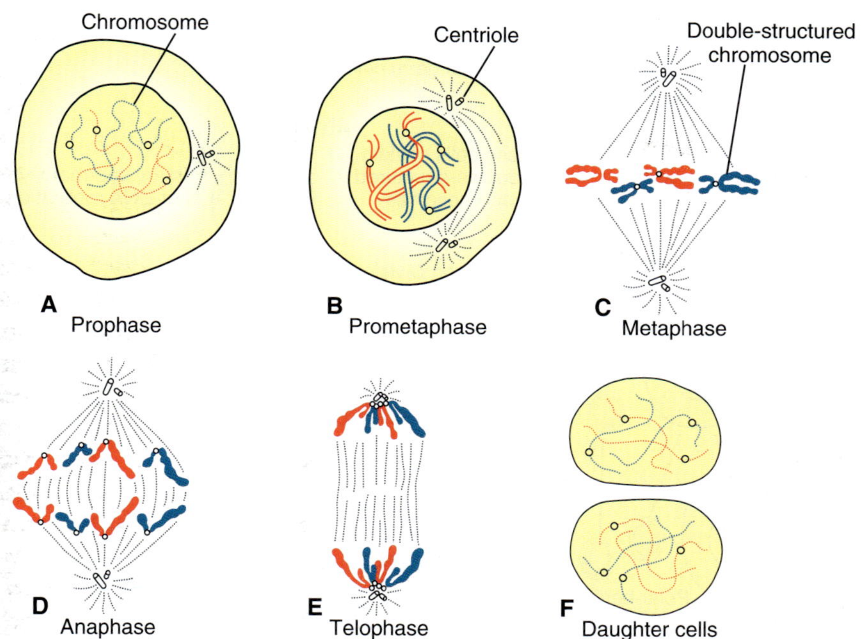


**FIGURE 2.3** Various stages of mitosis. In prophase, chromosomes are visible as slender threads. Doubled chromatids become clearly visible as individual units during metaphase. At no time during division do members of a chromosome pair unite. *Blue*, paternal chromosomes; *red*, maternal chromosomes.

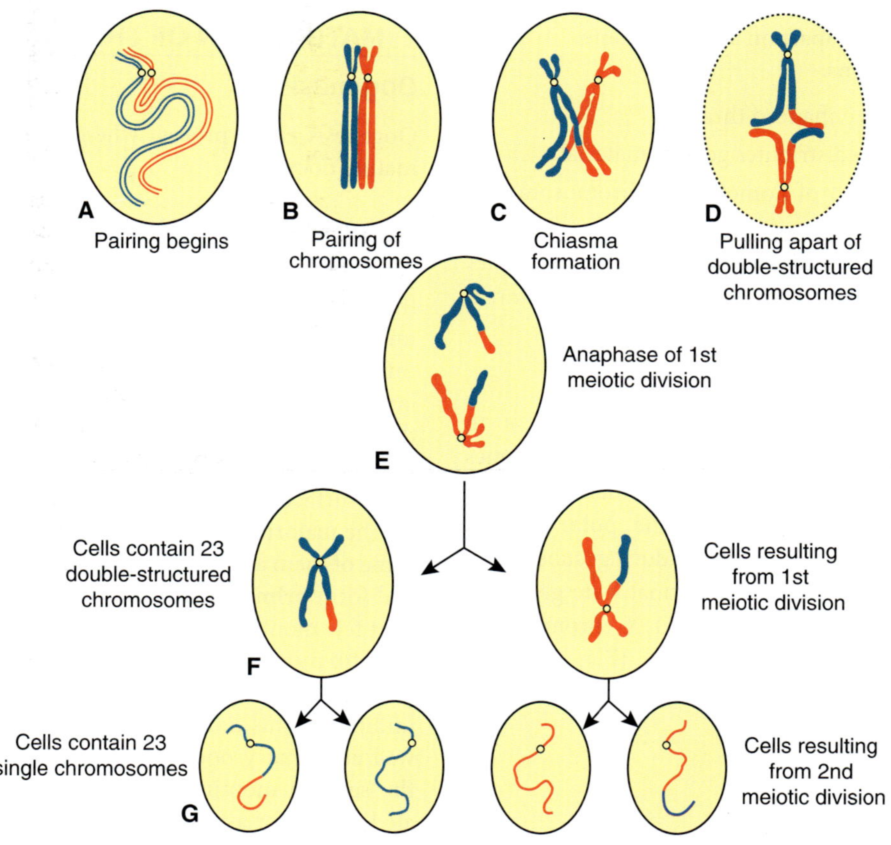


**FIGURE 2.4** First and second meiotic divisions. **A.** Homologous chromosomes approach each other. **B.** Homologous chromosomes pair, and each member of the pair consists of two chromatids. **C.** Intimately paired homologous chromosomes interchange chromatid fragments (crossover). Note the chiasma. **D.** Double-structured chromosomes pull apart. **E.** Anaphase of the first meiotic division. **F,G.** During the second meiotic division, the double-structured chromosomes split at the centromere. At completion of division, chromosomes in each of the four daughter cells are different from each other.

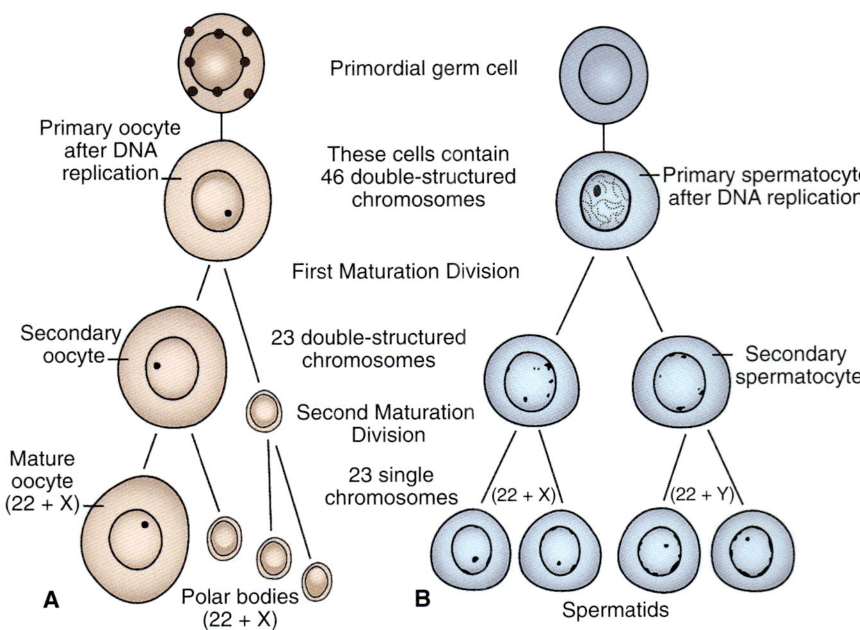


**FIGURE 2.5** Primordial germ cells and the events occurring during the first and second maturation divisions. **A.** Oogonia forming the primitive female germ cell (primary oocyte) produces only one mature gamete, the mature oocyte. **B.** Spermatogonia forming the primitive male germ cell (primary spermatocyte) produces four spermatids, all of which develop into spermatozoa.

chromosome) with each meiotic I division are most frequent between genes that are far apart on a chromosome.

**Result of meiotic divisions:**

- **Genetic variability** is enhanced through
  - Crossover, which redistributes genetic material
  - Random distribution of homologous chromosomes to the daughter cells
- Each germ cell contains a haploid number of chromosomes so that at fertilization, the diploid number of 46 is restored.

### *Polar Bodies*

Also during meiosis, one primary oocyte gives rise to four daughter cells, each with 22 plus 1 X chromosomes (Fig. 2.5*A*). Only one of these develops into a mature gamete, however, the oocyte; the other three, the **polar bodies,** receive little cytoplasm and degenerate during subsequent development. Similarly, one primary spermatocyte gives rise to four daughter cells, two with 22 plus 1 X chromosomes and two with 22 plus 1 Y chromosomes (Fig. 2.5*B*). In contrast to oocyte formation, however, all four develop into mature gametes.

### Gametogenesis

It is the process in which primordial germ cell of males, the spermatogonia, is converted to a spermatid (22+X and 22+Y chromosomes) and the primordial germ cell of females, oogonia, is converted to an oocyte. Both the gametes have haploid DNA and 22+X and 22+X chromosomes (Fig. 22.5).

## MORPHOLOGICAL CHANGES DURING MATURATION OF THE GAMETES

### Oogenesis

Oogenesis is the process whereby oogonia differentiate into mature oocytes.

#### *Maturation of Oocytes Begins Before Birth*

Once **PGCs** have arrived in the gonad of a genetic female, they differentiate into **oogonia** (Fig. 2.6*A,B*). These cells undergo a number of mitotic divisions, and by the end of the third month, they are arranged in clusters surrounded by a layer of flat epithelial cells (Figs. 2.7 and 2.8). Whereas all of the oogonia in one cluster are probably derived from a single cell, the flat epithelial cells, known as **follicular cells,** originate from surface epithelium covering the ovary.

The majority of oogonia continue to divide by mitosis, but some of them arrest their cell division in prophase of meiosis I and form **primary oocytes** (Figs. 2.6*C* and 2.7*A*). During the next few months, oogonia increase rapidly in number, and by the fifth month of prenatal development, the total number of germ cells in the ovary reaches its maximum, estimated at 7 million. At this time, cell death begins, and many oogonia as well as primary oocytes degenerate and become **atretic.** By the seventh month, the majority of oogonia have degenerated except for a few near the surface. All surviving primary oocytes have entered prophase of meiosis I, and most of them are individually surrounded by a layer of flat follicular epithelial cells (Fig. 2.7*B*). A primary oocyte, together with its surrounding flat epithelial cells, is known as a **primordial follicle** (Fig. 2.8*A*).

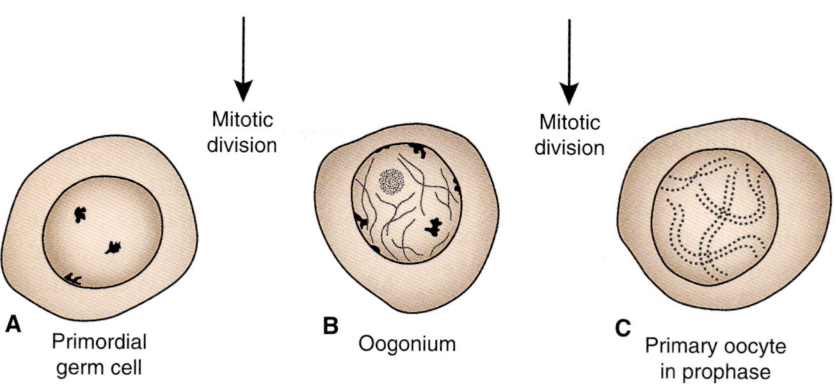


**FIGURE 2.6** Differentiation of PGCs into oogonia begins shortly after their arrival in the ovary. By the third month of development, some oogonia give rise to primary oocytes that enter prophase of the first meiotic division. This prophase may last 40 or more years and finishes only when the cell begins its final maturation. During this period, it carries 46 double-structured chromosomes.

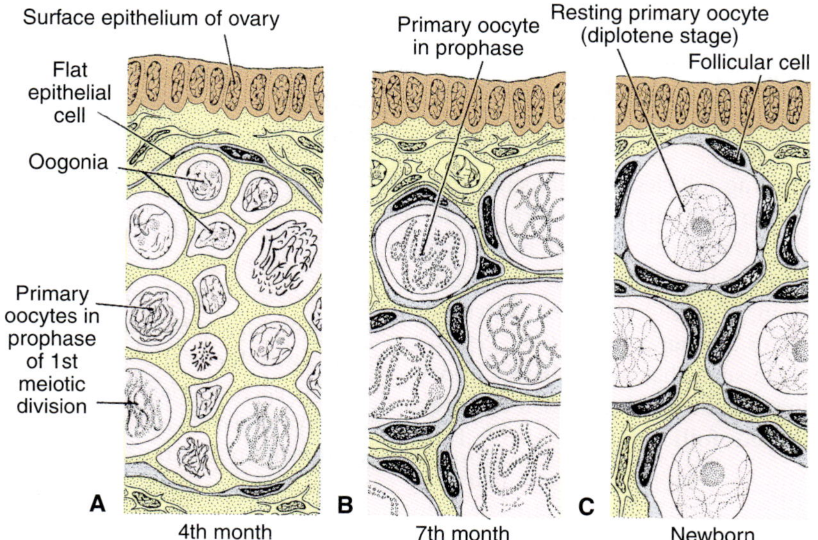


**FIGURE 2.7** Segment of the ovary at different stages of development. **A.** Oogonia are grouped in clusters in the cortical part of the ovary. Some show mitosis; others have differentiated into primary oocytes and entered prophase of the first meiotic division. **B.** Almost all oogonia are transformed into primary oocytes in prophase of the first meiotic division. **C.** There are no oogonia. Each primary oocyte is surrounded by a single layer of follicular cells, forming the primordial follicle. Oocytes have entered the diplotene stage of prophase, in which they remain until just before ovulation. Only then do they enter metaphase of the first meiotic division.

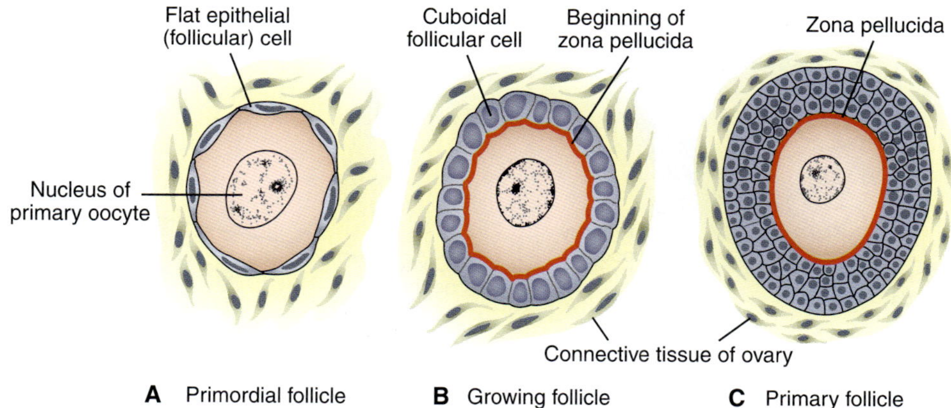


**FIGURE 2.8 A.** Primordial follicle consisting of a primary oocyte surrounded by a layer of flattened epithelial cells. **B.** Early primary or preantral stage follicle recruited from the pool of primordial follicles. As the follicle grows, follicular cells become cuboidal and begin to secrete the zona pellucida, which is visible in irregular patches on the surface of the oocyte. **C.** Mature primary (preantral) follicle with follicular cells forming a stratified layer of granulosa cells around the oocyte and the presence of a well-defined zona pellucida.

### *Maturation of Oocytes Continues at Puberty*

Near the time of birth, all primary oocytes have started prophase of meiosis I, but instead of proceeding into metaphase, they enter the **diplotene stage**, a resting stage during prophase that is characterized by a lacy network of chromatin (Fig. 2.7*C*). Primary oocytes remain arrested in prophase and do not finish their first meiotic division before puberty is reached. This arrested state is produced by **oocyte maturation inhibitor (OMI)**, a small peptide secreted by follicular cells. The total number of primary oocytes at birth is estimated to vary from 600,000 to 800,000. During childhood, most oocytes become atretic; only approximately 40,000 are present by the beginning of puberty, and fewer than 500 will be ovulated. Some oocytes that reach maturity late in life have been dormant in the diplotene stage of the first meiotic division for 40 years or more before ovulation. Whether the diplotene stage is the most suitable phase to protect the oocyte against environmental influences is unknown. The fact that the risk of having children with chromosomal abnormalities increases with maternal age indicates that primary oocytes are vulnerable to damage as they age.

At puberty, a pool of growing follicles is established and continuously maintained from the supply of primordial follicles. Each month, 15 to 20 follicles selected from this pool begin to mature. Some of these die, whereas others begin to accumulate fluid in a space called the **antrum**, thereby entering the **antral** or **vesicular stage** (Fig. 2.9*A*). Fluid continues to accumulate such that, immediately prior to ovulation, follicles are quite swollen and are called **mature vesicular follicles** or **graafian follicles** (Fig. 2.9*B*). The antral stage is the longest, whereas the mature vesicular stage encompasses approximately 37 hours prior to ovulation.

As primordial follicles begin to grow, surrounding follicular cells change from flat to cuboidal and proliferate to produce a stratified epithelium of **granulosa cells**, and the unit is called a **primary follicle** (Fig. 2.8*B,C*). Granulosa cells rest on a basement membrane separating them from surrounding ovarian connective tissue (stromal cells) that form the **theca folliculi**. Also, granulosa cells and the oocyte secrete a layer of glycoproteins on the surface of the oocyte, forming the **zona pellucida** (Fig. 2.8*C*). As follicles continue to grow, cells of the theca folliculi organize into an inner layer of secretory cells, the **theca interna**, and an outer fibrous capsule, the **theca externa**. Also, small, fingerlike processes of the follicular cells extend across the zona pellucida and interdigitate with microvilli of the plasma membrane of the oocyte. These processes are important for transport of materials from follicular cells to the oocyte.

As development continues, fluid-filled spaces appear between granulosa cells. Coalescence of these spaces forms the **antrum**, and the follicle is termed a **vesicular or an antral follicle**. Initially, the antrum is crescent-shaped, but with time, it enlarges (Fig. 2.9). Granulosa cells surrounding the oocyte remain intact and form the **cumulus oophorus**. At maturity, the **mature vesicular (graafian) follicle** may be 25 mm or more in diameter. It is surrounded by the theca interna, which is composed of cells having characteristics of steroid secretion, rich in blood vessels, and the theca externa, which gradually merges with the ovarian connective tissue (Fig. 2.9).

With each ovarian cycle, a number of follicles begin to develop, but usually, only one reaches full maturity. The others degenerate and become atretic. When the secondary follicle

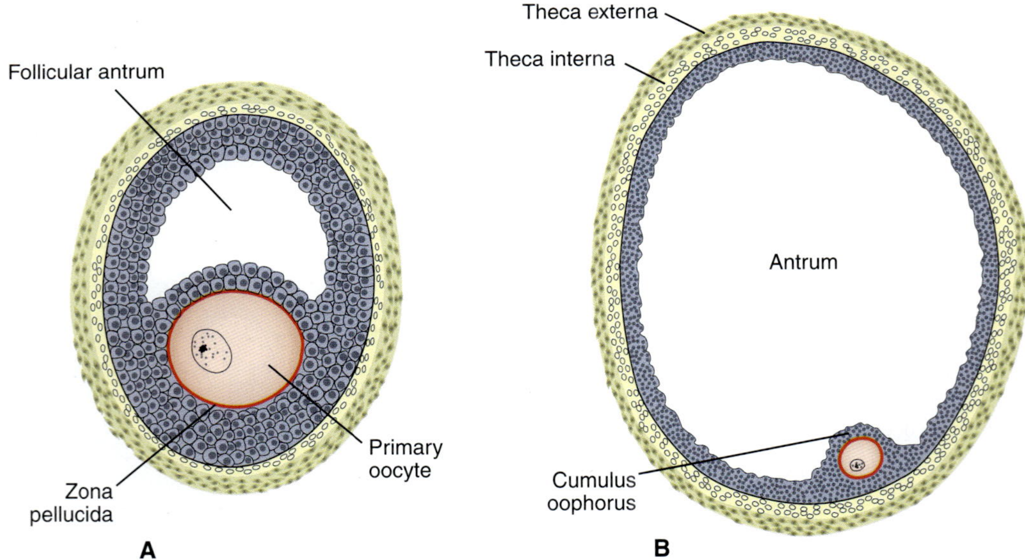


**FIGURE 2.9 A.** Vesicular (antral) stage follicle. The oocyte, surrounded by the zona pellucida, is off center; the antrum has developed by fluid accumulation between intercellular spaces. Note the arrangement of cells of the theca interna and the theca externa. **B.** Mature vesicular (graafian) follicle. The antrum has enlarged considerably, is filled with follicular fluid, and is surrounded by a stratified layer of granulosa cells. The oocyte is embedded in a mound of granulosa cells, the cumulus oophorus.

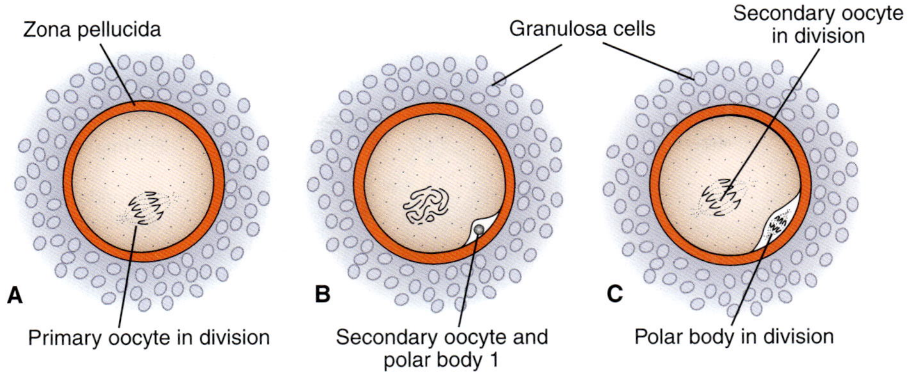


**FIGURE 2.10** Maturation of the oocyte. **A.** Primary oocyte showing the spindle of the first meiotic division. **B.** Secondary oocyte and first polar body. The nuclear membrane is absent. **C.** Secondary oocyte showing the spindle of the second meiotic division. The first polar body is also dividing.



is mature, a surge in **luteinizing hormone (LH)** induces the preovulatory growth phase. Meiosis I is completed, resulting in formation of two daughter cells of unequal size, each with 23 double-structured chromosomes (Fig. 2.10*A*,*B*). One cell, the **secondary oocyte**, receives most of the cytoplasm; the other, the **first polar** body, receives practically none. The first polar body lies between the zona pellucida and the cell membrane of the secondary oocyte in the perivitelline space (Fig. 2.10*B*). The cell then enters meiosis II but arrests in metaphase approximately 3 hours before ovulation. Meiosis II is completed only if the oocyte is fertilized; otherwise, the cell degenerates approximately 24 hours after ovulation. The first polar body may undergo a second division (Fig. 2.10*C*).

The timeline and events taking place during oogenesis are discussed in Table 2.1.

## Spermatogenesis

### *Maturation of Sperm Begins at Puberty*

**Spermatogenesis**, which begins at puberty, includes all of the events by which **spermatogonia** are transformed into **spermatozoa**. At birth, germ cells in the male infant can be recognized in the sex cords of the testis as large, pale cells surrounded by supporting cells (Fig. 2.11*A*). Supporting cells, which are derived from the surface epithelium of the testis in the same manner as follicular cells, become **sustentacular cells** or **Sertoli cells** (Fig. 2.11*B*).

Shortly before puberty, the sex cords acquire a lumen and become the **seminiferous tubules**. At about the same time, PGCs give rise to spermatogonial stem cells. At regular intervals, cells emerge from this stem cell population to form **type A spermatogonia**, and their production marks the initiation

**Table 2.1 Timeline and Events Taking Place During Oogenesis**

| Time | Number | Cell Type | Events |
|---|---|---|---|
| 3-month prenatal | | Primordial germ cells | Migrate from yolk sac to gonadal ridge |
| 5-month prenatal | 7,000,000 approximately | Primary oocytes are enclosed by surface epithelial cells of gonadal ridge | Lot of mitosis and some oocytes have started meiosis I; arrest in prophase |
| 7-month prenatal | | Primary oocyte surrounded by follicular cells forms the primordial follicle | Degeneration with loss of germ cells. Oocytes in prophase |
| Birth | 600,000 to 800,000 approximately | Primary oocyte; primordial follicle | All oocytes enter meiosis I and arrest in diplotene or prophase I (resting state); oocytes lie toward surface of ovary |
| Puberty | 40,000 out of which only 500 ovulate during the reproductive span | Secondary oocyte complete meiosis I and the release of first polar body | Meiosis II is incomplete; stops 3 hours before ovulation |
| Fertilization | One secondary oocyte | Zygote | Fertilization of secondary oocyte occurs with sperm; completion of meiosis II |

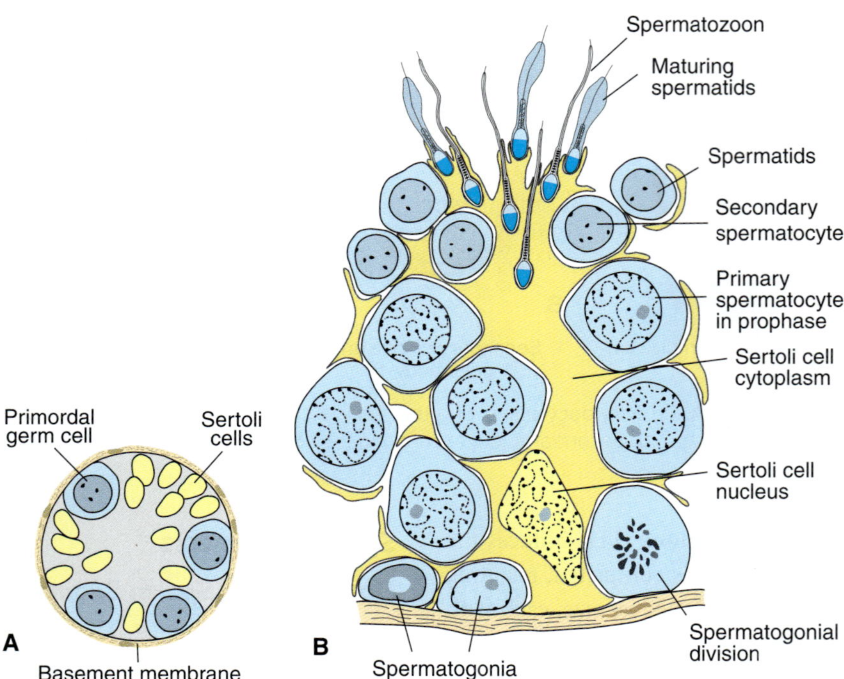


**FIGURE 2.11** **A.** Cross section through primitive sex cords of a newborn boy showing PGCs and their supporting Sertoli cells. **B.** Cross section through a seminiferous tubule at puberty. Note the different stages of spermatogenesis and that developing sperm cells are embedded in the cytoplasmic processes of a supporting Sertoli cell.

of spermatogenesis. Type A cells undergo a limited number of mitotic divisions to form clones of cells. The last cell division produces **type B spermatogonia**, which then divide to form **primary spermatocytes** (Figs. 2.11*B* and 2.12). Primary spermatocytes then enter a prolonged prophase (22 days) followed by rapid completion of meiosis I and formation of **secondary spermatocytes**. During the second meiotic division, these cells immediately begin to form haploid **spermatids** (Figs. 2.11*B*, 2.12, 2.13). Throughout this series of events, from the time type A cells leave the stem cell population to formation of spermatids, cytokinesis is incomplete so that successive cell generations are joined by cytoplasmic bridges. Thus, the progeny of a single type A spermatogonium form a clone of germ cells that maintain contact throughout differentiation (Fig. 2.12). Furthermore, spermatogonia and spermatids remain embedded in deep recesses of Sertoli cells throughout their development (Fig. 2.11*B*). In this manner, Sertoli cells support and protect the germ cells, participate in their nutrition, and assist in the release of mature spermatozoa.

Spermatogenesis is regulated by LH production by the pituitary gland. LH binds to receptors on Leydig cells and stimulates testosterone production, which in turn binds to Sertoli cells to promote spermatogenesis. **Follicle-stimulating hormone (FSH)** is also essential because its binding to Sertoli cells stimulates testicular fluid production and synthesis of intracellular androgen receptor proteins.

The differences between oogenesis and spermatogenesis are discussed in Tables 2.2 and 2.3.

### Spermiogenesis

The series of changes resulting in the transformation of spermatids into spermatozoa is **spermiogenesis**. These changes include (1) formation of the **acrosome**, which covers half of the nuclear surface and contains enzymes to assist in penetration of the egg and its surrounding layers during fertilization (Fig. 2.14); (2) condensation of the nucleus; (3) formation of neck, middle piece, and tail; and (4) shedding of most of the cytoplasm as residual bodies that are phagocytized by Sertoli cells. In humans, the time required for a spermatogonium to develop into a mature spermatozoon is approximately 74 days, and approximately 300 million sperm cells are produced daily.

When fully formed, spermatozoa enter the lumen of seminiferous tubules. From there, they are pushed toward the epididymis by contractile elements in the wall of the seminiferous tubules. Although initially only slightly motile, spermatozoa obtain full motility in the epididymis.

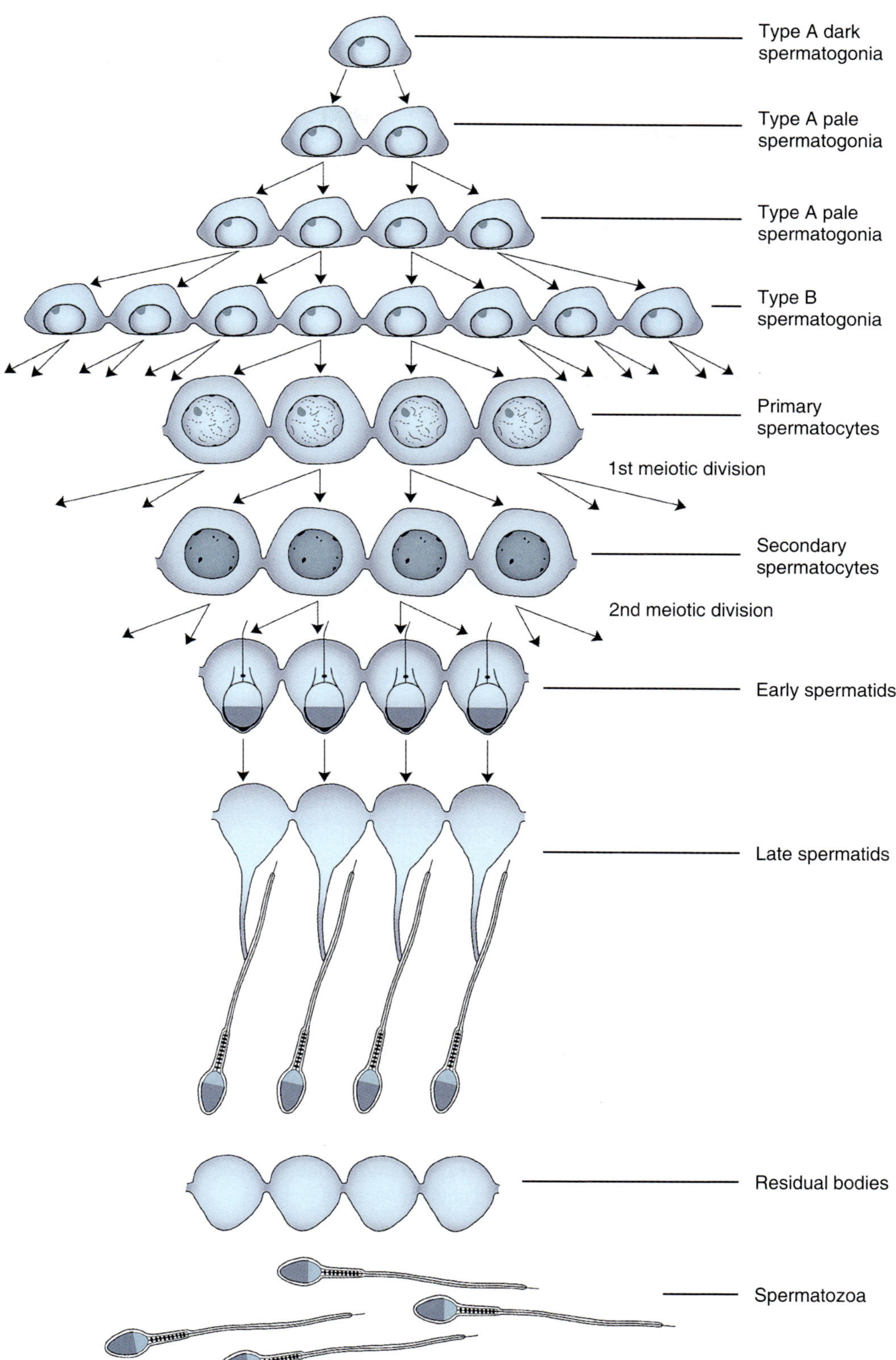


**FIGURE 2.12** Type A spermatogonia, derived from the spermatogonial stem cell population, represent the first cells in the process of spermatogenesis. Clones of cells are established, and cytoplasmic bridges join cells in each succeeding division until individual sperm are separated from residual bodies. In fact, the number of individual interconnected cells is considerably greater than depicted in this figure.

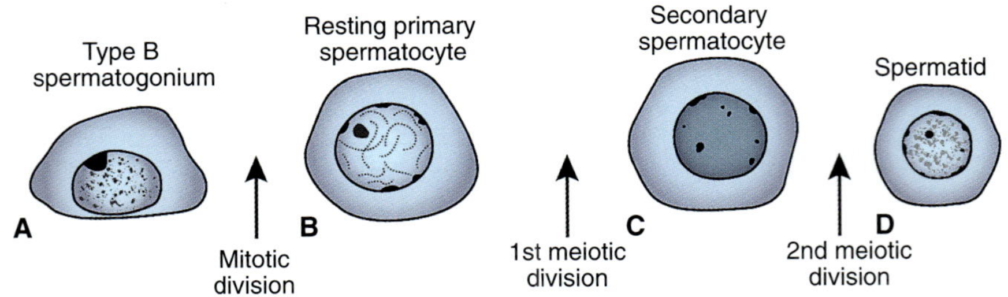


**FIGURE 2.13** The products of meiosis during spermatogenesis in humans.

**Table 2.2 Differences Between Oogenesis and Spermatogenesis From Primordial Germ Cells to Mature Gametes**

| Events | Time | Oogenesis | Spermatogenesis |
|---|---|---|---|
| Primordial germ cell (PGC) and gonad | Migrates from the yolk sac to the gonadal ridge in the second to third month of intrauterine life | Ovary developing in absence of testis-determining Factor | Testis develops under influence of testis-determining factor |
| Meiosis | At birth | Primary oocyte arrested in diplotene of prophase of meiosis I under influence of oocyte maturation inhibitor (OMI) | PGC and Sertoli cells lining the seminiferous tubules |
| | At puberty | Ovulation begins. Primary oocyte divides to form secondary oocyte | Primary spermatocyte forms secondary spermatocyte. It forms spermatids that undergo spermiogenesis to form mature spermatozoa |
| | | Final completion of meiosis II will happen only at time of fertilization | Entire process of meiosis is completed without any arrest phase |
| Location | | Inside the ovary, but completion of meiosis II happens in fallopian tube (ampulla) | Inside the testis |
| Cell division | Cell division | Unequal | Equal |
| End result | | 1 haploid ovum and 3 polar bodies | 4 haploid sperms |
| | | Produces non-motile cells | Produces motile cells |
| | | No major change in cell structure | Cellular restructuring: Reduction of cytoplasm and nuclear condensation |
| | | Size of ovum larger than that of oogonium | Size of spermatozoa smaller than that of spermatogonium |
| Time span | | Begins in fetal life, and then arrested until puberty. Resumes at puberty and continues until menopause | Begins at puberty and continues throughout life |
| | | Cyclical process: Once a month | Continues on a daily basis |
| | | Approximately 500 oocytes ovulate during the reproductive time span | Millions of spermatozoa develop; 2 to 3 million sperms released in each ejaculation |

**Table 2.3 Differences Between Spermatogenesis and Oogenesis**

| Oogenesis | Spermatogenesis |
|---|---|
| Once-a-month cycle in reproductive age | Continuous process from puberty to death |
| • Around 500 oocytes mature during the reproductive phase<br>• Every month, 20 to 30 follicles mature | One ejaculate has 2 to 3 million sperms |
| Ova viable for 3 to 4 days | Sperm viable for 24 to 72 hours in female reproductive tract |
| One germ cell: One oocyte (gamete) | One germ cell: Four sperms (gamete) |

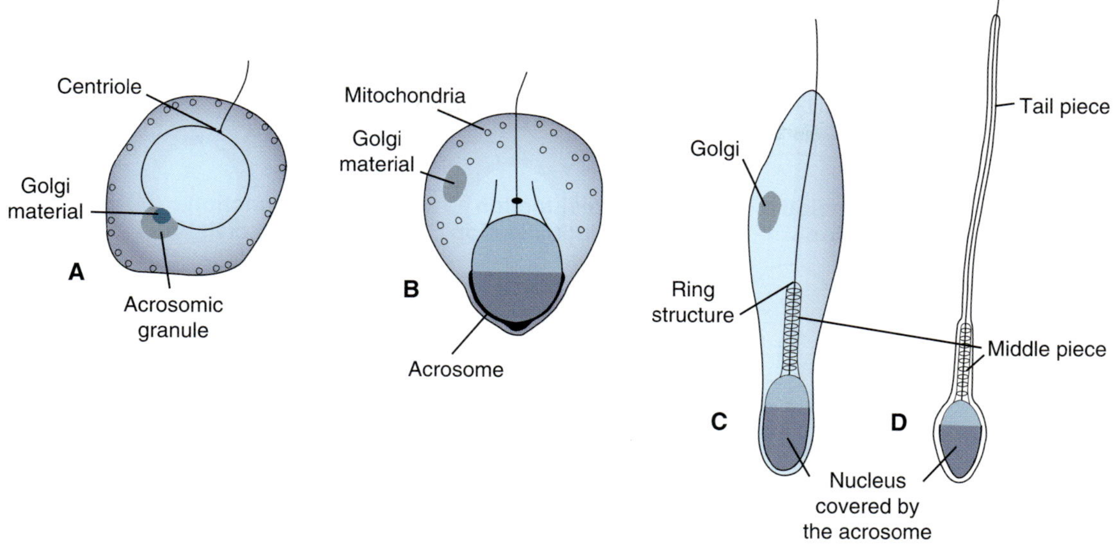


**FIGURE 2.14** Important stages in transformation of the human spermatid into the spermatozoon.



## ■ GENETIC COUNSELING

Parents need to be counseled in a few conditions like if the mother has had a repeated episode of abortion, family history of genetic defects, elderly mother, sibling with a congenital defect, or any physical ailment or mental health issues with the parents.

The parents are explained about the consequences of planning a child and advised according to the situation.

## *Clinical Correlates*

Any abnormality during cell division can lead to a number of defects which are described in the subsequent text. These defects can lead to spontaneous abortions.

### Birth Defects and Spontaneous Abortions: Chromosomal and Genetic Factors

**Chromosomal abnormalities**, which may be **numerical** or **structural**, are important causes of birth defects and spontaneous abortions. It is estimated that 50% of conceptions end in spontaneous abortion and that 50% of these abortuses have major chromosomal abnormalities. Thus, approximately 25% of conceptuses have a major chromosomal defect. The most common chromosomal abnormalities in abortuses are 45,X (Turner syndrome), triploidy, and trisomy 16. Chromosomal abnormalities account for 10% of major birth defects, and **gene mutations** account for an additional 8%.

#### *Numerical Abnormalities*

The normal human somatic cell contains 46 chromosomes; the normal gamete contains 23. Normal somatic cells are **diploid**, or **2*n***; normal gametes are **haploid**, or ***n***. **Euploid** refers to any exact multiple of *n* (e.g., diploid or triploid). **Aneuploid** refers to any chromosome number that is not euploid; it is usually applied when an extra chromosome is present (**trisomy**) or when one is missing (**monosomy**). Abnormalities in chromosome number may originate during meiotic or mitotic divisions. In **meiosis**, two members of a pair of homologous chromosomes normally separate during the first meiotic division so that each daughter cell receives one member of each pair (Fig. 2.15*A*). Sometimes, however, separation does not occur (**nondisjunction**), and both members of a pair move into one cell (Fig. 2.15*B*,*C*). As a result of nondisjunction of the chromosomes, one cell receives 24 chromosomes, and the other receives 22 instead of the normal 23. When, at fertilization, a gamete having 23 chromosomes fuses with a gamete having 24 or 22 chromosomes, the result is an individual with either 47 chromosomes (trisomy) or 45 chromosomes (monosomy). Nondisjunction, which occurs during either the first or the second meiotic division of the germ cells, may involve the autosomes or sex chromosomes. In women, the incidence of chromosomal abnormalities, including nondisjunction, increases with age, especially at 35 years and older.

Sometimes, chromosomes break, and pieces of one chromosome attach to another. Such **translocations** may be **balanced**, in which case breakage and reunion occur between two chromosomes, but no critical genetic material is lost and individuals are normal; or they may be **unbalanced**, in which case part of one chromosome is lost, and an altered phenotype is produced. For example, unbalanced translocations between the long arms of chromosomes 14 and 21 during meiosis I or II produce gametes with an extra copy of chromosome 21, one of the causes of Down syndrome (Fig. 2.16). Translocations are particularly common between chromosomes 13, 14, 15, 21, and 22 because they cluster during meiosis.

(*Continued*)

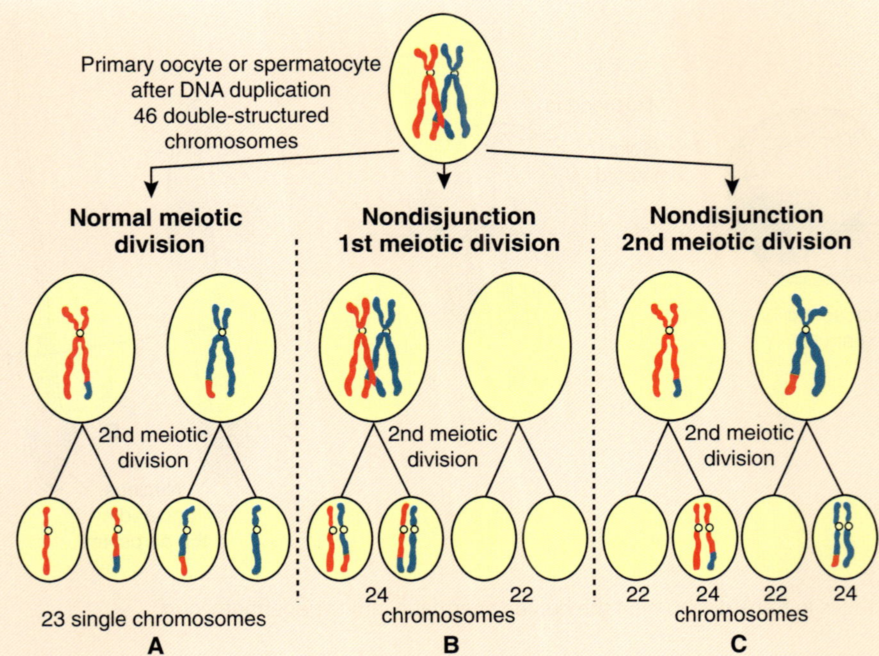


**FIGURE 2.15** **A.** Normal maturation divisions. **B.** Nondisjunction in the first meiotic division. **C.** Nondisjunction in the second meiotic division.

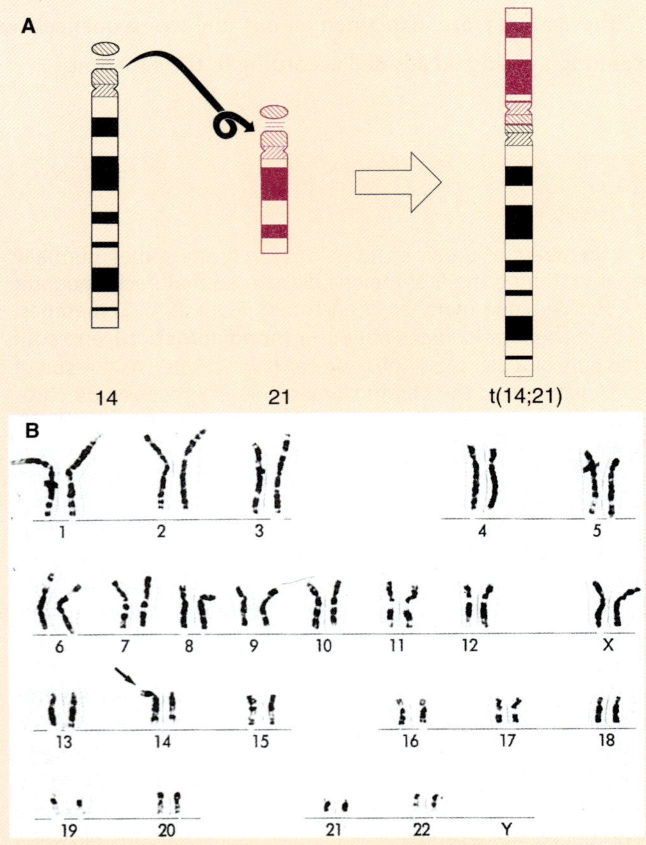


**FIGURE 2.16** **A.** Translocation of the long arms of chromosomes 14 and 21 at the centromere. Loss of the short arms is not clinically significant, and these individuals are clinically normal, although they are at risk for producing offspring with unbalanced translocations. **B. Karyotype** of translocation of chromosome 21 onto 14, resulting in Down syndrome.

### Trisomy 21 (Down Syndrome)

**Down syndrome** is caused by an extra copy of **chromosome 21 (trisomy 21)** (Fig. 2.17). Features of children with Down syndrome include growth retardation; varying degrees of intellectual disability; craniofacial abnormalities, including upward slanting eyes, epicanthal folds (extra skin folds at the medial corners of the eyes), flat facies, and small ears; cardiac defects; and hypotonia (Fig. 2.18). These individuals also have an increased chance of developing leukemia, infections, thyroid dysfunction, and premature aging. Furthermore, an increased frequency and earlier onset of Alzheimer disease is observed among persons with Down syndrome. In 95% of cases, the syndrome is caused by trisomy 21 resulting from meiotic nondisjunction, and in 75% of these instances, nondisjunction occurs during **oocyte formation**. The incidence of Down syndrome is approximately 1 in 2,000 conceptuses for women under age 25 years. This risk increases with maternal age to 1 in 300 at age 35 years and 1 in 100 at age 40 years.

In approximately 4% of cases of Down syndrome, there is an unbalanced translocation between chromosome 21 and chromosomes 13, 14, 15, or 21 (Fig. 2.16). The final 1% is caused by mosaicism resulting from a trisomic conception followed by the loss of the extra chromosome in some cells during mitosis. These individuals have **mosaicism**, with some cells having a normal chromosome number and some having trisomy. They may exhibit few or many of the characteristics of Down syndrome.

### Trisomy 18 (Edward Syndrome)

Patients with **trisomy 18** show the following features: intellectual disability, congenital heart defects, low-set ears, and flexion of fingers and hands (Fig. 2.19). In addition, patients frequently show micrognathia, renal anomalies, syndactyly, and malformations of the skeletal system. The incidence of this condition is approximately 1 in 5,000 newborns. Eighty-five percent are lost between 10 weeks of gestation and term, whereas those born alive usually die by 2 months of age. Approximately 5% live beyond 1 year.

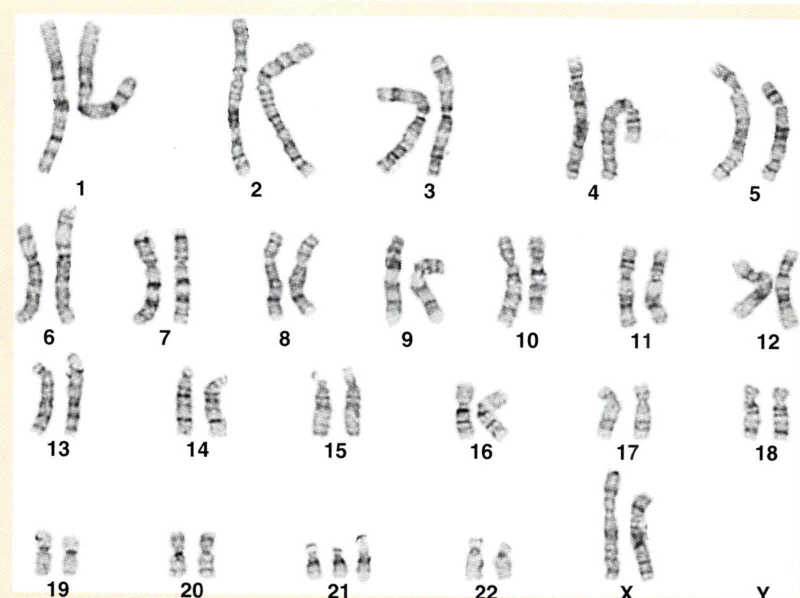


**FIGURE 2.17** Karyotype of trisomy 21, Down syndrome.

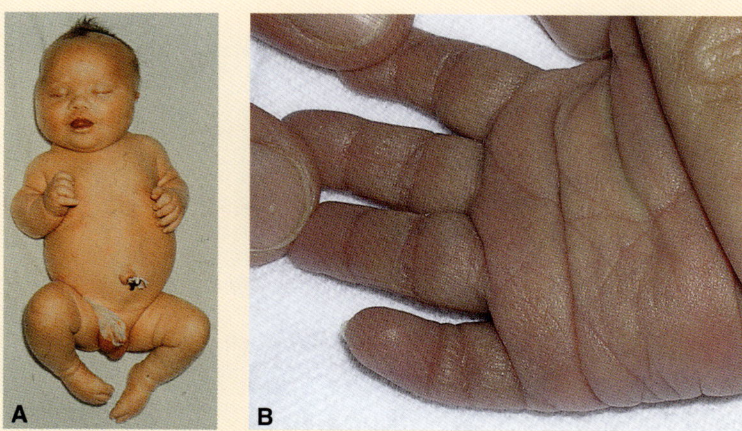


**FIGURE 2.18** **A.** Child with Down syndrome. Note the flat broad face, oblique palpebral fissures, and protruding tongue. Children with Down syndrome usually have some degree of intellectual disability and many have cardiac defects. **B.** Another characteristic of these children is a broad hand with a single transverse (simian) crease.

### Trisomy 13 (Patau Syndrome)

The main abnormalities of **trisomy 13** are intellectual disability, holoprosencephaly, congenital heart defects, deafness, cleft lip and palate, and eye defects, such as microphthalmia, anophthalmia, and coloboma (Fig. 2.20). The incidence of this abnormality is approximately 1 in 20,000 live births, and more than 90% of the infants die in the first month after birth. Approximately 5% live beyond 1 year.

### Klinefelter Syndrome

The clinical features of **Klinefelter syndrome**, found only in males and usually detected by amniocentesis, are sterility, testicular atrophy, hyalinization of the seminiferous tubules, and usually gynecomastia. The cells have 47 chromosomes with a sex chromosomal complement of the XXY type, and a **sex chromatin (Barr) body** is found in 80% of cases. (**Barr body**: formed by condensation of an inactivated X chromosome; a Barr body is also present in normal females because one of the X chromosomes is normally inactivated). The incidence is approximately 1 in 500 males. Nondisjunction of the XX homologues is the most common causative event. Occasionally, patients with Klinefelter syndrome have 48 chromosomes: 44 autosomes and 4 sex chromosomes (48,XXXY). Although intellectual disability is not generally part of the syndrome, the more X chromosomes there are, the more likely there will be some degree of cognitive impairment.

### Turner Syndrome

**Turner syndrome**, with a 45,X karyotype, is the only monosomy compatible with life. Even then, 98% of all fetuses with the syndrome are spontaneously aborted. The few that survive are unmistakably female in appearance (Fig. 2.21) and are characterized by the absence of ovaries (**gonadal dysgenesis**) and short stature.

(*Continued*)

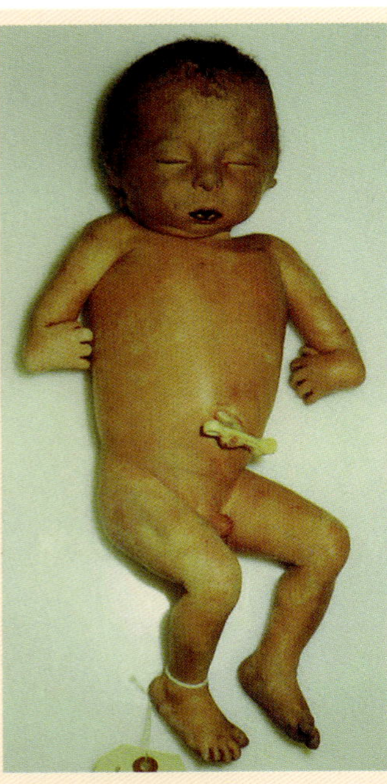

**FIGURE 2.19** Child with trisomy 18. Note the low-set ears, small mouth, deficient mandible (micrognathia), flexion of the hands, and absent and/or hypoplasia of the radius and ulna.

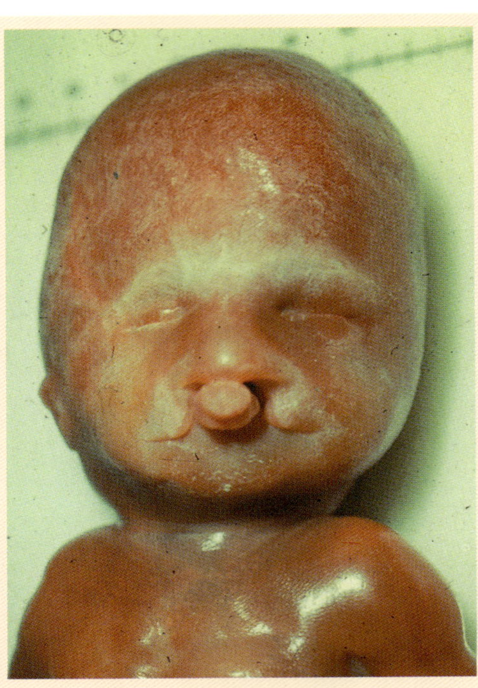

**FIGURE 2.20** Child with trisomy 13. Note the bilateral cleft lip, the sloping forehead, and anophthalmia.

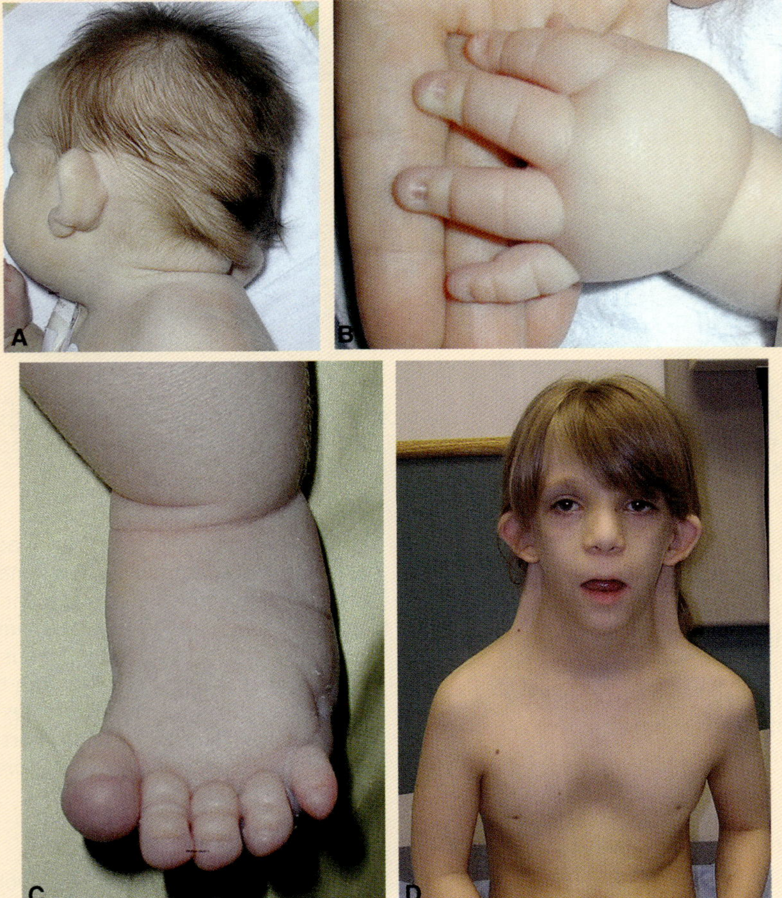

**FIGURE 2.21** Patient with Turner syndrome. **A.** At birth. Note the loose skin at the posterior of the neck caused by the remains of a cystic hygroma (fluid-filled cyst), the short neck, malformed ears, and swelling in the hand **(B)** and the foot **(C)** caused by lymphedema. **D.** At 6 years of age, the webbed neck is prominent, and the nipples are widely spaced with a broad chest.

Other common associated abnormalities are webbed neck, lymphedema of the extremities, skeletal deformities, and a broad chest with widely spaced nipples. Approximately 55% of affected females are monosomic for the X and chromatin body negative because of nondisjunction. In 80% of these females, nondisjunction in the **male gamete** is the cause. In the remainder of females, structural abnormalities of the X chromosome or mitotic nondisjunction resulting in mosaicism is the cause.

#### Triple X Syndrome

Patients with **triple X syndrome (47,XXX)** often go undiagnosed because of their mild physical features. However, these girls frequently have problems with speech and self-esteem. They have two sex chromatin bodies in their cells.

### *Structural Abnormalities*

**Structural chromosome abnormalities**, which involve one or more chromosomes, usually result from chromosome breakage. It has been suggested that breaks are caused by environmental factors, such as viruses, radiation, and drugs, but the evidence is inconclusive. The result of breakage depends on what happens to the broken pieces. In some cases, the broken piece of a chromosome is lost, and the infant with partial **deletion** of a chromosome is abnormal. A well-known syndrome, caused by partial deletion of the short arm of chromosome 5, is the **cri-du-chat syndrome**. Affected infants have a cat-like cry, microcephaly (small head), intellectual disability, and congenital heart disease. Many other relatively rare syndromes are known to result from a partial chromosome deletion.

**Microdeletions**, spanning only a few **contiguous genes**, may result in **microdeletion syndrome** or **contiguous gene syndrome**. Sites where these deletions occur, called **contiguous gene complexes**, are usually identified by **fluorescence in situ hybridization** (**FISH**; see p. 22). An example of a microdeletion occurs on the long arm of chromosome 15 (15q11–15q13). (Note: Chromosomes have a long arm, designated "q," and a short arm, designated "p," based on the position of the centromere.) When the microdeletion occurs on the maternal chromosome, it results in **Angelman syndrome**, and the children have intellectual disability, cannot speak, exhibit poor motor development, and are prone to unprovoked and prolonged periods of laughter (Fig. 2.22). If the microdeletion occurs on the paternal chromosome, **Prader-Willi syndrome** results. Affected individuals are characterized by hypotonia, obesity, intellectual disability, hypogonadism, and undescended testes (Fig. 2.23). Characteristics that are differentially expressed depending upon whether the genetic material is inherited from the mother or the father are examples of **genomic imprinting**. Other contiguous gene syndromes may be inherited from either parent, including **Miller-Dieker syndrome** (lissencephaly, developmental delay, seizures, and cardiac and facial abnormalities resulting from a deletion at 17p13) and most cases of **22q11 syndrome** (palatal defects, conotruncal heart defects, speech delay, learning disorders, and schizophrenia-like disorder resulting from a deletion in 22q11).

**Fragile sites** are regions of chromosomes that demonstrate a propensity to separate or break under certain cell manipulations. For example, fragile sites can be revealed by culturing lymphocytes from a patient in folate-deficient medium. Although numerous fragile sites have been defined and consist of **CGG repeats**, only those in the **FMRI** gene on the long arm of the X chromosome (Xq27) have been correlated

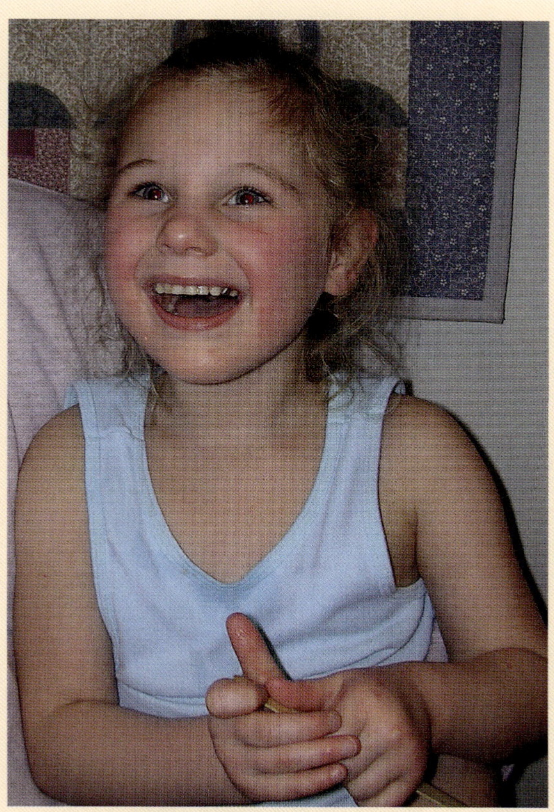

**FIGURE 2.22** Patient with Angelman syndrome resulting from a microdeletion on maternal chromosome 15. If the defect is inherited on the paternal chromosome, Prader-Willi syndrome occurs (Fig. 2.23).

with an altered phenotype that is called the **fragile X syndrome**. Greater than 200 repeats occur in the promoter region of the gene in affected individuals compared to 6 to 54 repeats in normal subjects. Fragile X syndrome is characterized by intellectual disability, large ears, prominent jaw, and large testes. The syndrome occurs in 1 per 5,000 individuals, and because it is an X-linked condition, males are affected almost exclusively, which may account for the preponderance of males among the cognitively impaired. Fragile X syndrome is second only to Down syndrome as a cause of intellectual disability due to genetic abnormalities.

### *Gene Mutations*

Many congenital malformations in humans are inherited, and some show a clear Mendelian pattern of inheritance. Many birth defects are directly attributable to a change in the structure or function of a single gene, hence the name **single gene mutation**. This type of defect is estimated to account for approximately 8% of all human malformations.

With the exception of the X and Y chromosomes in the male, genes exist as pairs, or **alleles**, so that there are two doses for each genetic determinant: one from the mother and one from the father. If a mutant gene produces an abnormality in a single dose, despite the presence of a normal allele, it is a **dominant mutation**. If both alleles must be abnormal (double dose) or if the mutation is X-linked (occurs on the X chromosome) in the male, it is a **recessive mutation**. Variations in the effects of mutant genes may be a result of **modifying factors**.

(Continued)

Part 1

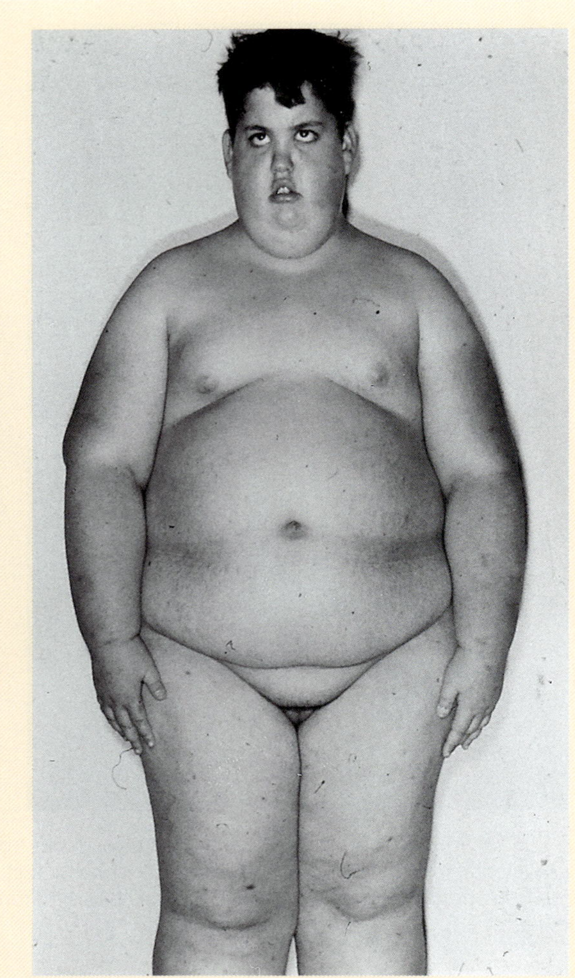

**FIGURE 2.23** Patient with Prader-Willi syndrome resulting from a microdeletion on paternal chromosome 15. If the defect is inherited on the maternal chromosome, Angelman syndrome occurs (Fig. 2.22).

In some cases, mutations occur in a cell as an embryo is developing. If the mutation occurs in a somatic cell, the individual will have **mosaicism** (having more than one genetically distinct cell line) with some cells having the mutation and some not. If the mutation occurs in a germ line cell (egg or sperm), the result is germ line mosaicism. In this case, the parent does not express an abnormality or disease because his or her somatic cells are normal. However, the parent can transmit the defect to multiple offspring.

**Chimerism** (chimera) is similar to mosaicism in that it is defined by the presence of two genetically distinct cell lines. However, in the case of chimerism, there is fusion of two different zygotes within a single embryo. Chimerism is often recognized because there are both 46,XX and 46,XY cell lines, which sometimes manifest clinically, but are readily discernable cytogenetically. Cytogenetic analysis is unable to detect chimerism without a difference in sex chromosome constitution between the two cell lines. Detection in these cases requires molecular analysis if chimerism is suspected. The use of a genome-wide SNP array, a novel technique, makes the differentiation of chimerism and mosaicism possible, as the additional presence of extra genotypes in the chimeras is readily detectable.

The application of molecular biological techniques has increased our knowledge of genes responsible for normal development. In turn, genetic analysis of human syndromes has shown that mutations in many of these same genes are responsible for some congenital abnormalities and childhood diseases. Thus, the link between key genes in development and their role in clinical syndromes is becoming clearer.

In addition to causing congenital malformations, mutations can result in **inborn errors of metabolism**. These diseases, among which **phenylketonuria**, **homocystinuria**, and **galactosemia** are the best known, may be accompanied by or cause various degrees of intellectual disability if proper diets and medical care are not instituted.

## Diagnostic Techniques for Identifying Genetic Abnormalities

**Cytogenetic analysis** is used to assess chromosome number and integrity. The technique requires dividing cells, which usually means establishing cell cultures that are arrested in metaphase by chemical treatment. Chromosomes are **Giemsa-stained** to reveal light and dark banding patterns (G-bands; Fig. 2.16) unique for each chromosome. Each band represents 5 to $10 \times 10^6$ base pairs of DNA, which may include a few to several hundred genes. Recently, **high-resolution metaphase banding techniques** have been developed that demonstrate greater numbers of bands representing even smaller pieces of DNA, thereby facilitating diagnosis of small deletions.

**Molecular** techniques, such as **fluorescent in situ hybridization (FISH)**, use specific DNA probes to identify ploidy for a few selected chromosomes and for detecting microdeletions. Fluorescent probes are hybridized to chromosomes or genetic loci using cells on a slide, and the results are visualized with a fluorescence microscope (Fig. 2.24).

**Microarrays** use spots of specific DNA sequences (probes) attached to a solid surface, usually glass or silicon (Affymetrix chips). These probes may be a short sequence from a gene or other DNA element that are used to hybridize a cDNA or cRNA sample (the target sample). Hybridization of probe-target sequences are detected and quantified using fluorescence or other reporter techniques. Results can detect single nucleotide polymorphisms, mutations, and changes in expression levels. Some companies now offer such techniques commercially for anyone who wants their genome tested or sequenced.

**Exome sequencing** represents a new approach to finding **mutations** and **polymorphisms** (single nucleotide changes [SNPs] in a DNA sequence) responsible for birth defects and diseases. With this technique, only the coding regions (exons) in the genome are sequenced. Together, these coding regions make up the **exome** and represent only 1% of the entire human genome, thereby making sequencing them more practical than trying to sequence all of the genome. Because most genetic variants lie within the coding regions for proteins, the technique is an efficient way to discover these differences. The technique is also superior to older approaches that relied on linkage studies followed by positional cloning (searching for candidate genes in specific regions of chromosomes) because these techniques required large numbers of affected individuals within a family and were not applicable to studying affected individuals from different families. In contrast, exome sequencing can find a causative mutation in a single affected individual if the exomes from both parents can also be sequenced. Even

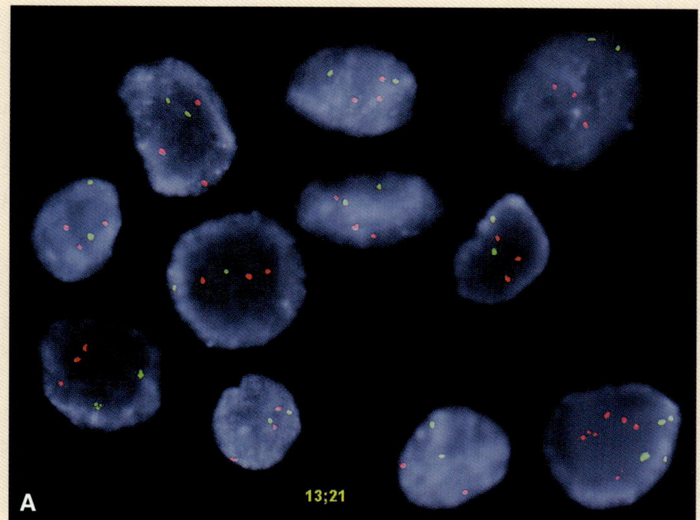


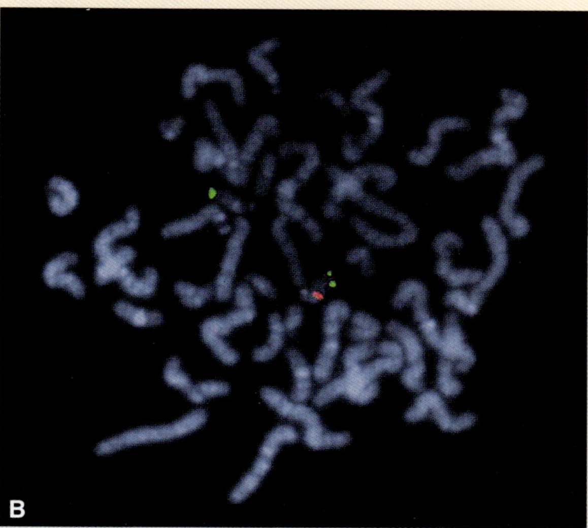


**FIGURE 2.24** **A.** FISH, using a probe for chromosome 21 (*red dots*). Note that there are three *red dots* in each cell, indicating trisomy 21 (Down syndrome). The *green dots* represent a control probe for chromosome 13. Two cells are superimposed on the lower right, giving the impression of the presence of multiple probes. **B.** FISH analysis of 22q11 deletion syndrome. The green signals identify chromosome 22; the red signal represents FISH probe N25, which is in the q11 region. It is present on only one of the pairs of chromosome 22 indicating the other has the 22q11 deletion.

sequencing-affected individuals from different families regardless of kinship can be successful. It must be remembered, however, that exome sequencing can only identify variants in the coding regions of genes that alter proteins. Other genetic causes of birth defects that lie outside the coding region will have to be identified by whole genome sequencing, but for now, the expense and time required to conduct these studies is prohibitive.

## *Clinical Correlates*

### Abnormal Gametes

In humans, and in most mammals, one ovarian follicle occasionally contains two or three clearly distinguishable primary oocytes (Fig. 2.25*A*). Although these oocytes may give rise to twins or triplets, they usually degenerate before reaching maturity. In rare cases, one primary oocyte contains two or even three nuclei (Fig. 2.25*B*). Such binucleated or trinucleated oocytes die before reaching maturity.

In contrast to atypical oocytes, abnormal spermatozoa are seen frequently, and up to 10% of all spermatozoa have observable defects. The head or the tail may be abnormal, spermatozoa may be giants or dwarfs, and sometimes, they are joined (Fig. 2.25*C*). Sperm with morphologic abnormalities lack normal motility and probably do not fertilize oocytes.

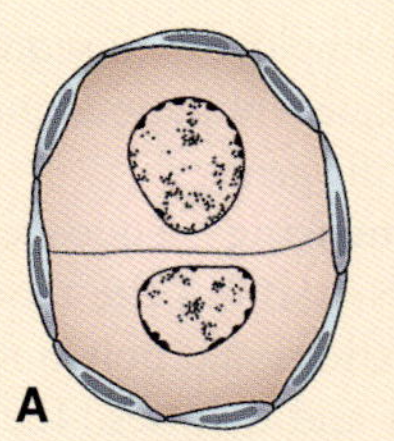


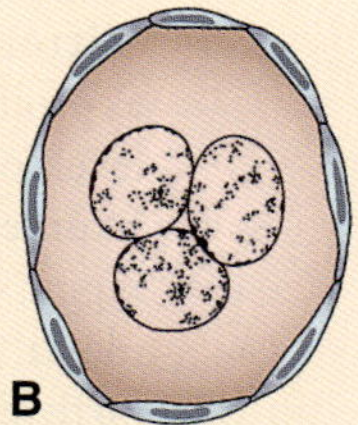


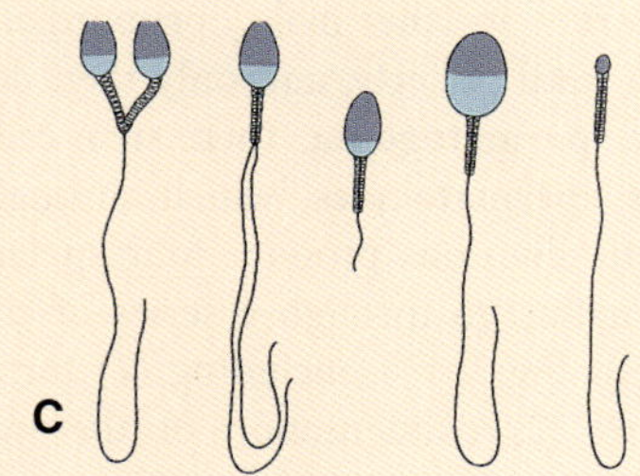


**FIGURE 2.25** Abnormal germ cells. **A.** Primordial follicle with two oocytes. **B.** Trinucleated oocyte. **C.** Various types of abnormal spermatozoa.

## SUMMARY

- **Primordial germ cells (PGCs)** are derived from the epiblast during gastrulation.
- PGCs migrate to the wall of the yolk sac in the fourth week.
- PGCs reach the indifferent gonad (Fig. 2.1), where they arrive at the end of the fifth week.
- In preparation for fertilization, both male and female germ cells undergo **gametogenesis**, which includes **meiosis** and **cytodifferentiation**.
- During meiosis I, **homologous chromosomes pair** and **exchange genetic material**.
- During meiosis II, cells fail to replicate DNA, and each cell is thus provided with a **haploid** number of chromosomes and half the amount of DNA of a normal somatic cell (Fig. 2.4).
- The mature male and female gametes have 22 plus X or 22 plus Y chromosomes, respectively.
- **Oogenesis**
  - **In the female**, maturation from primitive germ cell to mature gamete, which is called **oogenesis, begins before birth**.
  - In the female, PGCs form **oogonia**.
  - After repeated mitotic divisions, some of these arrest in prophase of meiosis I to form **primary oocytes**. By the seventh month, many oogonia have become atretic, and only primary oocytes remain surrounded by a layer of **follicular cells** derived from the surface epithelium of the ovary (Fig. 2.7).
  - Together, they form the **primordial follicle**. At puberty, a pool of growing follicles is recruited and maintained from the finite supply of primordial follicles. Thus, every month, 15 to 20 follicles begin to grow, and as they mature, they pass through three stages: (1) **primary** or **preantral**, (2) **vesicular or antral**, and (3) **mature vesicular or graafian follicle**. The primary oocyte remains in prophase of the first meiotic division until the secondary follicle is mature. At this point, a surge in **luteinizing hormone (LH)** stimulates preovulatory growth: Meiosis I is completed, and secondary oocyte and polar body are formed. Then, the secondary oocyte is arrested in metaphase of meiosis II approximately 3 hours before ovulation and will not complete this cell division until fertilization.
- **Spermatogenesis**
  - **In the male**, it is called **spermatogenesis**, and it **begins at puberty**. In the male, primordial cells remain dormant until puberty, and only then do they differentiate into **spermatogonia**. These stem cells give rise to **primary spermatocytes**, which through two successive meiotic divisions produce four **spermatids** (Fig. 2.5). Spermatids go through a series of changes (**spermiogenesis**) (Fig. 2.14), including (1) formation of the acrosome; (2) condensation of the nucleus; (3) formation of the neck, middle piece, and tail; and (4) shedding of most of the cytoplasm. The time required for a spermatogonium to become a mature spermatozoon is approximately 74 days.
- **Birth defects:** These may arise through abnormalities in **chromosome number** or **structure** and from **single gene mutations**. Approximately 10% of major birth defects are a result of chromosome abnormalities, and 8% are a result of gene mutations.
  - *Numerical abnormalities*
    - **Trisomies** (an extra chromosome) and **monosomies** (loss of a chromosome) arise during mitosis or meiosis. During meiosis, homologous chromosomes normally pair and then separate.
    - If separation fails (**nondisjunction**), however, one cell receives too many chromosomes, and one receives too few (Fig. 2.15). The incidence of abnormalities of chromosome number increases with age of the mother, particularly with mothers aged 35 years and older.
  - *Structural abnormalities*
    - Chromosomes include large **deletions (cri-du-chat syndrome)** and **microdeletions.**
    - Microdeletions involve **contiguous genes** that may result in defects such as **Angelman syndrome** (maternal deletion, chromosome 15q11–15q13) or **Prader-Willi syndrome** (paternal deletion, chromosome 15q11–15q13). Because these syndromes depend on whether the affected genetic material is inherited from the mother or the father, they are also an example of **imprinting**.
    - Gene mutations may be **dominant** (only one gene of an allelic pair has to be affected to produce an alteration) or **recessive** (both allelic gene pairs must be mutated). Mutations responsible for many birth defects affect genes involved in normal embryological development.
- **Diagnostic techniques** for identifying genetic abnormalities include the following:
  - **Cytogenetics** is used to test for chromosome numbers (**ploidy**) and for **high-resolution metaphase banding** techniques to test for small deletions.
  - **Fluorescent in situ hybridization (FISH)** uses fluorescent DNA probes to identify specific chromosomes or regions of chromosomes to determine deletions, translocations, and ploidy.
  - **Microarrays** employ small sequences of DNA on chips as probes to detect mutations and changes in expression levels of specific genes.
  - **Exome sequencing** sequences the protein-coding region of DNA (1% of the total DNA; the **exome**) to identify mutations and polymorphisms responsible for birth defects and diseases. The technique is accurate, timely, and cost-effective compared to sequencing the entire genome.

## Self-Assessment

### Comprehensive Questions

1. What is the most common cause of abnormal chromosome number? Give an example of a clinical syndrome involving abnormal numbers of chromosomes.
2. In addition to numerical abnormalities, what types of chromosomal alterations occur?
3. What is mosaicism, and how does it occur?
4. List the differences between oogenesis and spermatogenesis.

### Problem Solving Questions

1. Elderly mothers are prone to have a child with Down syndrome. Explain the embryological basis.
2. At the age of 16 years, a phenotypically female has not attained menarche. What is the most possible reason?
3. What are linked genes?
4. Discuss the genetic basis of Prader-Willi syndrome.

### Multiple Choice Questions

1. All of the following statements are true for primordial germ cell except
   (a) It is formed in epiblast in the second week post-fertilization.
   (b) It migrates to the primitive streak in the third week.
   (c) It moves to the wall of the yolk sac at the fourth week.
   (d) It reaches the genital ridge at 30 weeks.
2. Origin of teratoma tumor is from which source?
   (a) Pluripotent
   (b) Multipotent
   (c) Oligopotent
   (d) Unipotent
3. Two cell lines derived from two different zygotes are known as
   (a) Chimerism
   (b) Mosaicism
   (c) Segregation
   (d) Pseudodominance
4. At birth, oocyte is in which stage in a female child?
   (a) Anaphase
   (b) Prophase
   (c) Maturation
   (d) Primordial germ cell
5. All of the following are true for Turner syndrome except
   (a) Gonadal dysgenesis
   (b) Phenotypically female
   (c) Karyotype 45XO
   (d) Long neck and tall stature
6. Results of meiotic division are which of the following?
   (a) During crossover, redistribution of genetic material occurs.
   (b) Sequential distribution of genetic material occurs in both the daughter cells.
   (c) Germ cells divide with diploid number of chromosomes.
   (d) Meiosis occurs at puberty in both male and female germ cells.
7. Aneuploidy results due to
   (a) Mosaicism
   (b) Nondisjunction
   (c) Mutations
   (d) Translocations
8. Which of the following statements is true for Prader-Willi syndrome?
   (a) It occurs due to microdeletions in contiguous genes in males.
   (b) It occurs due to microdeletions in noncontiguous genes in males.
   (c) It is identified by karyotyping.
   (d) It occurs due to microdeletions in contiguous genes in females.
9. During spermiogenesis, all of the following statements are true except
   (a) Acrosome formation occurs which covers the anterior aspect of the head.
   (b) Condensation of nucleus occurs to form the head.
   (c) Tail detaches from the head.
   (d) Shedding of most of the cytoplasm occurs.
10. Time taken for a spermatogonium to form a sperm is approximately
   (a) 50 days
   (b) 62 days
   (c) 74 days
   (d) 90 days

### Answers

1. (d) 2. (a) 3. (a) 4. (b) 5. (d) 6. (a) 7. (b) 8. (a) 9. (c) 10. (c)

CHAPTER

# 3 Female Reproductive Cycle, First Week of Development: Ovulation to Implantation

Part 1

## Specific Learning Objectives

- Female reproductive cycle
- Oocyte transport
- Menstrual cycle and uterus at the time of implantation
- Capacitation of sperm
- Stages of fertilization and result of fertilization
- Embryonic period first 8 days: Fertilization, cleavage, and blastocyst formation
- Stem cells
- Clinical correlates
- Contraceptive methods
- Infertility and in vitro fertilization
- Surrogacy

## Competencies Covered

AN77.1 Describe the uterine changes occurring during the menstrual cycle.
AN77.2 Describe the synchrony between the ovarian and menstrual cycles.
AN77.4 Describe the stages and consequences of fertilization.
AN77.5 Enumerate and describe the anatomical principles underlying contraception.
AN77.6 Describe fertility and sterility and surrogate motherhood.
AN78.1 Describe cleavage and formation of a blastocyst.

## FEMALE REPRODUCTIVE CYCLE

The ovary is the female gonad which releases the mature oocyte for fertilization. The oocyte and sperm fertilize in the uterine tube and the fertilized zygote is transported to the uterine cavity where implantation takes place. All the events in a woman's reproductive tract are under the hormonal control. The monthly menstrual cycles which involve the changes in the uterine endometrium along with the maturation of the oocyte are hormone-dependent. The next sections of the chapter will discuss the ovarian cycle, ovulation, and the correlation with the menstrual cycle along with the hormonal control.

## OVARIAN CYCLE

At puberty, the female begins to undergo regular monthly cycles. These **sexual cycles** are controlled by the hypothalamus. **Gonadotropin-releasing hormone (GnRH)**, produced by the hypothalamus, acts on cells of the anterior lobe (adenohypophysis) of the pituitary gland, which in turn secrete **gonadotropins**. These hormones, **follicle-stimulating hormone (FSH)** and **luteinizing hormone (LH)**, stimulate and control cyclic changes in the ovary.

At the beginning of each ovarian cycle, 15 to 20 primary-stage (preantral) follicles are stimulated to grow under the influence of FSH. (The hormone is not necessary to promote development of primordial follicles to the primary follicle stage, but without it, these primary follicles die and become atretic.) Thus, FSH rescues 15 to 20 of these cells from a pool of continuously forming primary follicles (Figs. 3.1 and 3.2). Under normal conditions, only one of these follicles reaches full maturity, and only one oocyte is discharged; the others degenerate and become atretic. In the next cycle, another group of primary follicles is recruited, and again, only one follicle reaches maturity. Consequently, most follicles degenerate without ever reaching full maturity. When a follicle becomes atretic, the oocyte and surrounding follicular cells degenerate and are replaced by connective tissue, forming a **corpus atreticum**. FSH also stimulates maturation of **follicular (granulosa)** cells surrounding the oocyte. In turn, proliferation of these cells is mediated by growth differentiation factor 9, a member of the transforming growth factor-β (TGF-β) family. In cooperation, theca interna and granulosa cells produce estrogens: Theca interna cells produce androstenedione and testosterone, and granulosa cells convert these hormones to estrone and 17 β-estradiol. As a result of this estrogen production:

- The uterine endometrium enters the follicular or proliferative phase.
- Thinning of the cervical mucus occurs to allow passage of sperm.
- The anterior lobe of the pituitary gland is stimulated to secrete LH.

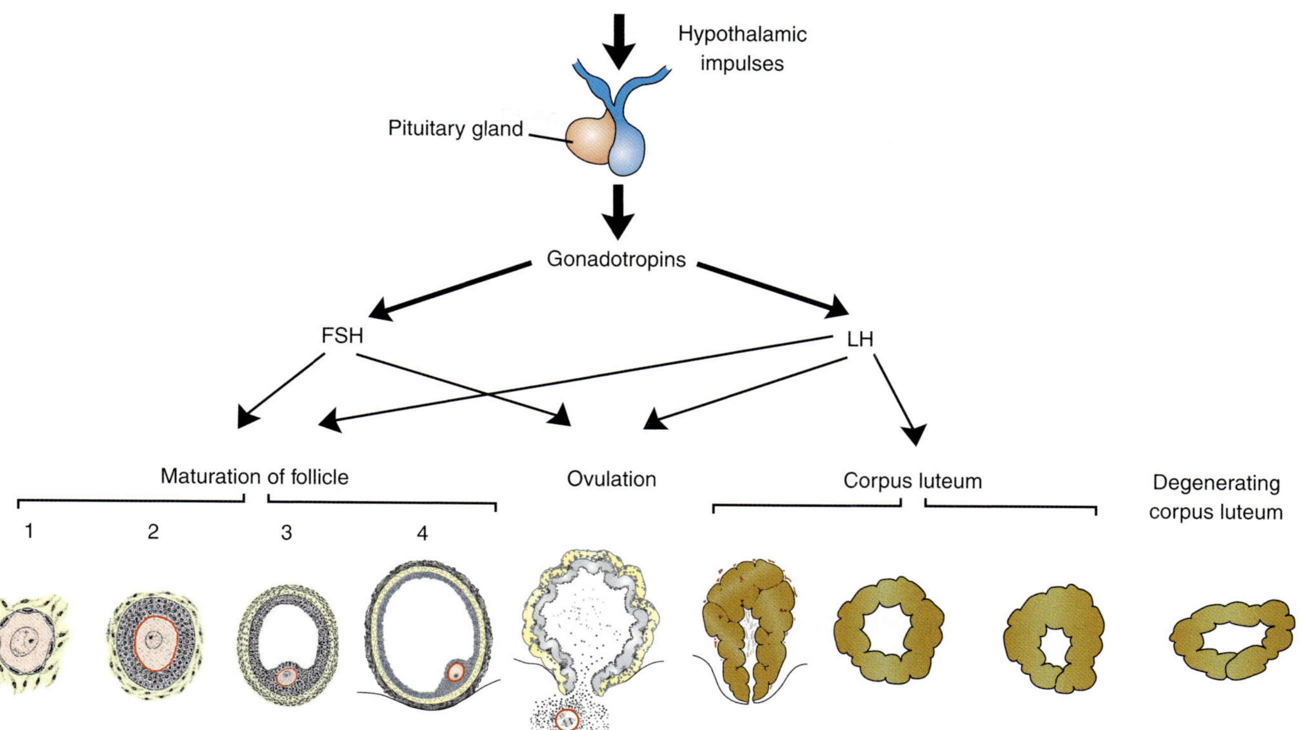


**FIGURE 3.1** Drawing showing the role of the hypothalamus and pituitary gland in regulating the ovarian cycle. Under the influence of GnRH from the hypothalamus, the pituitary releases the gonadotropins, FSH, and LH. Follicles are stimulated to grow by FSH and to mature by FSH and LH. Ovulation occurs when concentrations of LH surge to high levels. LH also promotes development of the corpus luteum. *1*, primordial follicle; *2*, growing follicle; *3*, vesicular follicle; *4*, mature vesicular (graafian) follicle.

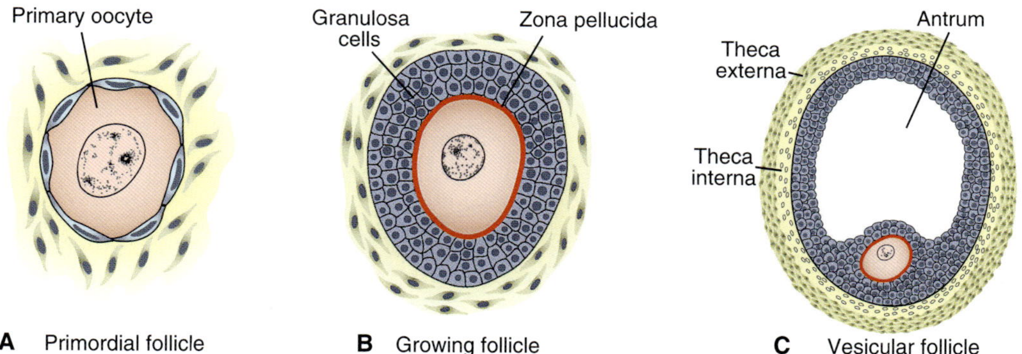


**FIGURE 3.2 A.** Primordial follicle. **B.** Growing follicle. **C.** Vesicular follicle. Every day from the pool of primordial follicles **(A)**, some begin to develop into growing follicles **(B)**, and this growth is independent of FSH. Then, as the cycle progresses, FSH secretion recruits growing follicles to begin development into vesicular (antral) follicles **(C)**. During the last few days of maturation of vesicular follicles, estrogens, produced by follicular and thecal cells, stimulate increased production of LH by the pituitary gland (Fig. 3.1), and this hormone causes the follicle to enter the mature vesicular (graafian) stage, to complete meiosis I, and to enter meiosis II, where it is arrested in metaphase approximately 3 hours before ovulation.

At midcycle, there is an LH surge that:

- Elevates concentrations of maturation-promoting factor, causing oocytes to complete meiosis I and initiate meiosis II
- Stimulates production of progesterone by follicular stromal cells (luteinization)
- Causes follicular rupture and ovulation

## Ovulation

In the days immediately preceding ovulation, under the influence of FSH and LH, the vesicular follicle grows rapidly to a diameter of 25 mm to become a mature vesicular (graafian) follicle. Coincident with final development of the vesicular follicle, there is an abrupt increase in LH that causes the

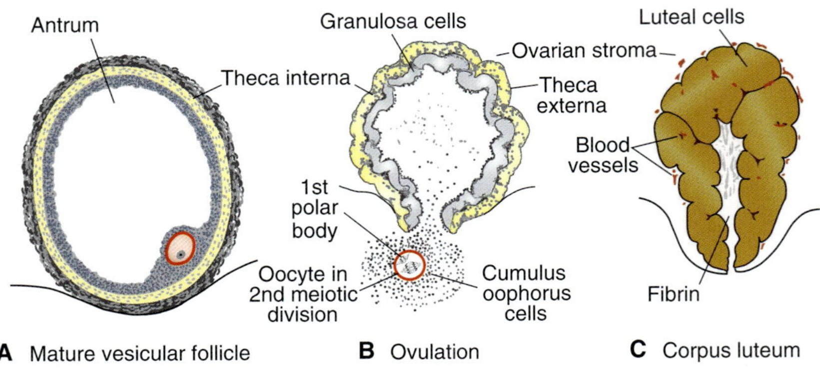


**FIGURE 3.3 A.** Mature vesicular follicle bulging at the ovarian surface. **B.** Ovulation. The oocyte, in metaphase of meiosis II, is discharged from the ovary together with a large number of cumulus oophorus cells. Follicular cells remaining inside the collapsed follicle differentiate into lutein cells. **C.** Corpus luteum. Note the large size of the corpus luteum, caused by hypertrophy and accumulation of lipid in granulosa and theca interna cells. The remaining cavity of the follicle is filled with fibrin.

primary oocyte to complete meiosis I and the follicle to enter the preovulatory mature vesicular stage. Meiosis II is also initiated, but the oocyte is arrested in metaphase approximately 3 hours before ovulation. In the meantime, the surface of the ovary begins to bulge locally, and at the apex, an avascular spot, the **stigma**, appears. The high concentration of LH increases collagenase activity, resulting in digestion of collagen fibers surrounding the follicle. Prostaglandin levels also increase in response to the LH surge and cause local muscular contractions in the ovarian wall. Those contractions extrude the oocyte, which together with its surrounding granulosa cells from the region of the cumulus oophorus breaks free (**ovulation**) and floats out of the ovary (Fig. 3.3). Some of the cumulus oophorus cells then rearrange themselves around the zona pellucida to form the **corona radiata** (Figs. 3.3*B*–3.6).

## *Clinical Correlates*

### Ovulation

During ovulation, some women feel a slight pain, called mittelschmerz (German for "middle pain") because it normally occurs near the middle of the menstrual cycle. Ovulation is also generally accompanied by a rise in basal temperature, which can be monitored to aid couples in becoming pregnant or preventing pregnancy. Some women fail to ovulate because of a low concentration of gonadotropins. In these cases, administration of an agent to stimulate gonadotropin release, and hence ovulation, can be employed. Although such drugs are effective, they often produce multiple ovulations so that the likelihood of multiple pregnancies is 10 times higher in these women than in the general population.

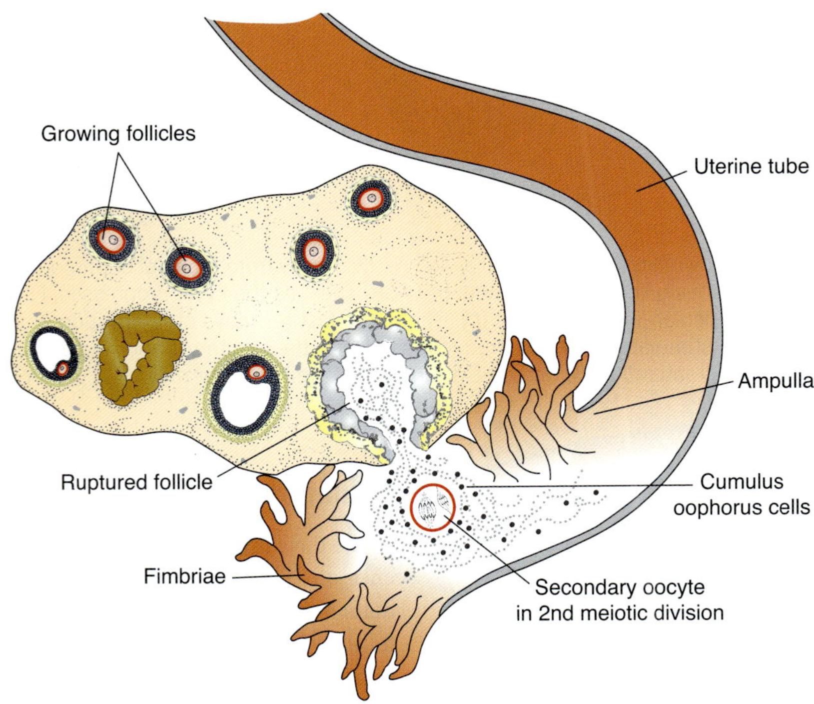


**FIGURE 3.4** Relation of fimbriae and ovary. Fimbriae collect the oocyte and sweep it into the uterine tube.

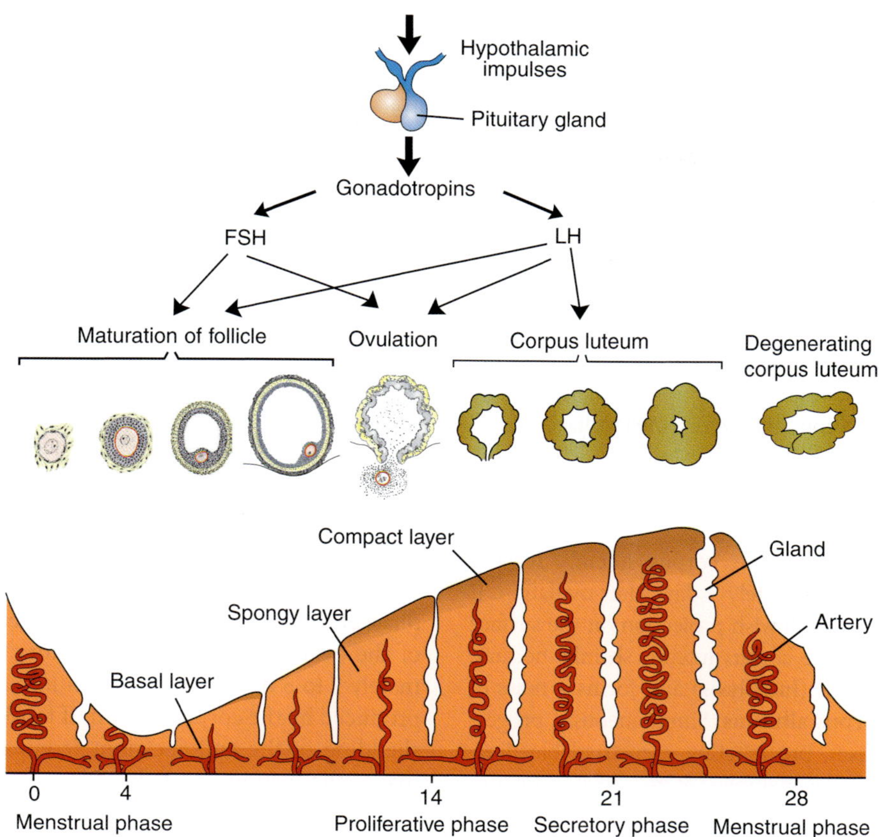


**FIGURE 3.5** Changes in the uterine mucosa (endometrium) and corresponding changes in the ovary during a regular menstrual cycle without fertilization.

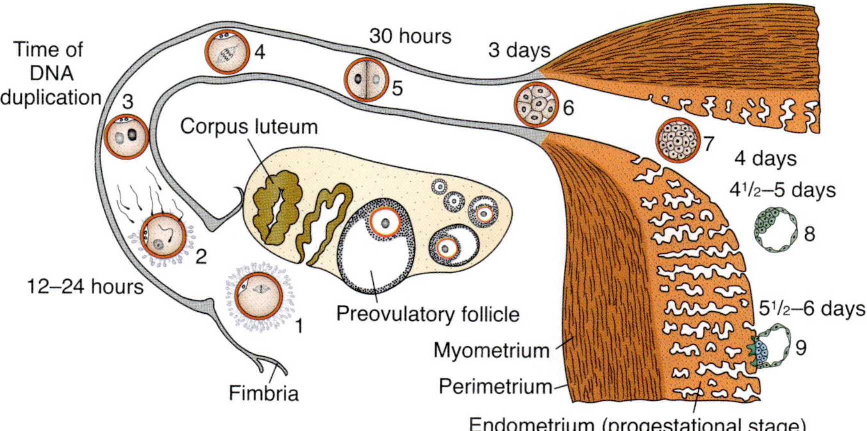


**FIGURE 3.6** Events during the first week of human development. *1*, oocyte immediately after ovulation; *2*, fertilization, approximately 12 to 24 hours after ovulation; *3*, stage of the male and female pronuclei; *4*, spindle of the first mitotic division; *5*, two-cell stage (approximately 30 hours of age); *6*, morula containing 12 to 16 blastomeres (approximately 3 days of age); *7*, advanced morula stage reaching the uterine lumen (approximately 4 days of age); *8*, early blastocyst stage (approximately 4.5 days of age; the zona pellucida has disappeared); *9*, early phase of implantation (blastocyst approximately 6 days of age). The ovary shows stages of transformation between a primary follicle and a preovulatory follicle as well as a corpus luteum. The uterine endometrium is shown in the progestational stage.

## Corpus Luteum

After ovulation, granulosa cells remaining in the wall of the ruptured follicle, together with cells from the theca interna, are vascularized by surrounding vessels. Under the influence of LH, these cells develop a yellowish pigment and change into **lutein cells**, which form the **corpus luteum** and secrete estrogens and **progesterone** (Fig. 3.3*C*). Progesterone, together with some estrogen, causes the uterine mucosa to enter the **progestational** or **secretory stage** in preparation for implantation of the embryo.

## Oocyte Transport

Shortly before ovulation, fimbriae of the uterine tube sweep over the surface of the ovary, and the tube itself begins to contract rhythmically. It is thought that the oocyte, surrounded by some granulosa cells (Fig. 3.6), is carried into the tube by these sweeping movements of the fimbriae and by motion of cilia on the epithelial lining. Once in the tube, cumulus cells withdraw their cytoplasmic processes from the zona pellucida and lose contact with the oocyte.

Once the oocyte is in the uterine tube, it is propelled by peristaltic muscular contractions of the tube and by cilia in the tubal mucosa with the rate of transport regulated by the endocrine status during and after ovulation. In humans, the fertilized oocyte reaches the uterine lumen in approximately 3 to 4 days.

## Corpus Albicans

If fertilization does not occur, the corpus luteum reaches maximum development approximately 9 days after ovulation. It can easily be recognized as a yellowish projection on the surface of the ovary. Subsequently, the corpus luteum shrinks because of degeneration of lutein cells (**luteolysis**) and forms a mass of fibrotic scar tissue, the **corpus albicans**. Simultaneously, progesterone production decreases, precipitating menstrual bleeding. If the oocyte is fertilized, degeneration of the corpus luteum is prevented by **human chorionic gonadotropin**, a hormone secreted by the syncytiotrophoblast of the developing embryo. The corpus luteum continues to grow and forms the **corpus luteum of pregnancy (corpus luteum graviditatis)**. By the end of the third month, this structure may be one-third to one-half of the total size of the ovary. Yellowish luteal cells continue to secrete progesterone until the end of the fourth month; thereafter, they regress slowly as secretion of progesterone by the trophoblastic component of the placenta becomes adequate for maintenance of pregnancy. Removal of the corpus luteum of pregnancy before the fourth month usually leads to abortion.

# THE MENSTRUAL CYCLE AND UTERUS AT THE TIME OF IMPLANTATION

The wall of the uterus consists of three layers:

1. **Endometrium** or mucosa lining the inside wall
2. **Myometrium**, a thick layer of smooth muscle
3. **Perimetrium**, the peritoneal covering lining the outside wall (Fig. 3.7)

From puberty (11 to 13 years) until menopause (45 to 50 years), the endometrium undergoes changes in a cycle of approximately 28 days under hormonal control by the ovaries. During this menstrual cycle, the uterine endometrium passes through three stages:

1. **Follicular** or **proliferative phase**
2. **Secretory** or **progestational phase**
3. **Menstrual phase** (Figs. 3.5 and 3.7)

The proliferative phase begins at the end of the menstrual phase, is under the influence of estrogen, and parallels growth of the ovarian follicles. The secretory phase begins approximately 2 to 3 days after ovulation in response to progesterone produced by the corpus luteum. If fertilization does not occur, shedding of the endometrium (compact and spongy layers) marks the beginning of the menstrual phase. If fertilization does occur, the endometrium assists in implantation and contributes to the formation of the placenta. Later in gestation, the placenta assumes the role of hormone production, and the corpus luteum degenerates.

At the time of implantation, the mucosa of the uterus is in the secretory phase (Fig. 3.7), during which time uterine glands and arteries become coiled and the tissue becomes succulent. As a result, three distinct layers can be recognized in the endometrium: a superficial **compact layer**, an intermediate **spongy layer**, and a thin **basal layer** (Fig. 3.7). Normally, the human blastocyst implants in the endometrium along the anterior

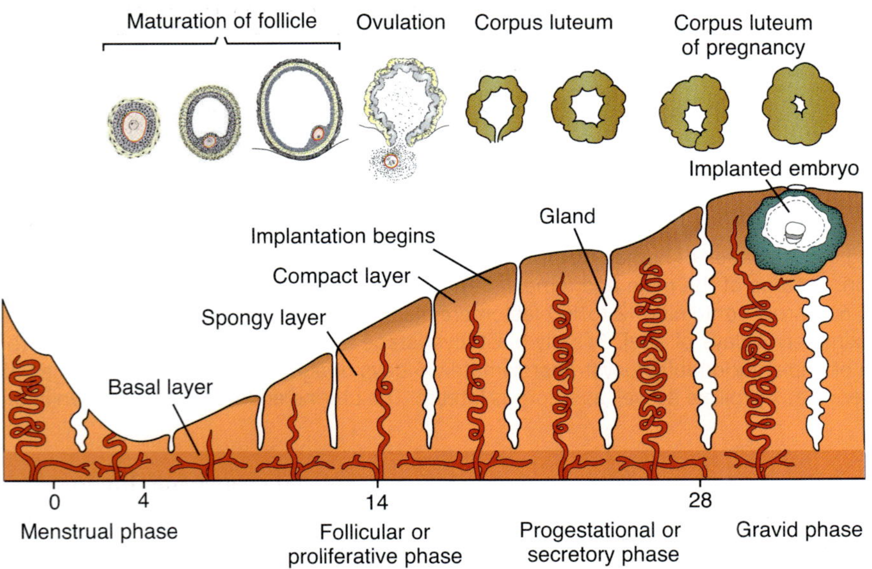


**FIGURE 3.7** Changes in the uterine mucosa correlated with those in the ovary. Implantation of the blastocyst has caused development of a large corpus luteum of pregnancy. Secretory activity of the endometrium increases gradually as a result of large amounts of progesterone produced by the corpus luteum of pregnancy.

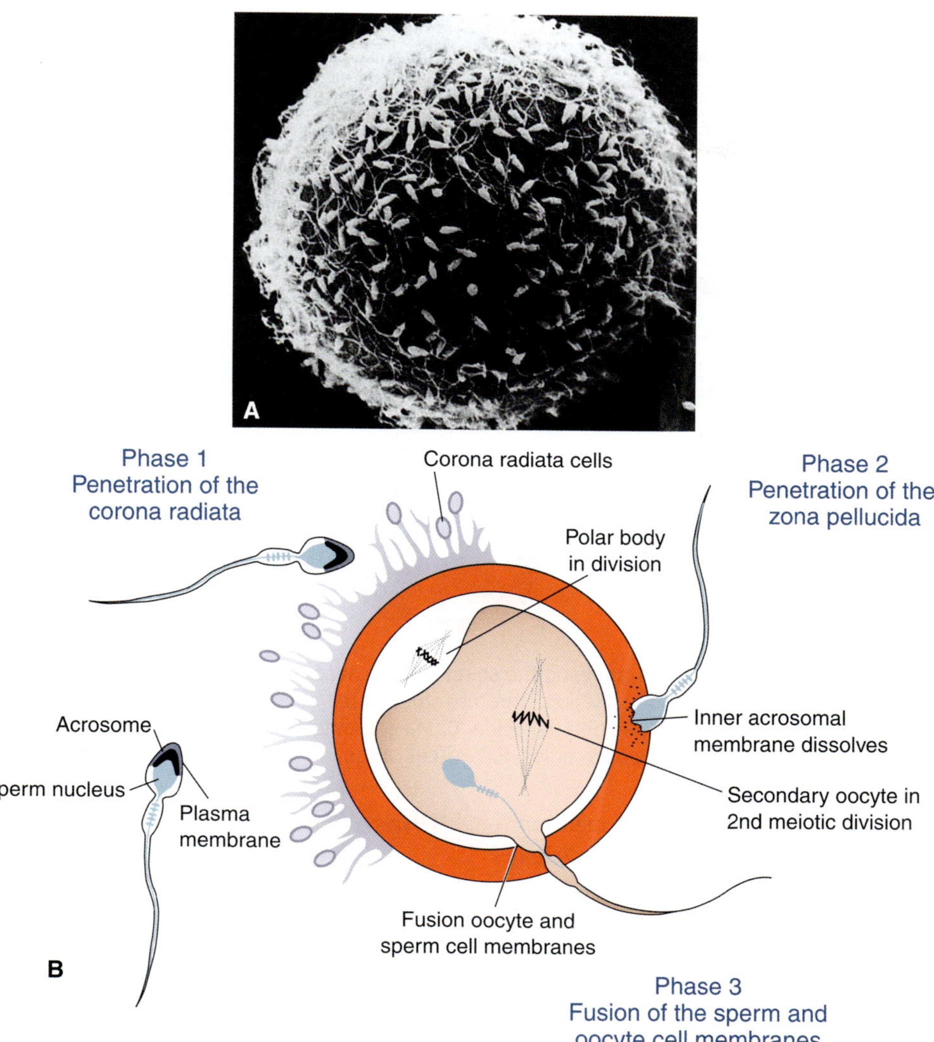


**FIGURE 3.8** **A.** Scanning electron micrograph of sperm binding to the zona pellucida. **B.** The three phases of oocyte penetration. In phase 1, spermatozoa pass through the corona radiata barrier; in phase 2, one or more spermatozoa penetrate the zona pellucida; and in phase 3, one spermatozoon penetrates the oocyte membrane while losing its own plasma membrane. *Inset* shows normal spermatocyte with acrosomal head cap.

or posterior wall of the body of the uterus, where it becomes embedded between the openings of the glands (Fig. 3.7).

If the oocyte is not fertilized, venules and sinusoidal spaces gradually become packed with blood cells, and an extensive diapedesis of blood into the tissue is seen. When the **menstrual phase** begins, blood escapes from superficial arteries, and small pieces of stroma and glands break away. During the following 3 or 4 days, the compact and spongy layers are expelled from the uterus, and the basal layer is the only part of the endometrium that is retained (Fig. 3.7). This layer, which is supplied by its own arteries, the **basal arteries**, functions as the regenerative layer in the rebuilding of glands and arteries in the **proliferative phase** (Fig. 3.7).

## FERTILIZATION

Fertilization, the process by which male and female gametes fuse, occurs in the **ampullary region of the uterine tube**. This is the widest part of the tube and is close to the ovary (Fig. 3.8). Spermatozoa may remain viable in the female reproductive tract for several days.

Only 1% of sperm deposited in the vagina enter the cervix, where they may survive for many hours. Movement of sperm from the cervix to the uterine tube occurs by muscular contractions of the uterus and uterine tube and very little by their own propulsion. The trip from cervix to oviduct can occur as rapidly as 30 minutes or as slow as 6 days. After reaching the isthmus, sperm become less motile and cease their migration. At ovulation, sperm again become motile, perhaps because of chemoattractants produced by cumulus cells surrounding the egg, and swim to the ampulla where fertilization usually occurs.

**Priming of the male gamete:** Spermatozoa are not able to fertilize the oocyte immediately upon arrival in the female genital tract. The following steps take place for the spermatozoa to fertilize the female gamete:

1. **Capacitation**
2. **Acrosome reaction**

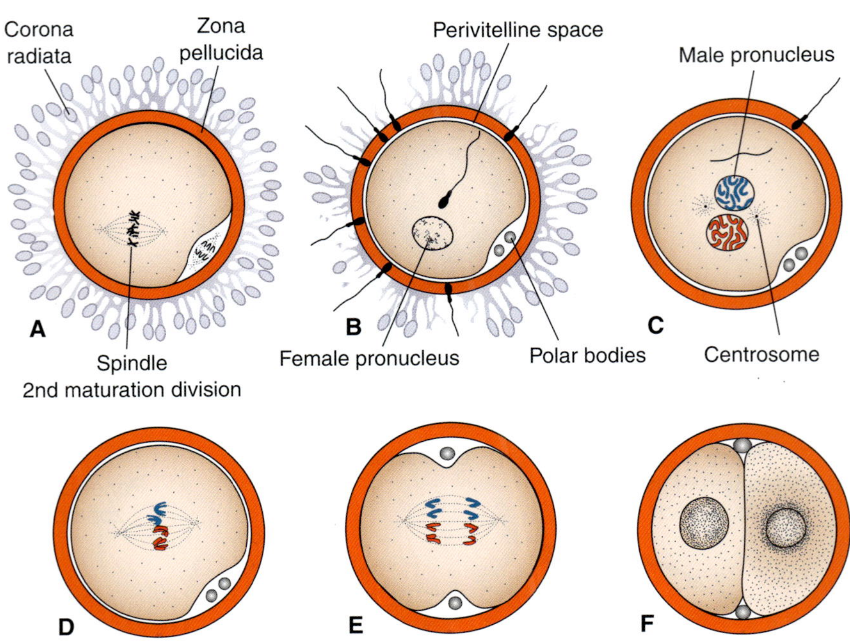


**FIGURE 3.9** **A.** Oocyte immediately after ovulation, showing the spindle of the second meiotic division. **B.** A spermatozoon has penetrated the oocyte, which has finished its second meiotic division. Chromosomes of the oocyte are arranged in a vesicular nucleus, the female pronucleus. Heads of several sperm are stuck in the zona pellucida. **C.** Male and female pronuclei. **D,E.** Chromosomes become arranged on the spindle, split longitudinally, and move to opposite poles. **F.** Two-cell stage.

**Capacitation** is a period of conditioning in the female reproductive tract that in the human lasts approximately 7 hours. Thus, speeding to the ampulla is not an advantage because capacitation has not yet occurred and such sperm are not capable of fertilizing the egg. Much of this conditioning during capacitation occurs in the uterine tube and involves epithelial interactions between the sperm and the mucosal surface of the tube. During this time, a glycoprotein coat and seminal plasma proteins are removed from the plasma membrane that overlies the acrosomal region of the spermatozoa. Only capacitated sperm can pass through the corona cells and undergo the acrosome reaction.

The **acrosome reaction**, which occurs after binding to the zona pellucida, is induced by zona proteins. This reaction culminates in the release of enzymes needed to penetrate the zona pellucida, including acrosin- and trypsin-like substances (Fig. 3.9).

**The phases of fertilization include the following:**

- Phase 1, penetration of the corona radiata
- Phase 2, penetration of the zona pellucida
- Phase 3, fusion of the oocyte and sperm cell membranes

## Phase 1: Penetration of the Corona Radiata

Of the 200 to 300 million spermatozoa normally deposited in the female genital tract, only 300 to 500 reach the site of fertilization. Only one of these fertilizes the egg. It is thought that the others aid the fertilizing sperm in penetrating the barriers protecting the female gamete. Capacitated sperm pass freely through corona cells (Fig. 3.9).

## Phase 2: Penetration of the Zona Pellucida

The zona is a glycoprotein shell surrounding the egg that facilitates and maintains sperm binding and induces the acrosome reaction. Both binding and the acrosome reaction are mediated by the ligand ZP3, a zona protein. Release of acrosomal enzymes (acrosin) allows sperm to penetrate the zona, thereby coming in contact with the plasma membrane of the oocyte (Fig. 3.5). Permeability of the zona pellucida changes when the head of the sperm comes in contact with the oocyte surface. This contact results in release of lysosomal enzymes from **cortical granules** lining the plasma membrane of the oocyte. In turn, these enzymes alter properties of the zona pellucida (**zona reaction**) to prevent sperm penetration and inactivate species-specific receptor sites for spermatozoa on the zona surface. Other spermatozoa have been found embedded in the zona pellucida, but only one seems to be able to penetrate the oocyte (Fig. 3.9).

## Phase 3: Fusion of the Oocyte and Sperm Cell Membranes

The initial adhesion of sperm to the oocyte is mediated in part by the interaction of integrins on the oocyte and their ligands, disintegrins, on sperm. After adhesion, the plasma membranes of the sperm and egg fuse (Fig. 3.9). Because the plasma membrane covering the acrosomal head cap disappears during the acrosome reaction, actual fusion is accomplished between the oocyte membrane and the membrane that covers the posterior region of the sperm head (Fig. 3.9). In the human, both the head and the tail of the spermatozoon enter the cytoplasm of the oocyte, but the plasma membrane is left behind on the

## Clinical Correlates

### Contraceptive Methods

**Barrier methods** of contraception include the male condom, made of latex and often containing chemical spermicides, which fits over the penis, and the female condom, made of polyurethane, which lines the vagina. Other barriers placed in the vagina include the diaphragm, the cervical cap, and the contraceptive sponge.

**Hormonal methods** are another commonly used form of contraception. These approaches provide the female hormones estrogen and/or progestin. These hormones produce their effects by inhibiting ovulation (by preventing the release of FSH and LH from the pituitary gland), changing the lining of the uterus, and thickening cervical mucus, making it difficult for sperm to enter the uterus. Hormonal contraception can be provided through birth control pills, a skin patch, vaginal ring, injection, or implant. There are two types of contraceptive pills: The first is a combination of estrogen and the progesterone analogue progestin; the second is composed of progestin alone. Both pills are effective, but one may suit some women better than others for various health-related issues.

A **male "pill"** has been developed and tested in clinical trials. It contains a synthetic androgen that prevents both LH and FSH secretion and either stops sperm production (70% to 90% of men) or reduces it to a level of infertility.

The **intrauterine device (IUD)** is a small T-shaped unit and there are two types: hormonal and copper. The hormonal device releases progestin that causes thickening of cervical mucus to prevent sperm from entering the uterus. Also, it may make sperm less active and both eggs and sperm less viable. The copper type releases copper into the uterus that prevents fertilization or inhibits attachment of the fertilized egg to the uterine wall. It also helps prevent sperm from entering the uterine tubes.

**Emergency contraceptive pills (ECPs)** are used as birth control measures that may prevent pregnancy if taken 120 hours after sexual intercourse. These pills may be administered as high doses of progestin alone or in combination with estrogen (Plan B). Other types of ECPs (mifepristone [RU-486] and ulipristal acetate) act as antihormonal agents. Also, mifepristone is effective as an abortifacient if taken after the time of implantation.

**Sterilization** is another form of birth control. The method for men is a vasectomy, which prevents the release of sperm by blocking the ductus deferens, the tube that transports sperm from the testes to the penis. The sterilization method for women is tubal sterilization in which the uterine tubes are blocked or ligated. These procedures for both men and women can be reversed in some cases.

### Infertility

**Infertility** is a problem for 14% to 15% of couples. Male infertility may be a result of insufficient numbers of sperm and/or poor motility. Normally, the ejaculate has a volume of 2 to 6 mL, with as many as 100 million sperm per milliliter. Men with 20 million sperm per milliliter or 50 million sperm per total ejaculate are usually fertile. Infertility in a woman may be due to a number of causes, including occluded uterine tubes (most commonly caused by pelvic inflammatory disease), hostile cervical mucus, immunity to spermatozoa, absence of ovulation, and others.

**Clomiphene citrate** is a drug used to increase FSH concentrations to stimulate ovulation. The drug is given early in the menstrual cycle to cause ovulation in women who do not ovulate or who ovulate irregularly. Also, it is given to stimulate egg development for use in in vitro fertilization procedures.

The three most crucial embryological events which determine the fate of assisted reproductive technology are the following: (1) a balance between hormonal axis regulation, (2) successful fertilization, and (3) implantation.

One percent to 2% of all pregnancies in the United States occur using **assisted reproductive technology (ART).** In a latest survey, for the National ART Registry, Indian Council of Medical Research (ICMR), the number of clinics is 125 in the capital city of India. There has been a higher demand of ART in India due to the availability of centers of excellence with a success rate of 30%. Offspring from these conceptions show increases in prematurity (<37 weeks' gestation), low birth weight (<2,500 g), very low birth weight (<1,500 g), and some types of birth defects. Most of these adverse outcomes are caused by increased rates of multiple births (twins, triplets, etc.), which occur more commonly among ART pregnancies. Recent studies indicate, however, that even among singleton births after ART, there are increases in preterm birth and malformed infants. Some of the approaches used for ART include **in vitro fertilization (IVF)** and **intracytoplasmic sperm injection (ICSI).**

**IVF** of human ova and embryo transfer is the standard procedure used by laboratories throughout the world. Follicle growth in the ovary is stimulated by administration of gonadotropins. Oocytes are recovered by laparoscopy from ovarian follicles with an aspirator just before ovulation when the oocyte is in the late stages of the first meiotic division. The egg is placed in a simple culture medium, and sperm are added immediately. Alternatively, a single sperm can be injected into an egg's cytoplasm to produce fertilization. This technique is called **ICSI** and can be used to circumvent male infertility (see the following discussion). With either approach, fertilized eggs are monitored to the eight-cell stage and then placed in the uterus to develop to term.

The success rate of IVF depends on maternal age. Approximately 30% of couples will conceive after one attempt if the woman is younger than 35 years. The rate drops to 25% for women aged 35 to 37 years, 17% for those aged 38 to 40 years, and to <5% for those older than 40 years. In addition to these relatively low success rates, the technique is also associated with a higher rate of birth defects. To increase chances of a successful pregnancy, four or five ova are collected, fertilized, and placed in the uterus. This approach sometimes leads to multiple births.

The frequency of multiple births depends on maternal age (with a higher incidence in younger women) and the number of embryos transferred. For a 20- to 29-year-old woman and three embryos transferred, the risk is 46%. Multiple births are a disadvantage because they have high rates of morbidity and mortality.

Severe **male infertility**, in which the ejaculate contains very few live sperm (**oligozoospermia**) or even no live sperm (**azoospermia**), can be overcome using **ICSI**. With this technique, a single sperm, which may be obtained from any point in the male reproductive tract, is injected into the cytoplasm of the egg to cause fertilization. This approach offers couples an alternative to using donor sperm for IVF. The technique carries an increased risk for fetuses to have Y chromosome deletions and appears to be associated with a higher incidence of birth defects than standard IVF techniques.

**Surrogacy** is a third party reproduction arrangement whereby a woman (surrogate mother) agrees to become pregnant for the purpose of gestating and giving birth to a child for others to raise. She may be the child's genetic mother (traditional surrogacy) or she may be implanted with someone else's fertilized egg (gestational surrogacy), depending on the type of arrangement.

oocyte surface. As soon as the spermatozoon has entered the oocyte, the egg responds in three ways:

1. **Cortical and zona reactions.** As a result of the release of cortical oocyte granules, which contain lysosomal enzymes, (1) the oocyte membrane becomes impenetrable to other spermatozoa, and (2) the zona pellucida alters its structure and composition to prevent sperm binding and penetration. These reactions prevent **polyspermy** (penetration of more than one spermatozoon into the oocyte).
2. **Resumption of the second meiotic division.** The oocyte finishes its second meiotic division immediately after entry of the spermatozoon. One of the daughter cells, which receives hardly any cytoplasm, is known as the **second polar body**; the other daughter cell is the **definitive oocyte**. Its chromosomes (22 plus X) arrange themselves in a vesicular nucleus known as the **female pronucleus** (Figs. 3.9 and 3.10).
3. **Metabolic activation of the egg.** The activating factor is probably carried by the spermatozoon. Activation encompasses the initial cellular and molecular events associated with early embryogenesis.

The spermatozoon, meanwhile, moves forward until it lies close to the female pronucleus. Its nucleus becomes swollen and forms the **male pronucleus** (Fig. 3.9); the tail detaches and degenerates. Morphologically, the male and female pronuclei are indistinguishable, and eventually, they come into close contact and lose their nuclear envelopes (Fig. 3.10*A*). During growth of male and female pronuclei (both haploid), each pronucleus must replicate its DNA. If it does not, each cell of the two-cell zygote has only half of the normal amount of DNA. Immediately after DNA synthesis, chromosomes organize on the spindle in preparation for a normal mitotic division. The 23 maternal and 23 paternal (double) chromosomes split longitudinally at the centromere, and sister chromatids move to opposite poles, providing each cell of the zygote with the normal diploid number of chromosomes and DNA (Fig. 3.9*D,E*). As sister chromatids move to opposite poles, a deep furrow appears on the surface of the cell, gradually dividing the cytoplasm into two parts (Figs. 3.9*F* and 3.10*B*).

**The main results of fertilization are as follows:**

- **Restoration of the diploid number of chromosomes,** half from the father and half from the mother. Hence, the zygote contains a new combination of chromosomes different from both parents.
- **Determination of the sex of the new individual.** An X-carrying sperm produces a female (XX) embryo, and a Y-carrying sperm produces a male (XY) embryo. Therefore, the chromosomal sex of the embryo is determined at fertilization.
- **Initiation of cleavage.** Without fertilization, the oocyte usually degenerates 24 hours after ovulation.

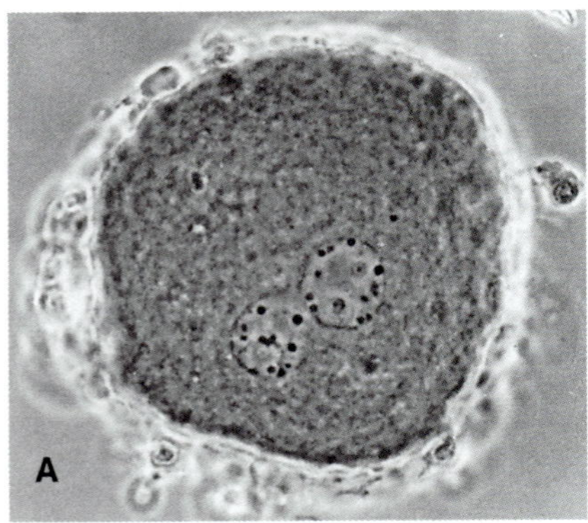


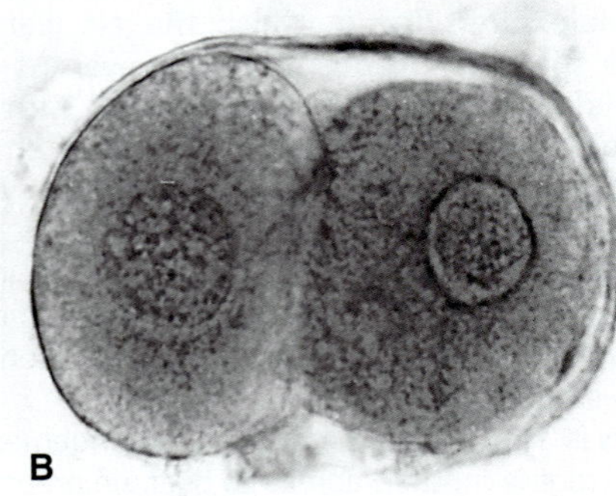


**FIGURE 3.10** **A.** Phase contrast view of the pronuclear stage of a fertilized human oocyte with male and female pronuclei. **B.** Two-cell stage of human zygote.

## CLEAVAGE

Once the zygote has reached the two-cell stage, it undergoes a series of mitotic divisions, increasing the numbers of cells. These cells, which become smaller with each cleavage division, are known as **blastomeres** (Fig. 3.11). Until the eight-cell stage, they form a loosely arranged clump (Fig. 3.12*A*). After the third cleavage, however, blastomeres maximize their contact with each other, forming a compact ball of cells held together by tight junctions (Fig. 3.12*B*). This process, **compaction**, segregates inner cells, which communicate extensively by gap junctions, from outer cells. Approximately 3 days after fertilization, cells of the compacted embryo divide again to form a 16-cell **morula** (mulberry). Inner cells of the morula constitute the **inner cell mass**, and surrounding cells

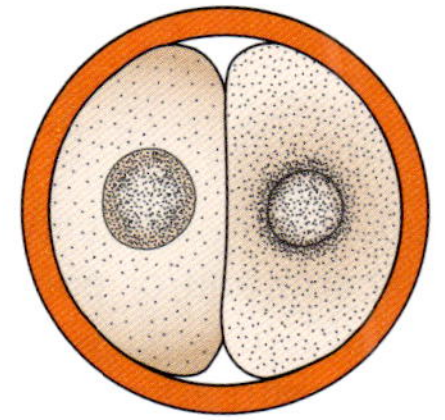


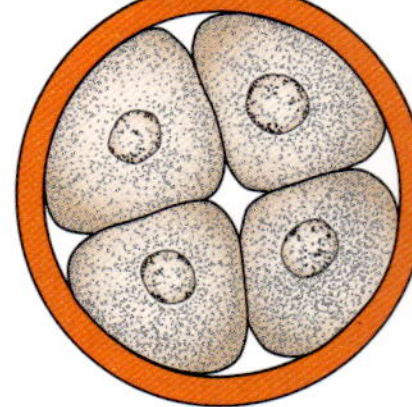


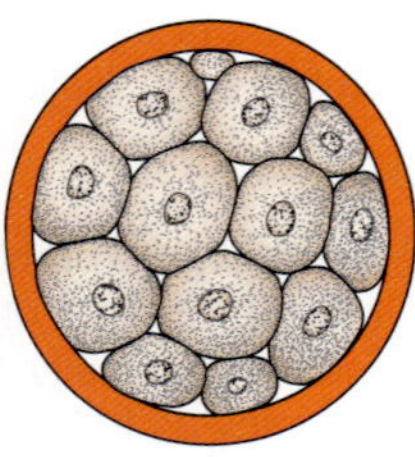


**FIGURE 3.11** Development of the zygote from the two-cell stage to the late morula stage. The two-cell stage is reached approximately 30 hours after fertilization; the four-cell stage is reached at approximately 40 hours; the 12- to 16-cell stage is reached at approximately 3 days; and the late morula stage is reached at approximately 4 days. During this period, blastomeres are surrounded by the zona pellucida, which disappears at the end of the fourth day.

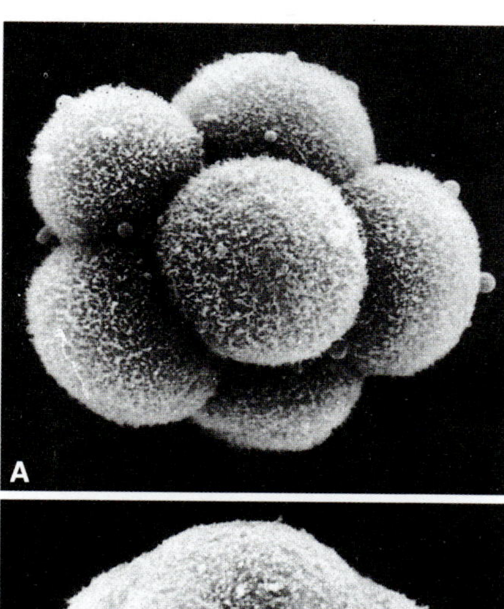


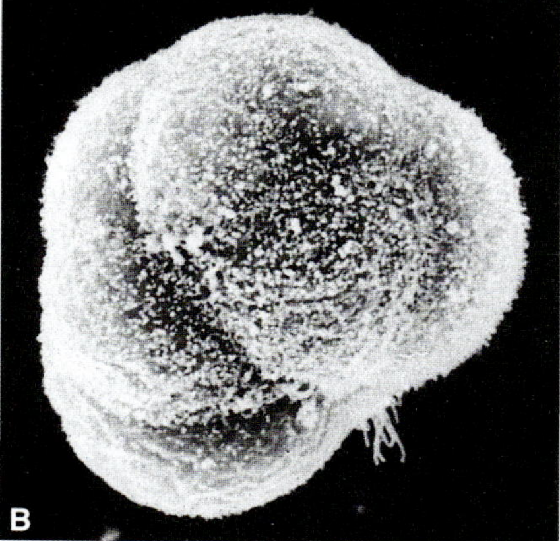


**FIGURE 3.12** Scanning electron micrographs of uncompacted **(A)** and compacted **(B)** eight-cell mouse embryos. In the uncompacted state, outlines of each blastomere are distinct, whereas after compaction, cell–cell contacts are maximized, and cellular outlines are indistinct.

compose the **outer cell mass**. The inner cell mass gives rise to tissues of the **embryo proper**, and the outer cell mass forms the **trophoblast**, which later contributes to the **placenta**.

## BLASTOCYST FORMATION

About the time the morula enters the uterine cavity, fluid begins to penetrate through the zona pellucida into the intercellular spaces of the inner cell mass. Gradually, the intercellular spaces become confluent, and finally, a single cavity, the **blastocele**, forms (Fig. 3.13*A,B*). At this time, the embryo is a **blastocyst**. Cells of the inner cell mass, now called the **embryoblast**, are at one pole, and those of the outer cell mass, or **trophoblast**, flatten and form the epithelial wall of the blastocyst (Fig. 3.13*A,B*). The zona pellucida has disappeared, allowing implantation to begin. In the human, trophoblastic cells over the embryoblast pole begin to penetrate between the epithelial cells of the uterine mucosa on about the sixth day (Fig. 3.13*C*). New studies suggest that **L-selectin** on trophoblast cells and its **carbohydrate receptors** on the uterine epithelium mediate initial attachment of the blastocyst to the uterus. Selectins are carbohydrate-binding proteins involved in interactions between leukocytes and endothelial cells that allow leukocyte "capture" from flowing blood. A similar mechanism is now proposed for "capture" of the blastocyst from the uterine cavity by the uterine epithelium. Following capture by selectins, further attachment and invasion by the trophoblast involve integrins, expressed by the trophoblast and the extracellular matrix molecules laminin and fibronectin. Integrin receptors for laminin promote attachment, whereas those for fibronectin stimulate migration. These molecules also interact along signal transduction pathways to regulate trophoblast differentiation, so that implantation is the result of mutual trophoblastic and endometrial action. Hence, by the end of the first week of development, the human zygote has passed through the morula and blastocyst stages and has begun implantation in the uterine mucosa.



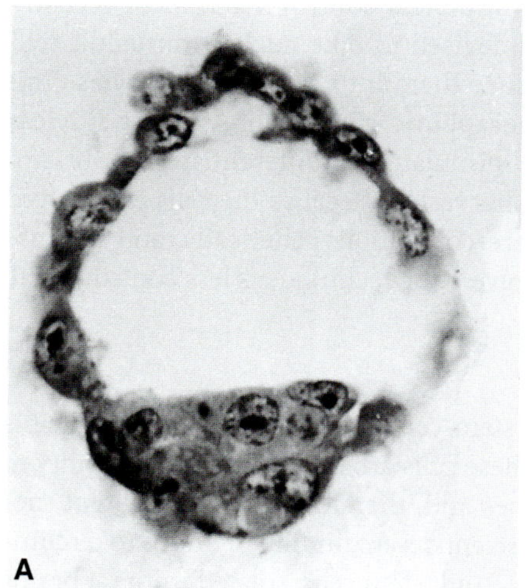


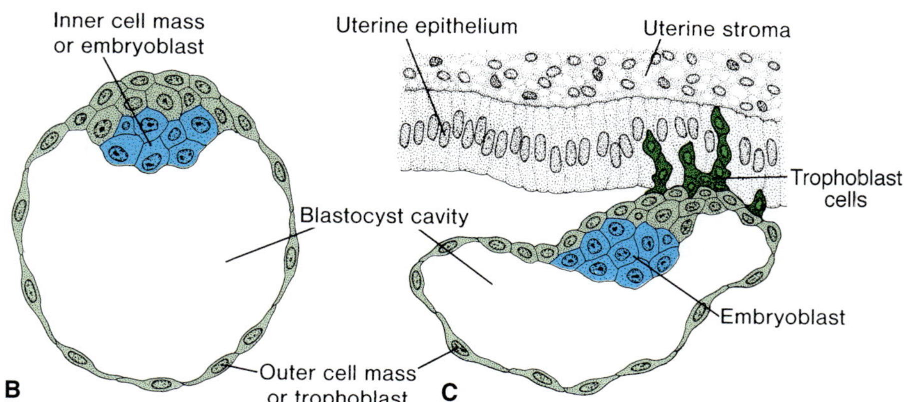


**FIGURE 3.13** **A.** Section of a 107-cell human blastocyst showing inner cell mass and trophoblast cells. **B.** Schematic representation of a human blastocyst recovered from the uterine cavity at approximately 4.5 days. *Blue*, inner cell mass or embryoblast; *green*, trophoblast. **C.** Schematic representation of a blastocyst at the sixth day of development showing trophoblast cells at the embryonic pole of the blastocyst penetrating the uterine mucosa. The human blastocyst begins to penetrate the uterine mucosa by the sixth day of development.

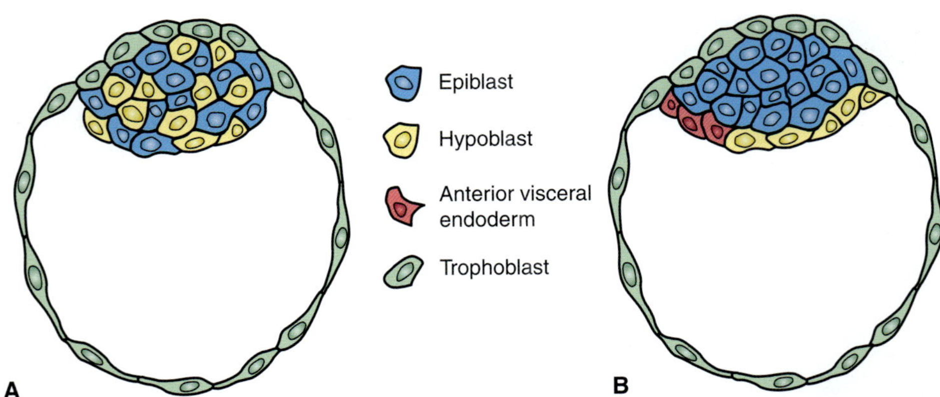


**FIGURE 3.14** **A.** At the early blastocyst stage, cells are specified to form epiblast and hypoblast cells, which are scattered in the embryoblast. **B.** Near the time of implantation (5.5 to 6 days), hypoblast cells move to form a layer ventral to the epiblast and adjacent to the blastocyst cavity. In addition, some cells in the hypoblast form the anterior visceral endoderm (AVE), and these cells migrate to the future cranial end of the embryo. Here, they will signal nearby epiblast cells to form cranial structures. Notice that formation and positioning of the hypoblast and AVE establishes the dorsal–ventral and cranial–caudal embryonic axes, respectively.

## EPIBLAST, HYPOBLAST, AND AXIS FORMATION

Under the influence of fibroblast growth factors (FGFs) at the early blastocyst stage, cells in the embryoblast differentiate into **epiblast** and **hypoblast** cells (Fig. 3.14*A*). Initially, these cells are scattered in the embryoblast, but near the time of implantation, they segregate according to their specification to become a layer of epiblast cells dorsally and hypoblast cells ventrally, adjacent to the blastocyst cavity (blastocele; Fig. 3.14*B*). Thus, a dorsal–ventral polarity is established in the embryo. In addition, some of the hypoblast cells are specified to form the **anterior visceral endoderm (AVE)**, and these cells migrate to what will become the cranial end of the embryo (Fig. 3.14*B*). AVE cells are classified as endoderm (as is the entire hypoblast) and are responsible for secreting nodal antagonists, including cerberus and lefty1, that act on adjacent epiblast cells to specify the cranial end of the embryo. In the absence of these inhibitors, nodal establishes the primitive streak at the caudal end of the embryo. In this manner, the cranial–caudal embryonic axis is established near the time of implantation (days 5.5 to 6).

## STEM CELLS

Stem cells have the remarkable potential to develop into many different cell types in the body during early life and growth. When a stem cell divides, each new cell has the potential either to remain a stem cell or to become another type of cell with a more specialized function, such as a muscle cell, a red blood cell, or a brain cell.

### Embryonic Stem Cells

**Embryonic stem cells (ES cells)** are derived from the inner cell mass of the embryo. Because these cells are **pluripotent** and can form virtually any cell or tissue type, they have the potential for curing a variety of diseases, including diabetes, Alzheimer and Parkinson diseases, anemias, spinal cord injuries, and many others. Using animal model research with stem cells has been encouraging. For example, mouse ES cells in culture have been induced to form insulin-secreting cells, muscle and nerve stem cells, and glial cells. In whole animals, ES cells have been used to alleviate the symptoms of Parkinson disease and to improve motor ability in rats with spinal cord injuries.

ES cells may be obtained from embryos after **IVF**, a process called **reproductive cloning**. This approach has the disadvantage that the cells may cause immune rejection because they would not be genetically identical to their hosts. The cells could be modified to circumvent this problem, however. Another issue with this approach is based on ethical considerations, as the cells are derived from viable embryos.

As the field of stem cell research progresses, scientific advances will provide more genetically compatible cells, and the approaches will be less controversial. Most recently, techniques have been devised to take nuclei from adult cells (e.g., skin) and introduce them into enucleated oocytes. This approach is called **therapeutic cloning** or **somatic nuclear transfer**. Oocytes are stimulated to differentiate into blastocysts, and ES cells are harvested. Because the cells are derived from the host, they are compatible genetically, and because fertilization is not involved, the technique is less controversial.

### Adult Stem Cells

Adult tissues contain stem cells that may also prove valuable in treating diseases. These cells are restricted in their ability to form different cell types and, therefore, are **multipotent**, not pluripotent, although scientists are finding methods to circumvent this disadvantage. Adult stem cells isolated from rat brains have been used to cure Parkinson disease in rats, suggesting that the approach has promise. Disadvantages of the approach include the slow rates of cell division characteristic of these cells and their scarcity, which makes them difficult to isolate in sufficient numbers for experiments.

## CLASSIFICATION OF STEM CELLS ACCORDING TO THEIR POTENCY AND THEIR CHARACTERISTICS

According to the potency and characteristics, stem cells are classified as follows:

- Totipotent: A cell that can give rise to the entire organism including the extraembryonic membranes. *Example:* A fertilized egg or a zygote up to the 8-cell or preimplantation stage.
- Pluripotent: A highly plastic cell that can differentiate into cell types of any of the three germ layers of the embryo, when given favorable conditions, but cannot give rise to the entire embryo. *Example:* Embryonic stem cells, inner cell mass cells of the blastocyst.
- Multipotent: Stem cell that has limited capabilities for specialization, normally within a specific tissue type, and can give rise to cells of the same system, when exposed to appropriate conditions. *Example:* Adult stem cells such as chondroblasts can convert into osteoblasts and vice versa with changing oxygen conditions.
- Unipotent: A highly differentiated cell that has the capacity to give rise to only one type of tissue/cell type. It is different from the terminally differentiated non-stem cells because of its property of self-renewal. *Example:* Hepatocytes (regeneration of liver), skin cells (renewal), gastric gland cells (renewal and repair).

### Abnormal Zygotes

The exact number of **abnormal zygotes** formed is unknown because they are usually lost within 2 to 3 weeks of fertilization, before the woman realizes she is pregnant, and therefore, are not detected. Estimates indicate that as many as **50% of pregnancies end in spontaneous abortion** and that half of these losses are a result of chromosomal abnormalities. These abortions are a natural means of screening embryos for defects, reducing the incidence of congenital malformations. Without this phenomenon, approximately 12% instead of 2% to 3% of infants would have birth defects.

With the use of a combination of IVF and **polymerase chain reaction**, molecular screening of embryos for genetic defects is being conducted. Single blastomeres from early-stage embryos can be removed, and their DNA can be amplified for analysis. As the Human Genome Project provides more sequencing information, and as specific genes are linked to various syndromes, such procedures will become more commonplace.

Part 1

## SUMMARY

- With each ovarian cycle, a number of primary follicles begin to grow, but usually only one reaches full maturity, and only one oocyte is discharged at **ovulation**.
- At ovulation, the oocyte is in **metaphase** of the **second meiotic division** and is surrounded by the zona pellucida and some granulosa cells (Fig. 3.4).
- The sweeping action of tubal fimbriae carries the oocyte into the uterine tube.

The following table depicts the events taking place in the reproductive organs during the monthly reproductive cycle:

| Changes | Uterine Endometrium | Fallopian Tube | Cervix | Hormonal Influence |
|---|---|---|---|---|
| Proliferative phase | Re-establishment of endometrium with straight uterine glands and lengthening of spiral arteries | Epithelial cell hypertrophy, increase in secretions, and ciliogenesis | Thinning of cervical mucus occurs to allow passage of sperm | Estrogen |
| Ovulatory phase | Deposition of nutrients and thickness of endometrium increases for implantation of oocyte | Oocyte is propelled by peristaltic muscular contractions and cilia | Cervical glands are enlarged | LH surge |
| Secretory phase | Edematous (glycogen deposition), tortuous uterine glands, and vascularity increases | Deciliation and reduction in secretions | Highly viscous mucus plug to hinder the passage of sperm | Progesterone |

- Before spermatozoa can fertilize the oocyte, they must undergo:
  - **Capacitation**, during which time a glycoprotein coat and seminal plasma proteins are removed from the spermatozoon head
  - The **acrosome reaction**, during which acrosin- and trypsin-like substances are released to penetrate the zona pellucida
- During fertilization, the spermatozoon must penetrate:
  - The **corona radiata**
  - The **zona pellucida**
  - The **oocyte cell membrane** (Fig. 3.7)
- As soon as the spermatocyte has entered the oocyte:
  - The oocyte finishes its second meiotic division and forms the **female pronucleus.**
  - The zona pellucida becomes impenetrable to other spermatozoa.
  - The head of the sperm separates from the tail, swells, and forms the **male pronucleus** (Figs. 3.5 and 3.10).

(Continued)

- After both pronuclei have replicated their DNA, paternal and maternal chromosomes intermingle, split longitudinally, and go through a mitotic division, giving rise to the two-cell stage.
- The **results of fertilization** are as follows:
  - **Restoration of the diploid number of chromosomes**
  - **Determination of chromosomal sex**
  - **Initiation of cleavage**
- **Cleavage** is a series of mitotic divisions that results in an increase in cells, **blastomeres**, which become smaller with each division. After three divisions, blastomeres undergo **compaction** to become a tightly grouped ball of cells with inner and outer layers. Compacted blastomeres divide to form a 16-cell **morula**. As the morula enters the uterus on the third or fourth day after fertilization, a cavity begins to appear, and the **blastocyst** forms.
- The **inner cell mass**, which is formed at the time of compaction and will develop into the embryo proper, is at one pole of the blastocyst.
- The **outer cell mass**, which surrounds the inner cells and the blastocyst cavity, will form the trophoblast.
- The uterus at the time of implantation is in the secretory phase.
- The blastocyst implants in the endometrium along the anterior or posterior wall (Fig. 3.7).
- If fertilization does not occur, then the menstrual phase begins, and the spongy and compact endometrial layers are shed. The basal layer remains to regenerate the other layers during the next cycle (Fig. 3.7).

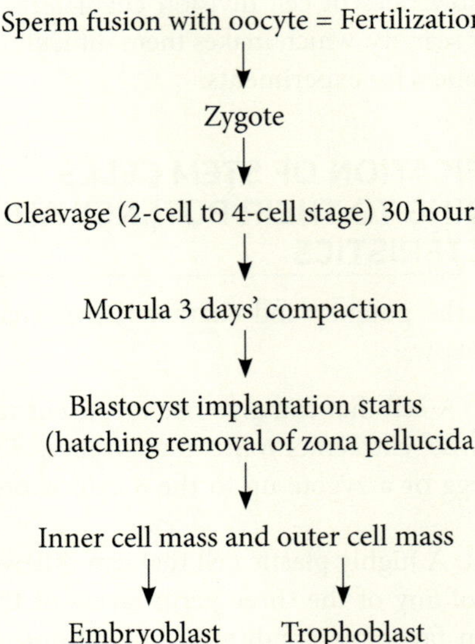


- **Infertility** is a problem for 15% to 30% of couples and can be overcome using **assisted reproductive technology (ART). In vitro fertilization** (**IVF**) involves fertilizing eggs in a culture medium and placing them in the uterus at the eight-cell stage. In some cases, eggs are fertilized by **intracytoplasmic sperm injection (ICSI)**, whereby a single sperm is injected into an egg's cytoplasm. These in vitro techniques are associated with an increased risk for birth defects, prematurity, low birth weight, and multiple births. Approximately 1% to 2% of all live births in the United States occur through ART. In a latest survey, for the National ART Registry, Indian Council of Medical Research (ICMR), the number of clinics is 125 in the capital city of India. There has been a higher demand of ART in India due to the availability of centers of excellence with a success rate of 30%.

## Self-Assessment

### Comprehensive Questions

1. What is the role of the corpus luteum, and what is its origin?
2. What are the three phases of fertilization, and what reactions occur once fusion of the sperm and oocyte membranes takes place?
3. What are the primary causes of infertility in men and women?
4. What are the differences between adult and embryonic stem cells?

### Problem Solving Questions

1. A woman has had several bouts of pelvic inflammatory disease and now wants to have children; however, she has been having difficulty becoming pregnant. What is likely to be the problem, and what would you suggest?
2. A couple have been married for 2 years and are not able to conceive a child. There are no physical or functional problems in the couple. How would you advise them to plan a conception?
3. A young 17-year-old girl fears to have been pregnant. Next day she comes to the OPD. What are the emergency contraception that you can advise?

### Multiple Choice Questions

1. The first week of human development is characterized by the formation of
   (a) Neural tube
   (b) Inner cell mass
   (c) Epiblast
   (d) Hypoblast
2. The phases of fertilization include all of the following except
   (a) Penetration of corona radiata
   (b) Penetration of zona pellucida
   (c) Completion of the first meiotic division
   (d) Fusion of male and female pronuclei
3. What does the inner cell mass form during blastocyst formation?
   (a) Cytotrophoblast
   (b) Syncytiotrophoblast
   (c) Embryoblast
   (d) Blastocele

4. Fertilization takes place in which part of the fallopian tube?
   (a) Ampulla
   (b) Infundibulum
   (c) Isthmus
   (d) Fimbria
5. Capacitation of sperm takes place in the female reproductive tract and is ready for fertilization ideally in
   (a) 30 minutes
   (b) 1 hour
   (c) 6 to 7 hours
   (d) 24 hours
6. Compaction occurs during which stage?
   (a) Zygote
   (b) Blastomeres to form morula
   (c) Blastocyst
   (d) Primitive streak formation
7. During ovulation, oocyte is in
   (a) Prophase
   (b) Metaphase of the first meiotic division
   (c) Metaphase of the second meiotic division
   (d) Telophase of the first meiotic division
8. The endometrium is under the influence of which of the following hormones during the secretory phase of the reproductive cycle?
   (a) LH
   (b) FSH
   (c) Progesterone
   (d) Estrogen

**Answers**

1. (b) 2. (c) 3. (c) 4. (a) 5. (c) 6. (b) 7. (c) 8. (c)

CHAPTER

# 4 Second Week of Development: Bilaminar Germ Disc



### Specific Learning Objectives

- Formation of the bilaminar disc from the inner cell mass
- Formation and differentiation of the trophoblast from the outer cell mass
- Initiation of the uteroplacental circulation
- Formation of the embryonic cavity and chorionic cavity
- Ectopic pregnancy

### Competencies Covered

AN78.2 Describe the development of trophoblast.
AN78.3 Describe the process of implantation and common abnormal sites of implantation.
AN78.4 Describe the formation of extraembryonic mesoderm and coelom, bilaminar disc, and prochordal plate.
AN78.5 Describe in brief abortion, decidual reaction, and pregnancy test.

This chapter gives a day-by-day account of the major events of the second week of development; however, embryos of the same fertilization age do not necessarily develop at the same rate. Indeed, considerable differences in rate of growth have been found even at these early stages of development.

## DAY 8

At the eighth day of development, the blastocyst is partially embedded in the endometrial stroma. In the area over the embryoblast, the trophoblast has differentiated into two layers: (1) an inner layer of mononucleated cells, the **cytotrophoblast**, and (2) an outer multinucleated zone without distinct cell boundaries, the **syncytiotrophoblast** (Figs. 4.1 and 4.2). Mitotic figures are found in the cytotrophoblast but not in the syncytiotrophoblast. Thus, cells in the cytotrophoblast divide and migrate into the syncytiotrophoblast, where they fuse and lose their individual cell membranes.

Cells of the inner cell mass or embryoblast also differentiate into two layers: (1) a layer of small cuboidal cells adjacent

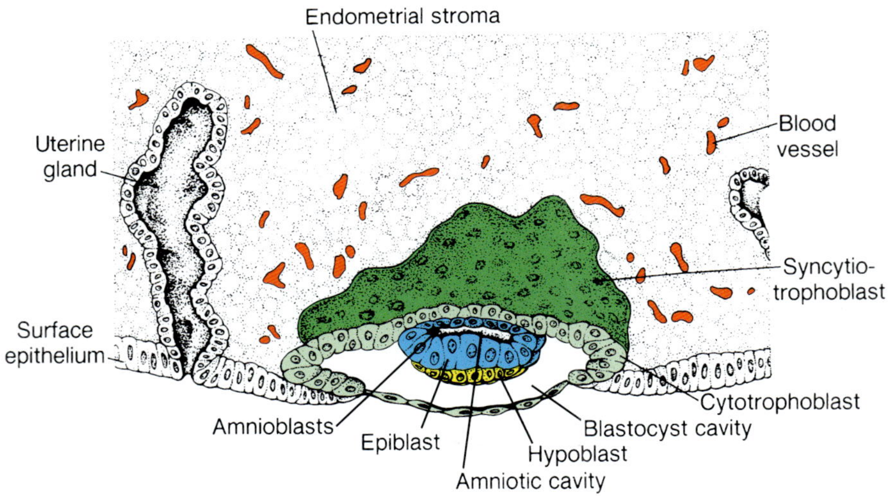


**FIGURE 4.1** A 7.5-day human blastocyst, partially embedded in the endometrial stroma. The trophoblast consists of an inner layer with mononuclear cells, the cytotrophoblast, and an outer layer without distinct cell boundaries, the syncytiotrophoblast. The embryoblast is formed by the epiblast and hypoblast layers. The amniotic cavity appears as a small cleft.

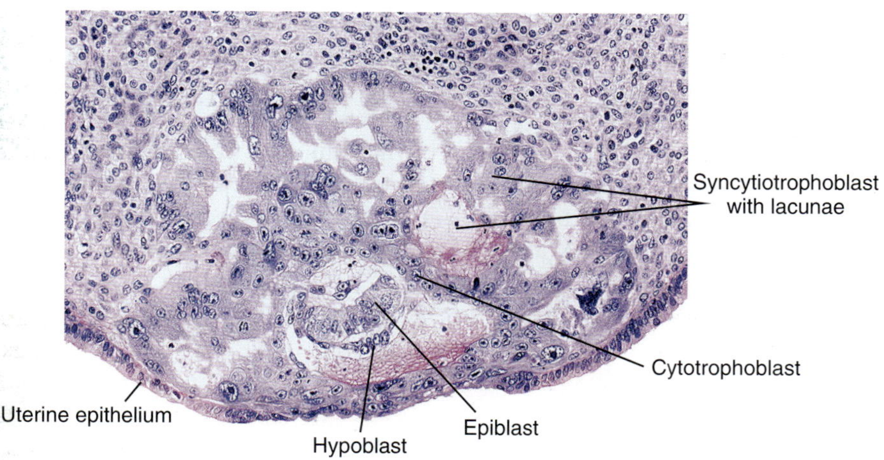


**FIGURE 4.2** Section of a 7.5-day human blastocyst (×100). Note the multinucleated appearance of the syncytiotrophoblast, large cells of the cytotrophoblast, and slit-like amniotic cavity.



to the blastocyst cavity, known as the **hypoblast layer**, and (2) a layer of high columnar cells adjacent to the amniotic cavity, the **epiblast layer** (Figs. 4.1 and 4.2).

Together, the layers form a flat disc. At the same time, a small cavity appears within the epiblast. This cavity enlarges to become the **amniotic cavity**. Epiblast cells adjacent to the cytotrophoblast are called **amnioblasts**; together with the rest of the epiblast, they line the amniotic cavity (Figs. 4.1 and 4.3). The endometrial stroma adjacent to the implantation site is edematous and highly vascular. The large, tortuous glands secrete abundant glycogen and mucus.

## DAY 9

The blastocyst is more deeply embedded in the endometrium, and the penetration defect in the surface epithelium is closed by a fibrin coagulum (Fig. 4.3). The trophoblast shows considerable progress in development, particularly at the embryonic pole, where vacuoles appear in the syncytium. When these vacuoles fuse, they form large lacunae, and this phase of trophoblast development is thus known as the **lacunar stage** (Fig. 4.3).

At the abembryonic pole, meanwhile, flattened cells probably originating from the hypoblast form a thin membrane, the exocoelomic (Heuser) membrane that lines

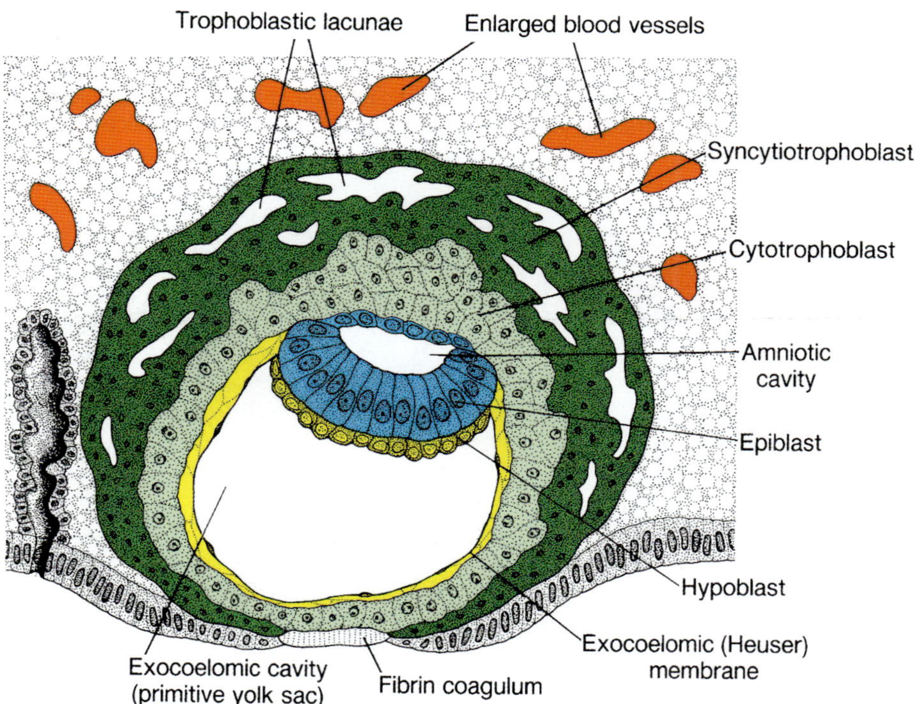


**FIGURE 4.3** A 9-day human blastocyst. The syncytiotrophoblast shows a large number of lacunae. Flat cells form the exocoelomic membrane. The bilaminar disc consists of a layer of columnar epiblast cells and a layer of cuboidal hypoblast cells. The original surface defect is closed by a fibrin coagulum.

the inner surface of the cytotrophoblast (Fig. 4.3). This membrane, together with the hypoblast, forms the lining of the **exocoelomic cavity**, or **primitive yolk sac**.

## DAYS 11 AND 12

By the 11th to the 12th day of development, the blastocyst is completely embedded in the endometrial stroma, and the surface epithelium almost entirely covers the original defect in the uterine wall (Figs. 4.4 and 4.5). The blastocyst now produces a slight protrusion into the lumen of the uterus. The trophoblast is characterized by lacunar spaces in the syncytium that form an intercommunicating network. This network is particularly evident at the embryonic pole; at the abembryonic pole, the trophoblast still consists mainly of cytotrophoblastic cells (Figs. 4.4 and 4.5).

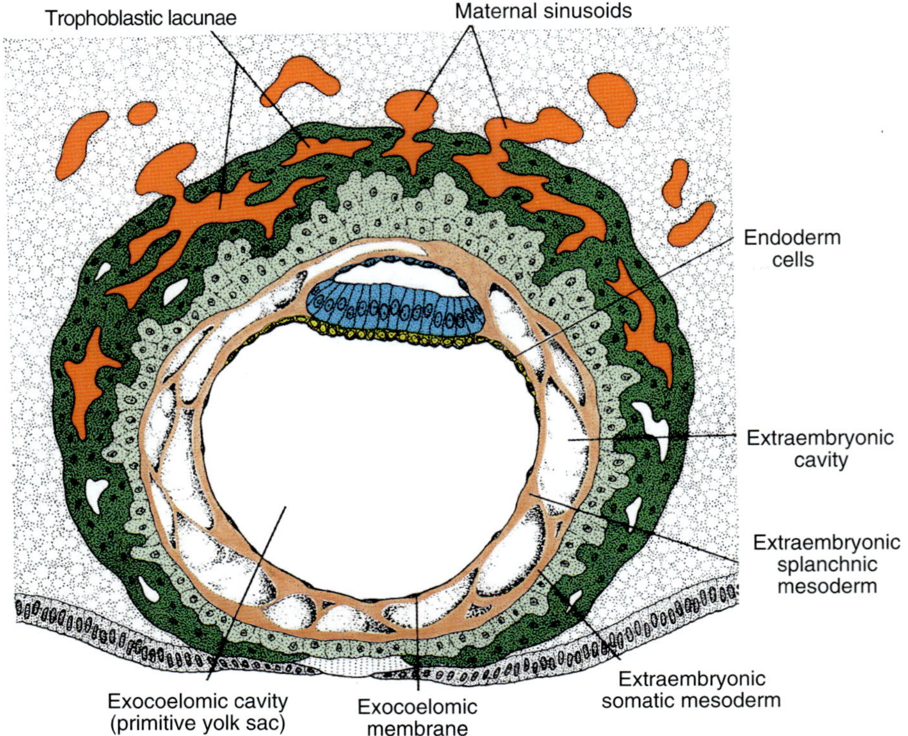


**FIGURE 4.4** Human blastocyst of approximately 12 days. The trophoblastic lacunae at the embryonic pole are in open connection with maternal sinusoids in the endometrial stroma. Extraembryonic mesoderm proliferates and fills the space between the exocoelomic membrane and the inner aspect of the trophoblast.

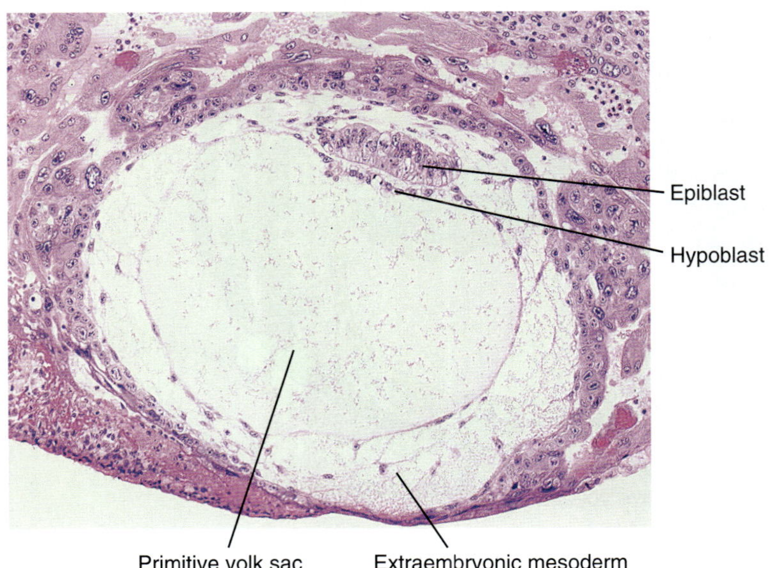


**FIGURE 4.5** Fully implanted 12-day human blastocyst (×100). Note maternal blood cells in the lacunae, the exocoelomic membrane lining the primitive yolk sac, and the hypoblast and epiblast.

Concurrently, cells of the syncytiotrophoblast penetrate deeper into the stroma and erode the endothelial lining of the maternal capillaries. These capillaries, which are congested and dilated, are known as **sinusoids**. The syncytial lacunae become continuous with the sinusoids, and maternal blood enters the lacunar system (Fig. 4.4). As the trophoblast continues to erode more and more sinusoids, maternal blood begins to flow through the trophoblastic system, establishing the **uteroplacental circulation**.

In the meantime, a new population of cells appears between the inner surface of the cytotrophoblast and the outer surface of the exocoelomic cavity. These cells, derived from yolk sac cells, form a fine, loose connective tissue, the **extraembryonic mesoderm**, which eventually fills all of the space between the trophoblast externally and the amnion and exocoelomic membrane internally (Figs. 4.4 and 4.5). Soon, large cavities develop in the extraembryonic mesoderm, and when these become confluent, they form a new space known as the **extraembryonic cavity**, or **chorionic cavity** (Fig. 4.4). This space surrounds the primitive yolk sac and amniotic cavity, except where the germ disc is connected to the trophoblast by the connecting stalk (Fig. 4.6). The extraembryonic mesoderm lining the cytotrophoblast and amnion is called the **extraembryonic somatic mesoderm**; the lining covering the yolk sac is known as the **extraembryonic splanchnic mesoderm** (Fig. 4.4).

Growth of the bilaminar disc is relatively slow compared with that of the trophoblast; consequently, the disc remains very small (0.1 to 0.2 mm). Cells of the endometrium, meanwhile, become polyhedral and loaded with glycogen and lipids; intercellular spaces are filled with extravasate, and the tissue is edematous. These changes, known as the **decidua reaction**, at first, are confined to the area immediately surrounding the implantation site but soon occur throughout the endometrium.

## DAY 13

By the 13th day of development, the surface defect in the endometrium has usually healed. Occasionally, however, bleeding occurs at the implantation site as a result of increased blood flow into the lacunar spaces. Because this bleeding occurs near the 28th day of the menstrual cycle, it may be confused with normal menstrual bleeding and, therefore, may cause inaccuracy in determining the expected delivery date.

The trophoblast is characterized by villous structures. Cells of the cytotrophoblast proliferate locally and penetrate into the



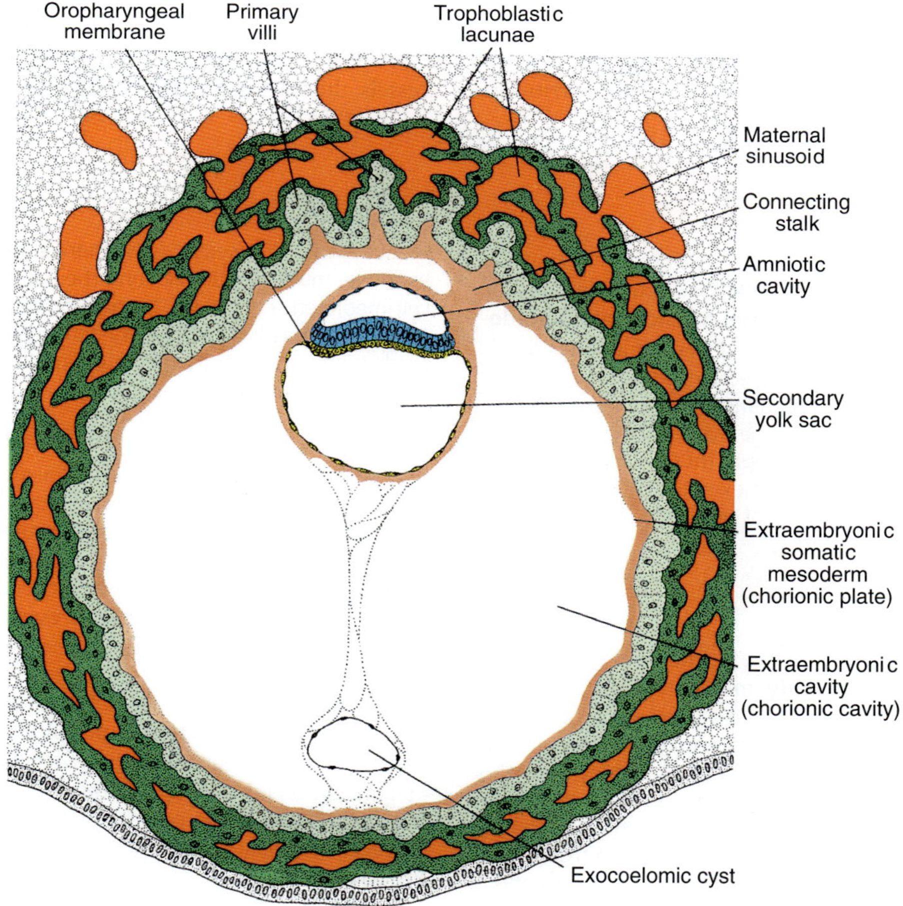


**FIGURE 4.6** A 13-day human blastocyst. Trophoblastic lacunae are present at the embryonic as well as the abembryonic pole, and the uteroplacental circulation has begun. Note the primary villi and the extraembryonic coelom or chorionic cavity. The secondary yolk sac is entirely lined with endoderm.

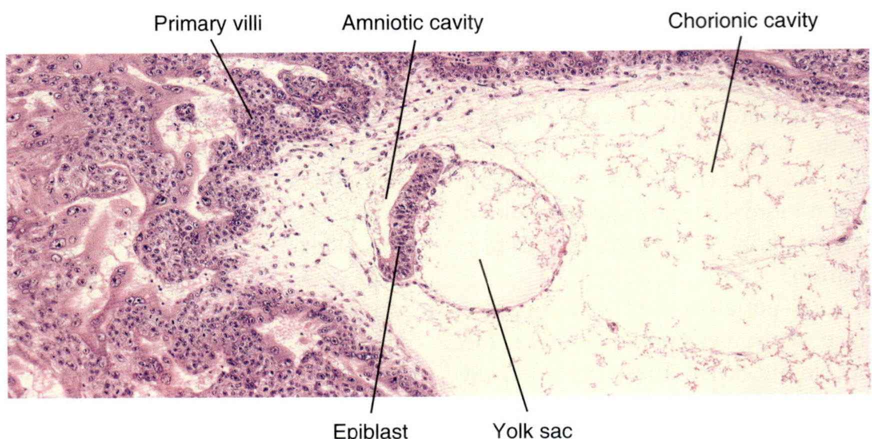


**FIGURE 4.7** Section through the implantation site of a 13-day embryo. Note the amniotic cavity, yolk sac, and chorionic cavity. Most of the lacunae are filled with blood.



syncytiotrophoblast, forming cellular columns surrounded by syncytium. Cellular columns with the syncytial covering are known as **primary villi** (Figs. 4.6 and 4.7) (see Chapter 5, p. 55).

In the meantime, the hypoblast produces additional cells that migrate along the inside of the exocoelomic membrane (Fig. 4.4). These cells proliferate and gradually form a new cavity within the exocoelomic cavity. This new cavity is known as the **secondary yolk sac** or **definitive yolk sac** (Figs. 4.6 and 4.7). This yolk sac is much smaller than the original exocoelomic cavity, or primitive yolk sac. During its formation, large portions of the exocoelomic cavity are pinched off. These portions are represented by **exocoelomic cysts**, which are often found in the extraembryonic coelom or **chorionic cavity** (Fig. 4.6).

Meanwhile, the extraembryonic coelom expands and forms a large cavity, the **chorionic cavity**. The extraembryonic mesoderm lining the inside of the cytotrophoblast is then known as the **chorionic plate**. The only place where extraembryonic mesoderm traverses the chorionic cavity is in the **connecting stalk** (Fig. 4.6). With development of blood vessels, the stalk becomes the **umbilical cord**.

## *Clinical Correlates*

### Pregnancy Test

The syncytiotrophoblast is responsible for hormone production (see Chapter 8, p. 96), including **human chorionic gonadotropin (hCG)**. By the end of the second week, quantities of this hormone are sufficient to be detected by radioimmunoassays, which serve as the basis for pregnancy testing. Hence, during the first 2 months of pregnancy, the syncytiotrophoblast produces **human chorionic gonadotropin (hCG)**, which maintains the corpus luteum. This hormone is excreted by the mother in the urine, and in the early stages of gestation, its presence is used as an indicator of pregnancy.

### *Immune System of the Mother: Why the Fetus Is Not Rejected by the Mother*

Since 50% of the implanting embryo's genome is derived from the father, it is a **foreign body** that potentially should be rejected by the maternal system, similar to rejection of a transplanted organ. A pregnant woman's immune system needs to change in order for her to tolerate the pregnancy. How this occurs is not well understood, but it appears that a shift from cell-mediated immunity to humoral (antibody-mediated) immunity occurs and that this shift protects the embryo from rejection. However, the immune system alterations place pregnant women at increased risk for certain infections, such as influenza, which explains the increased risk of death from these infections in pregnant women. In addition, manifestations of autoimmune disease may change during pregnancy. For example, multiple sclerosis and rheumatoid arthritis, primarily cell-mediated conditions, show improvement during pregnancy, whereas women with systemic lupus erythematosus (a predominantly antibody-mediated immune disorder) are more severely affected when pregnant.

### *Abnormal Implantation: Ectopic Pregnancy*

Abnormal implantation sites sometimes occur even within the uterus. Normally, the human blastocyst implants along the anterior or posterior wall of the body of the uterus. Occasionally, the blastocyst implants close to the internal os (opening) (Fig. 4.8) of the cervix so that later in development, the placenta bridges the opening (**placenta previa**) and causes severe, even life-threatening bleeding in the second part of pregnancy and during delivery.

Occasionally, implantation takes place outside the uterus, resulting in an **extrauterine pregnancy**, or **ectopic pregnancy**. Ectopic pregnancies may occur at any place in the abdominal cavity, ovary, or uterine tube (Fig. 4.8). Ninety-five percent of ectopic pregnancies occur in the uterine tube, however, and most of these are in the ampulla (80%; Fig. 4.9). In the abdominal cavity, the blastocyst most frequently attaches itself to the peritoneal lining of the **rectouterine cavity**, or **pouch of Douglas** (Fig. 4.10). The blastocyst may also attach itself to the peritoneal covering of the intestinal tract or to the

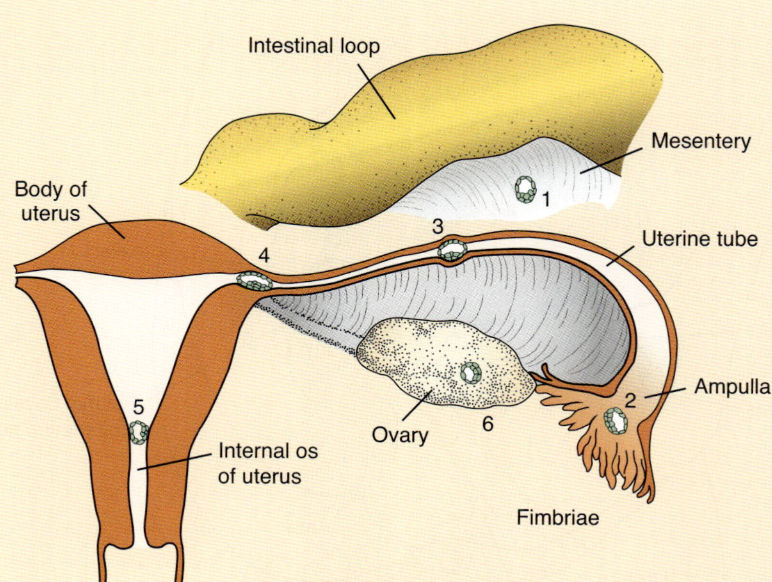


**FIGURE 4.8** Abnormal implantation sites of the blastocyst. *1*, implantation in the abdominal cavity (1.4%; the ovum most frequently implants in the rectouterine cavity [pouch of Douglas; Fig. 4.10] but may implant at any place covered by peritoneum); *2*, implantation in the ampullary region of the tube (80%); *3*, tubal implantation (12%); *4*, interstitial implantation (0.2%; e.g., in the narrow portion of the uterine tube); *5*, implantation in the region of the internal os, frequently resulting in placenta previa (0.2%); and *6*, ovarian implantation (0.2%).

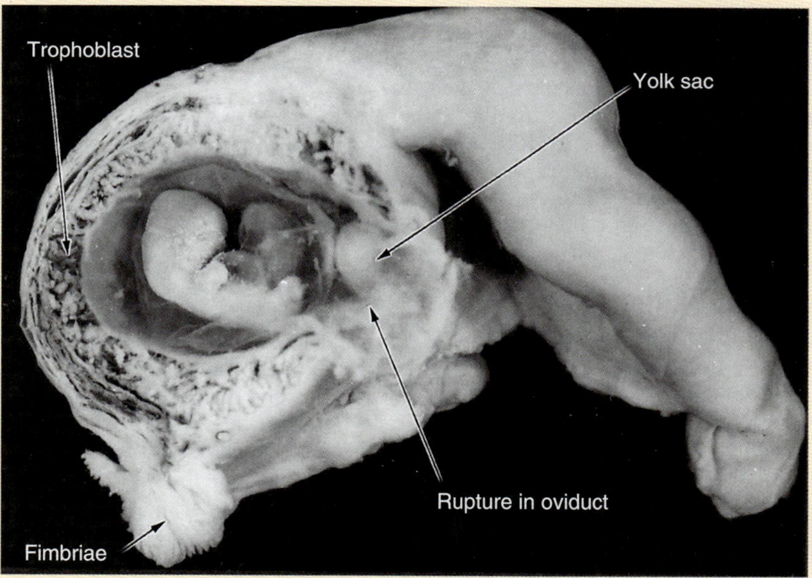


**FIGURE 4.9** Tubal pregnancy. Embryo is approximately 2 months old and is about to escape through a rupture in the tubal wall.

omentum. Sometimes, the blastocyst develops in the ovary proper, causing a **primary ovarian pregnancy**. Ectopic pregnancies occur in 2% of all pregnancies and account for 9% of all pregnancy-related deaths for the mother. In most ectopic pregnancies, the embryo dies about the second month of gestation and may result in severe hemorrhaging in the mother.

Abnormal blastocysts are common. For example, in a series of 26 implanted blastocysts varying in age from 7.5 to 17 days recovered from patients of normal fertility, 9 (34.6%) were abnormal. Some consisted of syncytium only; others showed varying degrees of trophoblastic hypoplasia. In 2, the embryoblast was absent, and in some, the germ disc showed an abnormal orientation.

It is likely that most abnormal blastocysts would not have produced any sign of pregnancy because their trophoblast was so inferior that the corpus luteum could not have persisted. These embryos probably would have been aborted with the next menstrual flow and, therefore, pregnancy would not have been detected. In some cases, however, the trophoblast develops and forms placental membranes, although little or no embryonic tissue is present. Such a condition is known as a **hydatidiform mole**. Moles secrete high levels of hCG and may produce benign or malignant (**invasive mole, choriocarcinoma**) tumors.

(Continued)

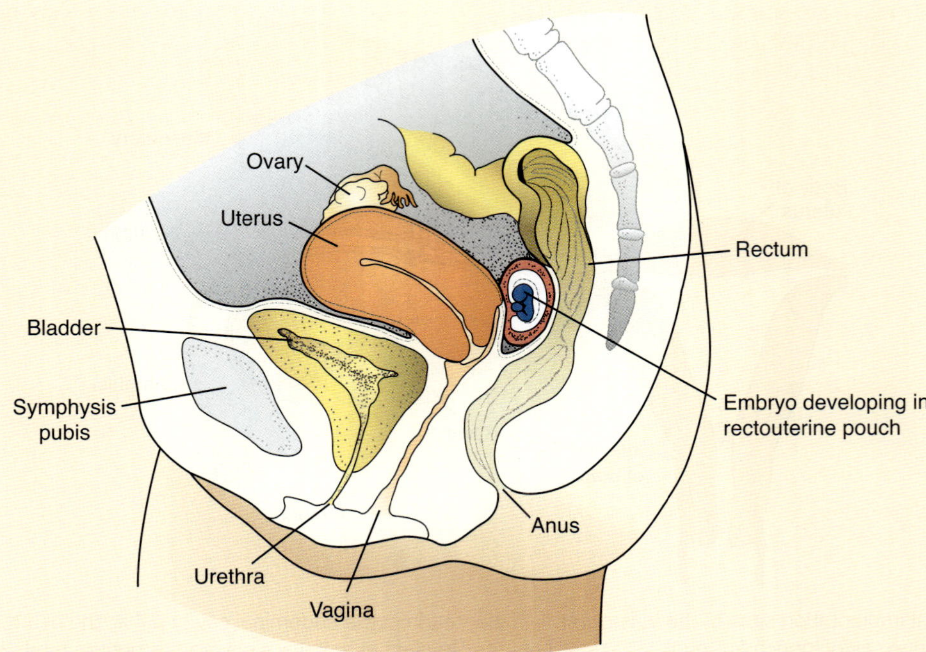


**FIGURE 4.10** Midline section of bladder, uterus, and rectum shows an abdominal pregnancy in the rectouterine (Douglas) pouch.

Genetic analysis of hydatidiform moles indicates that although male and female pronuclei may be genetically equivalent, they may be different functionally. This evidence is derived from the fact that although cells of moles are diploid, their entire genome is paternal. Thus, most moles arise from fertilization of an oocyte lacking a nucleus followed by duplication of the male chromosomes to restore the diploid number. These results also suggest that paternal genes regulate most of the development of the trophoblast because in moles this tissue differentiates even in the absence of a female pronucleus.

### *Genomic Imprinting*

Other examples of functional differences in maternal and paternal genes are provided by the observation that certain genetic diseases depend on whether the defective or missing gene is inherited from the father or the mother. This phenomenon, in which there is differential modification and/or expression of homologous alleles or chromosome regions depending on the parent from whom the genetic material is derived, is known as **genomic imprinting**. Less than 1% of human genes are believed to be imprinted (see Chapter 2, p. 21).

### *Abortion*

When a fetus is expelled from the uterine cavity before term, it is known as abortion. Abortions can be spontaneous. Spontaneous abortions occur due to genetic, maternal, or environmental factors. The couple who have repeated abortions should go for counseling. Sometimes when an abnormality is seen in the antenatal period, the pregnancies are terminated as the baby born will not be viable or it may be having serious congenital anomalies. These children do not survive and if they do for some time, they are very much dependent on the parents. In India, unwanted pregnancies can be terminated before 20 weeks of gestation under the MTP Act (1971).

Preimplantation and postimplantation reproductive failure occurs often. Even in some fertile women under optimal conditions for pregnancy, 15% of oocytes are not fertilized, and 10% to 15% start cleavage but fail to implant. Of the 70% to 75% that implant, only 58% survive until the second week, and 16% of those are abnormal. Hence, when the first expected menstruation is missed, only 42% of the eggs exposed to sperm are surviving. Of this percentage, a number will be aborted during subsequent weeks, and a number will be abnormal at the time of birth.

## SUMMARY


- At the beginning of the second week, the blastocyst is partially embedded in the endometrial stroma.
- The **trophoblast** differentiates into (1) an inner, actively proliferating layer, the **cytotrophoblast**, and (2) an outer layer, the **syncytiotrophoblast**, which erodes maternal tissues (Fig. 4.1).
- By day 9, lacunae develop in the syncytiotrophoblast. Subsequently, maternal sinusoids are eroded by the syncytiotrophoblast, maternal blood enters the lacunar network.
- By the end of the second week, a primitive **uteroplacental circulation** begins (Fig. 4.6).
- The cytotrophoblast, meanwhile, forms cellular columns penetrating into and surrounded by the syncytium. These columns are **primary villi**.
- By the end of the second week, the blastocyst is completely embedded, and the surface defect in the mucosa has healed (Fig. 4.6).

- The **inner cell mass** or **embryoblast**, meanwhile, differentiates into (1) the **epiblast** and (2) the **hypoblast**, together forming a **bilaminar disc** (Fig. 4.6).
- Epiblast cells give rise to **amnioblasts** that line the **amniotic cavity** superior to the epiblast layer.
- Hypoblast cells are continuous with the **exocoelomic membrane**, and together, they surround the **primitive yolk sac** (Fig. 4.4).
- By the end of the second week, extraembryonic mesoderm fills the space between the trophoblast and the amnion and exocoelomic membrane internally.
- When vacuoles develop in this tissue, the **extraembryonic coelom** or **chorionic cavity** forms (Fig. 4.6). **Extraembryonic mesoderm** lining the cytotrophoblast and amnion is **extraembryonic somatic mesoderm**; the lining surrounding the yolk sac is **extraembryonic splanchnic mesoderm** (Fig. 4.6).
- The second week of development is known as the **week of 2's**:
  - The trophoblast differentiates into two layers: the cytotrophoblast and syncytiotrophoblast.
  - The embryoblast forms two layers: the epiblast and hypoblast.
  - The extraembryonic mesoderm splits into two layers: the somatic and splanchnic layers.
  - Two cavities form: the amniotic and yolk sac cavities.
- **Implantation** occurs at the end of the first week. Trophoblast cells invade the epithelium and underlying endometrial stroma with the help of proteolytic enzymes.
- Implantation may also occur outside the uterus, such as in the rectouterine pouch, on the mesentery, in the uterine tube, or in the ovary (**ectopic pregnancies**).

Part 1

## Self-Assessment

### Comprehensive Questions

1. Write a short note on ectopic pregnancy.
2. The second week of development is known as the week of 2's. Formation of what structures supports this statement?
3. Discuss about the formation of amniotic cavity.

### Problem Solving Questions

1. During implantation, the trophoblast is invading maternal tissues, and because it contains approximately 50% paternal genes, it is a foreign body. Why is the conceptus not rejected by an immunologic response from the mother's system?
2. A woman who believes she is pregnant complains of edema and vaginal bleeding. Examination reveals high plasma hCG concentrations and placental tissue but no evidence of an embryo. How would you explain this condition?
3. A young woman who has missed two menstrual periods complains of intense abdominal pain. What might an initial diagnosis be, and how would you confirm it?
4. A young woman has missed her cycle and she is under stress. What is the earliest method by which she can confirm her pregnancy and what is the scientific basis of this test?

### Multiple Choice Questions

1. Amniotic cavity develops at
   (a) Day 5
   (b) Day 6
   (c) Day 7
   (d) Day 8
2. Hormone detected in urine and responsible for a positive pregnancy test is
   (a) hCG
   (b) Estrogen
   (c) Progesterone
   (d) LH
3. What is the normal site of implantation of blastocyst?
   (a) Endometrium and myometrium
   (b) Functional layer of the endometrium
   (c) Basal layer of the endometrium
   (d) Myometrium
4. What does the inner cell mass form during blastocyst formation?
   (a) Cytotrophoblast
   (b) Syncytiotrophoblast
   (c) Embryoblast
   (d) Blastocele
5. First week of human development is characterized by the formation of
   (a) Neural tube
   (b) Inner cell mass
   (c) Epiblast
   (d) Hypoblast
6. Primitive uteroplacental circulation starts at what stage of development?
   (a) First week
   (b) Second week
   (c) Third week
   (d) Fourth week
7. Implantation is complete at which day postfertilization?
   (a) 6
   (b) 7
   (c) 8
   (d) 9
8. Common site for ectopic pregnancy is
   (a) Uterine tube
   (b) Rectouterine pouch
   (c) Ovary
   (d) Mesentery
9. Bilaminar germ disc is formed by
   (a) Cytotrophoblast and syncytiotrophoblast
   (b) Ectoderm and endoderm
   (c) Epiblast and hypoblast
   (d) Amniogenic cells and epiblast

### Answers

1. (d) 2. (a) 3. (b) 4. (c) 5. (b) 6. (b) 7. (c) 8. (a) 9. (c)

CHAPTER

# 5 Third Week of Development: Trilaminar Germ Disc



## Specific Learning Objectives

- Process of gastrulation which occurs during the third week of intrauterine life
- Formation of primitive streak
- Establishment of the trilaminar germ disc
- Formation of notochord
- Establishment of body axis
- Formation of primary secondary and tertiary villi
- Differentiation of decidua
- Formation of connecting stalk

## Competencies Covered

AN79.1 Describe the formation and fate of the primitive streak.
AN79.2 Describe the formation and fate of the notochord.

## GASTRULATION: FORMATION OF EMBRYONIC MESODERM AND ENDODERM

The most characteristic event occurring during the third week of gestation is **gastrulation**, the process that establishes all three **germ layers** (**ectoderm**, **mesoderm**, and **endoderm**) in the embryo. Gastrulation begins with formation of the **primitive streak** on the surface of the epiblast (Figs. 5.1 and 5.2). Initially, the streak is vaguely defined (Fig. 5.1), but in a 15- to 16-day embryo, it is clearly visible as a narrow groove with slightly bulging regions on either side. The cephalic end of the streak, the **primitive node**, consists of a slightly elevated area surrounding the small **primitive pit** (Fig. 5.2). Cells of the epiblast migrate toward the primitive streak (Fig. 5.2). Upon arrival in the region of the streak, they become flask-shaped, detach from the epiblast, and slip beneath it (Fig. 5.2*B*,*C*). This inward movement is known as **invagination**. Cell migration and specification are controlled by **fibroblast growth factor 8 (FGF8)**, which is synthesized by streak cells themselves. This growth factor controls cell movement by downregulating E-cadherin, a protein that normally binds epiblast cells together. FGF8 then controls cell specification into the mesoderm by regulating *BRACHYURY (T)* expression. Once the cells have invaginated, some displace the hypoblast, creating the embryonic **endoderm**, and others come to lie between the epiblast and newly created endoderm to form **mesoderm**. Cells remaining in the epiblast then form **ectoderm**. Thus, the epiblast, through the process of gastrulation, is the source of all of the germ layers (Fig. 5.2*B*), and cells in these layers will give rise to all of the tissues and organs in the embryo.

As more and more cells move between the epiblast and hypoblast layers, they begin to spread laterally and cranially in the embryonic disc (Fig. 5.2). Gradually, they migrate beyond the margin of the disc and establish contact with the extraembryonic mesoderm covering the yolk sac and amnion. In the cephalic direction, they pass on each side of the **prechordal plate**. The prechordal plate itself forms between the tip of the notochord and the **oropharyngeal membrane** and is derived from some of the first cells that migrate through the node in the midline and move in a cephalic direction. Later, the prechordal plate will be important for induction of the forebrain (Figs. 5.2 and 5.3). The oropharyngeal membrane at the cranial end of the disc consists of a small region of tightly adherent ectoderm and endoderm cells that represents the future opening of the oral cavity.

## FORMATION OF THE NOTOCHORD

**Prenotochordal cells** invaginating in the primitive node move forward cranially in the midline until they reach the **prechordal plate** (Fig. 5.3). These prenotochordal cells become intercalated in the hypoblast so that for a short time, the midline of the embryo consists of two cell layers that form the **notochordal plate** (Fig. 5.3*B*). As the hypoblast is replaced by endoderm cells moving in at the streak, cells of the notochordal plate proliferate and detach from the endoderm. They then form a solid cord of cells, the **definitive notochord** (Fig. 5.3*C*), which underlies the neural tube and is a signaling center for inducing the axial skeleton. Because elongation of the notochord is a dynamic process, the cranial end forms first, and caudal regions are added as the primitive streak assumes a more caudal position. The notochord and prenotochordal cells extend cranially to the prechordal plate (an area just caudal to the oropharyngeal membrane) and caudally to the primitive pit. At the point where the pit forms an indentation in the epiblast, the **neurenteric canal** temporarily connects the amniotic and yolk sac cavities (Fig. 5.3*A*).

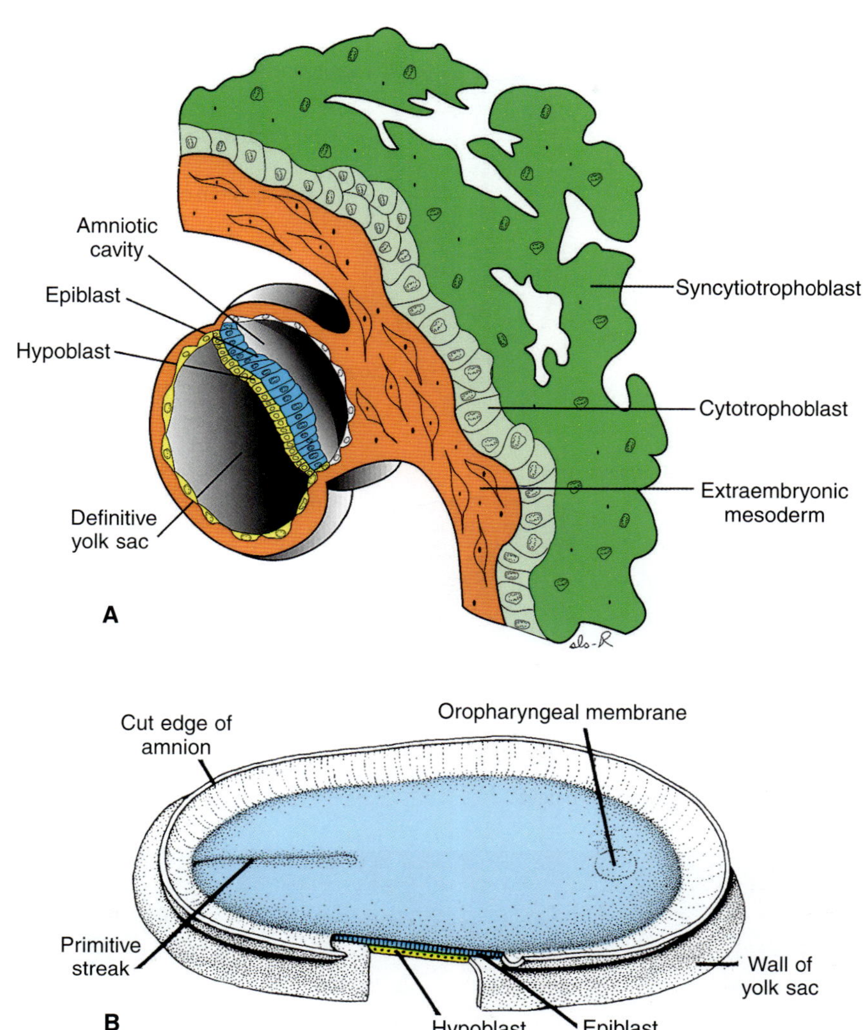


**FIGURE 5.1** **A.** Implantation site at the end of the second week. **B.** Representative view of the germ disc at the end of the second week of development. The amniotic cavity has been opened to permit a view of the dorsal side of the epiblast. The hypoblast and epiblast are in contact with each other, and the primitive streak forms a shallow groove in the caudal region of the embryo.

The **cloacal membrane** is formed at the caudal end of the embryonic disc (Fig. 5.2*A*). This membrane, which is similar in structure to the oropharyngeal membrane, consists of tightly adherent ectoderm and endoderm cells with no intervening mesoderm. When the cloacal membrane appears, the posterior wall of the yolk sac forms a small diverticulum that extends into the connecting stalk. This diverticulum, the **allantoenteric diverticulum**, or **allantois**, appears around the 16th day of development (Fig. 5.3*A*). Although in some lower vertebrates, the allantois serves as a reservoir for excretion products of the renal system, in humans, it remains rudimentary but may be involved in abnormalities of bladder development (see Chapter 16, p. 218).

## ■ ESTABLISHMENT OF THE BODY AXES

Establishment of the **body axes, anterior–posterior (A–P; craniocaudal)**, **dorso–ventral (D–V)**, and **left–right (L–R)**, occurs early in embryogenesis and is probably initiated during the late morula to blastocyst stages of development with the A–P and D–V axes specified prior to the L–R (see Chapter 3, p. 36). By the blastocyst stage, the A–P axis is determined and cells that are destined to form the **anterior visceral endoderm (AVE)** at the cranial end of the endoderm layer of the bilaminar disc (Fig. 5.4) migrate toward what will become the head region.

### Molecular Regulation for Establishment of Body Axis

At this bilaminar disc stage, cells in the *AVE* express genes essential for head formation, including the transcription factors *OTX2*, *LIM1*, and *HESX1*, and the secreted factors **cerberus** and **lefty1** (members of the TGF-β family), which inhibit **nodal** (a member of the TGF-β family) activity, thereby establishing the cranial end of the embryo. The absence of cerberus and lefty1 at the caudal end of the embryo allows nodal expression to continue, and this signal establishes and maintains the primitive streak (Fig. 5.4). Once the streak is formed, *NODAL* upregulates a number of genes

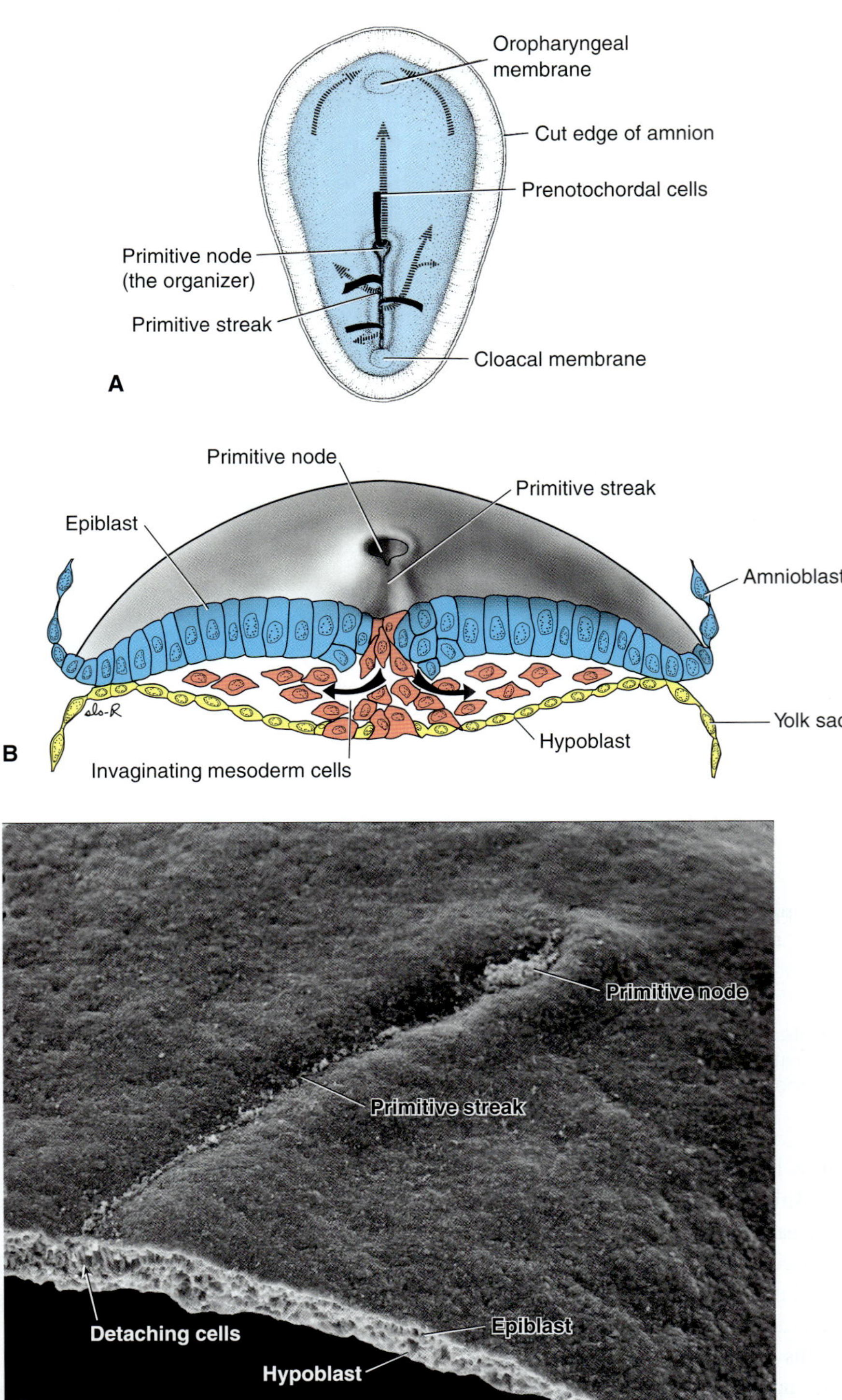


**FIGURE 5.2** **A.** Dorsal side of the germ disc from a 16-day embryo indicating the movement of surface epiblast cells (*solid black lines*) through the primitive streak and node and the subsequent migration of cells between the hypoblast and epiblast (*broken lines*). **B.** Cross section through the cranial region of the streak at 15 days showing invagination of epiblast cells. The first cells to move inward displace the hypoblast to create the definitive endoderm. Once definitive endoderm is established, inwardly moving epiblast forms mesoderm. **C.** Dorsal view of an embryo showing the primitive node and streak and a cross section through the streak. The view is similar to the illustration in **B**; *arrow*, detaching epiblast cells in the primitive streak.

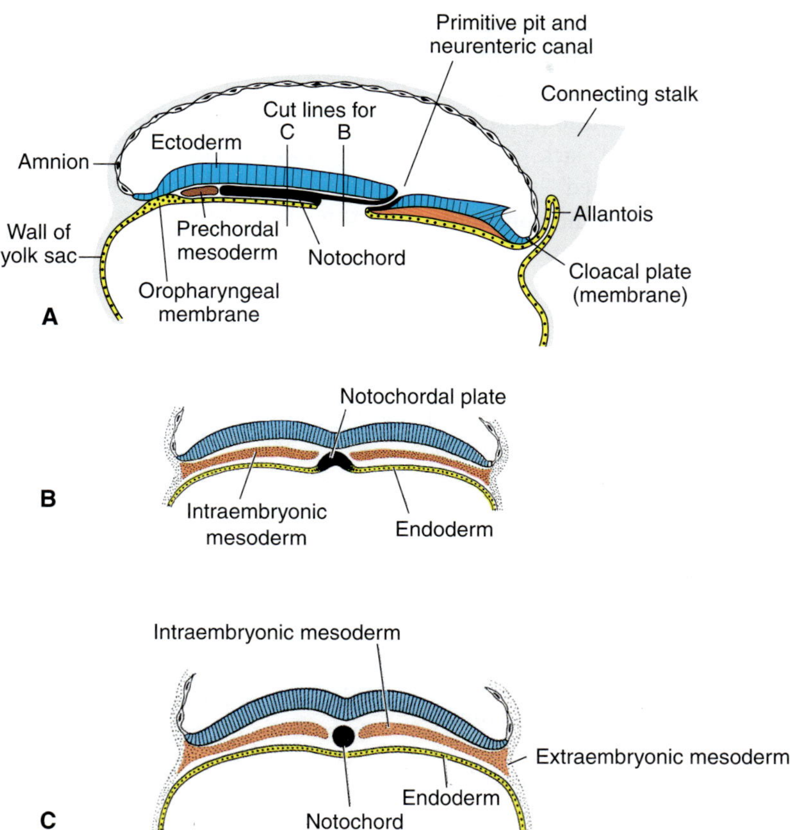


**FIGURE 5.3** Schematic views illustrating formation of the notochord, whereby prenotochordal cells migrate through the primitive streak, become intercalated in the endoderm to form the notochordal plate, and finally detach from the endoderm to form the definitive notochord. Because these events occur in a cranial-to-caudal sequence, portions of the definitive notochord are established in the head region first. **A.** Drawing of a sagittal section through a 17-day embryo. The most cranial portion of the definitive notochord has formed, whereas prenotochordal cells caudal to this region are intercalated into the endoderm as the notochordal plate. *Note that some cells migrate ahead of the notochord. These mesoderm cells form the prechordal plate that will assist in forebrain induction.* **B.** Schematic cross section through the region of the notochordal plate. Soon, the notochordal plate will detach from the endoderm to form the definitive notochord. **C.** Schematic view showing the definitive notochord.

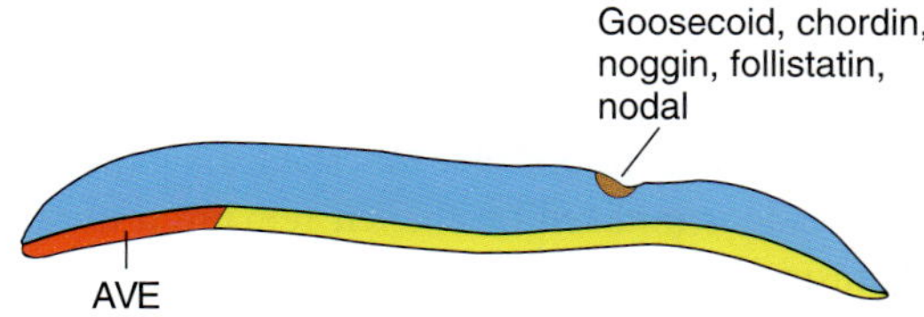


**FIGURE 5.4** Sagittal section through the node and primitive streak showing the expression pattern of genes regulating the craniocaudal and dorsoventral axes. Cells at the prospective cranial end of the embryo in the *AVE* express the transcription factors *OTX2*, *LIM1*, and *HESX1* and the secreted factor cerberus that contribute to head development and establish the cephalic region. Once the streak is formed and gastrulation is progressing, BMP4 is secreted throughout the bilaminar disc and acts with FGF to ventralize mesoderm into intermediate and lateral plate mesoderm. *GOOSECOID*, expressed in the node, regulates *CHORDIN* expression, and this gene product, together with noggin and follistatin, antagonizes the activity of BMP4, dorsalizing mesoderm into notochord and paraxial mesoderm for the head region. Later, expression of the *BRACHYURY (T)* gene antagonizes BMP4 to dorsalize mesoderm into notochord and paraxial mesoderm in caudal regions of the embryo.

responsible for formation of dorsal and ventral mesoderm and head and tail structures.

Another member of the TGF-β family, **bone morphogenetic protein 4 (BMP4)**, is secreted throughout the embryonic disc (Fig. 5.4). In the presence of this protein and **FGF**, mesoderm will be ventralized to contribute to kidneys (intermediate mesoderm), blood, and body wall mesoderm (lateral plate mesoderm). In fact, all mesoderm would be ventralized if the activity of BMP4 were not blocked by other genes expressed in the node. For this reason, the node is the **organizer**. It was given that designation by Hans Spemann, who first described this activity in the dorsal lip of the blastopore, a structure analogous to the node, in *Xenopus* embryos. Thus, ***CHORDIN*** (activated by the transcription factor ***GOOSECOID***), **noggin**, and **follistatin** antagonize the activity of BMP4. As a result, cranial mesoderm is dorsalized into notochord, somites, and somitomeres (Fig. 5.4). Later, these three genes are expressed in the notochord and are important in neural induction in the cranial region.

As mentioned, **Nodal** is involved in initiating and maintaining the primitive streak. Similarly, ***HNF-3β*** maintains the node and later induces regional specificity in the forebrain and midbrain areas. Without *HNF-3β*, embryos fail to gastrulate properly and lack forebrain and midbrain structures. As mentioned previously, *GOOSECOID* activates inhibitors of BMP4 and contributes to regulation of head development. Over- or underexpression of this gene in laboratory animals results in severe malformations of the head region, including duplications, similar to some types of conjoined twins (Fig. 5.5).

Regulation of dorsal mesoderm formation in middle and caudal regions of the embryo is controlled by the ***BRACHYURY (T)* gene** expressed in the node, notochord precursor cells, and notochord. This gene is essential for cell migration through the primitive streak. ***BRACHYURY*** encodes a sequence-specific DNA-binding protein that functions as a transcription factor. The DNA-binding domain is called the **T-box**, and there are more than 20 genes in the T-box family. Thus, mesoderm formation in these regions depends on this gene product, and its absence results in shortening of the embryonic axis (caudal dysgenesis). The degree of shortening depends on the time at which the protein becomes deficient.

**Laterality (L–R sidedness)** also is established early in development. Normally, many organs exhibit asymmetries, including the heart, lungs, gut, spleen, stomach, liver, and others. Positioning these organs and establishing their asymmetries is orchestrated by a cascade of signal molecules and genes. When the primitive streak appears, **FGF8** is secreted by cells in the node and primitive streak, and this growth factor induces expression of ***NODAL*** (Fig. 5.6*A*). *NODAL* expression is then restricted to the left side of the embryo by the accumulation of **serotonin (5-HT)** on the left side. These high concentrations of 5-HT on the left activate expression of the transcription factor *MAD3* that restricts *NODAL* expression to the left side of the primitive node (Fig. 5.6*B*). Midline genes like *SONIC HEDGEHOG* (*SHH*), *LEFTY1*, and *ZIC3* (a gene on the X chromosome that codes for a zinc finger transcription factor) are not only involved in establishing the midline but also involved in preventing *NODAL* expression from crossing over to the right side. Ultimately, Nodal protein in the left lateral plate mesoderm initiates a signaling cascade that includes *LEFTY2* to upregulate ***PITX2*** (Fig. 5.6*B*). *PITX2* is a homeobox-containing transcription factor that is a "master gene" responsible for establishing left-sidedness, and its expression is repeated on the left side of the heart, stomach, and gut primordia as these organs are assuming their normal asymmetrical body positions. If the gene is expressed ectopically (e.g., on the right side), this abnormal expression results in **laterality defects**, including *situs inversus* and dextrocardia (placement of the heart to the right side; see "Clinical Correlates," p. 54).

Note that the neurotransmitter **5-HT** also plays a critical role in this signaling cascade that establishes laterality. 5-HT is concentrated on the left side, which activates *MAD3* and restricts Nodal signaling to the left side (Fig. 5.6*B*). Animal studies show that altering 5-HT signaling can result in *situs inversus*, dextrocardia, heart malformations, and a variety of laterality-related birth defects called heterotaxy, whereas epidemiology studies indicate that similar malformations occur in humans when 5-HT signaling is disrupted by pharmaceutical agents (see "Clinical Correlates," p. 54).

Genes regulating right-sided development are not as well-defined, although expression of the transcription factor ***SNAIL*** is restricted to the right lateral plate mesoderm and probably regulates effector genes responsible for establishing the right side. Why the cascade is initiated on the left remains a mystery, but the mechanism may involve **cilia** on cells in the node that beat to create a gradient of Nodal toward the left or by a signaling gradient established by **gap junctions** and small ion transport.

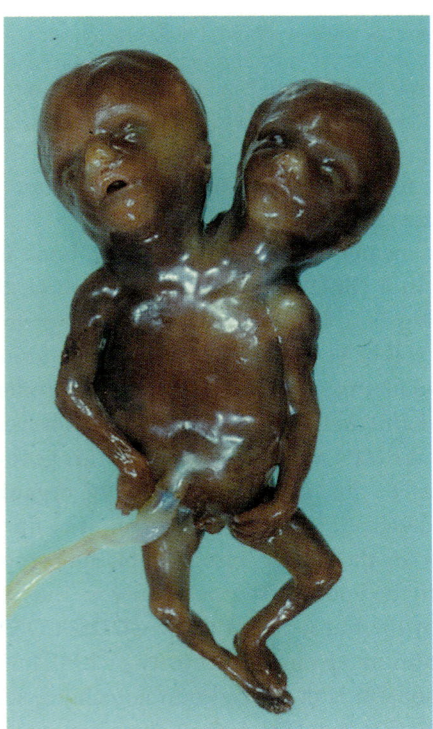

**FIGURE 5.5** Conjoined twins. If the gene *GOOSECOID* is overexpressed in frog embryos, the result is a two-headed tadpole. Perhaps, overexpression of this gene explains the origin of this type of conjoined twins.

## FATE MAP ESTABLISHED DURING GASTRULATION

Regions of the epiblast that migrate and ingress through the primitive streak have been mapped, and their ultimate fates have been determined (Fig. 5.7). For example, cells that ingress through the cranial region of the node become prechordal plate and notochord, those migrating at the lateral edges of the node and from the cranial end of the streak become **paraxial mesoderm**, cells migrating through the midstreak region become **intermediate mesoderm**, those migrating through the more caudal part of the streak form **lateral plate mesoderm**, and cells migrating through the caudalmost part of the streak

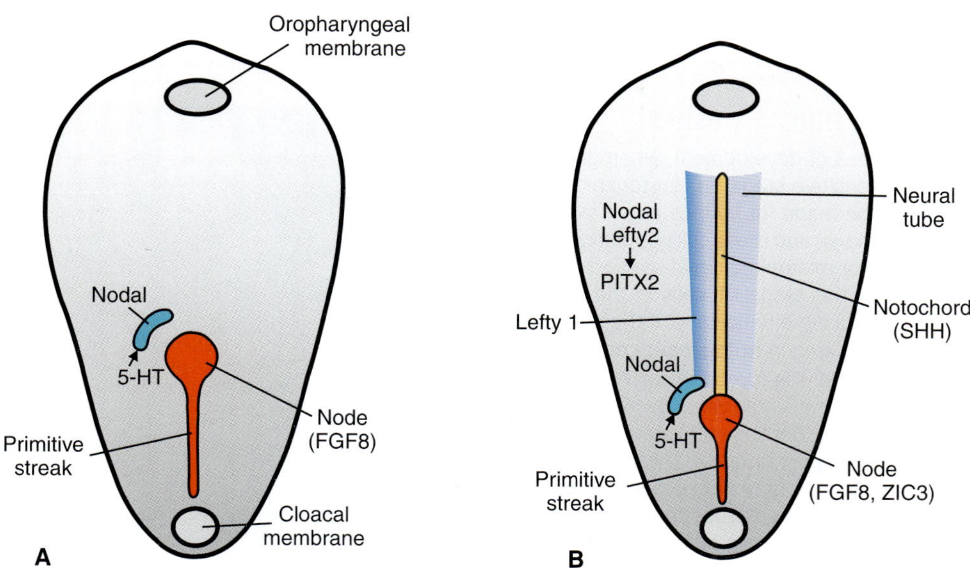


**FIGURE 5.6** Dorsal views of the germ disc showing gene expression patterns responsible for establishing the left–right body axis. **A.** FGF8, secreted by the node and primitive streak, establishes expression of *Nodal*, a member of the TGF-β superfamily. **B.** The neurotransmitter, serotonin (5-HT), increases in concentration on the left side and signals through the transcription factor *MAD3* to restrict *Nodal* expression to the left side of the node. The 5-HT degrading enzyme monoamine oxidase (MAO) is expressed on the right side of the node and helps to keep 5-HT concentrations lower on that side. *Nodal* then initiates a signaling cascade that ends in expression of the master gene for left-sidedness, a transcription factor called *PITX2*. *LEFTY1* and *SONIC HEDGEHOG* are expressed more toward the midline in the lateral plate mesoderm and notochord, respectively, and may serve as midline barriers and also represses expression of left-sided genes on the right. Genes involved in establishing the right side are largely unknown, but the transcription factor *SNAIL* may regulate downstream genes important for this process.



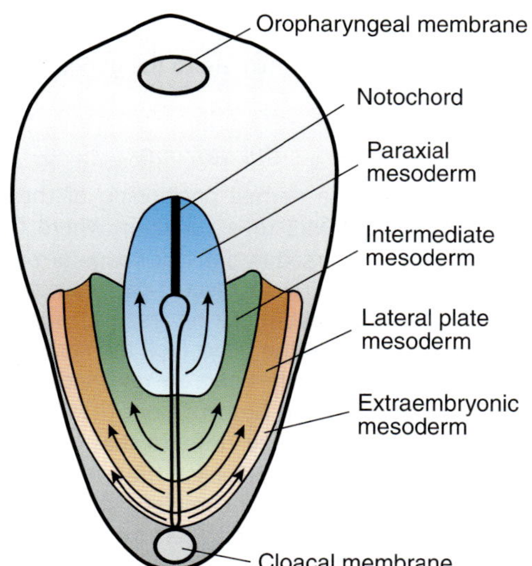


**FIGURE 5.7** Dorsal view of the germ disc showing the primitive streak and a fate map for epiblast cells. Epiblast cells migrate through specific parts of the node and streak, and their path of migration determines what type of mesoderm they will form. Thus, cells migrating through the cranialmost part of the node form the notochord, those migrating more posteriorly through the node and the cranialmost aspect of the streak form paraxial mesoderm (somites and somitomeres), those migrating through the next portion of the streak form intermediate mesoderm (urogenital system), those migrating through more caudal regions of the streak form lateral plate mesoderm (body wall), and those migrating through the caudalmost part of the streak contribute to formation of extraembryonic mesoderm (chorion).

contribute to extraembryonic mesoderm (the other source of this tissue is the primitive yolk sac [hypoblast]).

## GROWTH OF THE EMBRYONIC DISC

The embryonic disc, initially flat and almost round, gradually becomes elongated, with a broad cephalic and a narrow caudal end (Fig. 5.2A). Expansion of the embryonic disc occurs mainly in the cephalic region; the region of the primitive streak remains more or less the same size. Growth and elongation of the cephalic part of the disc are caused by a continuous migration of cells from the primitive streak region in a cephalic direction. Invagination of surface cells in the primitive streak and their subsequent migration forward and laterally continues until the end of the fourth week. At that stage, the primitive streak shows regressive changes, rapidly shrinks, and soon disappears.

That the primitive streak at the caudal end of the disc continues to supply new cells until the end of the fourth week has an important bearing on development of the embryo.

In the cephalic part, germ layers begin their specific differentiation by the middle of the third week.

In the caudal part, differentiation begins by the end of the fourth week.

Thus, gastrulation, or formation of the germ layers, continues in caudal segments while cranial structures are differentiating, causing the embryo to develop cephalocaudally.

## Clinical Correlates

### Teratogenesis Associated with Gastrulation

The beginning of the third week of development, when gastrulation is initiated, is a highly sensitive stage for teratogenic insult. At this time, fate maps can be made for various organ systems, such as the eyes and brain anlage, and these cell populations may be damaged by teratogens. For example, animal studies indicate that high doses of alcohol at this stage kill cells in the anterior midline of the germ disc, producing a deficiency of the midline in craniofacial structures and resulting in **holoprosencephaly** (see Chapter 17, p. 251). In such a child, the forebrain is small, the two lateral ventricles often merge into a single ventricle, and the eyes are close together (hypotelorism). Because this stage is reached 2 weeks after fertilization, it is approximately 4 weeks from the last menses. Therefore, the woman may not recognize that she is pregnant, having assumed that menstruation is late and will begin shortly. Consequently, she may not take precautions she would normally consider if she knew she was pregnant.

Gastrulation itself may be disrupted by genetic abnormalities and toxic insults. In **caudal dysgenesis (sirenomelia)**, insufficient mesoderm is formed in the caudalmost region of the embryo. Because this mesoderm contributes to formation of the lower limbs, urogenital system (intermediate mesoderm), and lumbosacral vertebrae, abnormalities in these structures ensue.

Affected individuals exhibit a variable range of defects, including hypoplasia and fusion of the lower limbs, vertebral abnormalities, renal agenesis, imperforate anus, and anomalies of the genital organs (Fig. 5.8*A,B*). In humans, the condition is associated with maternal diabetes and other causes. In mice, abnormalities of *BRACHYURY (T)*, *WNT*, and *ENGRAILED* genes produce a similar phenotype.

### Tumors Associated with Gastrulation

Sometimes, remnants of the primitive streak persist in the sacrococcygeal region. These clusters of pluripotent cells proliferate and form tumors, known as **sacrococcygeal teratomas**, which commonly contain tissues derived from all three germ layers (Fig. 5.9). This is the most common tumor in newborns, occurring with a frequency of 1 in 37,000. Teratomas may also arise from **primordial germ cells** that fail to migrate to the gonadal ridge (see Chapter 2, p. 8).

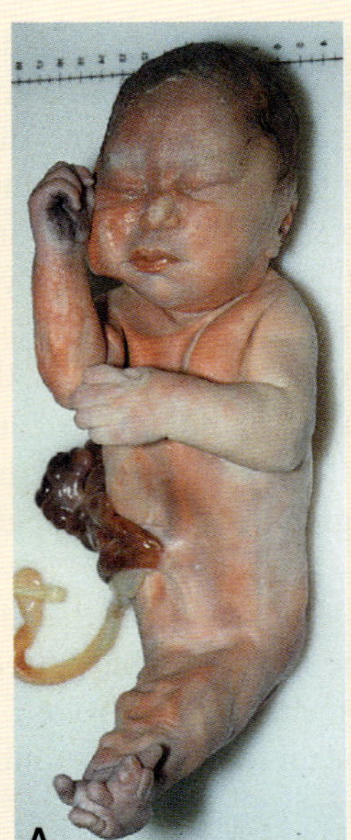

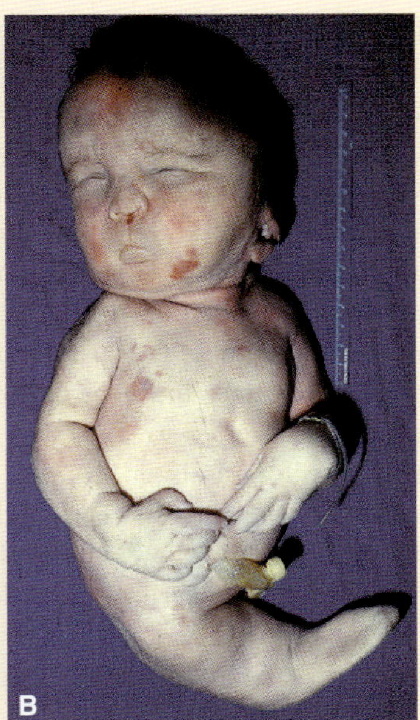

**FIGURE 5.8 A,B.** Two examples of sirenomelia (caudal dysgenesis). Loss of mesoderm in the lumbosacral region has resulted in fusion of the limb buds and other defects.

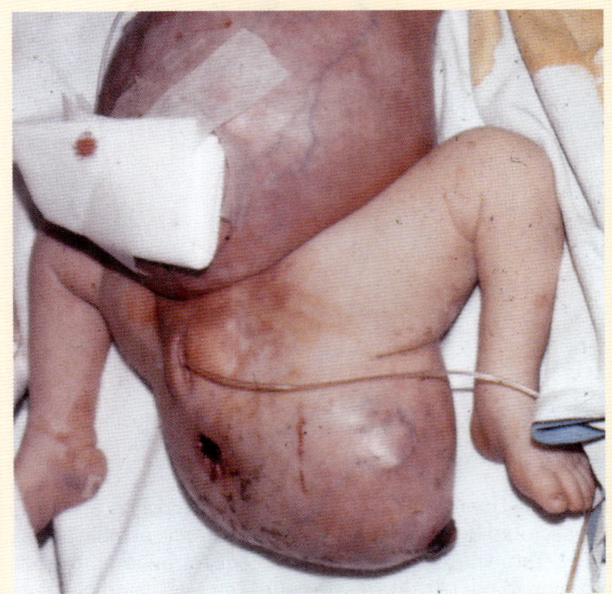

**FIGURE 5.9** Sacrococcygeal teratoma probably resulting from remnants of the primitive streak. These tumors may become malignant and are most common in female fetuses.

### *Birth Defects Associated with Laterality*

***Situs solitus*** refers to the normal positioning of the internal organs. ***Situs inversus*** refers to a condition where the positioning of all organs is reversed in a mirror image arrangement. Discordant organ positioning with respect to symmetry, where one or more organs are abnormally reversed in position or if isomerisms (i.e., both atria in the heart look the same) or inversions (i.e., the two ventricles in the heart are reversed) are present is called ***situs ambiguus*** or **heterotaxy**. These individuals are considered to have **laterality defects** that have occurred because of a failure to properly establish the L–R axis. Patients with these conditions do not have complete *situs inversus* but appear to be predominantly bilaterally left-sided or right-sided. The spleen reflects the differences: Those with left-sided bilaterality have polysplenia, and those with right-sided bilaterality have asplenia or hypoplastic spleen.

Individuals with *situs inversus* do not have a high risk for having other congenital abnormalities (although they have a slightly greater risk of having a heart defect), but their progeny have an increased risk for having laterality defects and an even higher risk for having a severe cardiac malformation. Also, approximately 20% of patients with complete *situs inversus* have bronchiectasis and chronic sinusitis because of abnormal cilia (**Kartagener syndrome**). Interestingly, cilia are normally present on the ventral surface of the primitive node and may be involved in L–R patterning.

In contrast, patients with ***situs ambiguous* (heterotaxy)** have a high risk of having a wide variety of other birth defects, including midline malformations, such as neural tube defects, cleft palate, anal atresia, etc. Furthermore, 90% of these individuals will have complex congenital heart defects. The heart exhibits more laterality than most organs and perhaps that explains its increased susceptibility when the L-R signaling pathway is disrupted. Mutations in the zinc finger transcription factor ***ZIC3***, a gene located on the X chromosome, cause **X-linked heterotaxy**. These individuals have a variety of birth defects, including neural tube defects, limb abnormalities, and omphalocele, and most also have severe heart malformations. The association between laterality and midline defects (neural tube defects, cleft palate, etc.) suggests that signaling pathways establishing the A–P and L–R axes must interact to specify the correct positioning of the body's organs and other structures. Because the body axes start to be specified late in the first week of development, the possibility that birth defects can be caused by disruption of these patterning events means that congenital malformations can be induced even earlier in gestation than previously thought.

The **neurotransmitter serotonin (5-HT)** is an important signal molecule for establishing laterality, and animal studies show that disrupting 5-HT signaling results in cases of situs inversus, heterotaxy, dextrocardia, and a wide variety of heart defects (see Chapter 13). Epidemiology studies show that children born to mothers who take antidepressants from the class of drugs called **selective serotonin reuptake inhibitors (SSRIs)** (**fluoxetine, paroxetine, sertraline, escitalopram, citalopram**, etc.) have an increased risk of having many different types of heart malformations and multiple other birth defects, thus providing additional evidence for 5-HT's importance in establishing laterality.

Part 1

## FURTHER DEVELOPMENT OF THE TROPHOBLAST

By the beginning of the third week, the trophoblast is characterized by **primary villi** that consist of a cytotrophoblastic core covered by a syncytial layer (Figs. 5.10 and 5.11). During further development, mesodermal cells penetrate the core of primary villi and grow toward the decidua. The newly formed structure is known as a **secondary villus** (Fig. 5.11).

By the end of the third week, mesodermal cells in the core of the villus begin to differentiate into blood cells and small blood vessels, forming the villous capillary system (Fig. 5.11). The villus is now known as a **tertiary villus** or a **definitive placental villus.** Capillaries in tertiary villi make contact with capillaries developing in the mesoderm of the chorionic plate and in the connecting stalk (Figs. 5.12 and 5.13). These vessels, in turn, establish contact with the intraembryonic circulatory system, connecting the placenta and the embryo.

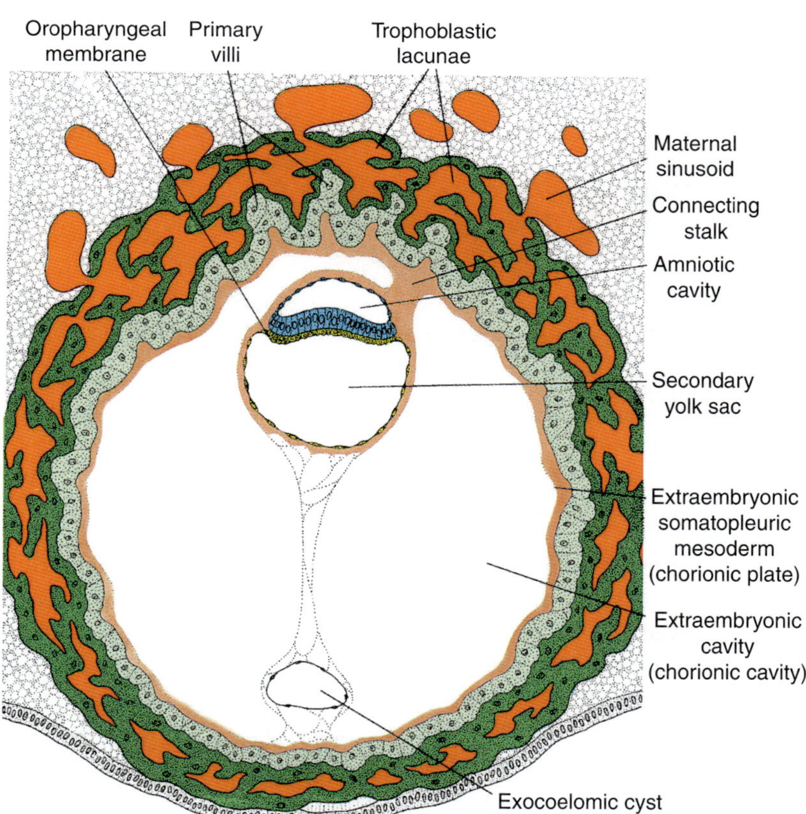


**FIGURE 5.10** A 13-day-old implantation site showing primary villi of the trophoblastic shell just beginning to be invaded by mesoderm from the chorionic plate.

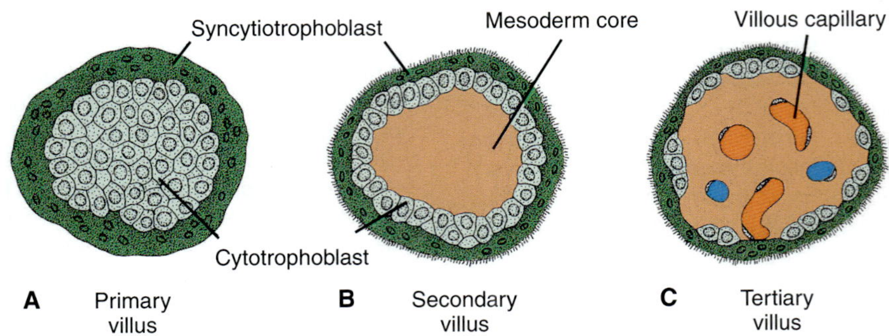


**FIGURE 5.11** Development of a villus. **A.** Transverse section of a primary villus showing a core of cytotrophoblastic cells covered by a layer of syncytium. **B.** Transverse section of a secondary villus with a core of mesoderm covered by a single layer of cytotrophoblastic cells, which in turn is covered by syncytium. **C.** Mesoderm of the villus showing a number of capillaries and venules.

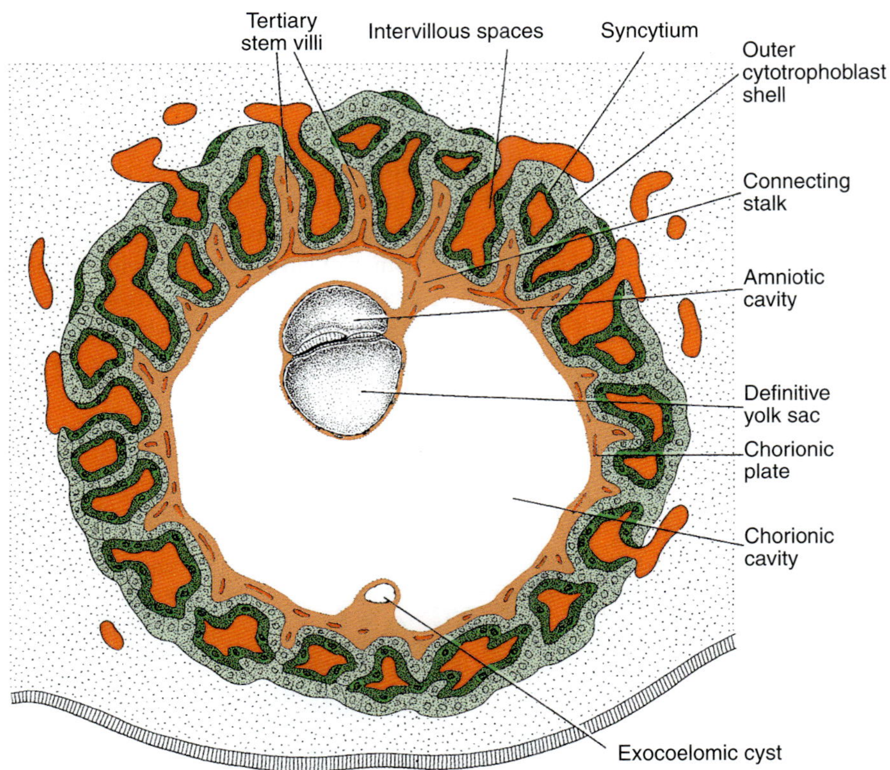


**FIGURE 5.12** Presomite embryo and the trophoblast at the end of the third week. Tertiary and secondary stem villi give the trophoblast a characteristic radial appearance. Intervillous spaces, which are found throughout the trophoblast, are lined with syncytium. Cytotrophoblastic cells surround the trophoblast entirely and are in direct contact with the endometrium. The embryo is suspended in the chorionic cavity by means of the connecting stalk.

Hence, when the heart begins to beat in the fourth week of development, the villous system is ready to supply the embryo with proper essential nutrients and oxygen.

Meanwhile, cytotrophoblastic cells in the villi penetrate progressively into the overlying syncytium until they reach the maternal endometrium. Here, they establish contact with similar extensions of neighboring villous stems, forming a thin **outer cytotrophoblast shell** (Figs. 5.12 and 5.13). This shell gradually surrounds the trophoblast entirely and attaches the chorionic sac firmly to the maternal endometrial tissue (Fig. 5.12). Villi that extend from the **chorionic plate** to the **decidua basalis** (**decidual plate**: the part of the endometrium where the placenta will form; see Chapter 8) are called **stem** or **anchoring villi**. Those that branch from the sides of stem villi are **free (terminal) villi**, through which exchange of nutrients and other factors will occur.

The chorionic cavity, meanwhile, becomes larger, and by the 19th or the 20th day, the embryo is attached to its trophoblastic shell by a narrow **connecting stalk** (Fig. 5.12). The connecting stalk later develops into the **umbilical cord**, which forms the connection between the placenta and embryo.

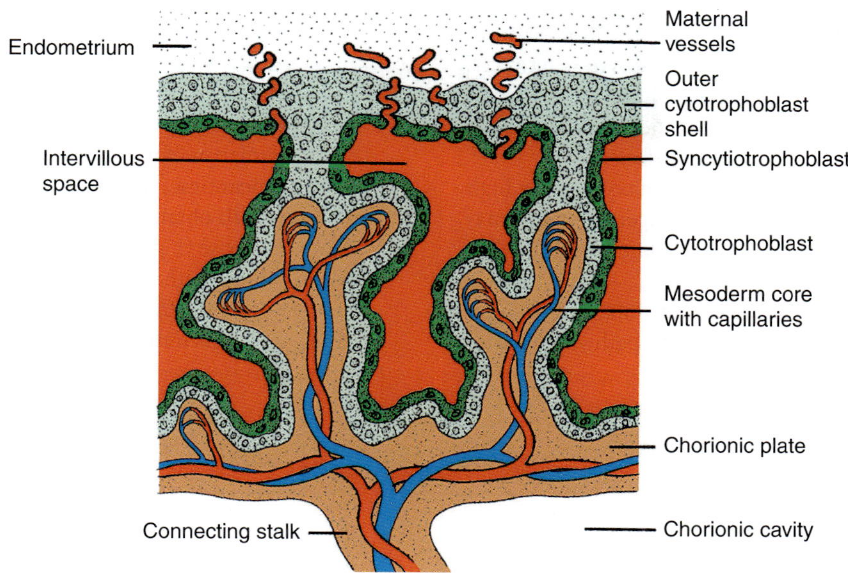


**FIGURE 5.13** Longitudinal section through a villus at the end of the fourth week of development. Maternal vessels penetrate the cytotrophoblastic shell to enter intervillous spaces, which surround the villi. Capillaries in the villi are in contact with vessels in the chorionic plate and in the connecting stalk, which in turn are connected to intraembryonic vessels.



## SUMMARY

- The most characteristic event occurring during the third week is **gastrulation**, which begins with the appearance of the **primitive streak**, which has at its cephalic end the **primitive node**.
- In the region of the node and streak, **epiblast** cells move inward (**invaginate**) to form new cell layers, **endoderm** and **mesoderm**.
- Cells that do not migrate through the streak but remain in the epiblast form **ectoderm**.
- Epiblast gives rise to all three **germ layers** in the embryo, **ectoderm**, **mesoderm**, and **endoderm**, and these layers form all of the tissues and organs (Figs. 5.2 and 5.3).
- **Prenotochordal cells** invaginating in the primitive pit move forward until they reach the **prechordal plate**.
- Prenotochordal cells intercalate in the endoderm as the **notochordal plate** (Fig. 5.3).
- With further development, the plate detaches from the endoderm, and a solid cord, the **notochord**, is formed.
- It forms a midline axis, which will serve as the basis of the axial skeleton (Fig. 5.3).
- Cephalic and caudal ends of the embryo are established before the primitive streak is formed.
- By the end of the third week, three basic **germ layers**, consisting of **ectoderm**, **mesoderm**, and **endoderm**, are established in the head region, and the process continues to produce these germ layers for more caudal areas of the embryo until the end of the fourth week. Tissue and organ differentiation has begun, and it occurs in a cephalocaudal direction as gastrulation continues.
- Epiblast cells moving through the node and streak are predetermined by their position to become specific types of mesoderm and endoderm. Thus, it is possible to construct a fate map of the epiblast showing this pattern (Fig. 5.7).
- Molecular pathways
  - The, cells in the hypoblast (endoderm) at the cephalic margin of the disc form the *AVE*, which expresses head-forming genes, including ***OTX2***, ***LIM1***, and ***HESX1*** and the secreted factor **cerberus**.
    - *NODAL*, a member of the *TGF-β* family of genes, is then activated and initiates and maintains the integrity of the node and streak.
    - In the presence of **FGF**, **BMP4** ventralizes mesoderm during gastrulation so that it forms intermediate and lateral plate mesoderm.
    - **Chordin**, **noggin**, and **follistatin** antagonize BMP4 activity and dorsalize mesoderm to form the notochord and somitomeres in the head region.
    - Formation of these structures in more caudal regions is regulated by the ***BRACHYURY (T)*** **gene** (Fig. 5.4A).
    - Laterality (L–R asymmetry) is regulated by a cascade of signaling molecules and genes. **FGF8**, secreted by cells in the node and streak, induces *NODAL* and ***LEFTY2*** expression on the left side, and these genes upregulate ***PITX2***, a transcription factor and master gene for left-sidedness (Fig. 5.6).
    - The **neurotransmitter serotonin (5-HT)** also plays a role in establishing laterality by restricting ***NODAL*** expression to the left side.
    - Normal L–R positioning of the organs is called ***situs solitus***, whereas their complete reversal is called ***situs inversus***.

(Continued)

- When one or more organs are abnormally positioned, the condition is called ***situs ambiguus*** or **heterotaxy**. Individuals with ***situs inversus*** have a low risk of having other birth defects, but their children have a higher risk, especially for heart defects.
- In contrast, patients with heterotaxy are at a high risk of having many types of congenital malformations, and almost all will have some type of cardiac abnormality.
- Disruption of 5-HT levels or misexpression of genes in the laterality signaling pathway, such as ***PITX2***, results in laterality defects, such as dextrocardia, situs inversus, and cardiac abnormalities. Mutations in the zinc finger transcription factor ***ZIC3*** cause **X-linked heterotaxy**, with severe cardiac malformations and other defects.
- In the meantime, the trophoblast progresses rapidly. **Primary villi** obtain a mesenchymal core in which small capillaries arise (Fig. 5.12). When these villous capillaries make contact with capillaries in the chorionic plate and connecting stalk, the villous system is ready to supply the embryo with its nutrients and oxygen (Fig. 5.13).

## Self-Assessment

### Comprehensive Questions

1. Write briefly about the formation of notochord.
2. Discuss about gastrulation.
3. Explain the molecular regulation of the formation of body axis.

### Problem Solving Questions

1. A 22-year-old woman consumes large quantities of alcohol at a party and loses consciousness; 3 weeks later, she misses her second consecutive period. A pregnancy test is positive. Should she be concerned about the effects of her binge-drinking episode on her baby?
2. An ultrasound scan detects a large mass near the sacrum of a 28-week female fetus. What might the origin of such a mass be, and what type of tissue might it contain?
3. On ultrasound examination, it was determined that a fetus had well-developed facial and thoracic regions, but caudal structures were abnormal. Kidneys were absent, lumbar and sacral vertebrae were missing, and the hind limbs were fused. What process may have been disturbed to cause such defects?
4. A child has polysplenia and abnormal positioning of the heart. How might these two abnormalities be linked developmentally, and when would they have originated? Should you be concerned that other defects might be present? What genes might have caused this event, and when during embryogenesis would it have been initiated?
5. A young woman arrives at your obstetrics clinic and says that she is depressed and things are not going well, including her attempts to start a family. She indicates that her friend is taking one of the new SSRI antidepressants and she wonders if she should be taking one as well. How do you respond?

### Multiple Choice Questions

1. Gastrulation begins with the formation of
   (a) Primitive node
   (b) Primitive streak
   (c) Primitive pit
   (d) Neural crest
2. The chief gene to establish laterality is
   (a) 5-HT
   (b) PITX2
   (c) FGF-8
   (d) BMP
3. Which of the following structures is the primary organizer or inducer during organogenesis?
   (a) Notochord
   (b) Primitive node
   (c) Primitive streak
   (d) Primitive pit
4. The adult derivative of notochord is
   (a) Vertebral column
   (b) Intervertebral disc
   (c) Nucleus pulposus of the intervertebral disc
   (d) Annulus fibrosus of the intervertebral disc
5. The anterior–posterior axis is determined at which stage?
   (a) During early embryogenesis in the first week of gestation
   (b) During the formation of primitive streak
   (c) During the formation of notochord
   (d) During the trilaminar disc formation
6. The cranial end of the developing embryo is formed due to secretion of
   (a) Nodal
   (b) Cerberus
   (c) PITX2
   (d) Lefty

### Answers

1. (a) 2. (b) 3. (b) 4. (c) 5. (a) 6. (b)

CHAPTER

# 6 Third to Eighth Weeks: The Embryonic Period

Part 1

## Specific Learning Objectives

- Embryonic period: Third week to eighth week—the period of organogenesis
- Formation of three germ layers
- Derivatives of ectoderm, mesoderm, and endoderm
- Neurulation and molecular regulation
- Derivatives of neural crest
- Division of mesoderm into paraxial, intermediate, and lateral plate mesoderm
- Concept of somite, their molecular regulations and their derivatives
- Patterning of the anteroposterior axis: Regulation by homeobox genes
- Major birth defects during this time period

## Competencies Covered

AN79.3 Describe the process of neurulation.
AN79.4 Describe the development of somites and intraembryonic coelom.
AN79.5 Explain the embryological basis of congenital malformations, nucleus pulposus, sacrococcygeal teratomas, and neural tube defects.

The **embryonic period**, or period of **organogenesis**, occurs from the **third to the eighth weeks** of development and is the time when each of the three germ layers, **ectoderm**, **mesoderm**, and **endoderm**, gives rise to a number of specific tissues and organs. By the end of the embryonic period, the main organ systems have been established, rendering the major features of the external body form recognizable by the end of the second month.

The third to eighth weeks are also cited as the time when the majority of birth defects are induced; prior to this time, any insult to the embryo results in its death and spontaneous abortion. Although this tenet holds true for many insults to normal development, it is important to note that **axis formation** begins late in the **first week** at the blastocyst stage (see Chapter 3, p. 36) and that a great variety of birth defects can be attributed to disruptions in cell signaling during specification of the cranial–caudal and left–right axes. Furthermore, not all embryos are lost if an environmental or genetic insult occurs during this critical time period.

## DERIVATIVES OF THE ECTODERMAL GERM LAYER

At the beginning of the third week of development, the ectodermal germ layer has the shape of a disc that is broader in the cephalic than in the caudal region (Fig. 6.1). Appearance of the notochord and prechordal mesoderm induces the overlying ectoderm to thicken and form the **neural plate** (Fig. 6.2*A,B*). Cells of the plate make up the **neuroectoderm**, and their induction represents the initial event in the process of **neurulation**.

### Neurulation

Neurulation is the process whereby the neural plate forms the neural tube. One of the key events in this process is lengthening of the neural plate and body axis by the phenomenon of convergent extension, whereby there is a lateral to medial movement of cells in the plane of the ectoderm and mesoderm. The process is regulated by signaling through the planar cell polarity pathway which makes the tissue longer and narrower (see Chapter 22, p. 312) and is essential for neural tube development. As the neural plate lengthens, its lateral edges elevate to form **neural folds**, and the depressed midregion forms the **neural groove** (Fig. 6.2). Gradually, the neural folds approach each other in the midline, where they fuse (Fig. 6.3*A,B*). Fusion begins in the cervical region (fifth somite) and proceeds cranially and caudally (Fig. 6.3*C,D*). As a result, the **neural tube** is formed. Until fusion is complete, the cephalic and caudal ends of the neural tube communicate with the amniotic cavity by way of the **anterior (cranial)** and **posterior (caudal) neuropores**, respectively (Figs. 6.3*C,D* and 6.4*A*).

Closure of the cranial neuropore occurs at approximately day 25 (18- to 20-somite stage), whereas the posterior neuropore closes at day 28 (25-somite stage) (Fig. 6.4*B*).

Neurulation is then complete, and the central nervous system is represented by a closed tubular structure with a narrow caudal portion, the **spinal cord**, and a much broader cephalic portion characterized by a number of dilations, the brain vesicles (see Chapter 18).

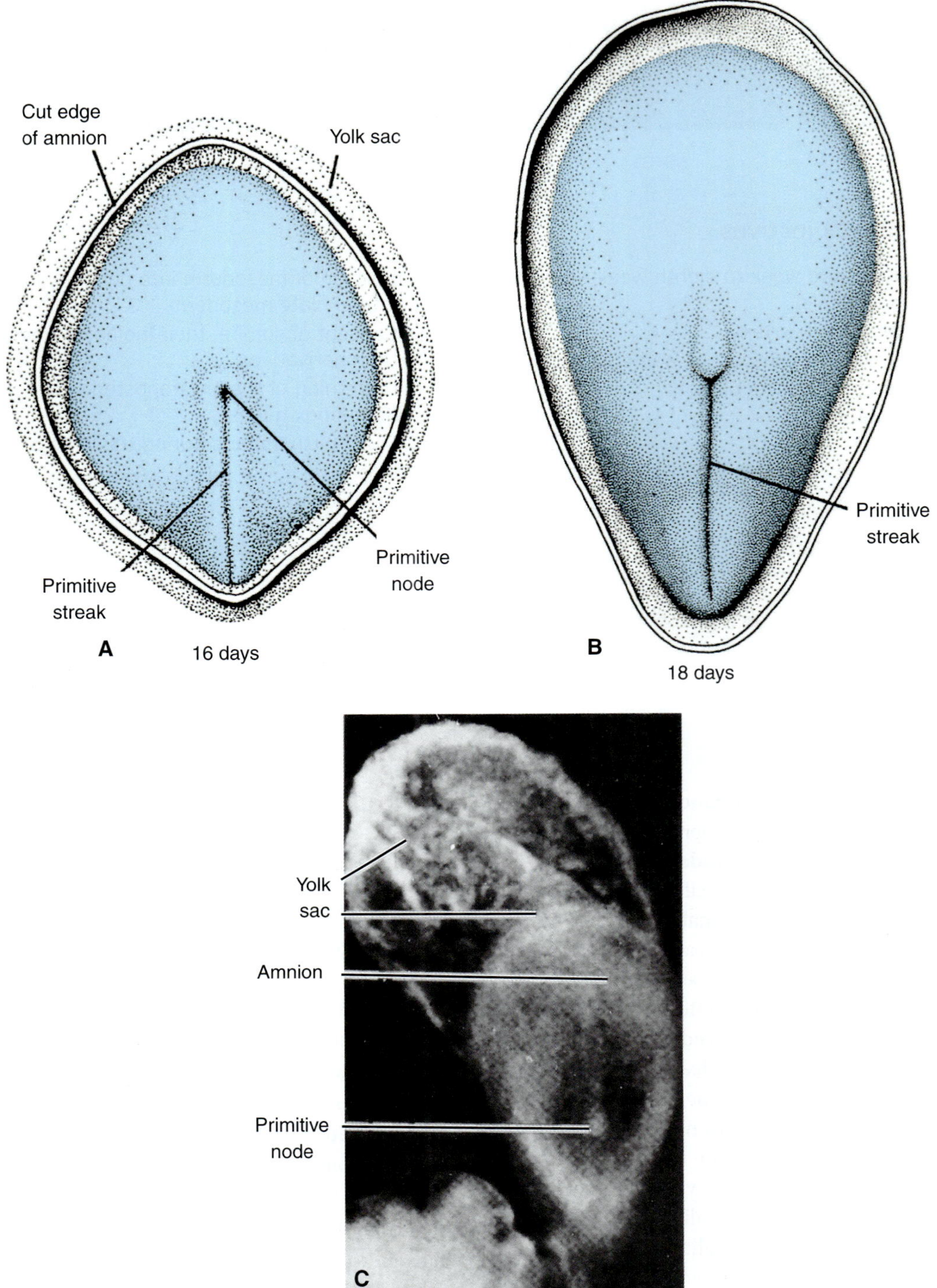


**FIGURE 6.1** **A.** Dorsal view of a 16-day presomite embryo. The primitive streak and primitive node are visible. **B.** Dorsal view of an 18-day presomite embryo. The embryo is pear-shaped, with its cephalic region somewhat broader than its caudal end. **C.** Dorsal view of an 18-day human embryo. Note the primitive node and, extending forward from it, the notochord. The yolk sac has a somewhat mottled appearance. The length of the embryo is 1.25 mm, and the greatest width is 0.68 mm.

## Molecular Regulation of Neural Induction

Upregulation of **fibroblast growth factor (FGF)** signaling together with inhibition of the activity of **bone morphogenetic protein 4 (BMP4)**, a **transforming growth factor-β** (TGF-β) family member responsible for ventralizing ectoderm and mesoderm, causes induction of the neural plate. FGF signaling probably promotes a neural pathway by an unknown mechanism while it represses *BMP* transcription and upregulates expression of ***CHORDIN*** and ***NOGGIN***, which inhibit BMP activity. In the presence of BMP4, which permeates the mesoderm and ectoderm of the gastrulating embryo, ectoderm is induced to form epidermis; and mesoderm forms intermediate and lateral plate mesoderm. If ectoderm is protected

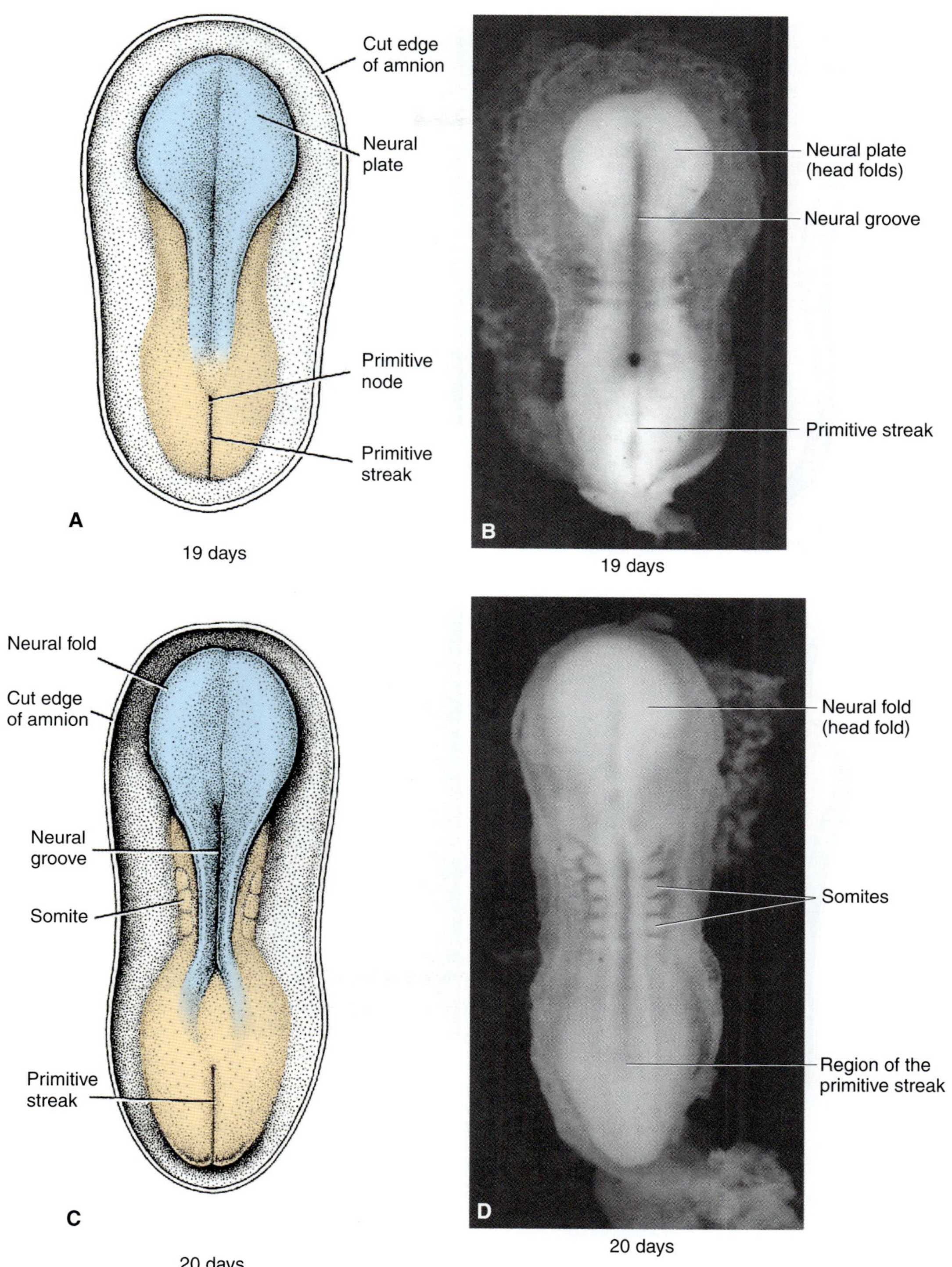


**FIGURE 6.2** **A.** Dorsal view of a late presomite embryo (approximately 19 days). The amnion has been removed, and the neural plate is clearly visible. **B.** Dorsal view of a human embryo at 19 days. **C.** Dorsal view of an embryo at approximately 20 days showing somites and formation of the neural groove and neural folds. **D.** Dorsal view of a human embryo at 20 days.

from exposure to BMPs, its "default state" is to become neural tissue. Secretion of three other molecules, **noggin**, **chordin**, and **follistatin**, inactivates BMP. These three proteins are present in the organizer (primitive node), notochord, and prechordal mesoderm. They neuralize ectoderm by inhibiting BMP and cause mesoderm to become notochord and paraxial mesoderm (dorsalizes mesoderm); however, these neural inducers induce only forebrain and midbrain types of tissues. Induction of caudal neural plate structures (hindbrain and spinal cord) depends on two secreted proteins, **WNT3a** and **FGF**. In addition, **retinoic acid (RA)** appears to play a role in organizing the cranial-to-caudal axis because it can cause respecification of cranial segments into more caudal ones by regulating expression of **homeobox genes** (see p. 75).

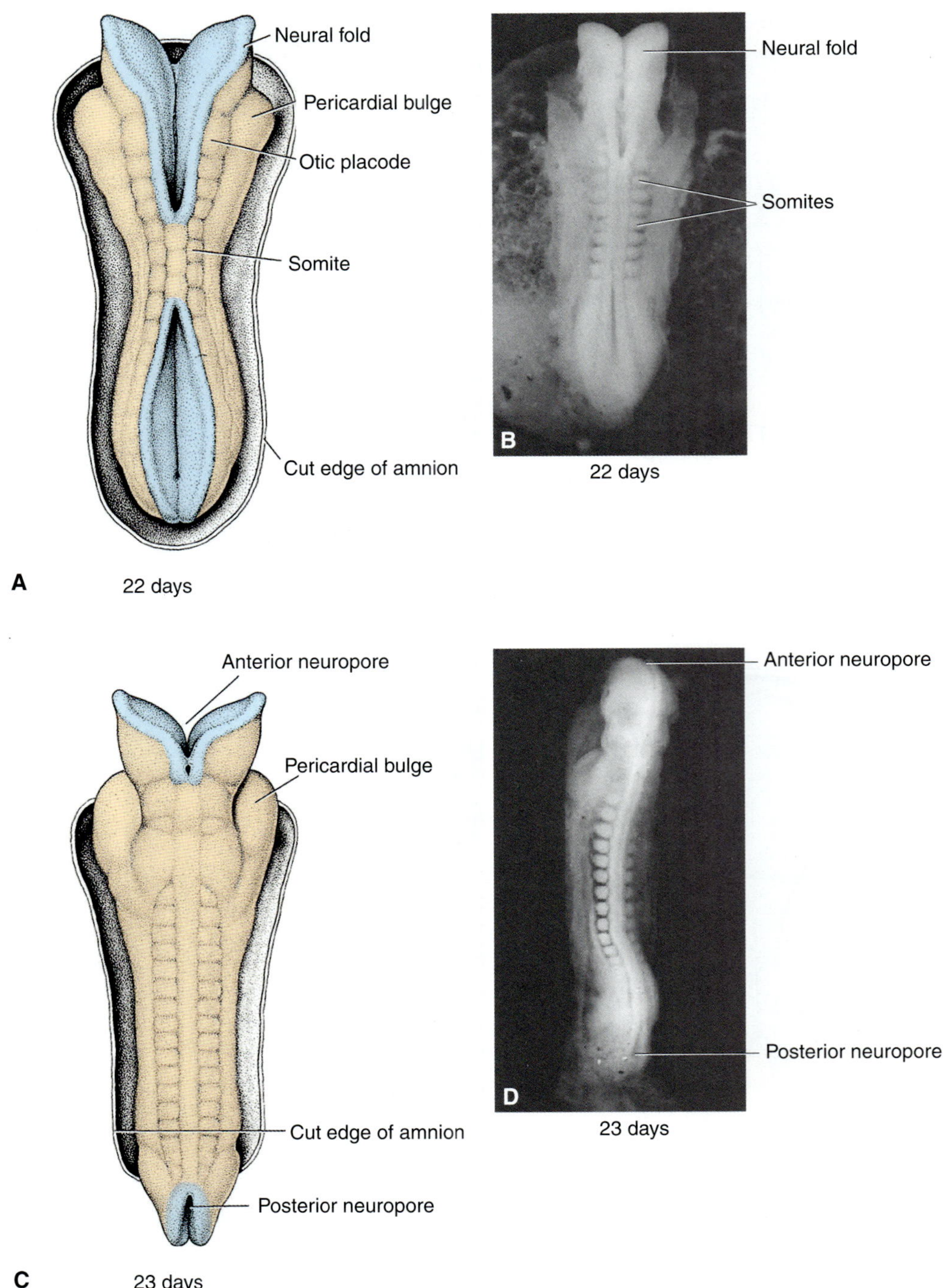


**FIGURE 6.3** **A.** Dorsal view of an embryo at approximately day 22. Seven distinct somites are visible on each side of the neural tube. **B.** Dorsal view of a human embryo at 22 days. **C.** Dorsal view of an embryo at approximately day 23. Note the pericardial bulge on each side of the midline in the cephalic part of the embryo. **D.** Dorsal view of a human embryo at 23 days.

## Neural Crest Cells

As the neural folds elevate and fuse, cells at the lateral border or crest of the neuroectoderm begin to dissociate from their neighbors. This cell population, the **neural crest** cells (NCC; Figs. 6.5 and 6.6), undergoes an **epithelial-to-mesenchymal transition** as it leaves the neuroectoderm by active migration and displacement to enter the underlying mesoderm. (**Mesoderm** refers to cells derived from the epiblast and extraembryonic tissues. **Mesenchyme** refers to loosely organized embryonic connective tissue regardless of origin.)

Neural crest cells from the trunk region leave the neuroectoderm **after closure** of the neural tube and migrate along the dorsal and ventral pathways.

1. They migrate along a dorsal pathway through the dermis, where they will enter the ectoderm through holes in the basal lamina to form **melanocytes** in the skin and hair follicles.

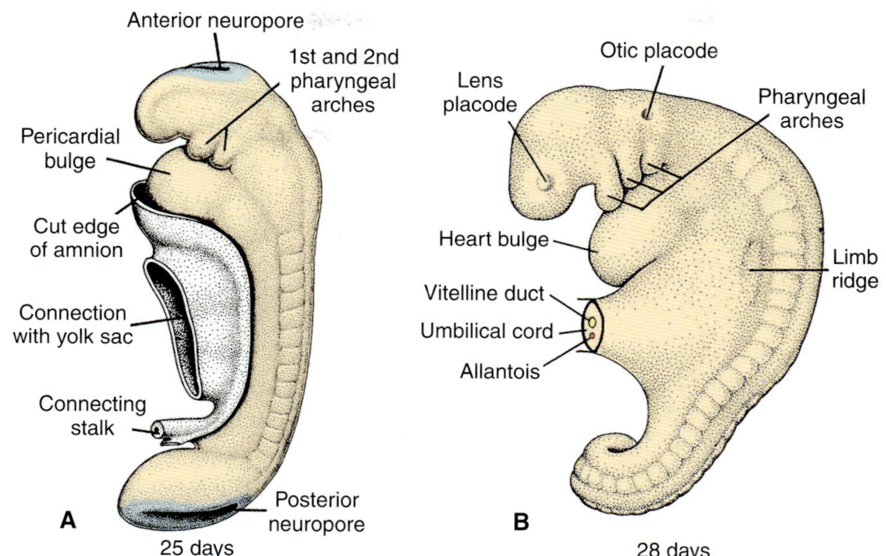


**FIGURE 6.4 A.** Lateral view of a 14-somite embryo (approximately 25 days). Note the bulging pericardial area and the first and second pharyngeal arches. **B.** The left side of a 25-somite embryo approximately 28 days old. The first three pharyngeal arches and lens and otic placodes are visible.

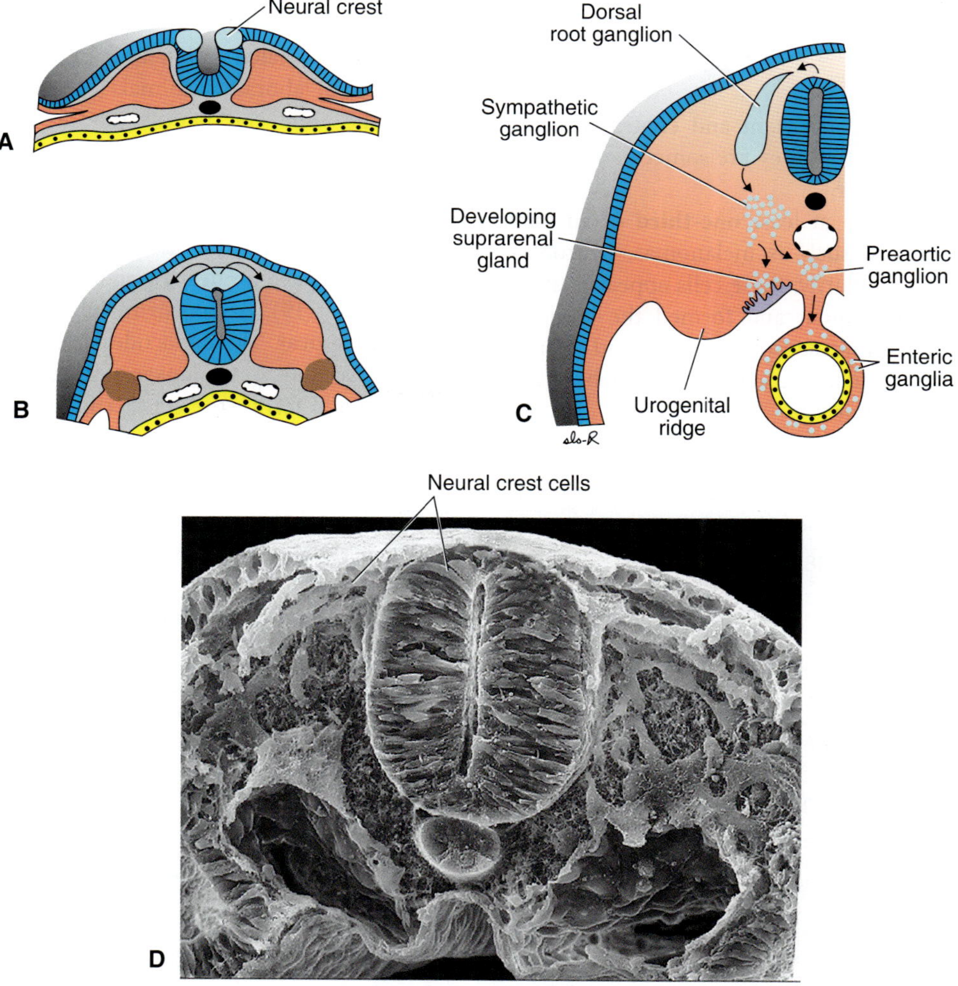


**FIGURE 6.5** Formation and migration of neural crest cells in the spinal cord. **A,B.** Crest cells form at the tips of neural folds and do not migrate away from this region until neural tube closure is complete. **C.** After migration, crest cells contribute to a heterogeneous array of structures, including dorsal root ganglia, sympathetic chain ganglia, adrenal medulla, and other tissues (Table 6.1, p. 64). **D.** In a scanning electron micrograph, crest cells at the top of the closed neural tube can be seen migrating away from this area.

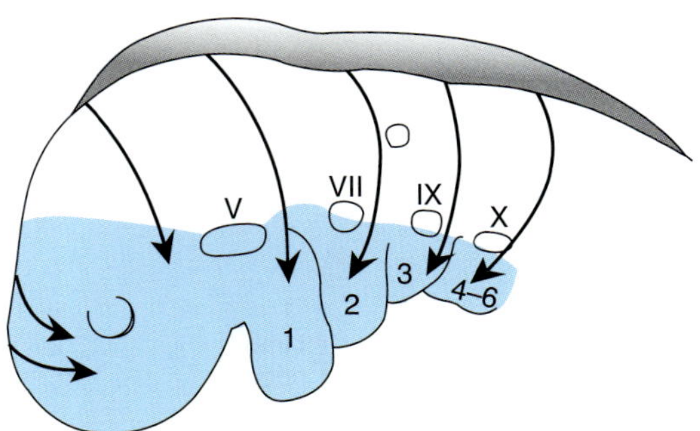


**FIGURE 6.6** Drawing shows the migratory paths of neural crest cells in the head region. These cells leave the crests of the neural folds prior to neural tube closure and migrate to form structures in the face and neck (*blue area*). *1 to 6*, pharyngeal arches; *V*, *VII*, *IX*, and *X*, epipharyngeal placodes.

2. They migrate along a ventral pathway through the anterior half of each somite to become **sensory ganglia**, **sympathetic** and **enteric neurons**, **Schwann cells**, and **cells of the adrenal medulla** (Fig. 6.5).
3. NCC also form and migrate from cranial neural folds, leaving the neural tube **before closure** in this region (Fig. 6.6). These cells contribute to the **craniofacial skeleton** as well as **neurons for cranial ganglia**, **glial cells**, **melanocytes**, and other cell types (Table 6.1).
4. NCC are fundamentally important and contribute to so many organs and tissues that they are sometimes referred to as the **fourth germ layer**.

They are also involved in at least **one-third** of all birth defects and many cancers, such as melanomas, neuroblastomas, and others. Evolutionarily, these cells appeared at the dawn of vertebrate development and formed the basis for vertebrate features, including sensory ganglia and craniofacial structures that expanded the success of vertebrates by perfecting a predatory lifestyle.

| Table 6.1 Neural Crest Derivatives |
|---|
| Connective tissue and bones of the face and skull |
| Cranial nerve ganglia (see Table 18.3, p. 268) |
| C cells of the thyroid gland |
| Conotruncal septum in the heart |
| Odontoblasts |
| Dermis in face and neck |
| Spinal (dorsal root) ganglia |
| Sympathetic chain and preaortic ganglia |
| Parasympathetic ganglia of the gastrointestinal tract |
| Adrenal medulla |
| Schwann cells |
| Glial cells |
| Meninges (forebrain) |
| Melanocytes |
| Smooth muscle cells to blood vessels of the face and forebrain |

### *Molecular Regulation of Neural Crest Induction*

Induction of NCC requires an interaction at the junctional border of the neural plate and surface ectoderm (epidermis) (Fig. 6.5*A*). Intermediate concentrations of BMPs are established at this boundary compared to neural plate cells that are exposed to very low levels of BMPs and surface ectoderm cells that are exposed to very high levels. The proteins noggin and chordin regulate these concentrations by acting as BMP inhibitors. The intermediate concentrations of BMPs, together with FGF and WNT proteins, induce *PAX3* and other transcription factors that "specify" the neural plate border (Fig. 6.5*A*). In turn, these transcription factors induce a second wave of transcription factors, including *SNAIL* and *FOXD3*, which specify cells as neural crest, and *SLUG*, which promotes crest cell migration from the neuroectoderm. Thus, the fate of the entire ectodermal germ layer depends on BMP concentrations: High levels induce epidermis formation; intermediate levels, at the border of the neural plate and surface ectoderm, induce the neural crest; and very low concentrations cause formation of neural ectoderm. BMPs, other members of the TGF-β family, and FGFs regulate NCC migration, proliferation, and differentiation, and abnormal concentrations of these proteins have been associated with neural crest defects in the craniofacial region of laboratory animals (see Chapter 17).

By the time the neural tube is closed, two bilateral **ectodermal thickenings**, the **otic placodes** and the **lens placodes**, become visible in the cephalic region of the embryo (Fig. 6.4*B*). During further development, the otic placodes invaginate and form the **otic vesicles**, which will develop into structures needed for hearing and maintenance of equilibrium (see Chapter 19). At approximately the same time, the **lens placodes** appear. These placodes also invaginate and, during the fifth week, form the **lenses** of the eyes (see Chapter 20).

In general terms, the ectodermal germ layer gives rise to organs and structures that maintain contact with the outside world:

- The central nervous system
- The peripheral nervous system
- The sensory epithelium of the ear, nose, and eye
- The epidermis, including the hair and nails

In addition, it gives rise to the following:

- The subcutaneous glands
- The mammary glands
- The pituitary gland
- Enamel of the teeth

## ■ DERIVATIVES OF THE MESODERMAL GERM LAYER

Initially, cells of the mesodermal germ layer form a thin sheet of loosely woven tissue on each side of the midline (Fig. 6.8). By approximately the 17th day, however, cells close to the midline proliferate and form a thickened plate of tissue known as **paraxial mesoderm** (Fig. 6.8). More laterally, the

## Clinical Correlates

### Neural Tube Defects

**Neural tube defects (NTDs)** result when neural tube closure fails to occur. If the neural tube fails to close in the cranial region, then most of the brain fails to form, and the defect is called **anencephaly** (Fig. 6.7*A*). If closure fails anywhere from the cervical region caudally, then the defect is called **spina bifida** (Fig. 6.7*B,C*). When the spinal cord is intact and the vertebral arches do not fuse its **spina bifida occulta,** if there is protrusion of the meninges through the gap its a **menigocele** and if the brain tissue protrudes it is **menigomyelocele**. The most common site for spina bifida to occur is in the lumbosacral region (Fig. 6.7*C*), suggesting that the closure process in this area may be more susceptible to genetic and/or environmental factors. Anencephaly is a lethal defect, and most of these cases are diagnosed prenatally and the pregnancies terminated. Children with spina bifida lose a degree of neurological function based on the spinal cord level of the lesion and its severity.

Occurrence of these types of defects is common and varies by different regions. For example, prior to fortification of enriched flour with folic acid in the United States, the overall rate was 1 in 1,000 births, but in North and South Carolina, the rate was 1 in 500 births. In parts of China, rates were as high as 1 in 200 births. In India, a survey showed the incidence to be 4.5 in 1000 live births, higher than the west. Various genetic and environmental factors apparently account for the variability. Genetic causes of NTDs remain elusive, although recently, mutations in the *VANGL* genes have been identified and associated with familial cases of these defects. The *VANGL* genes are part of the planar cell polarity pathway (see Chapter 22, p. 312) that regulates convergent extension, the process that lengthens the neural tube and is necessary for normal closure to occur.

Regardless of the region or country where NTDs occur, rates have been reduced significantly following **folic acid** administration. For example, rates throughout the United States are now approximately 1 in 1,500 births. It is estimated that 50% to 70% of NTDs can be prevented if women take **400 μg** of folic acid daily (the dose present in most multivitamins) beginning 3 months prior to conception and continuing throughout pregnancy. Because 50% of pregnancies are unplanned, it is recommended that all women of childbearing age take a multivitamin containing 400 μg of folic acid daily. If a woman has had a child with an NTD or if there is a history of such defects in her family, it is recommended that she take 400 μg of folic acid daily and then **4,000 μg** per day starting 1 month before she tries to become pregnant and continuing through the first 3 months of pregnancy.

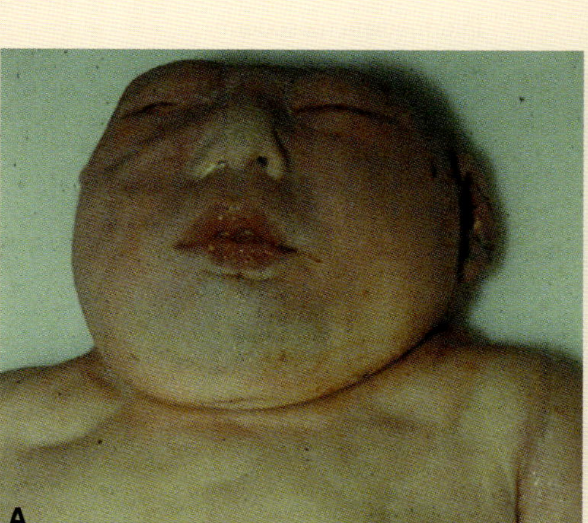
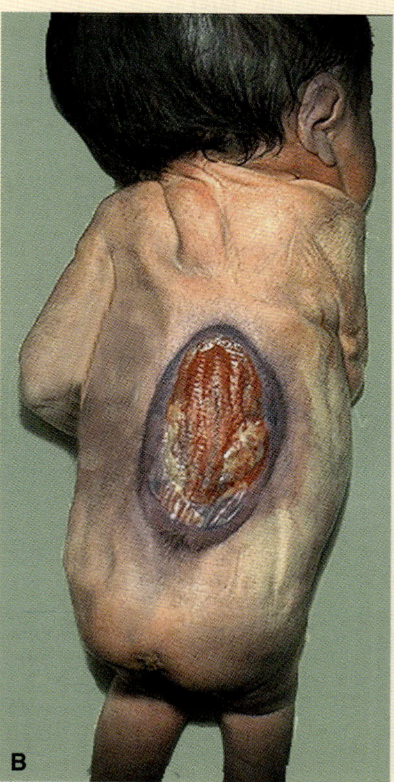
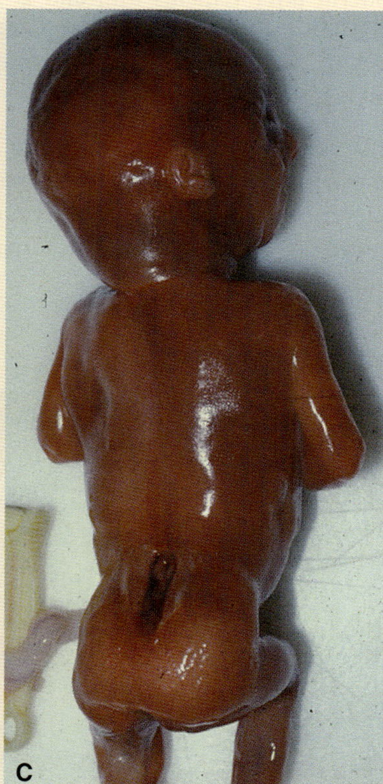

**FIGURE 6.7** Examples of NTDs, which occur when closure of the neural tube fails. **A.** Anencephaly. **B,C.** Infants with spina bifida. Most cases occur in the lumbosacral region. Fifty percent to 70% of all NTDs can be prevented by the vitamin folic acid.

Part 1

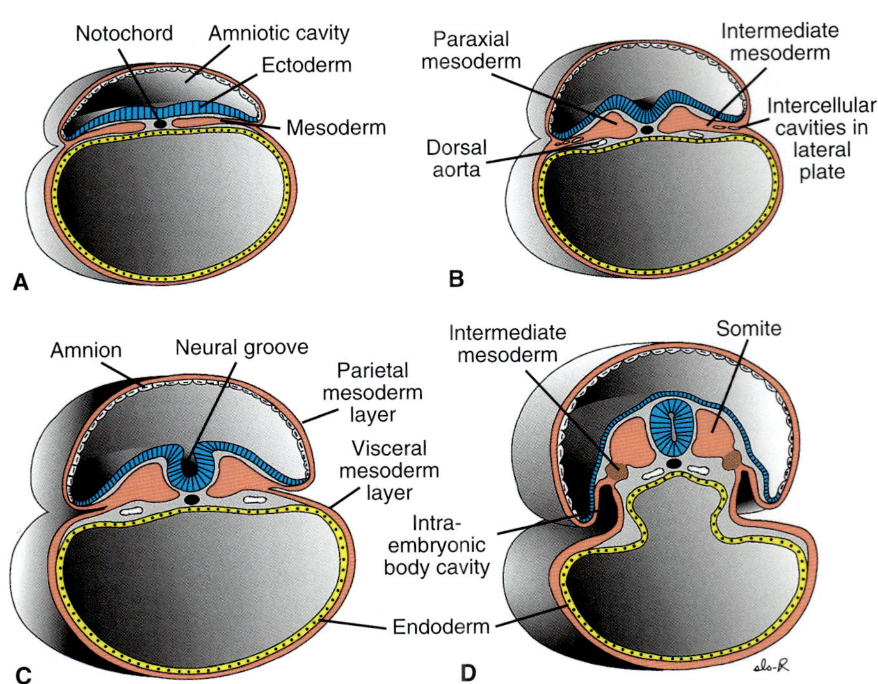


**FIGURE 6.8** Transverse sections showing development of the mesodermal germ layer. **A.** Day 17. **B.** Day 19. **C.** Day 20. **D.** Day 21. The thin mesodermal sheet gives rise to paraxial mesoderm (future somites), intermediate mesoderm (future excretory units), and the lateral plate, which is split into parietal and visceral mesoderm layers lining the intraembryonic cavity.

mesoderm layer remains thin and is known as the **lateral plate**. With the appearance and coalescence of intercellular cavities in the lateral plate, this tissue is divided into two layers (Fig. 6.8*B,C*):

- A layer continuous with mesoderm covering the amnion, known as the **somatic** or **parietal mesoderm layer**
- A layer continuous with mesoderm covering the yolk sac, known as the **splanchnic** or **visceral mesoderm layer** (Figs. 6.8*C,D* and 6.9)

Together, these layers line a newly formed cavity, the **intraembryonic cavity**, which is continuous with the extraembryonic cavity on each side of the embryo. **Intermediate mesoderm** connects paraxial and lateral plate mesoderm (Figs. 6.8*B,D* and 6.9).

## Paraxial Mesoderm

By the beginning of the third week, paraxial mesoderm begins to be organized into segments. These segments, known

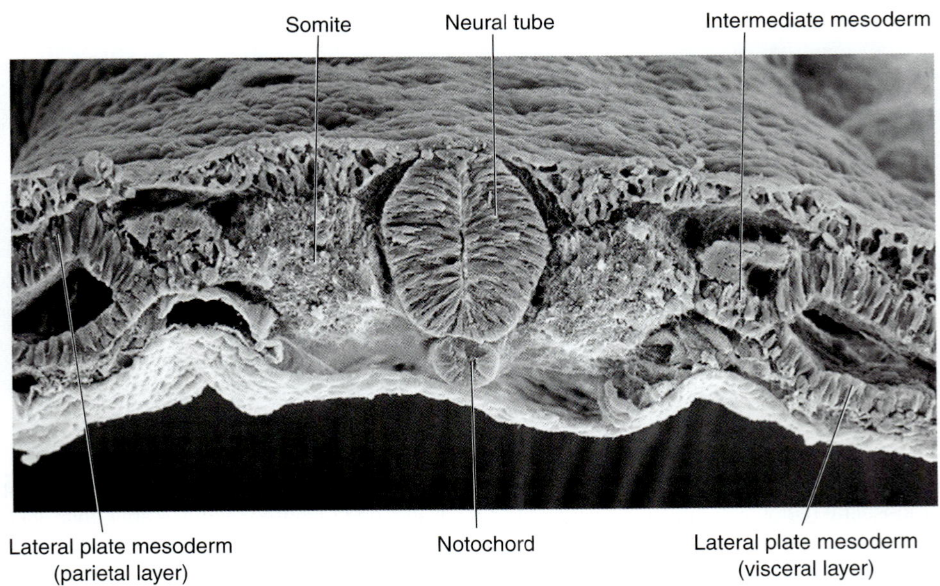


**FIGURE 6.9** Cross section through the somites and neural tube showing the organization of the paraxial mesoderm into somites and intermediate and lateral plate mesoderm.

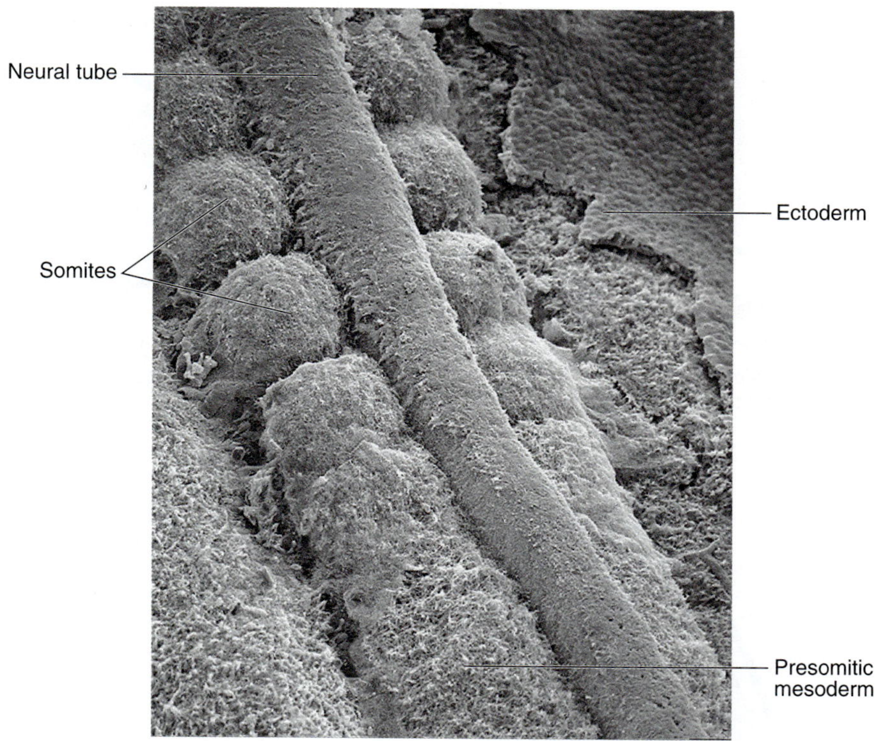


**FIGURE 6.10** Dorsal view of somites forming along the neural tube (the ectoderm has been partially removed). Somites form from unsegmented presomitic paraxial mesoderm caudally and become segmented in more cranially positioned regions.

as **somitomeres**, first appear in the cephalic region of the embryo, and their formation proceeds cephalocaudally. Each somitomere consists of mesodermal cells arranged in concentric whorls around the center of the unit. In the head region, somitomeres form in association with segmentation of the neural plate into **neuromeres** and contribute to mesenchyme in the head (see Chapter 17). From the occipital region caudally, somitomeres further organize into somites. The first pair of somites arises in the occipital region of the embryo at approximately the 20th day of development (Fig. 6.2*C,D*). From here, new somites appear in craniocaudal sequence (Fig. 6.10) at a rate of approximately three pairs per day until, at the end of the fifth week, 42 to 44 pairs are present (Figs. 6.4*B* and 6.10). There are 4 occipital, 8 cervical, 12 thoracic, 5 lumbar, 5 sacral, and 8 to 10 coccygeal pairs. The first occipital and the last five to seven coccygeal somites later disappear, whereas the remaining somites form the axial skeleton (see Chapter 10). Because somites appear with a specified periodicity, the age of an embryo can be accurately determined during this early time period by counting somites (Table 6.2).

**Table 6.2 Number of Somites Correlated to Approximate Age in Days**

| Approximate Age (d) | Number of Somites |
|---|---|
| 20 | 1–4 |
| 21 | 4–7 |
| 22 | 7–10 |
| 23 | 10–13 |
| 24 | 13–17 |
| 25 | 17–20 |
| 26 | 20–23 |
| 27 | 23–26 |
| 28 | 26–29 |
| 30 | 34–35 |

### *Somite Differentiation*

When somites first form from presomitic mesoderm, they exist as a ball of mesoderm (fibroblast-like) cells. These cells then undergo a process of **epithelization** and arrange themselves in a donut shape around a small lumen (Fig. 6.11). By the beginning of the fourth week, cells in the ventral and medial walls of the somite lose their epithelial characteristics, become mesenchymal (fibroblast-like) again, and shift their position to surround the neural tube and notochord. Collectively, these cells form the **sclerotome** that will differentiate into the vertebrae and ribs (see Chapter 10). Cells at the dorsomedial and ventrolateral edges of the upper region of the somite form precursors for muscle cells, whereas cells between these two groups form the dermatome (Fig. 6.11*B*). Cells from both muscle precursor groups become mesenchymal again and migrate beneath the dermatome to create the dermomyotome (Fig. 6.11*C,D*). In addition, cells from the ventrolateral edge migrate into the parietal layer of lateral plate mesoderm to form most of the musculature for the body wall (external

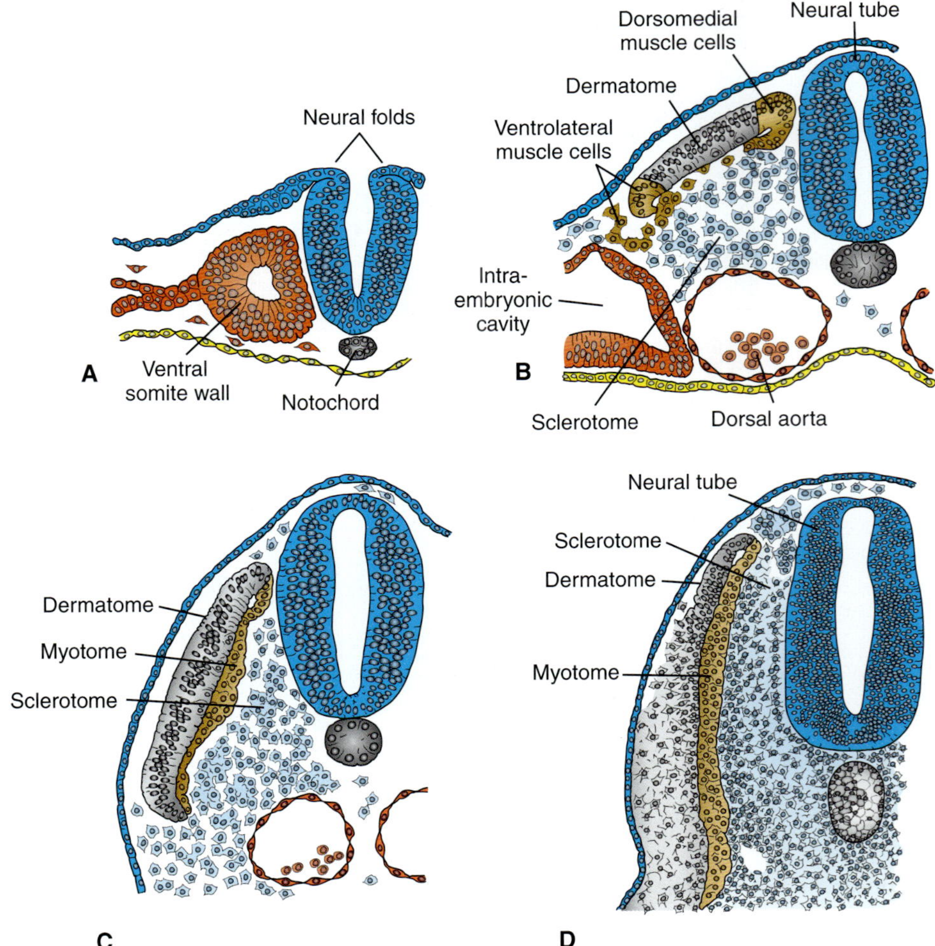


**FIGURE 6.11** Stages in the development of a somite. **A.** Mesoderm cells that have undergone epithelization are arranged around a small cavity. **B.** Cells from the ventral and medial walls of the somite lose their epithelial arrangement and migrate around the neural tube and notochord. Collectively, these cells constitute the sclerotome that will form the vertebrae and ribs. Meanwhile, cells at the dorsomedial and ventrolateral regions differentiate into muscle precursor cells, whereas cells that remain between these locations form the dermatome. **C.** Both groups of muscle precursor cells become mesenchymal and migrate beneath the dermatome to form the dermomyotome **(B,C)**, whereas some cells from the ventrolateral group also migrate into the parietal layer of lateral plate mesoderm. **D.** Eventually, dermatome cells also become mesenchymal and migrate beneath the ectoderm to form the dermis of the back **(D)**.

and internal oblique and transversus abdominis muscles) and most of the limb muscles (Fig. 6.11*B*; see Chapter 11). Cells in the dermomyotome ultimately form dermis for the skin of the back and muscles for the back, body wall (intercostal muscles), and some limb muscles (see Chapter 11).

Each myotome and dermatome retains its innervation from its segment of origin, no matter where the cells migrate. Hence, each somite forms its own **sclerotome** (the tendon cartilage and bone component), its own **myotome** (providing the segmental muscle component), and its own **dermatome**, which forms the dermis of the back. Each myotome and dermatome also has its own segmental nerve component.

## Molecular Regulation of Somite Formation

Formation of segmented somites from unsegmented presomitic (paraxial) mesoderm (Fig. 6.10) depends on a **segmentation clock** established by cyclic expression of a number of genes. The cyclic genes include members of the ***NOTCH*** and ***WNT*** signaling pathways that are expressed in an oscillating pattern in presomitic mesoderm. Thus, Notch protein accumulates in presomitic mesoderm destined to form the next somite and then decreases as that somite is established. The increase in Notch protein activates other segment-patterning genes that establish the somite. Boundaries for each somite are regulated by **retinoic acid (RA)** and a combination of **FGF8** and **WNT3a**. RA is expressed at high concentrations cranially and decreases in concentration caudally, whereas the combination of **FGF8** and **WNT3a** proteins is expressed at higher concentrations caudally and lower ones cranially. These overlapping expression gradients control the segmentation clock and activity of the NOTCH pathway.

## Molecular Regulation of Somite Differentiation

Signals for somite differentiation arise from surrounding structures, including the notochord, neural tube, epidermis,

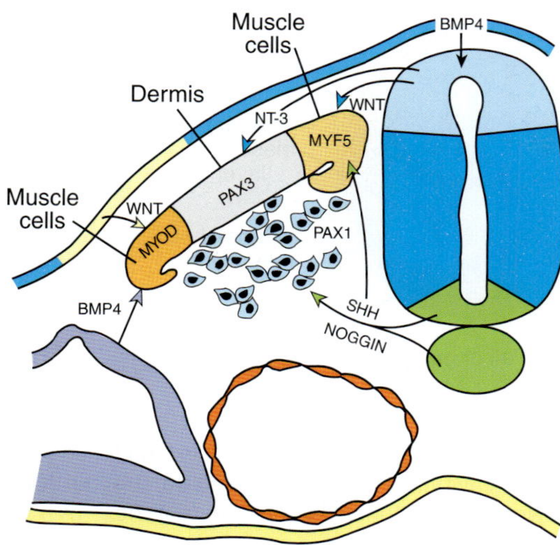


**FIGURE 6.12** Expression patterns of genes that regulate somite differentiation. Sonic hedgehog (*SHH*) and noggin, secreted by the notochord and floor plate of the neural tube, cause the ventral part of the somite to form sclerotome and to express *PAX1*, which in turn controls chondrogenesis and vertebrae formation. WNT proteins from the dorsal neural tube activate *PAX3*, which demarcates the dermomyotome. WNT proteins also direct the dorsomedial portion of the somite to differentiate into muscle precursor cells and to express the muscle-specific gene *MYF5*. The mid-dorsal portion of the somite is directed to become dermis by neurotrophin 3 (*NT-3*) expressed by the dorsal neural tube. Additional muscle precursor cells are formed from the dorsolateral portion of the somite under the combined influence of activating WNT proteins and inhibitory bone morphogenetic protein 4 (*BMP4*) protein, which together activate MyoD expression.

and lateral plate mesoderm (Fig. 6.12). The secreted protein products of the ***NOGGIN*** genes and **sonic hedgehog (SHH)**, produced by the notochord and floor plate of the neural tube, induce the ventromedial portion of the somite to become sclerotome. Once induced, sclerotome cells express the transcription factor ***PAX1***, which initiates the cascade of cartilage- and bone-forming genes for vertebral formation. Expression of ***PAX3***, regulated by **WNT** proteins from the dorsal neural tube, marks the dermomyotome region of the somite. WNT proteins from the dorsal neural tube also target the dorsomedial portion of the somite, causing it to initiate expression of the muscle-specific gene ***MYF5*** and to form primaxial muscle precursors. Interplay between the inhibiting protein **BMP4** (and probably **FGFs**) from the lateral plate mesoderm and activating WNT products from the epidermis direct the dorsolateral portion of the somite to express another muscle-specific gene, ***MYOD***, and to form primaxial and abaxial muscle precursors. The midportion of the dorsal epithelium of the somite is directed by **neurotrophin 3 (NT-3)**, secreted by the dorsal region of the neural tube, to form dermis.

## Intermediate Mesoderm

Intermediate mesoderm, which temporarily connects paraxial mesoderm with the lateral plate (Figs. 6.8*D* and 6.9), differentiates into urogenital structures. In cervical and upper thoracic regions, it forms segmental cell clusters (future **nephrotomes**), whereas more caudally, it forms an unsegmented mass of tissue, the **nephrogenic cord**. Excretory units of the urinary system and the gonads develop from this partly segmented, partly unsegmented intermediate mesoderm (see Chapter 16).

## Lateral Plate Mesoderm

**Lateral plate mesoderm** splits into **parietal** (**somatic**) and **visceral** (**splanchnic**) layers, which line the intraembryonic cavity and surround the organs, respectively (Figs. 6.8*C,D*, 6.9, and 6.13*A*).

- Mesoderm from the parietal layer, together with overlying ectoderm, forms the lateral body wall folds (Fig. 6.13*A*).
- These folds, together with the head (cephalic) and tail (caudal) folds, close the ventral body wall.
- The parietal layer of lateral plate mesoderm then forms the dermis of the skin in the body wall and limbs, the bones and connective tissue of the limbs, and the sternum.
- In addition, sclerotome and muscle precursor cells that migrate into the parietal layer of lateral plate mesoderm form the costal cartilages, limb muscles, and most of the body wall muscles (see Chapter 11).
- The visceral layer of lateral plate mesoderm, together with embryonic endoderm, forms the wall of the gut tube (Fig. 6.13*B*).
- Mesoderm cells of the parietal layer surrounding the intraembryonic cavity form thin membranes, the **mesothelial membranes**, or **serous membranes**, which will line the peritoneal, pleural, and pericardial cavities and secrete serous fluid (Fig. 6.13*B*). Mesoderm cells of the visceral layer form a thin serous membrane around each organ (see Chapter 7).

## Blood and Blood Vessels

Blood cells and blood vessels also arise from mesoderm. Blood vessels form in two ways: **vasculogenesis**, whereby vessels arise from blood islands (Fig. 6.14), and **angiogenesis**, which entails sprouting from existing vessels. The first blood islands appear in mesoderm surrounding the wall of the yolk sac at 3 weeks of development and slightly later in lateral plate mesoderm and other regions (Fig. 6.15). These islands arise from mesoderm cells that are induced to form **hemangioblasts**, a common precursor for vessel and blood cell formation.

Although the first blood cells arise in blood islands in the wall of the yolk sac, this population is transitory. The definitive **hematopoietic stem cells** are derived from mesoderm surrounding the aorta in a site near the developing mesonephric kidney called the **aorta-gonad-mesonephros region (AGM)**. These cells colonize the liver, which becomes the major hematopoietic organ of the embryo and fetus from

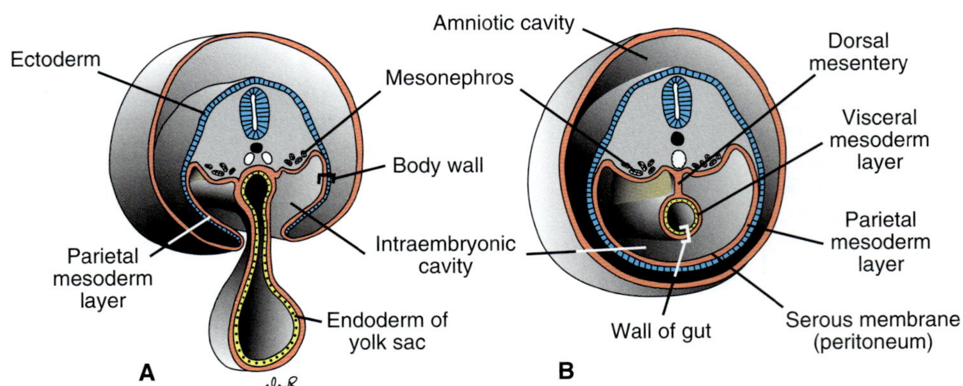


**FIGURE 6.13** **A.** Cross section through a 21-day embryo in the region of the mesonephros showing parietal and visceral mesoderm layers. The intraembryonic cavities communicate with the extraembryonic cavity (chorionic cavity). **B.** Section at the end of the fourth week. Parietal mesoderm and overlying ectoderm form the ventral and lateral body wall. Note the peritoneal (serous) membrane.

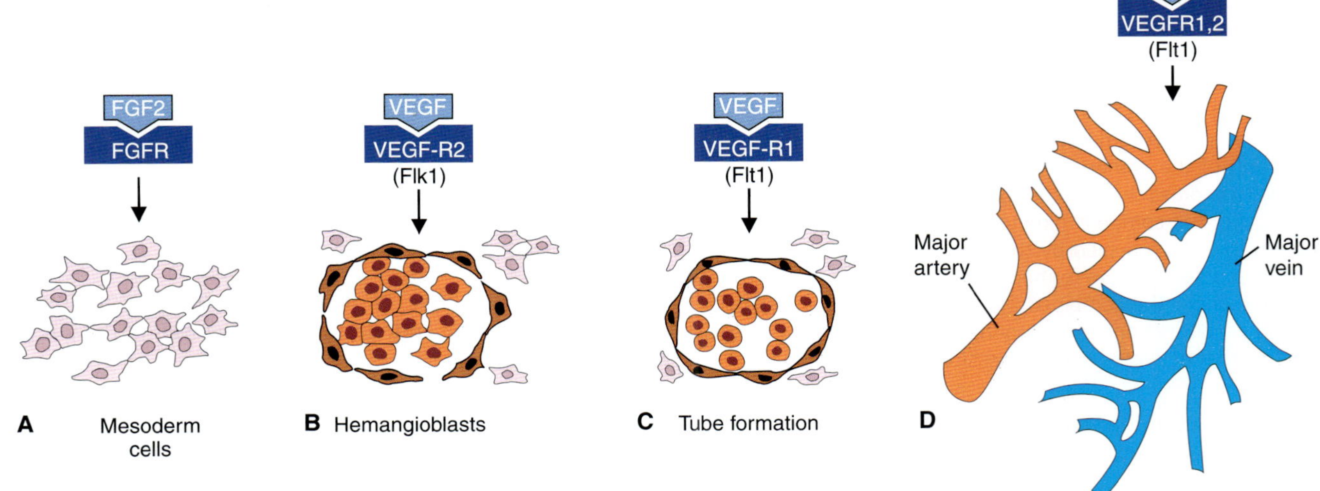


**FIGURE 6.14** Blood vessels form in two ways: vasculogenesis (**A–C**), in which vessels arise from blood island, and angiogenesis (**D**), in which new vessels sprout from existing ones. During vasculogenesis, fibroblast growth factor 2 (FGF2) binds to its receptor on subpopulations of mesoderm cells and induces them to form hemangioblasts. Then, under the influence of vascular endothelial growth factor (VEGF) acting through two different receptors, these cells become endothelial and coalesce to form vessels. Angiogenesis is also regulated by VEGF, which stimulates proliferation of endothelial cells at points where new vessels will sprout from existing ones. Final modeling and stabilization of the vasculature are accomplished by PDGF and TGF-β.

approximately the second to seventh months of development. Stem cells from the liver colonize the bone marrow, the definitive blood-forming tissue, in the seventh month of gestation; thereafter, the liver loses its blood-forming function.

## Molecular Regulation of Blood Vessel Formation

**FGF2** induces blood island development from competent mesoderm cells that form hemangioblasts. Hemangioblasts are directed to form blood cells and vessels by **vascular endothelial growth factor (VEGF)**, which is secreted by surrounding mesoderm cells. The signal to express VEGF may involve *HOXB5*, which upregulates the VEGF receptor **FLK1** (Fig. 6.14). Hemangioblasts in the center of blood islands form **hematopoietic stem cells**, the precursors of all blood cells, whereas peripheral hemangioblasts differentiate into **angioblasts**, the precursors to blood vessels. These angioblasts proliferate and are eventually induced to form endothelial cells by VEGF secreted by surrounding mesoderm cells (Fig. 6.14). This same factor then regulates coalescence of these endothelial cells into the first primitive blood vessels.

Once the process of vasculogenesis establishes a primary vascular bed, which includes the dorsal aorta and cardinal veins, additional vasculature is added by angiogenesis, the sprouting of new vessels (Fig. 6.14). This process is also mediated by VEGF, which stimulates proliferation of endothelial cells at points where new vessels are to be formed. Maturation and modeling of the vasculature are regulated by other growth factors, including **platelet-derived growth factor (PDGF)** and **TGF-β**, until the adult pattern is established. Specification of arteries, veins, and the lymphatic system occurs soon after angioblast induction. SHH, secreted by the notochord, induces

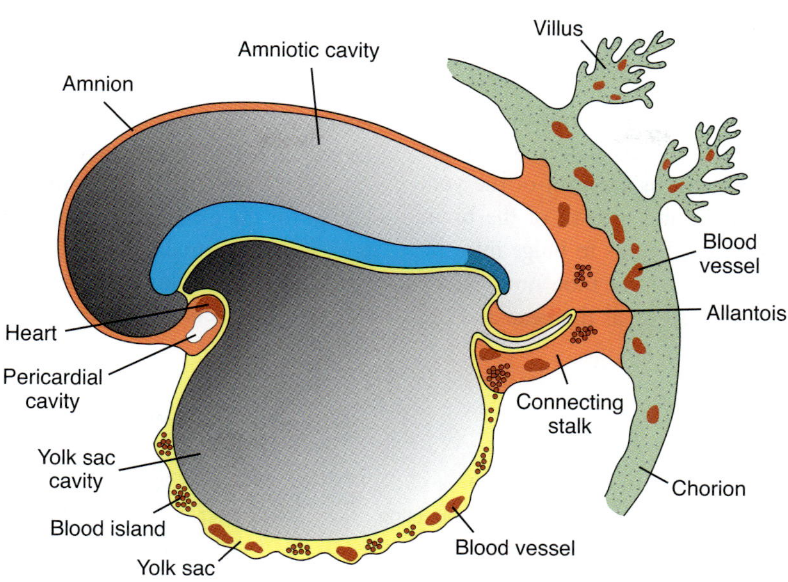


**FIGURE 6.15** Extraembryonic blood vessel formation in the villi, chorion, connecting stalk, and wall of the yolk sac in a presomite embryo of approximately 19 days.

surrounding mesenchyme to express *VEGF*. In turn, *VEGF* expression induces the **NOTCH pathway** (a transmembrane receptor pathway), which specifies arterial development through expression of ***EPHRINB2*** (ephrins are ligands that bind to **Eph receptors** in a pathway involving **tyrosine kinase signaling**). In addition to specifying arteries, expression of *EPHRINB2* suppresses venous cell fate. NOTCH signaling also upregulates expression of ***EPHB4***, a vein-specific gene, but how this gene and others specify venous development is not clear. On the other hand, ***PROX1***, a homeodomain-containing transcription factor, appears to be the master gene for lymphatic vessel differentiation. Vessel outgrowth is patterned, not random, and appears to involve guidance factors similar to those employed by the nervous system.

## Clinical Correlates

### Capillary Hemangiomas

**Capillary hemangiomas** are abnormally dense collections of capillary blood vessels that form the most common tumors of infancy, occurring in approximately 10% of all births. They may occur anywhere but are often associated with craniofacial structures (Fig. 6.16*A*). Facial lesions may be focal or diffuse, with diffuse lesions causing more secondary complications, including ulcerations, scarring, and airway obstruction (mandibular hemangiomas; Fig. 6.16*B*). Insulin-like growth factor 2 is highly expressed in the lesions and may be one factor promoting abnormal vessel growth. Whether or not VEGF plays a role has not been determined.

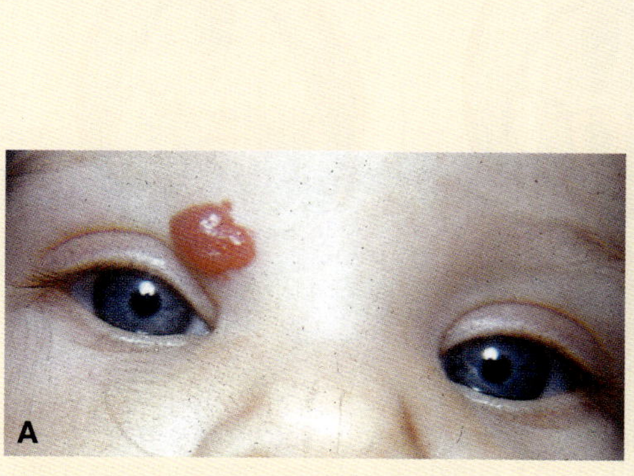


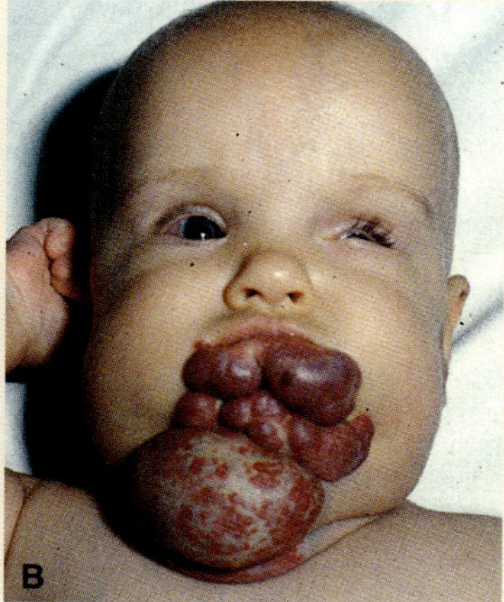


**FIGURE 6.16 A.** Focal capillary hemangioma. **B.** Diffuse capillary hemangioma involving the oral cavity.

## DERIVATIVES OF THE ENDODERMAL GERM LAYER

The gastrointestinal tract is the main organ system derived from the endodermal germ layer. This germ layer covers the ventral surface of the embryo and forms the roof of the yolk sac (Fig. 6.17*A*). With development and growth of the brain vesicles, however, the embryonic disc begins to bulge into the amniotic cavity. Lengthening of the neural tube now causes the embryo to curve into the fetal position as the head and tail regions (folds) move ventrally (Fig. 6.17). Simultaneously, two lateral body wall folds form and also move ventrally to close the ventral body wall (Fig. 6.18). As the head and tail and two lateral folds move ventrally, they pull the amnion down with them, such that the embryo lies within the amniotic cavity (Figs. 6.17 and 6.18). The ventral body wall closes completely except for the umbilical region where the connecting stalk and yolk sac duct remain attached (Figs. 6.17 and 6.19). Failure of the lateral body folds to close the body wall results in **ventral body wall defects** (see Chapter 7).

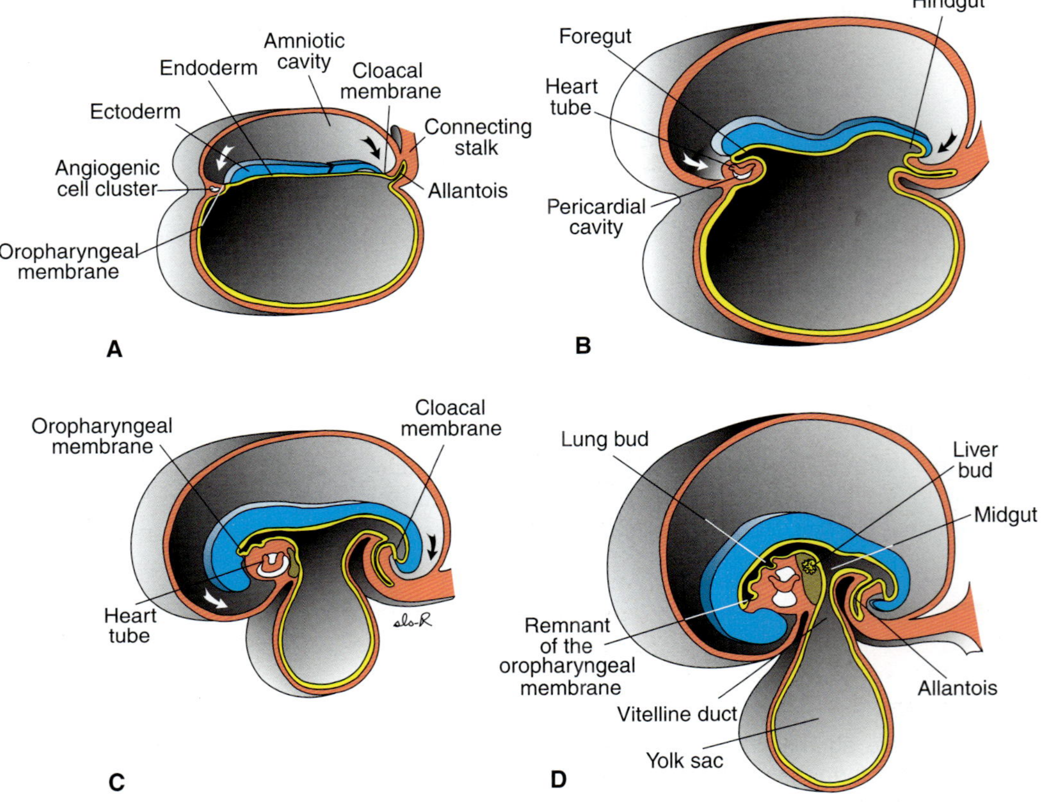


**FIGURE 6.17** Sagittal midline sections of embryos at various stages of development to demonstrate cephalocaudal folding and its effect on position of the endoderm-lined cavity. **A.** 17 days. **B.** 22 days. **C.** 24 days. **D.** 28 days. *Arrows*, head and tail folds.

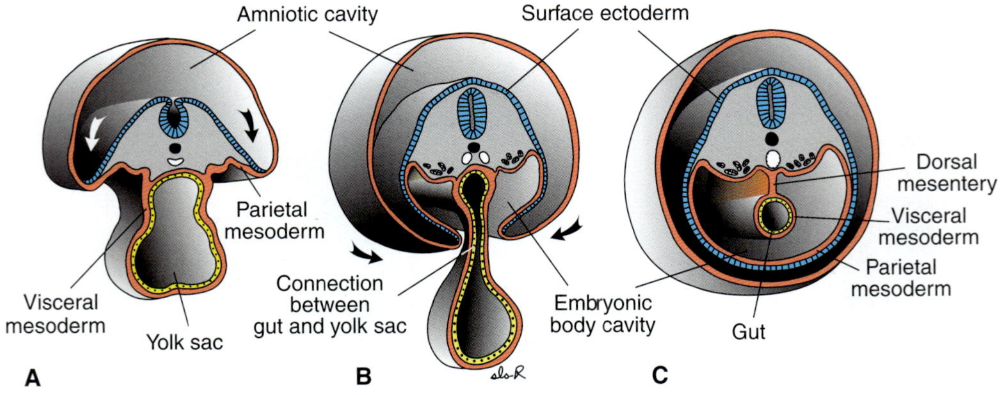


**FIGURE 6.18** Cross sections through embryos at various stages of development to show the effect of lateral folding on the endoderm-lined cavity. **A.** Folding is initiated. **B.** Transverse section through the midgut to show the connection between the gut and yolk sac. **C.** Section just below the midgut to show the closed ventral abdominal wall and gut suspended from the dorsal abdominal wall by its mesentery. *Arrows*, lateral folds.

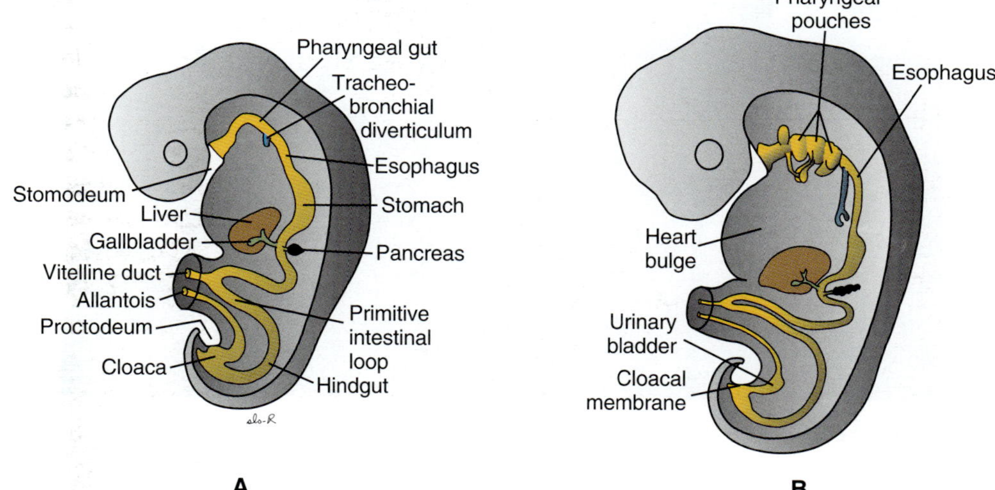


**FIGURE 6.19** Sagittal sections through embryos showing derivatives of the endodermal germ layer. **A.** The urinary bladder is derived from the cloaca and, at this stage of development, is in open connection with the allantois. **B.** Pharyngeal pouches, epithelial lining of the lung buds and trachea, liver, gallbladder, and pancreas.



As a result of cephalocaudal growth and closure of the lateral body wall folds, a continuously larger portion of the endodermal germ layer is incorporated into the body of the embryo to form the gut tube. The tube is divided into three regions: the **foregut**, **midgut**, and **hindgut** (Fig. 6.17*C*). The midgut communicates with the yolk sac by way of a broad stalk, the **vitelline (yolk sac) duct** (Fig. 6.17*D*). This duct is wide initially, but with further growth of the embryo, it becomes narrow and much longer (Figs. 6.17*D* and 6.18*B*).

At its cephalic end, the foregut is temporarily bounded by an ectodermal–endodermal membrane called the **oropharyngeal membrane** (Fig. 6.17*A,C*). This membrane separates the **stomodeum**, the primitive oral cavity derived from ectoderm, from the pharynx, a part of the foregut derived from endoderm. In the fourth week, the oropharyngeal membrane ruptures, establishing an open connection between the oral cavity and the primitive gut (Fig. 6.17*D*). The hindgut also terminates temporarily at an ectodermal–endodermal membrane, the **cloacal membrane** (Fig. 6.17*C*). This membrane separates the upper part of the anal canal, derived from endoderm, from the lower part, called the **proctodeum**, which is formed by an invaginating pit lined by ectoderm. The membrane breaks down in the seventh week to create the opening for the anus.

Another important result of cephalocaudal growth and lateral folding is partial incorporation of the allantois into the body of the embryo, where it forms the **cloaca** (Fig. 6.19*A*). The distal portion of the allantois remains in the connecting stalk. By the fifth week, the yolk sac duct, allantois, and umbilical vessels are restricted to the umbilical region (Fig. 6.19).

The role of the yolk sac is not clear. It may function as a nutritive organ during the earliest stages of development prior to the establishment of blood vessels. It also contributes some of the first blood cells, although this role is very transitory. One of its main functions is to house germ cells that reside in its posterior wall and later migrate to the gonads to form eggs and sperm (see Chapter 16).

Hence, the endodermal germ layer initially forms the epithelial lining of the primitive gut and the intraembryonic portions of the allantois and vitelline duct (Fig. 6.19*A*).

During further development, endoderm gives rise to the following:

- The epithelial lining of the respiratory tract
- The **parenchyma** of the thyroid, parathyroids, liver, and pancreas (see Chapters 15 and 17)
- The reticular stroma of the tonsils and the thymus
- The epithelial lining of the urinary bladder and the urethra (see Chapter 16)
- The epithelial lining of the tympanic cavity and auditory tube (see Chapter 19)

## EXTERNAL APPEARANCE DURING THE SECOND MONTH

At the end of the fourth week, when the embryo has approximately 28 somites, the main external features are the somites and pharyngeal arches (Fig. 6.20). The age of the embryo is therefore usually expressed in somites (Table 6.2, p. 67). Because counting somites becomes difficult during the second month of development, the age of the embryo is then indicated as the **crown-rump length (CRL)** and expressed in millimeters (Table 6.3). CRL is the measurement from the

**Table 6.3** Crown-Rump Length Correlated to Approximate Age in Weeks

| Crown-Rump Length (mm) | Approximate Age (wk) |
|---|---|
| 5–8 | 5 |
| 10–14 | 6 |
| 17–22 | 7 |
| 28–30 | 8 |

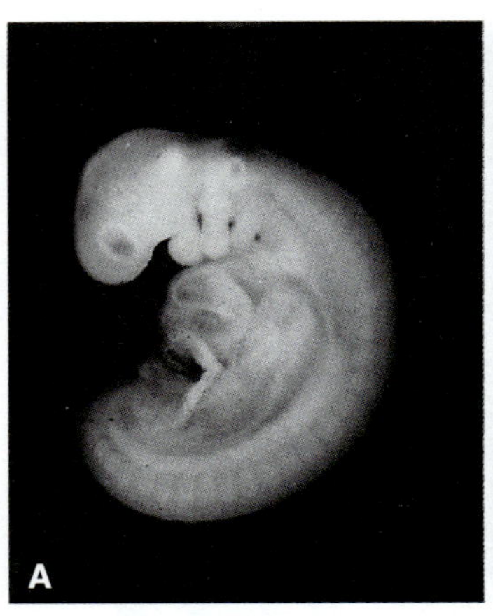


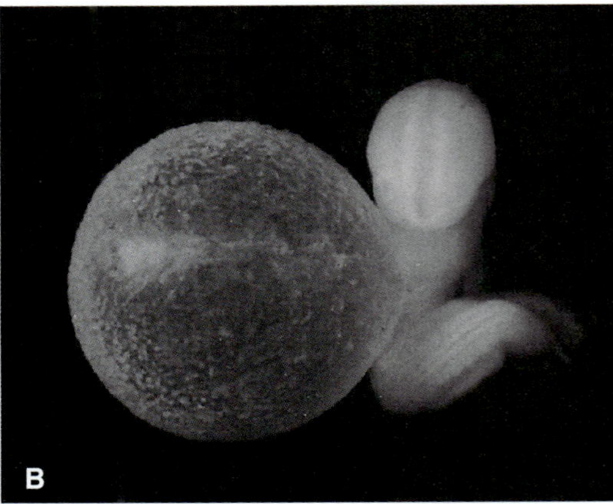


**FIGURE 6.20** **A.** Lateral view of a 28-somite human embryo. The main external features are the pharyngeal arches and somites. Note the pericardial liver bulge. **B.** The same embryo taken from a different angle to demonstrate the size of the yolk sac.



## Clinical Correlates

### Birth Defects

Most major organs and organ systems are formed during the **third to eighth weeks**. This period, which is critical for normal development, is therefore called the period of **organogenesis** or **embryogenesis**. Stem cell populations are establishing each of the organ primordia, and these interactions are sensitive to insult from genetic and environmental influences. Thus, **from the third to eighth weeks is the time when many gross structural birth defects are induced**. Unfortunately, the mother may not realize she is pregnant during this critical time, especially during the third and fourth weeks, which are particularly vulnerable. Consequently, she may not avoid harmful influences, such as cigarette smoking and alcohol. Understanding the main events of organogenesis is important for identifying the time that a particular defect was induced and, in turn, determining possible causes for the malformation (see Chapter 9).

vertex of the skull to the midpoint between the apices of the buttocks.

During the second month, the external appearance of the embryo is changed by an increase in head size and formation of the limbs, face, ears, nose, and eyes. By the beginning of the fifth week, forelimbs and hind limbs appear as paddle-shaped buds (Fig. 6.21). The former are located dorsal to the pericardial swelling at the level of the fourth cervical to the first thoracic somites, which explains their innervation by the **brachial plexus**. Hind limb buds appear slightly later just caudal to attachment of the umbilical stalk at the level of the lumbar and upper sacral somites. With further growth, the terminal portions of the buds flatten, and a circular constriction separates them from the proximal, more cylindrical segment (Fig. 6.22). Soon, four radial grooves separating five slightly thicker areas appear on the distal portion of the buds, foreshadowing formation of the digits (Fig. 6.22).

These grooves, known as **rays**, appear in the hand region first and shortly afterward in the foot, as the upper limb is slightly more advanced in development than the lower limb. While fingers and toes are being formed (Fig. 6.23), a second constriction divides the proximal portion of the buds into two segments, and the three parts characteristic of the adult extremities can be recognized (Fig. 6.24).

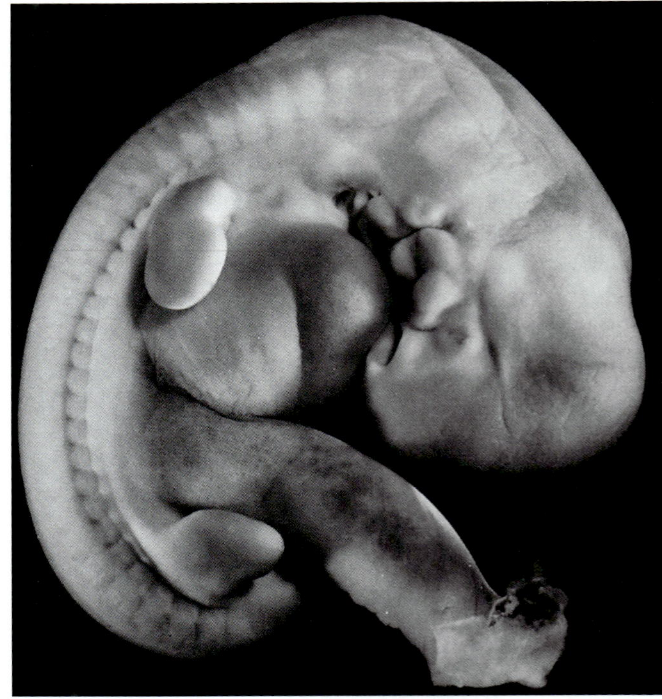

**FIGURE 6.21** Human embryo (CRL 9.8 mm, fifth week) (×29.9). The forelimbs are paddle-shaped.

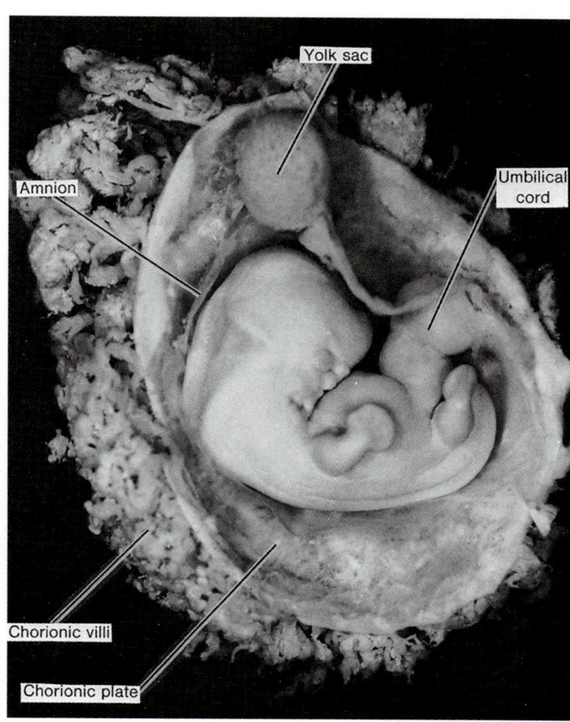


**FIGURE 6.22** Human embryo (CRL 13 mm, sixth week) showing the yolk sac in the chorionic cavity.

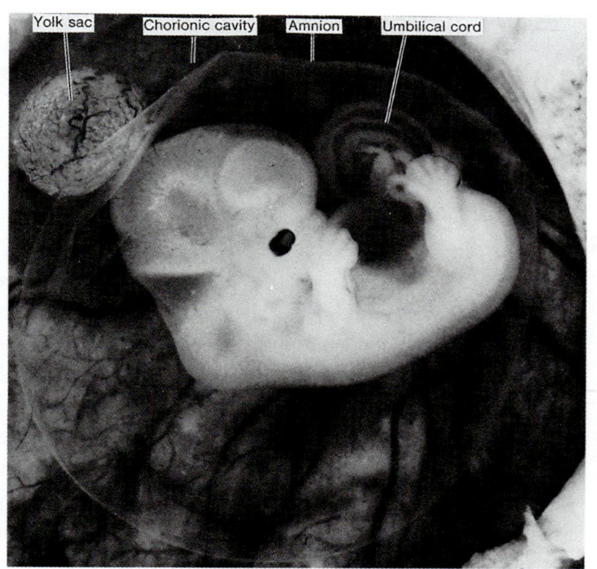


**FIGURE 6.23** Human embryo (CRL 21 mm, seventh week) (×4). The chorionic sac is open to show the embryo in its amniotic sac. The yolk sac, umbilical cord, and vessels in the chorionic plate of the placenta are clearly visible. Note the size of the head in comparison with the rest of the body.

## PATTERNING OF THE ANTEROPOSTERIOR AXIS: REGULATION BY HOMEOBOX GENES

**Homeobox** genes are known for their **homeodomain**, a DNA-binding motif, the **homeobox**. They code for

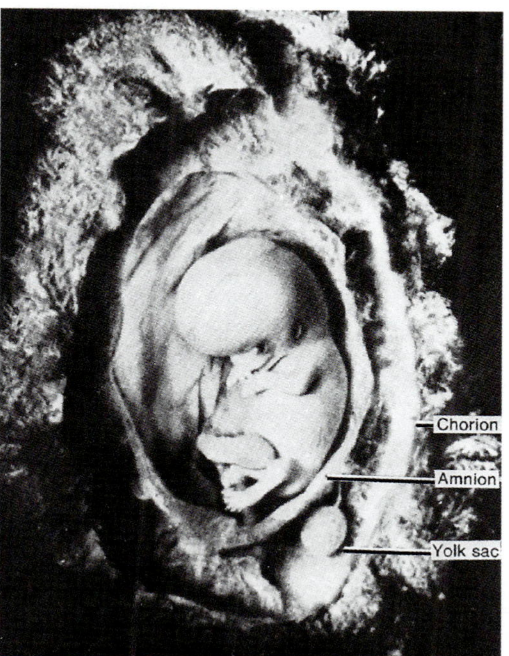


**FIGURE 6.24** Human embryo (CRL 25 mm, seventh to eighth weeks). The chorion and the amnion have been opened. Note the size of the head, the eye, the auricle of the ear, the well-formed toes, the swelling in the umbilical cord caused by intestinal loops, and the yolk sac in the chorionic cavity.

transcription factors that activate cascades of genes regulating phenomena such as segmentation and axis formation. Many homeobox genes are collected into **homeotic clusters**, although other genes also contain the homeodomain. An important cluster of genes specifying the craniocaudal axis is the homeotic gene complex ***Hom-C*** in *Drosophila*. These genes, which contain the ***Antennapedia*** and ***Bithorax*** classes of homeotic genes, are organized on a single chromosome as a functional unit. Thus, genes specifying more cranial structures lie at the 39 end of the DNA and are expressed first, with genes controlling posterior development expressed sequentially and lying increasingly toward the 59 end (Fig. 6.25). These genes are **conserved** in humans, existing as four copies—***HOXA, HOXB, HOXC,*** and ***HOXD***—which are arranged and expressed like those in *Drosophila*. Thus, each cluster lies on a separate chromosome, and the genes in each group are numbered 1 to 13 (Fig. 6.25). Genes with the same number, but belonging to different clusters, form a **paralogous** group, such as *HOXA4, HOXB4, HOXC4,* and *HOXD4*. The pattern of expression of these genes, along with evidence from **knockout** experiments in which mice are created that lack one or more of these genes, supports the hypothesis that they play a role in cranial-to-caudal patterning of the derivatives of all three germ layers. For example, an overlapping expression pattern of the *HOX* code exists in the somites and vertebrae, with genes located more toward the 39 end in each cluster being expressed in and regulating development of more cranial segments (Fig. 6.25).

Part 1

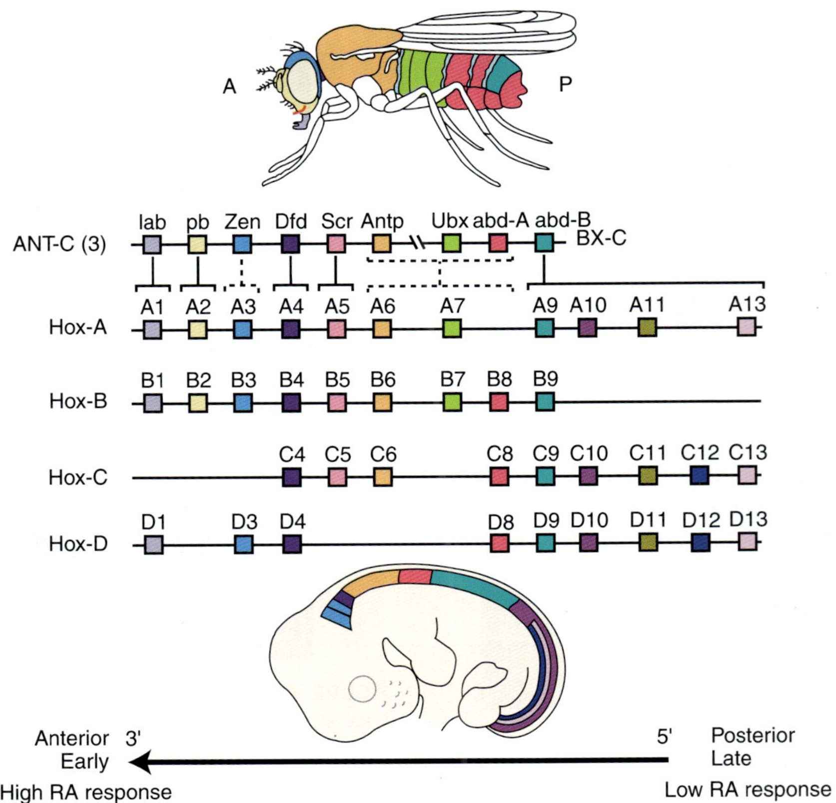


**FIGURE 6.25** Drawing showing the arrangement of homeobox genes of the *Antennapedia* (*ANT-C*) and *Bithorax* (*BX-C*) classes of *Drosophila* and conserved homologous genes of the same classes in humans. During evolution, these genes have been duplicated, such that humans have four copies arranged on four different chromosomes. Homology between *Drosophila* genes and those in each cluster of human genes is indicated by color. Genes with the same number, but positioned on different chromosomes, form a paralogous group. Expression of the genes is in a cranial-to-caudal direction from the 3′ (expressed early) to the 5′ (expressed later) end as indicated in the fly and mouse embryo diagrams. Retinoic acid (*RA*) modulates expression of these genes, with those at the 3′ end being more responsive to the compound.

## SUMMARY

- The **embryonic period**, which extends from the **third to the eighth weeks** of development, is the period during which each of the three germ layers, **ectoderm**, **mesoderm**, and **endoderm**, gives rise to its own tissues and organ systems. As a result of organ formation, major features of body form are established (Table 6.4).
- The **ectodermal germ layer** gives rise to the organs and structures that maintain contact with the outside world:
  - Central nervous system
  - Peripheral nervous system
  - Sensory epithelium of ear, nose, and eye
  - Skin, including hair and nails
  - Pituitary, mammary, and sweat glands and enamel of the teeth
- Induction of the **neural plate** is regulated by inactivation of the growth factor BMP4. In the cranial region, inactivation is caused by noggin, chordin, and follistatin secreted by the node, notochord, and prechordal mesoderm. Inactivation of BMP4 in the hindbrain and spinal cord regions is effected by WNT3a and FGF. In the absence of inactivation, BMP4 causes ectoderm to become epidermis and mesoderm to ventralize to form intermediate and lateral plate mesoderm.
- Important components of the mesodermal germ layer are **paraxial**, **intermediate**, and **lateral plate** mesoderm. Paraxial mesoderm forms **somitomeres**, which give rise to mesenchyme of the head and organize into **somites** in occipital and caudal segments.
- Somites give rise to the **myotome** (muscle tissue), **sclerotome** (cartilage and bone), and **dermatome** (dermis of the skin), which are **all supporting tissues of the body**.
- Signals for somite differentiation are derived from surrounding structures, including the notochord, neural tube, and epidermis.
- The notochord and floor plate of the neural tube secrete **SHH**, which induces the sclerotome.
- Two muscle-forming regions differentiate. One is induced in the dorsomedial region of the somite by **WNT proteins** secreted by the dorsal portion of the neural tube. The other is induced in the ventrolateral region of the somite by a combination of **BMP4** and **FGF**, secreted by lateral plate mesoderm, and by **WNT proteins**, secreted by the overlying ectoderm.
- The dorsal midportion of the somite becomes dermis under the influence of **NT-3**, secreted by the dorsal neural tube (Fig. 6.12).

**Table 6.4 Summary of Key Events During the Embryonic Period**

| Days | Somites | Length (mm) | Figure | Characteristic Features |
|---|---|---|---|---|
| 14–15 | 0 | 0.2 | 6.1*A* | Appearance of primitive streak |
| 16–18 | 0 | 0.4 | 6.1*B* | Notochordal process appears; hemopoietic cells in yolk sac |
| 19–20 | 0 | 1.0–2.0 | 6.2*A* | Intraembryonic mesoderm spreads under cranial ectoderm; primitive streak continues; umbilical vessels and cranial neural folds begin to form. |
| 20–21 | 1–4 | 2.0–3.0 | 6.2*B,C* | Cranial neural folds elevated and deep neural groove established; embryo begins to bend. |
| 22–23 | 5–12 | 3.0–3.5 | 6.3*B,C* | Fusion of neural folds begins in cervical region; cranial and caudal neuropores open widely; visceral arches 1 and 2 present; heart tube begins to fold. |
| 24–25 | 13–20 | 3.0–4.5 | 6.4 | Cephalocaudal folding under way; cranial neuropore closing or closed; optic vesicles formed; otic placodes appear. |
| 26–27 | 21–29 | 3.5–5.0 | 6.4*B* | Caudal neuropore closing or closed; upper limb buds appear; three pairs of visceral arches |
| 28–30 | 30–35 | 4.0–6.0 | 6.20*A* | Fourth visceral arch formed; hind limb buds appear; otic vesicle and lens placode |
| 31–35 | | 7.0–10.0 | 6.21 | Forelimbs paddle-shaped; nasal pits formed; embryo tightly C-shaped |
| 36–42 | | 9.0–14.0 | 6.22 | Digital rays in hand and foot plates; brain vesicles prominent; external auricle forms from auricular hillocks; umbilical herniation initiated |
| 43–49 | | 13.0–22.0 | 6.23 | Pigmentation of retina visible; digital rays separate; nipples and eyelids formed; maxillary swellings fuse with medial nasal swellings as upper lip forms; prominent umbilical herniation |
| 50–56 | | 21.0–31.0 | 6.24 | Limbs long, bent at elbows, knees; fingers, toes free; face more humanlike; tail disappears; umbilical herniation persists to end of third month. |

- Mesoderm also gives rise to the **vascular system** (i.e., the heart, arteries, veins, lymph vessels, and all blood and lymph cells). Furthermore, it gives rise to the **urogenital system**: kidneys, gonads, and their ducts (but not the bladder). Finally, the **spleen** and **cortex of the suprarenal glands** are mesodermal derivatives.
- The **endodermal germ layer** provides the epithelial lining of the **gastrointestinal tract**, **respiratory tract**, and **urinary bladder**. It also forms the **parenchyma** of the **thyroid**, **parathyroids**, **liver**, and **pancreas**. Finally, the epithelial lining of the **tympanic cavity** and **auditory tube** originates in the endodermal germ layer.
- Craniocaudal patterning of the embryonic axis is controlled by **homeobox genes**. These genes, conserved from *Drosophila*, are arranged in four clusters—***HOXA***, ***HOXB***, ***HOXC***, and ***HOXD***—on four different chromosomes. Genes toward the 3′ end of the chromosome control development of more cranial structures; those more toward the 5′ end regulate differentiation of more posterior structures. Together, they regulate patterning of the hindbrain and axis of the embryo (Fig. 6.25).
- As a result of formation of organ systems and rapid growth of the central nervous system, the initial flat embryonic disc begins to lengthen and to form head and tail regions (folds) that cause the embryo to curve into the fetal position.
- The embryo also forms two **lateral body wall folds** that grow ventrally and close the ventral body wall. As a result of this growth and folding, the amnion is pulled ventrally and the embryo lies within the amniotic cavity (Fig. 6.17).
- Connection with the yolk sac and placenta is maintained through the **vitelline duct** and **umbilical cord**, respectively.

## Self-Assessment

### Comprehensive Questions

1. Describe the process of neurulation and include definitions for the terms *neural folds*, *neural tube*, and *neural tube closure*. Where is neural tube closure initiated, and how does it proceed? What week in gestation is the process completed? What happens if neural tube closure fails cranially? Caudally? What is an NTD, and how can most be prevented?
2. What is the embryological origin of NCC? Are they ectodermal, mesodermal, or endodermal in origin? To what structures do they contribute? What protein is primarily responsible for their induction?
3. From what germ layer are somites formed? How are they organized, and what tissues do they form?
4. What are the two ways that blood vessels arise? What growth factor plays a key role in early blood cell and vessel formation? What type of tumor is caused by abnormal proliferations of capillary blood vessels?

(*Continued*)

5. What are the major subdivisions of the gut tube, and what germ layer gives rise to these parts? What structure forms a connection from the midgut to the yolk sac? What membranes close the gut tube cranially and caudally?
6. Why are the third to eighth weeks of embryogenesis so important for normal development and a time for induction of structural defects?

## Problem Solving Questions

1. A-30-year-old multipara presented with 18 weeks of pregnancy. On her routine ultrasound, a spinal defect was noted in the lumbosacral region with herniation of neural elements through it. Explain the given condition.
2. At 20 weeks, a lady came for antenatal checkup. On routine ultrasound, the fetal head size was the same as that in the first trimester. What is the probable reason for this? At what trimester does the head increase in size?
3. A newborn baby is born with an imperforate anus. What is the membrane that ruptures to form the anal opening? How does the membrane form?

## Multiple Choice Questions

1. A clinical condition in which there is failure of closure of neural tube in the cranial region is called
   (a) Spina bifida
   (b) Anencephaly
   (c) Sacrococcygeal teratoma
   (d) Sirenomelia
2. Regression of gastrulation leads to
   (a) Sirenomelia
   (b) Anencephaly
   (c) Sacrococcygeal teratoma
   (d) Spina bifida
3. Anterior and posterior neuropore closure occurs at
   (a) 21st and 22nd days
   (b) 23rd and 24th days
   (c) 25th and 26th day s
   (d) 25th and 28th days
4. All of the following are neural crest cell derivatives except
   (a) Schwann cells
   (b) Glial cells
   (c) Ventral horn cells
   (d) Melanocytes
5. Neural crest cells develop during a process known as neurulation. These cells can ultimately form which of the following?
   (a) Melanocytes
   (b) Lymphocytes
   (c) Dermatome
   (d) Angioblasts
6. Which drug can be given to mothers to prevent neural tube defects?
   (a) Iron
   (b) Calcium
   (c) Folic acid
   (d) Vitamin A
7. Neural tube is a derivative of
   (a) Ectoderm
   (b) Mesoderm
   (c) Notochord
   (d) Endoderm
8. Somites are formed from
   (a) Lateral plate mesoderm
   (b) Paraxial mesoderm
   (c) Intermediate mesoderm
   (d) Notochord
9. Patterning of the anteroposterior axis is regulated by which of the following transcription factors?
   (a) TGF-β
   (b) Homeobox genes
   (c) SHH
   (d) PAX
10. Which of the following structures is not a derivative of endoderm?
   (a) Gastrointestinal epithelium
   (b) Urinary tract epithelium
   (c) Endothelium of blood vessels
   (d) Respiratory epithelium

### Answers

1. (b) 2. (a) 3. (d) 4. (c) 5. (a) 6. (c) 7. (a) 8. (b) 9. (b) 10. (c)

CHAPTER

# 7 The Gut Tube and the Body Cavities

**Specific Learning Objectives**

- Cephalocaudal and lateral folding of the embryo
- Formation of the body cavity
- Body wall defects
- Formation of the diaphragm and diaphragmatic hernia

**Competencies Covered**

AN52.4 Describe the development of the anterior abdominal wall.
AN52.5 Describe the development and congenital anomalies of the diaphragm.



## A TUBE ON TOP OF A TUBE

During the third and fourth weeks, the top layer (ectoderm) of the trilaminar embryonic disc forms the neural plate that rolls up into a tube to form the brain and spinal cord by the process called **neurulation** (see Chapter 6, p. 59). Almost simultaneously, the ventral layer (endoderm) rolls down to form the gut tube, such that the embryo consists of a tube on top of a tube: the neural tube dorsally and the gut tube ventrally (Fig. 7.1). The middle layer (mesoderm) holds the two tubes together and the lateral plate component of this mesoderm layer also splits into visceral (splanchnic) and parietal (somatic) layers. The visceral layer rolls ventrally and is intimately connected to the gut tube; the parietal layer, together with the overlying ectoderm, forms the **lateral body wall folds** (one on each side of the embryo), which move ventrally and meet in the midline to close the **ventral body wall** (Fig. 7.1). The space between visceral and parietal layers of lateral plate mesoderm is the **primitive body cavity**, which at this early stage is a continuous cavity, because it has not yet been subdivided into the pericardial, pleural, and abdominopelvic regions.

## FORMATION OF THE BODY CAVITY

At the end of the third week, **intraembryonic mesoderm** differentiates into **paraxial mesoderm**, which forms somitomeres and somites that play a major role in forming the skull and vertebrae; **intermediate mesoderm**, which contributes to the urogenital system; and **lateral plate mesoderm**, which is involved in forming the body cavity (Fig. 7.1). Soon after it forms as a solid mesodermal layer, clefts appear in the lateral plate mesoderm that coalesce to split the solid layer into two (Fig. 7.1*B*):

1. The **parietal (somatic)** layer adjacent to the surface ectoderm and continuous with the extraembryonic parietal mesoderm layer over the amnion. Together, the parietal (somatic) layer of lateral plate mesoderm and overlying ectoderm are called the **somatopleure**.
2. The **visceral (splanchnic)** layer adjacent to endoderm forming the gut tube and continuous with the visceral layer of extraembryonic mesoderm covering the yolk sac (Fig. 7.1*B*). Together, the visceral (splanchnic) layer of lateral plate mesoderm and underlying endoderm are called the **splanchnopleure**.

The space created between the two layers of lateral plate mesoderm constitutes the **primitive body cavity**.

During the fourth week, the sides of the embryo begin to grow ventrally forming two **lateral body wall folds** (Fig. 7.1*B,C*). These folds consist of the parietal layer of lateral plate mesoderm, overlying ectoderm, and cells from adjacent somites that migrate into the mesoderm layer across the lateral somitic frontier. As these folds progress, the endoderm layer also folds ventrally and closes to form the gut tube (Fig. 7.1*D,E*). By the end of the fourth week, the lateral body wall folds meet in the midline and fuse to close the ventral body wall (Fig. 7.1*C–E*).

This closure is aided by growth of the head and tail regions (folds) that cause the embryo to curve into the **fetal position** (Fig. 7.2). Closure of the ventral body wall is complete except in the region of the connecting stalk (future umbilical cord).

Similarly, closure of the gut tube is complete except for a connection from the midgut region to the yolk sac called the **vitelline (yolk sac) duct** (Fig. 7.2*D*). This duct is incorporated into the umbilical cord, becomes very narrow (Fig. 8.18), and degenerates with the yolk sac between the second and third months of gestation. (Note that throughout the process of body cavity and gut tube development, the parietal and

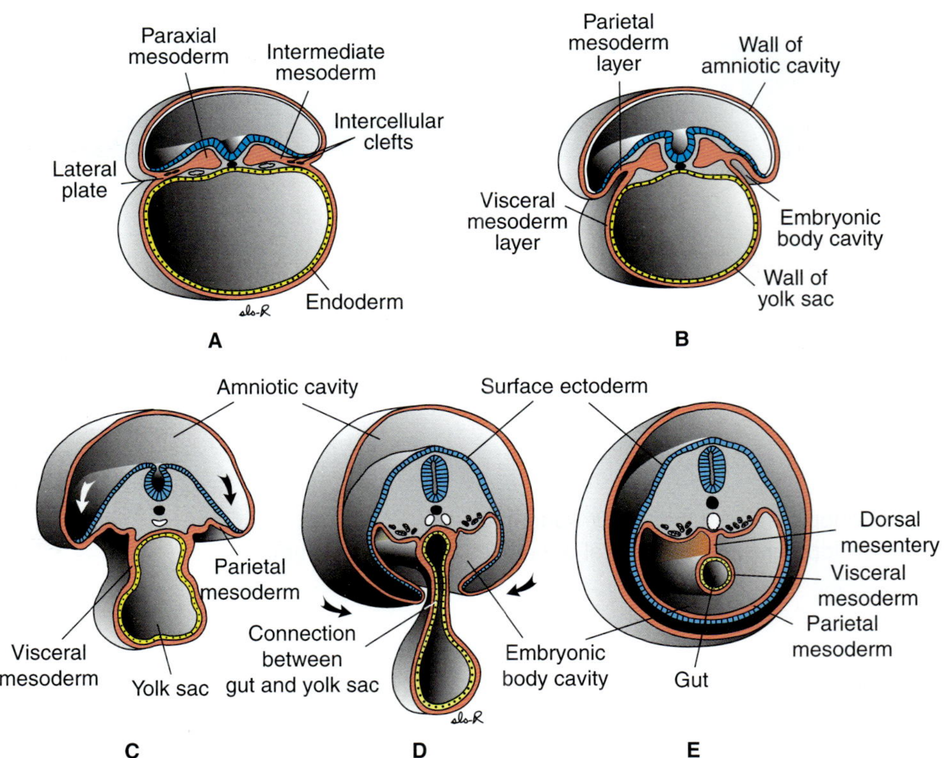


**FIGURE 7.1** Transverse sections through embryos at various stages of closure of the gut tube and ventral body wall. **A.** At approximately 19 days, intercellular clefts are visible in the lateral plate mesoderm. **B.** At 20 days, the lateral plate is divided into parietal and visceral mesoderm layers that line the primitive body cavity (intraembryonic cavity). **C.** By 21 days, the primitive body cavity (intraembryonic cavity) is still in open communication with the extraembryonic cavity. **D.** By 24 days, the lateral body wall folds, consisting of the parietal layer of lateral plate mesoderm and overlying ectoderm are approaching each other in the midline. **E.** At the end of the fourth week, visceral mesoderm layers are continuous with parietal layers as a double-layered membrane, the dorsal mesentery. Dorsal mesentery extends from the caudal limit of the foregut to the end of the hindgut.

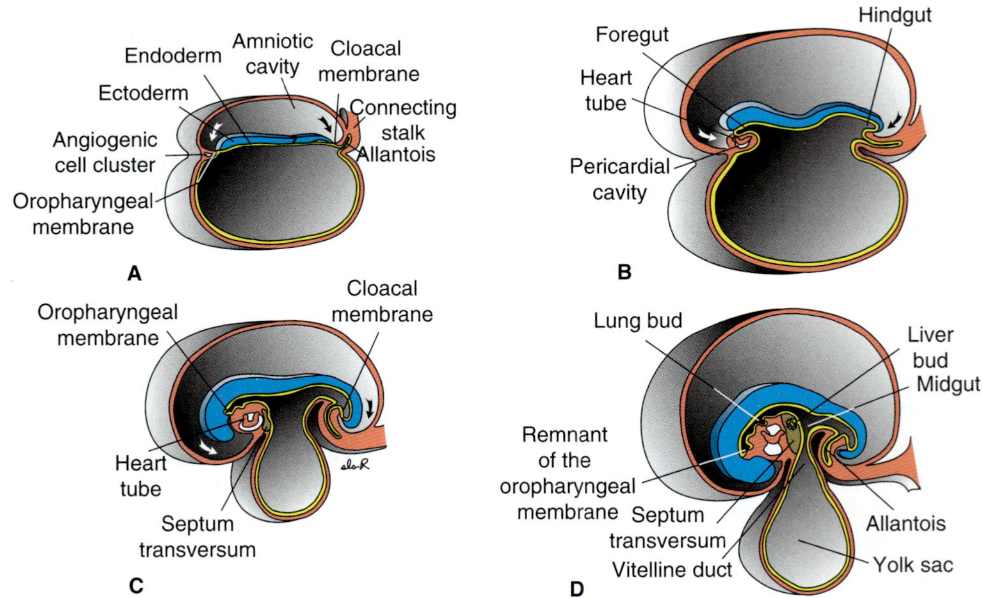


**FIGURE 7.2** Midsagittal sections of embryos at various stages of development showing cephalocaudal folding and its effects on position of the heart, septum transversum, yolk sac, and amnion. Note that as folding progresses, the opening of the gut tube into the yolk sac narrows until it forms a thin connection, the vitelline (yolk sac) duct, between the midgut and the yolk sac **(D)**. Simultaneously, the amnion is pulled ventrally until the amniotic cavity nearly surrounds the embryo. **A.** 17 days. **B.** 22 days. **C.** 24 days. **D.** 28 days. *Arrows*, head and tail folds.

visceral layers of lateral plate mesoderm are continuous with each other at the junction of the gut tube with the posterior body wall [Fig. 7.1*D,E*].)

## ■ SEROUS MEMBRANES

Some cells of the parietal layer of lateral plate mesoderm lining the body wall of the primitive embryonic cavity become mesothelial and form the **parietal layer of the serous membranes** lining the outside of the **peritoneal**, **pleural**, and **pericardial cavities**. In a similar manner, some cells of the visceral layer of lateral plate mesoderm form the **visceral layer of the serous membranes** covering the abdominal organs, lungs, and heart (Fig. 7.1*E*). Visceral and parietal layers are continuous with each other as the **dorsal mesentery** (Fig. 7.1*E*), which suspends the gut tube from the posterior body wall into the peritoneal cavity. Dorsal mesentery extends continuously from the caudal limit of the foregut to the end of the hindgut. **Ventral mesentery** exists only from the caudal foregut to the upper portion of the duodenum and results from thinning of mesoderm of the **septum transversum**, a block of mesoderm that forms connective tissue in the liver and forms a scaffold for formation of the diaphragm (see Figs. 7.2*D* and 7.5). These mesenteries are **double layers** of peritoneum that provide a pathway for blood vessels, nerves, and lymphatics to the organs.

Part 1

## *Clinical Correlates*

### Ventral Body Wall Defects

**Ventral body wall defects** occur in the thorax, abdomen, and pelvis and involve the heart (**ectopia cordis**), abdominal viscera (**gastroschisis**), and/or urogenital organs **bladder or cloacal exstrophy**), depending on the location and size of the abnormality. The malformations are due to a failure of the ventral body wall to close and probably involve the lateral body wall folds to a greater extent than the head and tail folds. Thus, one or both of the lateral body wall folds fail to progress ventrally or there are abnormalities in the fusion process once they meet in the midline (see p. 205).

**Ectopia cordis** occurs when lateral body wall folds fail to close the midline in the thoracic region causing the heart to lie outside the body cavity (Fig. 7.3*A*). Sometimes, the closure defect begins at the caudal end of the sternum and extends into the upper abdomen resulting in a spectrum of abnormalities called

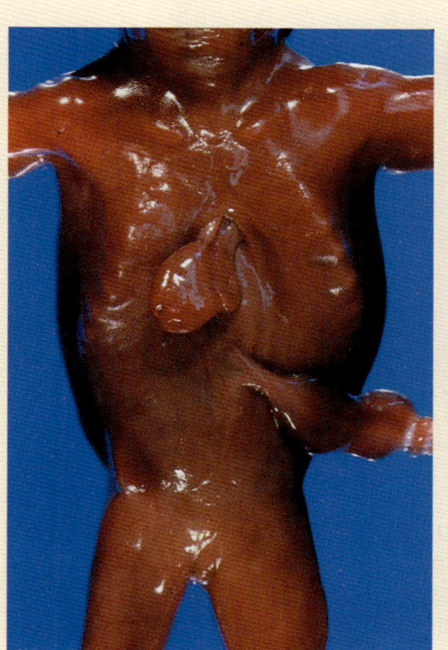
A

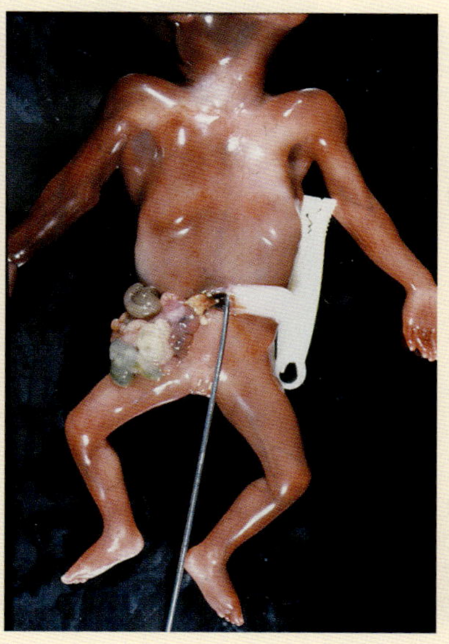
B

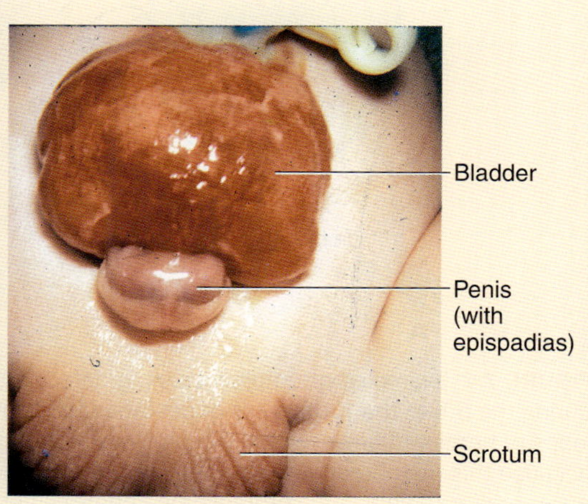

C

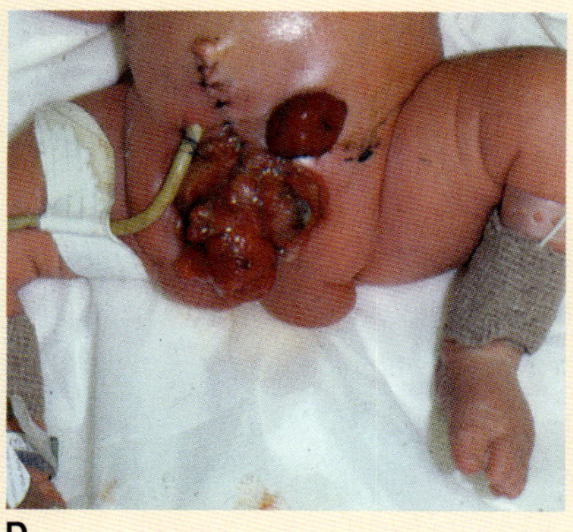
D

**FIGURE 7.3** Examples of ventral body wall defects due to failure of the ventral body wall to close. **A.** Ectopia cordis. The heart lies outside the thorax, and there is a cleft in the thoracic wall. **B.** Gastroschisis. Intestines have herniated through the abdominal wall to the right of the umbilicus, the most common location for this defect. **C.** Bladder exstrophy. Closure in the pelvic region has failed. In males, the defect usually includes a split in the dorsum of the penis, a defect called *epispadias*. **D.** Cloacal exstrophy. A larger closure defect in which most of the pelvic region has failed to close, leaving the bladder, part of the rectum, and the anal canal exposed.

(*Continued*)

**Cantrell pentalogy**. This spectrum includes ectopia cordis, defects in the anterior region of the diaphragm, absence of the pericardium, defects in the sternum, and abdominal wall defects including omphalocele and gastroschisis. (Note: Omphaloceles that may occur in Cantrell pentalogy are secondary to the body wall closure defect, not primary. The closure defect reduces the size of the abdominal cavity and prevents the return of the intestinal loops from the umbilical cord; see p. 205).

**Gastroschisis** occurs when body wall closure fails in the abdominal region (Fig. 7.3*B*). As a result, intestinal loops herniate into the amniotic cavity through the defect, which usually lies to the right of the umbilicus. The incidence of gastroschisis is increasing (3.5/10,000), and it is most common in infants from thin white women younger than 20 years of age. The defect can be detected by fetal ultrasound and by elevated α-fetoprotein (AFP) concentrations in maternal serum and the amniotic fluid. The malformation is not associated with chromosome abnormalities, but other defects occur in 15% of cases, including heart defects in 5%. Affected loops of bowel may be damaged by exposure to amniotic fluid, which has a corrosive effect, or by twisting around each other (volvulus) and compromising their blood supply.

**Bladder** or **cloacal exstrophy** results from abnormal body wall closure in the pelvic region. Bladder exstrophy represents a less severe closure defect in this region and only the bladder is exposed (Fig. 7.3*C*; in males, the penis may be involved and epispadias [a split in the dorsum of the penis; see Chapter 16, p. 228] is common). Cloacal exstrophy results from a more severe failure of body wall closure in the pelvis such that the bladder and rectum, which are derived from the cloaca (see Chapter 16, p. 220), are exposed (Fig. 7.3*D*).

**Omphalocele** represents another ventral body wall defect (Fig. 7.4), but it does not arise from a failure in body wall closure. Instead, it originates when portions of the gut tube (the midgut) that normally herniates into the umbilical cord during the 6th to the 10th weeks (**physiological umbilical herniation**) fails to return to the abdominal cavity (see Chapter 15, p. 205). Subsequently, loops of bowel, and other viscera, including the liver, may herniate into the defect. Because the umbilical cord is covered by a reflection of the amnion, the defect is covered by this epithelial layer. (In contrast, loops of bowel in gastroschisis are not covered by amnion because they herniate through the abdominal wall directly into the amniotic cavity.) Omphalocele, which occurs in 2.5/10,000 births, is associated with high mortality rates and severe malformations, including cardiac abnormalities and neural tube defects. Furthermore, chromosome abnormalities are present in 15% of cases. Like gastroschisis, omphaloceles are associated with elevated AFP concentrations. The differences between omphalocele and gastroschisis are listed in Table 7.1.

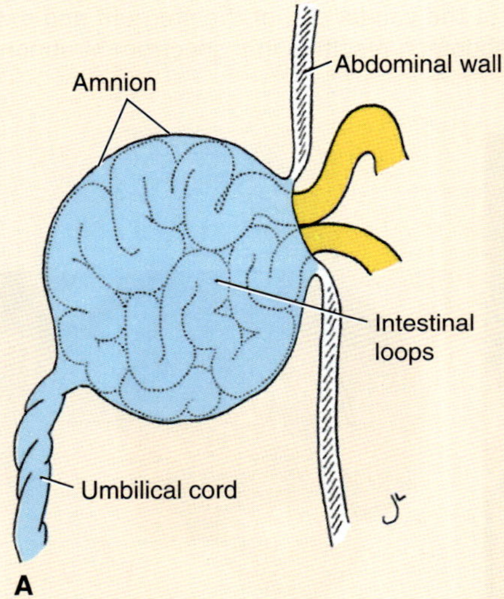


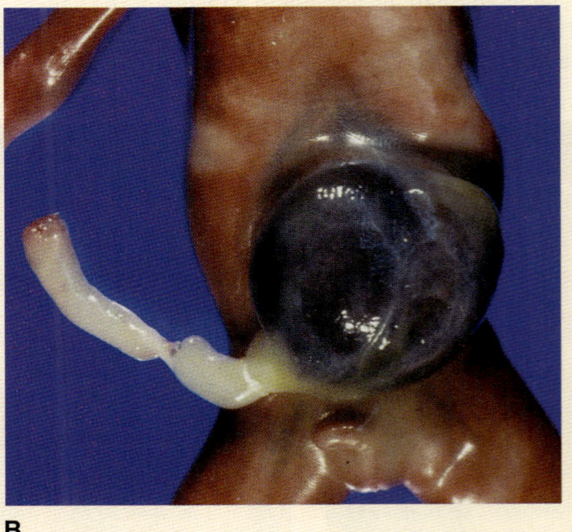


**FIGURE 7.4** Examples of omphaloceles, a defect that occurs when loops of bowel, which normally herniate into the umbilical cord during the 6th to the 10th weeks of gestation (physiological umbilical herniation), fail to return to the body cavity. **A.** Drawing showing loops of herniated bowel within the umbilical cord that have failed to return to the abdominal cavity. The bowel is covered by amnion because this membrane normally reflects onto the umbilical cord. **B.** Infant with an omphalocele. The defect is associated with other major malformations and chromosome abnormalities.

**Table 7.1 Differences Between Omphalocele and Gastroschisis**

| | Omphalocele | Gastroschisis |
|---|---|---|
| Cause | Failure of return of physiologically herniated loops of bowel to the body cavity in the 10th week | Failure of closure of lateral body wall folds in the abdominal region |
| Position of defect | Midline | Paramedian, right sided |
| Herniated viscera | Liver, intestines, stomach, spleen, or gallbladder | Mainly intestines and sometimes other organs |
| Amnion | Covered by amnion | Not covered by amnion |
| | 2.5/10,000 births | 1/10,000 births |
| Maternal age | – | Less maternal age (<20 years) |
| Associated defects | Cardiac (50%), neural tube defects (40%), chromosomal defects (15%) | Not associated with severe defects |

## DIAPHRAGM AND THORACIC CAVITY

The **septum transversum** is a thick plate of mesodermal tissue occupying the space between the thoracic cavity and the stalk of the yolk sac (Fig. 7.5*A*,*B*). The septum is derived from visceral (splanchnic) mesoderm surrounding the heart and assumes its position between the primitive thoracic and abdominal cavities when the cranial end of the embryo grows and curves into the fetal position (Fig. 7.2*B*–*D*). This septum does not separate the thoracic and abdominal cavities completely but leaves large openings, the **pericardioperitoneal canals**, on each side of the foregut (Fig. 7.5*B*).

When lung buds begin to grow, they expand caudolaterally within the pericardioperitoneal canals (Fig. 7.5*C*). As a result of the rapid growth of the lungs, the pericardioperitoneal canals become too small, and the lungs begin to expand into the mesenchyme of the body wall dorsally, laterally, and ventrally (Fig. 7.5*C*). Ventral and lateral expansion is posterior to the **pleuropericardial folds**. At first, these folds appear as small ridges projecting into the primitive undivided thoracic cavity (Fig. 7.5*C*). With expansion of the lungs, mesoderm of the body wall forms two components (Fig. 7.6): (1) the definitive wall of the thorax and (2) the **pleuropericardial membranes**, which are extensions of the pleuropericardial folds that contain the **common cardinal veins** and **phrenic nerves**. Subsequently, descent of the heart and positional changes of the sinus venosus shift the common cardinal veins toward the midline, and the pleuropericardial membranes are drawn out in mesentery-like fashion (Fig. 7.6*A*). Finally, they fuse with each other and with the root of the lungs, and the thoracic cavity is divided into the definitive **pericardial cavity** and two **pleural cavities** (Fig. 7.6*B*). In the adult, the pleuropericardial membranes form the **fibrous pericardium**.

## FORMATION OF THE DIAPHRAGM

Although the pleural cavities are separate from the pericardial cavity, they remain in open communication with the abdominal (peritoneal) cavity by way of the **pericardioperitoneal canals** (Fig. 7.5*B*). During further development, the opening between the prospective pleural and peritoneal cavities is partially closed by crescent-shaped folds, the **pleuroperitoneal folds**, which project into the caudal end of the pericardioperitoneal canals (Fig. 7.7*A*). By the seventh week, the folds become thinner to form the **pleuroperitoneal membranes** that grow medially to fuse with the mesentery of the esophagus that forms the **crura of the diaphragm** around the aorta (Fig. 7.7*A*,*B*). The pleuroperitoneal membranes then continue to grow until they fuse with each other and completely cover the septum transversum (Fig. 7.7*B*,*C*). The central region of these fused membranes forms the **central tendon of the diaphragm**, whereas their periphery forms connective tissue that serves as a scaffold and guide for migrating myoblasts (Fig. 7.7*C*). These muscle cells originate

Part 1

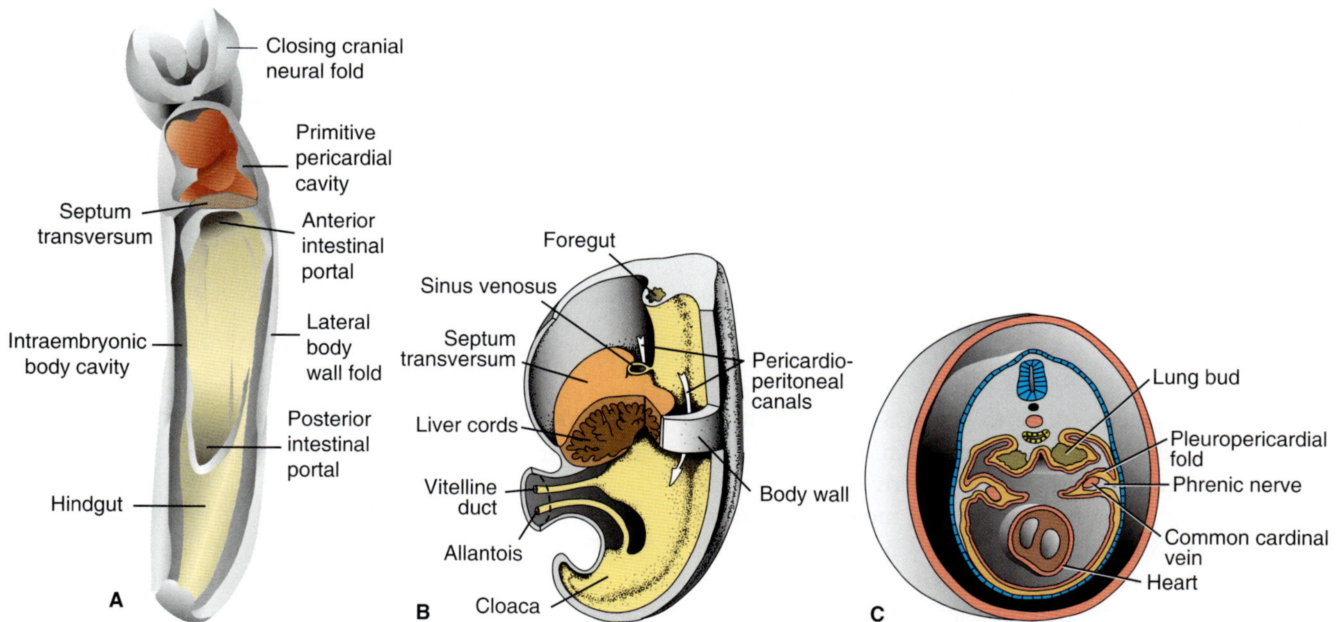


**FIGURE 7.5** **A.** Drawing showing the ventral view of an embryo at 24 days of gestation. The gut tube is closing, the anterior and posterior intestinal portals are visible, and the heart lies in the primitive pleuropericardial cavity, which is partially separated from the abdominal cavity by the septum transversum. **B.** Portion of an embryo at approximately 5 weeks with parts of the body wall and septum transversum removed to show the pericardioperitoneal canals. Note the size and thickness of the septum transversum and liver cords penetrating the septum. **C.** Growth of the lung buds into the pericardioperitoneal canals. Note the pleuropericardial folds.

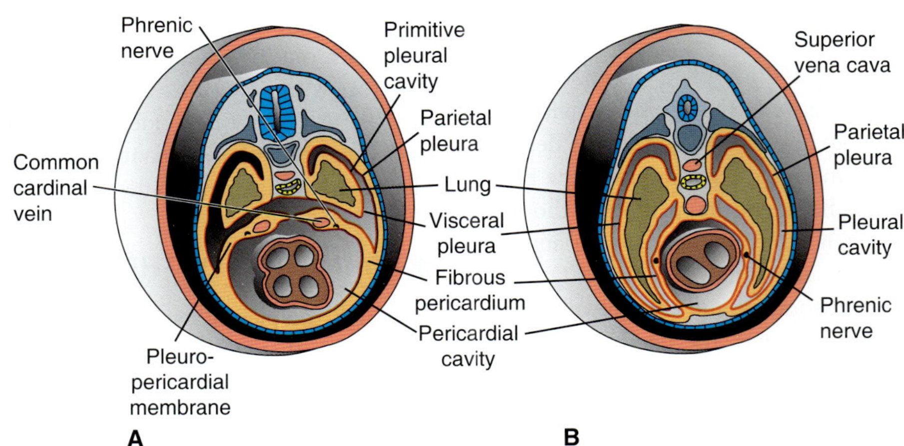


**FIGURE 7.6** **A.** Transformation of the pericardioperitoneal canals into the pleural cavities and formation of the pleuropericardial membranes. Note the pleuropericardial folds containing the common cardinal vein and phrenic nerve. Mesenchyme of the body wall forms the pleuropericardial membranes and definitive body wall. **B.** The thorax after fusion of the pleuropericardial folds with each other and with the root of the lungs. Note the position of the phrenic nerve, now in the fibrous pericardium. The right common cardinal vein has developed into the superior vena cava.

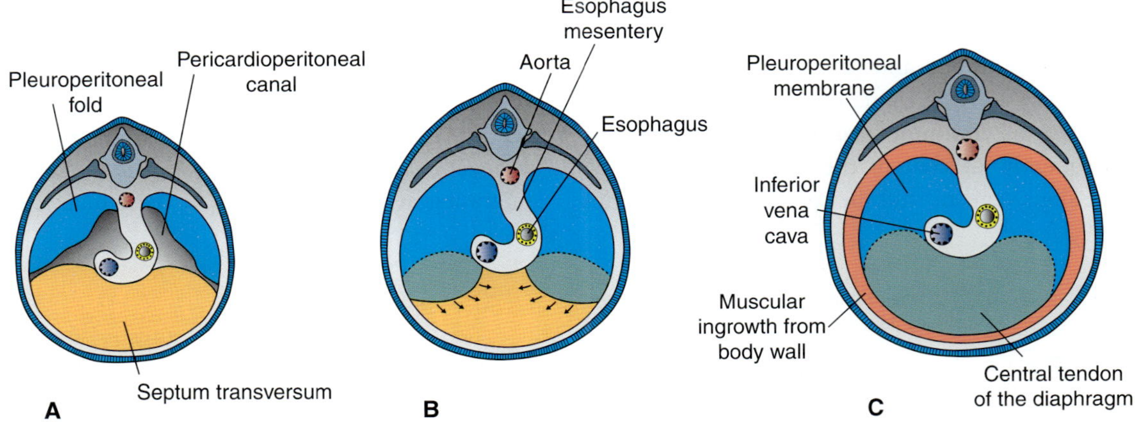


**FIGURE 7.7** Development of the diaphragm. **A.** Pleuroperitoneal folds appear at the beginning of the fifth week. **B.** By the seventh week, pleuroperitoneal membranes grow over the septum transversum, fuse with the mesentery of the esophagus, and continue to grow toward each other. **C.** Transverse section at the fourth month of development. The pleuroperitoneal membranes have fused and formed the central tendon of the diaphragm. On the periphery, they provide connective tissue scaffolding for migrating muscle cells arising from cervical segments three to five (C3–C5).

from **cervical segments three to five (C3–C5)** to form the musculature of the diaphragm. Innervation of the diaphragm is via the **phrenic nerves** that are derived from ventral primary rami of spinal nerves carrying motor and sensory fibers that also originate from C3 to C5. The reason that muscle cells and nerve fibers from cervical segments populate and innervate the diaphragm is because the cervical region is where diaphragm development originated in the fourth week. Later, in the sixth week, differential growth, whereby growth of the dorsal part of the embryo (brain and vertebral column) is greater than the ventral part, causes the diaphragm to move ventrally and caudally to its final location, resulting in the phrenic nerves taking a long course to reach their destination.

**In summary, the diaphragm is derived from the following structures:**

- Central tendon of diaphragm derived from septum transversum
- The two pleuroperitoneal membranes form the central tendon of the diaphragm and provide a connective tissue scaffold for muscle cells migrating in on the periphery.
- Muscular components from somites at cervical segments three to five
- The mesentery of the esophagus, in which the **crura** of the diaphragm develop

## Clinical Correlates

### Diaphragmatic Hernias

A **congenital diaphragmatic hernia**, one of the more common malformations in the newborn (1/2,000), may be caused by shortness of the foregut that keeps the stomach in the thoracic region. Initially, the gut tube is tightly adherent to the dorsal body wall (Fig. 7.1*D*), but thinning of the mesodermal attachment in this region causes formation of the dorsal mesentery. This mesentery suspends the gut tube in the body cavity (Fig. 7.1*E*) and allows the gut to grow longer. Failure to form the mesentery causes the gut to remain attached to the body wall and prevents its normal growth, resulting in the stomach protruding through the diaphragm into the thoracic cavity.

A more common mechanism for the origin of diaphragmatic hernias occurs when muscle cells fail to populate a region of the pleuroperitoneal membranes resulting in a weakened area and subsequent herniation of abdominal organs into the thoracic cavity (Fig. 7.8). The primary cause for the muscle deficiency appears to reside in fibroblasts in the pleuroperitoneal membranes that fail to provide the appropriate scaffolding and/or guidance cues for migrating myoblasts.

Regardless of the origin of the defects, those that are most severe allow abdominal organs, such as the stomach, intestines, liver, and/or spleen to enter the thoracic cavity. Eighty-five percent to 90% of severe defects occur on the left side due to failure of the muscle cells to properly invade and populate this region (Fig. 7.8*A*). The presence of abdominal organs in the thoracic cavity inhibits lung growth causing hypoplasia of the lungs and often results in death of the baby.

Occasionally, muscle tissue fails to develop in other smaller regions of the diaphragm providing additional sites for hernias to occur. Frequently, these smaller hernias arise in the **parasternal region** and a small peritoneal sac containing intestinal loops may enter the chest between the sternal and costal portions of the diaphragm (Fig. 7.8*A*). Sometimes, these smaller abnormalities can go undetected until later in life.

Another type of smaller diaphragmatic hernia, an **esophageal hernia**, is thought to be due to congenital shortness of the gut tube in the region of the lower esophagus. This defect represents a milder form of the gut shortening mentioned previously.

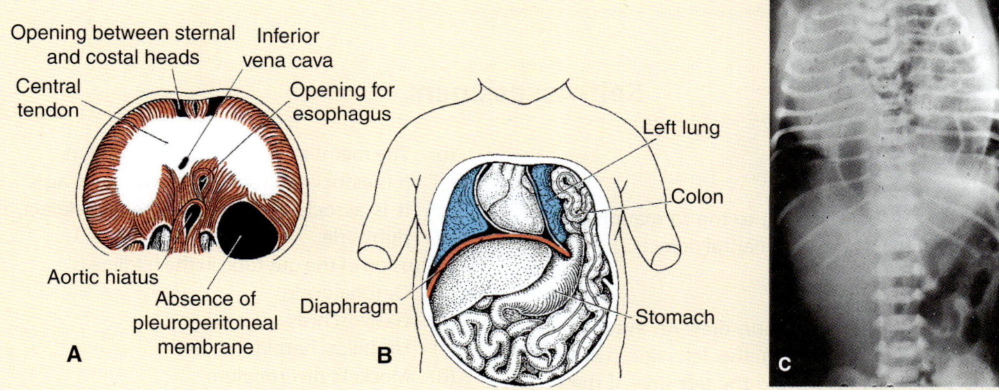


**FIGURE 7.8** Congenital diaphragmatic hernia. **A.** Abdominal surface of the diaphragm showing a large defect of the pleuroperitoneal membrane. **B.** Hernia of the intestinal loops and part of the stomach into the left pleural cavity. The heart and mediastinum are frequently pushed to the right, and the left lung is compressed. **C.** Radiograph of a newborn with a large defect in the left side of the diaphragm. Abdominal viscera have entered the thorax through the defect.

## SUMMARY

- At the end of the third week, the neural tube is elevating and closing dorsally.
- The gut tube is rolling and closing ventrally to create a "tube on top of a tube." Mesoderm holds the tubes together.
- The **lateral plate mesoderm** splits to form a **visceral (splanchnic) layer** associated with the gut and a **parietal (somatic) layer** that, together with overlying ectoderm, forms the **lateral body wall folds**.
- The space between the visceral and parietal layers of lateral plate mesoderm is the **primitive body cavity** (Fig. 7.1).
- When the lateral body wall folds move ventrally and fuse in the midline, the body cavity is closed, except in the region of the connecting stalk (Figs. 7.1 and 7.2).
- The gut tube maintains an attachment to the yolk sac as the **yolk sac (vitelline) duct**.
- The lateral body wall folds also pull the amnion with them so that the amnion surrounds the embryo and extends over the **connecting stalk**, which becomes the **umbilical cord** (Figs. 7.1*D* and 7.2*D*).
- Failure of the ventral body wall to close results in **ventral body wall defects**, such as the following:
  - **Ectopia cordis**
  - **Gastroschisis**
  - **Exstrophy of the bladder and cloaca** (Fig. 7.3)
- Parietal mesoderm will form the **parietal layer of serous membranes** lining the outside (walls) of the **peritoneal, pleural**, and **pericardial cavities**.

(*Continued*)

Part 1

- The **visceral layer** will form the **visceral layer of the serous membranes** covering the lungs, heart, and abdominal organs.
- These layers are continuous at the root of each organ as the organs lie in their respective cavities. (This relationship is similar to the picture created when you stick a finger [organ] into the side of a balloon: The layer of the balloon surrounding the finger [organ] being the visceral layer, and the rest of the balloon being the somatic or parietal layer. The space between is the "primitive body cavity." The two layers of the balloon are continuous at the base [root] of the finger.)
- In the gut, the layers form the **peritoneum** and in places suspend the gut from the body wall as double layers of peritoneum called **mesenteries** (Fig. 7.1*E*). Mesenteries provide a pathway for vessels, nerves, and lymphatics to the organs.
- Initially, the gut tube from the caudal end of the foregut to the end of the hindgut is suspended from the dorsal body wall by **dorsal mesentery** (Fig. 7.1*E*). **Ventral mesentery**, derived from the septum transversum, exists only in the region of the terminal part of the esophagus, the stomach, and the upper portion of the duodenum (see Chapter 15).
- The **diaphragm** divides the body cavity into the **thoracic** and **peritoneal cavities**.
- The **diaphragm** develops from three components:
  - **Pleuroperitoneal membranes form the central tendon as well as connective tissue in their periphery to provide scaffolding and guidance cues for migrating muscle cells.**
  - **Dorsal mesentery of the esophagus forms the crura.**
  - **Muscular components from somites are present at cervical levels three to five (C3–C5)** (Fig. 7.7).
- Because the diaphragm begins its development opposite cervical segments three to five and because muscle cells for the diaphragm originate from somites at these segments, the **phrenic nerve**, that innervates the diaphragm, also arises from these segments of the spinal cord (**C3, C4, and C5 keep the diaphragm alive**!).
- Congenital diaphragmatic hernias involving a defect of the pleuroperitoneal membrane on the left side occur frequently.
- The **thoracic cavity** is divided into the **pericardial cavity** and two **pleural cavities** for the lungs by the **pleuropericardial membranes** (Fig. 7.6).

## Self-Assessment

### Comprehensive Questions

1. Explain the formation of the pleural cavity.
2. Write down the components contributing to the formation of the diaphragm with a note on its developmental defects.

### Problem Solving Questions

1. A newborn infant cannot breathe and soon dies. An autopsy reveals a large diaphragmatic defect on the left side, with the stomach and the intestines occupying the left side of the thorax. Both lungs are severely hypoplastic. What is the embryological basis for this defect?
2. A child is born with a large defect lateral to the umbilicus. Most of the large and the small bowel protrude through the defect and are not covered by amnion. What is the embryological basis for this abnormality, and should you be concerned that other malformations may be present?
3. Explain why the phrenic nerve, which supplies motor and sensory fibers to the diaphragm, originates from cervical segments when most of the diaphragm is in the thorax. From which cervical segments does the nerve originate?

### Multiple Choice Questions

1. Body cavity is formed at
   (a) End of second week
   (b) End of third week
   (c) End of fourth week
   (d) End of fifth week
2. A 27-year-old primigravida presented with 19 weeks of amenorrhea in an obstetrics clinic. Her routine antenatal ultrasound revealed an abdominal swelling enclosed in a membrane with herniation of liver and intestinal loops. She was then admitted for termination of pregnancy. *Identify the **correct** statement regarding the anomaly in the given case.*
   (a) It results from failure of fusion of lateral body folds.
   (b) The membrane covering it is amnion.
   (c) It is associated with young maternal age.
   (d) It is associated with paramedian defect, usually on the right side.
3. Protrusion of the gut tube in the midline is
   (a) Omphalocele
   (b) Gastroschisis
   (c) Umbilical hernia
   (d) Meckel's diverticulum
4. Split in which mesoderm forms the primitive body cavity?
   (a) Paraxial mesoderm
   (b) Lateral plate mesoderm
   (c) Septum transversum
   (d) Intermediate mesoderm
5. Diaphragm is developed from all of the following except
   (a) Two pleuroperitoneal membranes
   (b) Somites of three to five thoracic segments
   (c) Mesentery of the esophagus
   (d) Septum transversum
6. In gastroschisis, the defect in the anterior abdominal wall is due to
   (a) Failure of fusion of the two lateral folds
   (b) Failure in reduction of physiological hernia
   (c) Defect in the septum transversum
   (d) Failure in fusion of the pleuroperitoneal membrane
7. A newborn baby comes with a discharge from the umbilicus (weeping umbilicus). What would be the most probable diagnosis?
   (a) Omphalocele
   (b) Patent vitellointestinal duct
   (c) Umbilical hernia
   (d) Failure of fusion of lateral body wall

### Answers

1. (b) 2. (b) 3. (a) 4. (b) 5. (b) 6. (a) 7. (b)

# CHAPTER 8

# Third Month to Birth: The Fetus and Placenta

Part 1

## Specific Learning Objectives

- Fetal growth from 8 weeks to birth
- Developmental horizons during fetal life
- Time of birth
- Low birth weight
- Placenta
  - Development of placenta: Changes in trophoblast and decidua
  - Structure of human placenta
  - Placental circulation and placental barriers
  - Function of placenta
- Amniotic fluid
- Umbilical cord
- Twinning
- Placental hormones and parturition

## Competencies Covered

AN80.1 Describe the formation, functions and fate of chorion: amnion, yolk sac, allantois, and decidua.
AN80.2 Describe the formation and structure of the umbilical cord.
AN80.3 Describe the formation of placenta, its physiological functions, fetomaternal circulation and placental barrier.
AN80.4 Describe the embryological basis of twinning in monozygotic and dizygotic twins.
AN80.5 Describe the role of placental hormones in uterine growth and parturition.
AN80.6 Explain the embryological basis of estimation of the fetal age.
AN80.7 Describe the various types of umbilical cord attachments.

## DEVELOPMENT OF THE FETUS

The period from the beginning of the ninth week to birth is known as the **fetal period**. It is characterized by maturation of tissues and organs and rapid growth of the body. The length of the fetus is usually indicated as the **crown-rump length (CRL)** (sitting height) or as the **crown-heel length (CHL)**, the measurement from the vertex of the skull to the heel (standing height). These measurements, expressed in centimeters, are correlated with the age of the fetus in weeks or months (Table 8.1). Growth in length is particularly striking during the third, fourth, and fifth months, whereas an increase in weight is most striking during the last 2 months of gestation. In general, **the length of pregnancy is considered to be 280 days, or 40 weeks after the onset of the last normal menstrual period (LNMP) or, more accurately, 266 days or 38 weeks after fertilization**. For the purposes of the following discussion, age is calculated from the time of fertilization and is expressed in weeks or calendar months.

**Table 8.1 Growth in Length and Weight During the Fetal Period**

| Age (wk) | CRL (cm) | Weight (g) |
|---|---|---|
| 9–12 | 5–8 | 10–45 |
| 13–16 | 9–14 | 60–200 |
| 17–20 | 15–19 | 250–450 |
| 21–24 | 20–23 | 500–820 |
| 25–28 | 24–27 | 900–1,300 |
| 29–32 | 28–30 | 1,400–2,100 |
| 33–36 | 31–34 | 2,200–2,900 |
| 37–38 | 35–36 | 3,000–3,400 |

*CRL*, crown-rump length.

### Monthly Changes

One of the most striking changes taking place during fetal life is the relative slowdown in growth of the head compared with the rest of the body. At the beginning of the third month, the head constitutes approximately half of the CRL (Figs. 8.1 and 8.2). By the beginning of the fifth month, the size of the head is about one-third of the CHL, and at birth, it is approximately one-quarter of the CHL (Fig. 8.2). Hence, over time, growth of the body accelerates but that of the head slows down.

During the **third month**, the face becomes more human looking (Figs. 8.3 and 8.4). The eyes, initially directed laterally, move to the ventral aspect of the face, and the ears come to lie close to their definitive position at the side of the head (Fig. 8.3). The limbs reach their relative length in comparison with the rest of the body, although the lower limbs are still a little shorter and less well developed than the upper

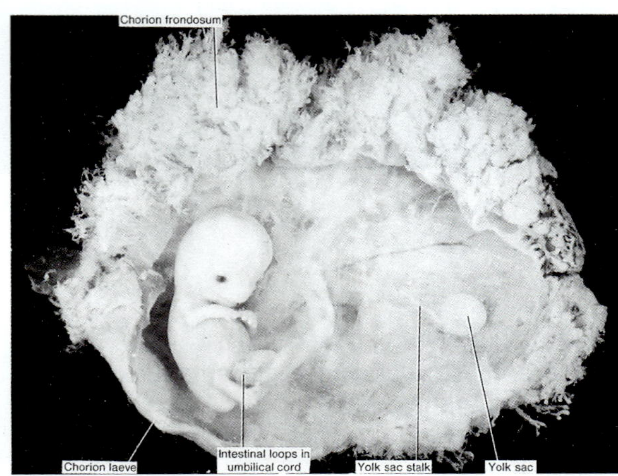


**FIGURE 8.1** A 9-week fetus. Note the large head size compared with that of the rest of the body. The yolk sac and long vitelline duct are visible in the chorionic cavity. Note the umbilical cord and herniation of intestinal loops. One side of the chorion has many villi (chorion frondosum), whereas the other side is almost smooth (chorion laeve).

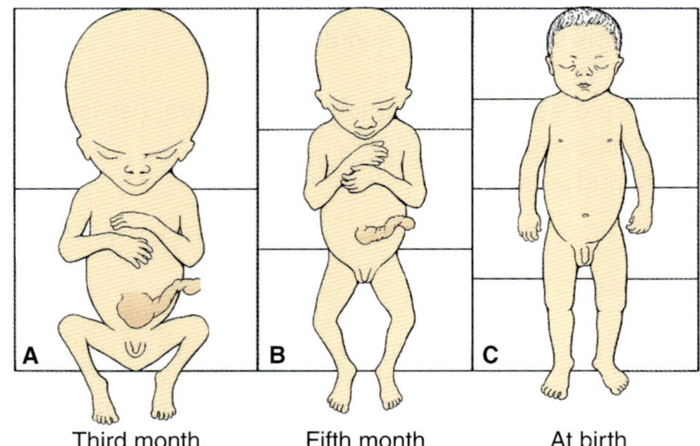


**FIGURE 8.2** Size of the head in relation to the rest of the body at various stages of development.

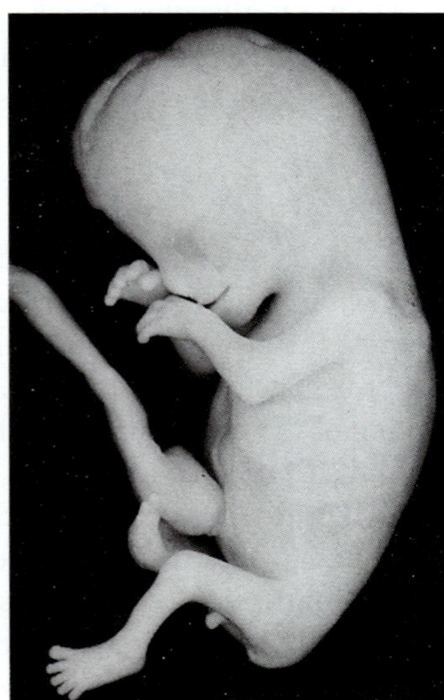

**FIGURE 8.3** An 11-week fetus. The umbilical cord still shows a swelling at its base, caused by herniated intestinal loops. The skull of this fetus lacks the normal smooth contours. Fingers and toes are well developed.

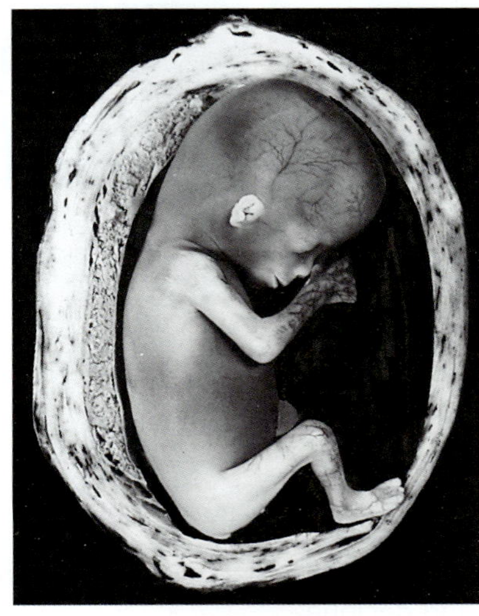

**FIGURE 8.4** A 12-week fetus in utero. Note the extremely thin skin and underlying blood vessels. The face has all of the human characteristics, but the ears are still primitive. Movements begin at this time but are usually not felt by the mother.

extremities. **Primary ossification centers** are present in the long bones and skull by the 12th week. Also, by the 12th week, external genitalia develop to such a degree that the sex of the fetus can be determined by external examination (ultrasound). During the 6th week, **intestinal loops cause a large swelling (herniation) in the umbilical cord**, but by the 12th week, the loops have withdrawn into the abdominal cavity. At the end of the third month, reflex activity can be evoked in aborted fetuses, indicating muscular activity.

During the **fourth** and **fifth months**, the fetus lengthens rapidly (Fig. 8.5 and Table 8.1), and at the end of the first half of intrauterine life, its CRL is approximately 15 cm, about half the total length of the newborn. The weight of the fetus increases little during this period and by the end of the fifth month is still <500 g. The fetus is covered with fine hair, called **lanugo**

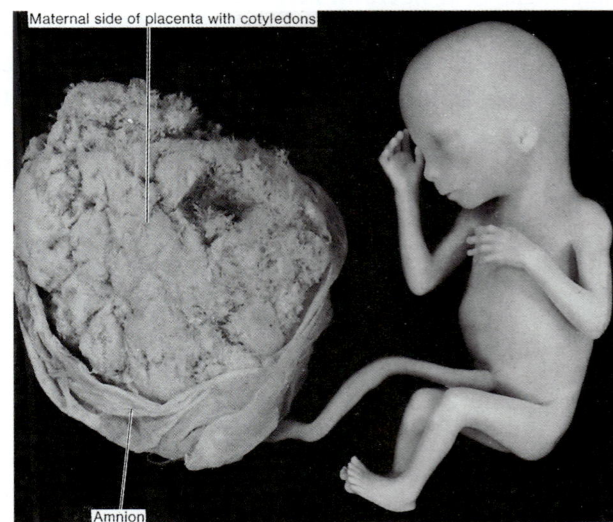


**FIGURE 8.5** An 18-week fetus connected to the placenta by its umbilical cord. The skin of the fetus is thin because of lack of subcutaneous fat. Note the placenta with its cotyledons and the amnion.

**hair**; eyebrows and head hair are also visible. **During the fifth month, movements of the fetus can be felt by the mother.**

During the **second half of intrauterine life**, weight increases considerably, particularly during the last 2.5 months, when 50% of the full-term weight (approximately 3,200 g) is added. During the **sixth month**, the skin of the fetus is reddish and has a wrinkled appearance because of the lack of underlying connective tissue. A fetus born early in the sixth month has great difficulty surviving. Although several organ systems are able to function, the respiratory system and the central nervous system have not differentiated sufficiently, and coordination between the two systems is not yet well established. By 6.5 to 7 months, the fetus has a CRL of about 25 cm and weighs approximately 1,100 g. If born at this time, the infant has a 90% chance of surviving. Some developmental events occurring during the first 7 months are indicated in Table 8.2.

During the last 2 months, the fetus obtains well-rounded contours as the result of deposition of subcutaneous fat (Fig. 8.6). By the end of intrauterine life, the skin is covered by a whitish, fatty substance (**vernix caseosa**) composed of secretory products from sebaceous glands.

**Table 8.2 Developmental Horizons During Fetal Life**

| Event | Age (wk) |
|---|---|
| Taste buds appear | 7 |
| Swallowing | 10 |
| Respiratory movements | 14–16 |
| Sucking movements | 24 |
| Some sounds can be heard | 24–26 |
| Eyes sensitive to light[a] | 28 |

[a]Recognition of form and color occurs postnatally.

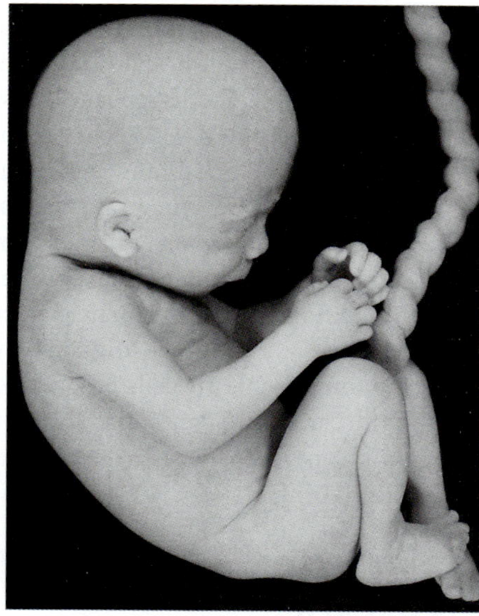

**FIGURE 8.6** A 7-month fetus. This fetus would be able to survive. It has well-rounded contours as a result of deposition of subcutaneous fat. Note the twisting of the umbilical cord.

At the end of the **ninth month**, the skull has the largest circumference of all parts of the body, an important fact with regard to its passage through the birth canal. At the time of birth, the weight of a normal fetus is 3,000 to 3,400 g, its CRL is about 36 cm, and its CHL is about 50 cm. Sexual characteristics are pronounced, and the testes should be in the scrotum.

## Time of Birth

The date of birth is most accurately indicated as 266 days, or 38 weeks, after fertilization. The oocyte is usually fertilized within 12 hours of ovulation; however, sperm deposited in the reproductive tract up to 6 days prior to ovulation can survive to fertilize oocytes. Thus, most pregnancies occur when sexual intercourse occurs within a 6-day period that ends on the day of ovulation. A pregnant woman usually will see her obstetrician when she has missed two successive menstrual bleeds. By that time, her recollection about coitus is usually vague, and it is readily understandable that the day of fertilization is difficult to determine.

The obstetrician calculates the date of birth as 280 days or 40 weeks from the first day of the LNMP. In women with regular 28-day menstrual periods, the method is fairly accurate, but when cycles are irregular, substantial miscalculations may be made. An additional complication occurs when the woman has some bleeding about 14 days after fertilization as a result of erosive activity by the implanting blastocyst (see Chapter 4, "Day 13," p. 43). Hence, the day of delivery is not always easy to determine. Most fetuses are born within 10 to 14 days of the calculated delivery date. If they are born much earlier, they are categorized as **premature**; if born later, they are considered **postmature**.

Occasionally, the age of an embryo or small fetus must be determined. By combining data on the onset of the last menstrual period with fetal length, weight, and other morphological characteristics typical for a given month of development, a reasonable estimate of the age of the fetus can be formulated. A valuable tool for assisting in this determination is **ultrasound**, which can provide an accurate (1 to 2 days) measurement of CRL during the 7th to 14th weeks. Measurements commonly used in the 16th to 30th weeks are **biparietal diameter (BPD)**, **head** and **abdominal circumference**, and **femur length**. An accurate determination of fetal size and age is important for managing pregnancy, especially if the mother has a small pelvis or if the baby has a birth defect.

# FETAL MEMBRANES AND PLACENTA

The placenta is the organ that facilitates nutrient and gas exchange between the maternal and fetal compartments. As the fetus begins the ninth week of development, its demands for nutritional and other factors increase, causing major changes in the placenta. Foremost among these is an increase in surface area between maternal and fetal components to facilitate exchange. The disposition of fetal membranes is also altered as production of amniotic fluid increases.

## Clinical Correlates

### Low Birth Weight

There is considerable variation in fetal length and weight, and sometimes, these values do not correspond with the calculated age of the fetus in months or weeks. Most factors influencing length and weight are genetically determined, but environmental factors also play an important role.

The average size of a newborn is 2,500 to 4,000 g (6 to 9 lb) with a length of 51 cm (20 in). The term **low birth weight (LBW)** refers to a weight <2,500 g, regardless of gestational age. Many infants weigh <2,500 g because they are **preterm** (born before 37 weeks of gestation). In contrast, the terms **intrauterine growth restriction (IUGR)** and **small for gestational age (SGA)** take into account gestational age.

**IUGR** is a term applied to infants who do not attain their optimal intrauterine growth. These infants are pathologically small and at risk for poor outcomes. Infants who are **SGA** have a birth weight that is below the 10th percentile for their gestational age. These babies may be pathologically small (they may have IUGR) or they may be constitutionally small (healthy but smaller in size). The challenge is to differentiate the two conditions so that healthy but small babies are not subjected to high-risk protocols used for babies with IUGR.

Approximately 1 in 10 babies have IUGR and therefore have an increased risk of neurological problems, congenital malformations, meconium aspiration, hypoglycemia, hypocalcemia, and respiratory distress syndrome (RDS). There are also long-term effects on these infants: In other words, what happens in the womb does not stay in the womb and adverse fetal exposures may predispose individuals to health problems as they get older. For example, babies with IUGR have been shown to have a greater chance as adults to develop a metabolic disorder later in life, such as obesity, hypertension, hypercholesterolemia, cardiovascular disease, and type 2 diabetes (called the **Barker hypothesis**).

The incidence of IUGR is higher in blacks than in whites. In India, the incidence of IUGR is almost 24%. Causative factors include chromosomal abnormalities; teratogens; congenital infections (rubella, cytomegalovirus, toxoplasmosis, and syphilis); poor maternal health (hypertension and renal and cardiac disease); the mother's nutritional status and socioeconomic level; her use of cigarettes, alcohol, and other drugs; placental insufficiency; and multiple births (e.g., twins, triplets).

The major growth-promoting factor during development before and after birth is **insulin-like growth factor 1 (IGF-1)**, which has **mitogenic and anabolic effects**. Fetal tissues express IGF-1, and serum levels are correlated with fetal growth. Mutations in the *IGF-1* gene result in IUGR, and this growth retardation is continued after birth. In contrast to the prenatal period, postnatal growth depends on **growth hormone (GH)**. This hormone binds to its receptor (growth hormone receptor [GHR]), activating a signal transduction pathway and resulting in synthesis and secretion of IGF-1. Mutations in the GHR result in **Laron dwarfism**, which is characterized by marked short stature, and sometimes blue sclera. These individuals show little or no IUGR because IGF-1 production does not depend on GH during fetal development.

### Changes in the Trophoblast

The fetal component of the placenta is derived from the trophoblast and extraembryonic mesoderm (the chorionic plate); the maternal component is derived from the uterine endometrium. By the beginning of the second month, the trophoblast is characterized by a great number of secondary and tertiary villi, which give it a radial appearance (Fig. 8.7). Stem (anchoring) villi extend from the mesoderm of the chorionic plate to the cytotrophoblast shell. The surface of the villi is formed by the syncytium, resting on a layer of cytotrophoblastic cells that in turn cover a core of vascular mesoderm (Fig. 8.8*A,C*). The capillary system developing in the core of the villous stems soon comes in contact with capillaries of the chorionic plate and connecting stalk, thus giving rise to the extraembryonic vascular system.

Maternal blood is delivered to the placenta by spiral arteries in the uterus. Erosion of these maternal vessels to release blood into intervillous spaces (Figs. 8.7 and 8.8) is accomplished by **endovascular invasion** by cytotrophoblast cells. These cells, released from the ends of anchoring villi (Figs. 8.7 and 8.8), invade the terminal ends of spiral arteries, where they replace maternal endothelial cells in the vessels' walls, creating hybrid vessels containing both fetal and maternal cells. To accomplish this process, cytotrophoblast cells undergo an epithelial-to-endothelial transition. Invasion of the spiral arteries by cytotrophoblast cells transforms these vessels from small-diameter, high-resistance vessels to larger diameter, low-resistance vessels that can provide increased quantities of maternal blood to intervillous spaces (Figs. 8.7 and 8.8).

During the following months, numerous small extensions grow out from existing stem villi and extend as **free villi** into the surrounding **lacunar** or **intervillous spaces**. Initially, these newly formed free villi are primitive (Fig. 8.8*C*), but by the beginning of the fourth month, cytotrophoblastic cells and some connective tissue cells disappear. The syncytium and endothelial wall of the blood vessels are then the only layers that separate the maternal and fetal circulations (Fig. 8.8*B,D*). Frequently, the syncytium becomes very thin, and large pieces containing several nuclei may break off and drop into the intervillous blood lakes. These pieces, known as **syncytial knots**, enter the maternal circulation and usually degenerate without causing any symptoms. Disappearance of cytotrophoblastic cells progresses from the smaller to larger villi, and although some always persist in large villi, they do not participate in the exchange between the two circulations.

## CHORION FRONDOSUM AND DECIDUA BASALIS

In the early weeks of development, villi cover the entire surface of the chorion (Fig. 8.7). As pregnancy advances, villi

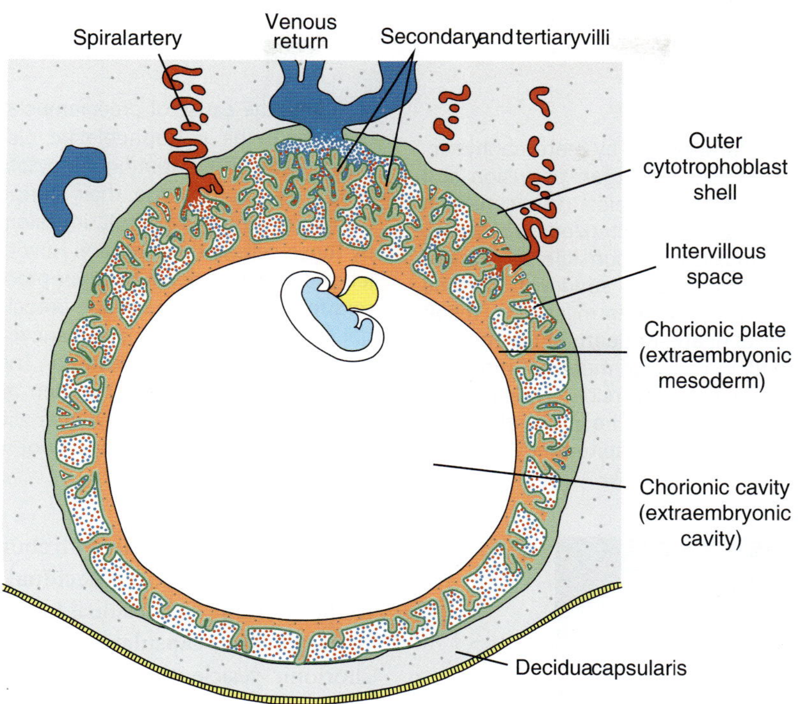


**FIGURE 8.7** Human embryo at the beginning of the second month of development. At the embryonic pole, villi are numerous and well formed; at the abembryonic pole, they are few in number and poorly developed.

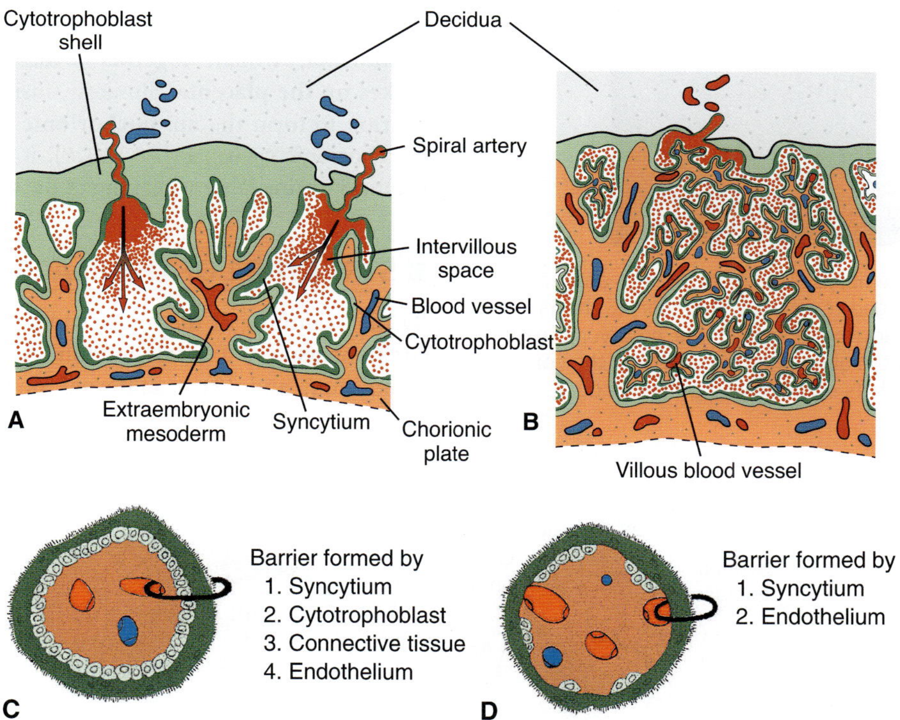


**FIGURE 8.8** Structure of villi at various stages of development. **A.** During the fourth week. The extraembryonic mesoderm penetrates the stem villi in the direction of the decidual plate. **B.** During the fourth month. In many small villi, the wall of the capillaries is in direct contact with the syncytium. **C,D.** Enlargement of the villus as shown in Figures 8.8*A,B*.

on the embryonic pole continue to grow and expand, giving rise to the **chorion frondosum** (bushy chorion). Villi on the abembryonic pole degenerate, and by the third month, this side of the chorion, now known as the **chorion laeve**, is smooth (Figs. 8.9 and 8.10*A*).

The difference between the embryonic and abembryonic poles of the chorion is also reflected in the structure of the **decidua**, the functional layer of the endometrium, which is shed during parturition. The decidua over the chorion frondosum, the **decidua basalis**, consists of a compact layer of

## Clinical Correlates

### Preeclampsia

**Preeclampsia** is a condition characterized by maternal hypertension and proteinuria due to reduced organ perfusion and occurs in approximately 5% of pregnancies. The condition may progress to eclampsia, which is characterized by seizures. In India, toxemia due to eclampsia is responsible for 10% of maternal mortality. Preeclampsia begins suddenly anytime from approximately 20 weeks' gestation to term and may result in fetal growth retardation, fetal death, or death of the mother. In fact, preeclampsia is a leading cause of maternal mortality in the United States and is completely reversible by delivery of the baby. However, delivery too early puts the infant at risk for complications related to preterm birth. Despite many years of research, the cause of preeclampsia is unknown. The condition appears to be a trophoblastic disorder related to failed or incomplete differentiation of cytotrophoblast cells, many of which do not undergo their normal epithelial-to-endothelial transformation. As a result, invasion of maternal blood vessels by these cells is rudimentary. How these cellular abnormalities lead to hypertension and other problems is not clear. Risk factors for preeclampsia include preeclampsia in a previous pregnancy, nulliparity (first pregnancy), obesity, family history of preeclampsia, multiple gestation (twins or more), and medical conditions, such as hypertension and diabetes. Preeclampsia also commonly occurs in women with hydatidiform moles (see Chapter 4, p. 45) in which case it occurs early in pregnancy.



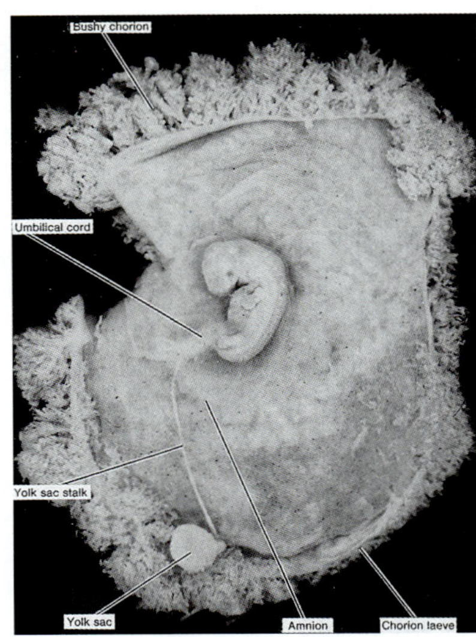


**FIGURE 8.9** A 6-week embryo. The amniotic sac and chorionic cavity have been opened to expose the embryo, showing the bushy appearance of the trophoblast at the embryonic pole in contrast to small villi at the abembryonic pole. Note the connecting stalk and yolk sac with its extremely long vitelline duct.

large cells, **decidual cells**, with abundant amounts of lipids and glycogen. This layer, the **decidual plate**, is tightly connected to the chorion. The decidual layer over the abembryonic pole is the **decidua capsularis** (Fig. 8.10*A*). With growth of the chorionic vesicle, this layer becomes stretched and degenerates. Subsequently, the chorion laeve comes into contact with the uterine wall (**decidua parietalis**) on the opposite side of the uterus, and the two fuse (Figs. 8.10, 8.11, and 8.12), obliterating the uterine lumen. Hence, the only portion of the chorion participating in the exchange process is the **chorion frondosum, which, together with the decidua basalis, makes up the placenta**. Similarly, fusion of the amnion and chorion to form the **amniochorionic membrane** obliterates the chorionic cavity (Fig. 8.10*A*,*B*). It is this membrane that ruptures during labor (breaking of the water).

## STRUCTURE OF THE PLACENTA

By the beginning of the fourth month, the placenta has two components: (1) a **fetal portion**, formed by the chorion frondosum, and (2) a **maternal portion**, formed by the

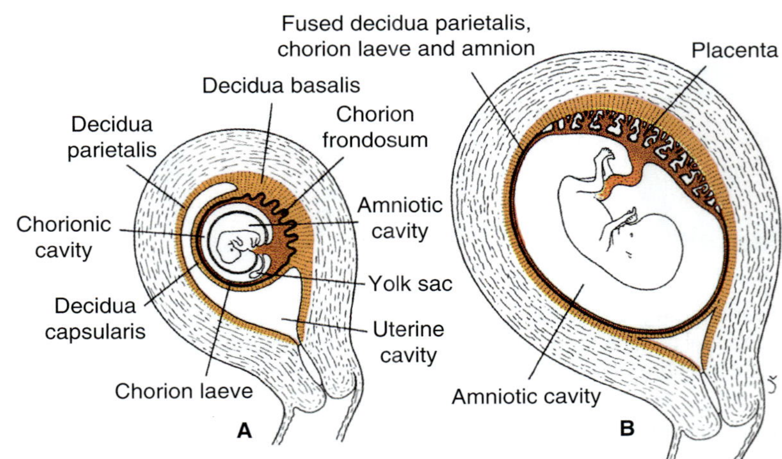


**FIGURE 8.10** Relation of fetal membranes to wall of the uterus. **A.** End of the second month. Note the yolk sac in the chorionic cavity between the amnion and chorion. At the abembryonic pole, villi have disappeared (chorion laeve). **B.** End of the third month. The amnion and chorion have fused, and the uterine cavity is obliterated by fusion of the chorion laeve and the decidua parietalis.

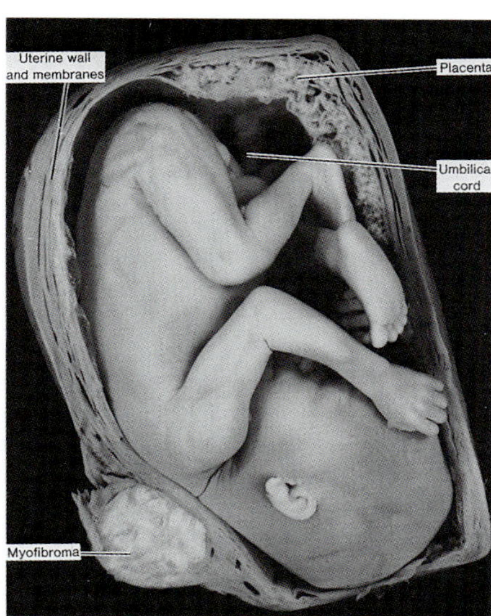


**FIGURE 8.11** A 19-week fetus in its natural position in the uterus, showing the umbilical cord and placenta. The lumen of the uterus is obliterated. In the wall of the uterus is a large growth, a myofibroma.

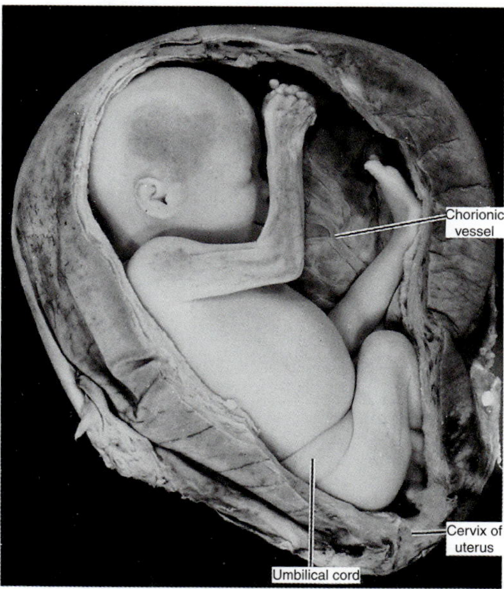


**FIGURE 8.12** A 23-week fetus in the uterus. Portions of the wall of the uterus and the amnion have been removed to show the fetus. In the background are placental vessels converging toward the umbilical cord. The umbilical cord is tightly wound around the abdomen, possibly causing abnormal fetal position in the uterus (breech position).

decidua basalis (Fig. 8.10*B*). On the fetal side, the placenta is bordered by the **chorionic plate** (Fig. 8.13); on its maternal side, it is bordered by the decidua basalis, of which the **decidual plate** is most intimately incorporated into the placenta. In the **junctional zone**, trophoblast and decidual cells intermingle. This zone, characterized by decidual and syncytial giant cells, is rich in amorphous extracellular material. By this time, most cytotrophoblast cells have degenerated. Between the chorionic and decidual plates are the intervillous spaces, which are filled with maternal blood. They are derived from lacunae in the syncytiotrophoblast and are lined with syncytium of fetal origin. The villous trees grow into the intervillous blood lakes (Figs. 8.8 and 8.13).

During the fourth and fifth months, the decidua forms a number of **decidual septa**, which project into intervillous spaces but do not reach the chorionic plate (Fig. 8.13). These septa have a core of maternal tissue, but their surface is covered by a layer of syncytial cells so that at all times, a syncytial layer separates maternal blood in intervillous lakes from fetal tissue of the villi. As a result of this septum formation, the placenta is divided into a number of compartments, or **cotyledons** (Fig. 8.14). Because the decidual septa do not reach the chorionic plate, contact between intervillous spaces in the various cotyledons is maintained.

As a result of the continuous growth of the fetus and expansion of the uterus, the placenta also enlarges. Its increase in surface area roughly parallels that of the expanding uterus, and throughout pregnancy, it covers approximately 15% to 30% of the internal surface of the uterus. The increase in thickness of the placenta results from arborization of existing villi and is not caused by further penetration into maternal tissues. The placenta is normally attached to the upper uterine segment. It

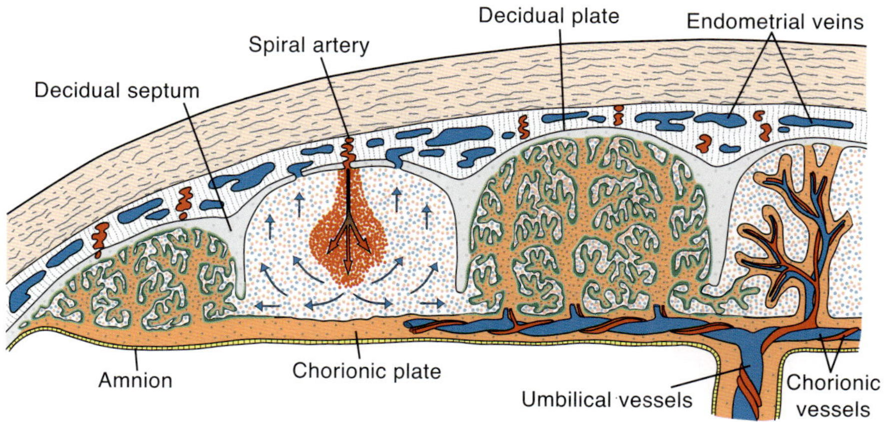


**FIGURE 8.13** The placenta in the second half of pregnancy. The cotyledons are partially separated by the decidual (maternal) septa. Most of the intervillous blood returns to the maternal circulation by way of the endometrial veins. A small portion enters neighboring cotyledons. The intervillous spaces are lined by syncytium.

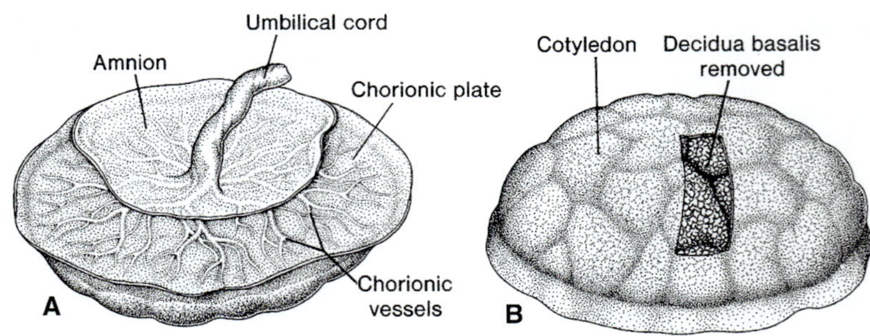


**FIGURE 8.14** A full-term placenta. **A.** Fetal side. The chorionic plate and umbilical cord are covered by amnion. **B.** Maternal side showing the cotyledons. In one area, the decidua has been removed. The maternal side of the placenta is always carefully inspected at birth, and frequently, one or more cotyledons with a whitish appearance are present because of excessive fibrinoid formation and infarction of a group of intervillous lakes.



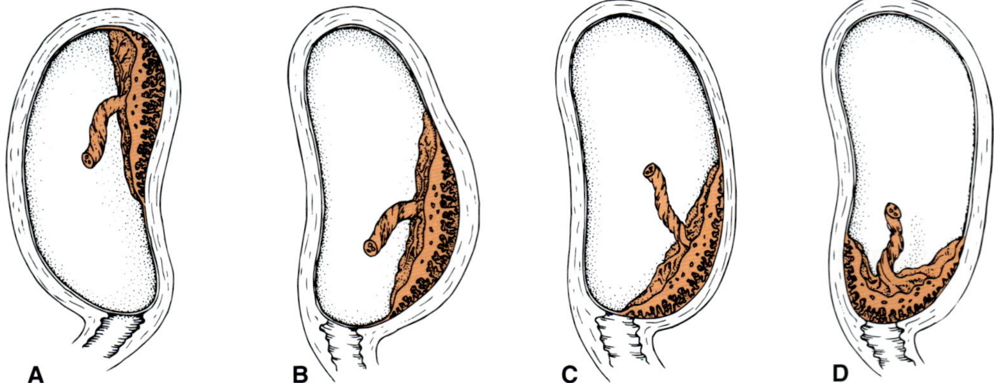


**FIGURE 8.15** Placenta previa. **A.** Normal. **B.** Low implantation. **C.** Partial placenta previa. **D.** Total placenta previa.

can sometimes have an abnormal implantation where it extends to the lower uterine segment, partially covering the internal os or completely covering the internal os where it is known as placenta previa (Fig. 8.15). This condition can lead to severe postpartum bleeding depending upon the site of implantation.

## Anomalies of Placenta Implantation (Fig. 8.16)

- **Decidua (normal):** The placenta attaches to the uterus until labor, when it separates with the help of contractions.

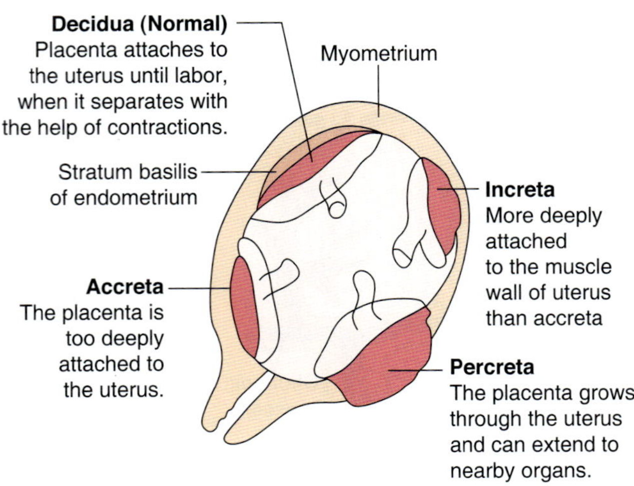


**FIGURE 8.16** Anomalies of placenta implantation in the uterus.

- **Accreta:** The placenta is too deeply attached to the uterus.
- **Increta:** The placenta is more deeply attached to the muscle wall of the uterus than in accreta.
- **Percreta:** The placenta grows through the uterus and can extend to the nearby organs.

## Full-Term Placenta

At full term, the placenta is discoid with a diameter of 15 to 25 cm, is approximately 3 cm thick, and weighs about 500 to 600 g. At birth, it is torn from the uterine wall and, approximately 30 minutes after birth of the child, is expelled from the uterine cavity as the afterbirth. When the placenta is viewed from the **maternal side**, 15 to 20 slightly bulging areas, the **cotyledons**, covered by a thin layer of decidua basalis, are clearly recognizable (Fig. 8.14*B*). Grooves between the cotyledons are formed by decidual septa.

The **fetal surface** of the placenta is covered entirely by the chorionic plate. A number of large arteries and veins, the **chorionic vessels**, converge toward the umbilical cord (Fig. 8.14*A*). The chorion, in turn, is covered by the amnion. Attachment of the **umbilical cord** is usually **eccentric** and occasionally even **marginal**. Rarely, however, does it insert into the chorionic membranes outside the placenta (**velamentous insertion**).

## Circulation of the Placenta

Cotyledons receive their blood through 80 to 100 spiral arteries that pierce the decidual plate and enter the intervillous spaces at more or less regular intervals (Fig. 8.13). Pressure in these arteries forces the blood deep into the intervillous spaces and bathes the numerous small villi of the villous tree in oxygenated blood. As the pressure decreases, blood flows back from the chorionic plate toward the decidua, where it enters the endometrial veins (Fig. 8.13). Hence, blood from the intervillous lakes drains back into the maternal circulation through the endometrial veins.

Collectively, the intervillous spaces of a mature placenta contain approximately 150 mL of blood, which is replenished about three or four times per minute. This blood moves along the chorionic villi, which have a surface area of 4 to 14 $m^2$. Placental exchange does not take place in all villi, however, only in those that have fetal vessels in intimate contact with the covering syncytial membrane. In these villi, the syncytium often has a brush border consisting of numerous microvilli, which greatly increases the surface area and, consequently, the exchange rate between maternal and fetal circulations (Fig. 8.8*D*). The **placental membrane**, which separates maternal and fetal blood, is initially composed of **four layers**: (1) the endothelial lining of fetal vessels, (2) the connective tissue in the villus core, (3) the cytotrophoblastic layer, and (4) the syncytium (Fig. 8.8*C*). From the **fourth month** on, the placental membrane thins because the endothelial lining of the vessels comes in intimate contact with the syncytial membrane, greatly increasing the rate of exchange (Fig. 8.8*D*). Sometimes called the **placental barrier**, the placental membrane is not a true barrier, as many substances pass through it freely. Because the maternal blood in the intervillous spaces is separated from the fetal blood by a chorionic derivative, the human placenta is considered to be of the **hemochorial** type. Normally, there is no mixing of maternal and fetal blood. However, small numbers of fetal blood cells occasionally escape across microscopic defects in the placental membrane.

## Function of the Placenta

Main functions of the placenta are (1) **exchange of metabolic and gaseous products** between maternal and fetal bloodstreams and (2) **production of hormones**.



### *Clinical Correlates*

#### Erythroblastosis Fetalis and Fetal Hydrops

Because some fetal blood cells escape across the placental barrier, there is a potential for these cells to elicit an antibody response by the mother's immune system. The basis for this response is the fact that more than 400 red blood cell antigens have been identified, and although most do not cause problems during pregnancy, some can stimulate a maternal antibody response against fetal blood cells. This process is an example of **isoimmunization**, and if the maternal response is sufficient, the antibodies will attack and hemolyze fetal red blood cells, resulting in **hemolytic disease of the fetus and newborn**. Previously, the disease was called **erythroblastosis fetalis** because in some cases, severe hemolysis stimulated an increase in production of fetal blood cells called **erythroblasts**. However, this severity of anemia occurs only in a few cases such that hemolytic disease of the fetus and newborn is a more appropriate terminology. In rare cases, the anemia becomes so severe that **fetal hydrops** (edema and effusions into the body cavities) occurs, leading to fetal death (Fig. 8.17). Most severe cases are caused by antigens from the **CDE (Rhesus)** blood group system. The D or **Rh antigen** is the most dangerous because immunization can result from a single exposure and occurs earlier and with greater severity with each succeeding pregnancy. The maternal antibody response occurs in cases when the fetus is D (Rh)-positive and the mother is D (Rh)-negative and is elicited when fetal red blood cells enter the maternal system because of small areas of bleeding at the surface of placental villi or at birth. This condition can be prevented by screening women at their first prenatal visit for Rh blood type and for the presence of anti-D antibodies to determine if she has been sensitized previously. In Rh-negative women without anti-D antibodies, recommendations include treatment with Rh immunoglobulin at 28 weeks' gestation; following times when fetal–maternal mixing of blood may have occurred (e.g., after amniocentesis or pregnancy loss); and after delivery if the newborn is found to be Rh-positive. Since the introduction of Rh immunoglobulin in 1968, hemolytic disease in the fetus and newborn in the United States has almost been eliminated. In India and China, the incidence is low.

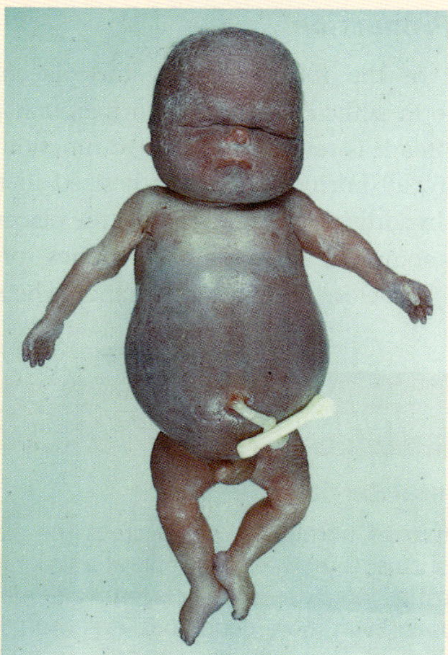

**FIGURE 8.17** Fetal hydrops caused by the accumulation of fluid in fetal tissues.

Antigens from the ABO blood group can also elicit an antibody response, but the effects are much milder than those produced by the CDE group. About 20% of all infants have an ABO maternal incompatibility, but only 5% will be clinically affected. These can be effectively treated postnatally.

### Exchange of Gases

Exchange of gases—such as oxygen, carbon dioxide, and carbon monoxide—is accomplished by simple diffusion. At term, the fetus extracts 20 to 30 mL of oxygen per minute from the maternal circulation, and even a short-term interruption of the oxygen supply is fatal to the fetus. Placental blood flow is critical to oxygen supply, as the amount of oxygen reaching the fetus primarily depends on delivery, not diffusion.

### Exchange of Nutrients and Electrolytes

Exchange of nutrients and electrolytes, such as amino acids, free fatty acids, carbohydrates, and vitamins, is rapid and increases as pregnancy advances.

### Transmission of Maternal Antibodies

Immunological competence begins to develop late in the first trimester, by which time the fetus makes all of the components of **complement**. Immunoglobulins consist almost entirely of **maternal immunoglobulin G (IgG)**, which begins to be transported from mother to fetus at approximately 14 weeks. In this manner, the fetus gains passive immunity against various infectious diseases. Newborns begin to produce their own IgG, but adult levels are not attained until the age of 3 years.

### Hormone Production

By the end of the fourth month, the placenta produces **progesterone** in sufficient amounts to maintain pregnancy if the corpus luteum is removed or fails to function properly. In all probability, all hormones are synthesized in the syncytial trophoblast. In addition to progesterone, the placenta produces increasing amounts of **estrogenic hormones**, predominantly **estriol**, until just before the end of pregnancy, when a maximum level is reached. These high levels of estrogens stimulate uterine growth and development of the mammary glands.

During the first 2 months of pregnancy, the syncytiotrophoblast also produces **human chorionic gonadotropin (hCG)**, which maintains the corpus luteum. This hormone is excreted by the mother in the urine, and in the early stages of gestation, its presence is used as an indicator of pregnancy. Another hormone produced by the placenta is **somatomammotropin** (formerly **placental lactogen**). It is a growth hormone–like substance that gives the fetus priority on maternal blood glucose and makes the mother somewhat diabetogenic. It also promotes breast development for milk production.

## AMNION AND UMBILICAL CORD

The oval line of reflection between the amnion and embryonic ectoderm (**amnio-ectodermal junction**) is the **primitive umbilical ring**. At the fifth week of development, the following structures pass through the ring (Fig. 8.19*A,C*): (1) the **connecting stalk**, containing the allantois and the umbilical vessels, consisting of two arteries and one vein; (2) the **yolk stalk (vitelline duct)**, accompanied by the vitelline vessels; and (3) the **canal connecting the intraembryonic and extraembryonic cavities** (Fig. 8.19*C*). The yolk sac proper occupies a space in the **chorionic cavity**, that is, the space between the amnion and chorionic plate (Fig. 8.19*B*).

During further development, the amniotic cavity enlarges rapidly at the expense of the chorionic cavity, and the amnion begins to envelop the connecting and yolk sac stalks, crowding them together and giving rise to the **primitive umbilical cord** (Fig. 8.19*B*). Distally, the cord contains the yolk sac stalk and umbilical vessels. More proximally, it contains some intestinal loops and the remnant of the allantois (Fig. 8.19*B,D*). The yolk sac, found in the chorionic cavity, is connected to the umbilical cord by its stalk. At the end of the third month, the

### Clinical Correlates

#### The Placental Barrier

Maternal steroidal hormones readily cross the placenta. Other hormones, such as thyroxine, do so only at a slow rate. Some synthetic progestins rapidly cross the placenta and may masculinize female fetuses. Even more dangerous was the use of the synthetic estrogen **diethylstilbestrol (DES)**, which easily crosses the placenta. This compound produced clear-cell carcinoma of the vagina and abnormalities of the cervix and uterus in females and in the testes of males in individuals who were exposed to the compound during their intrauterine life (see Chapter 9).

Although the placental barrier is frequently considered to act as a protective mechanism against damaging factors, many viruses–such as rubella, cytomegalovirus, coxsackie, variola, varicella, measles, and poliomyelitis virus–traverse the placenta without difficulty. Once in the fetus, some viruses cause infections, which may result in cell death and birth defects (see Chapter 9).

Unfortunately, most drugs and drug metabolites traverse the placenta without difficulty, and many cause serious damage to the embryo (see Chapter 9). In addition, maternal use of heroin and cocaine can cause habituation in the fetus.

#### Abnormal Types of Placenta

- **Placenta bilobata:** A placenta having two equal lobes connected with placental tissue (Fig. 8.18*A*).
- **Placenta succenturiata:** A placenta comprising a large lobe and a smaller lobe connected with a membrane (Fig. 8.18*B*).
- **Placenta circumvallate:** A circumvallate placenta (Fig. 8.18*C*) is one in which the membranes are folded back on the fetal surface of the placenta, exposing a ring of the fetal surface around the umbilical cord.
- **Velamentous insertion of cord:** In a placenta with a velamentous insertion of cord (Fig. 8.18*D*), the cord is inserted into the margin of the placenta.
- **Battledore placenta:** A battledore placenta (Fig. 8.18*E*) is a placenta in which the cord is inserted at the margin rather that at the center of the placenta as with a normal insertion.

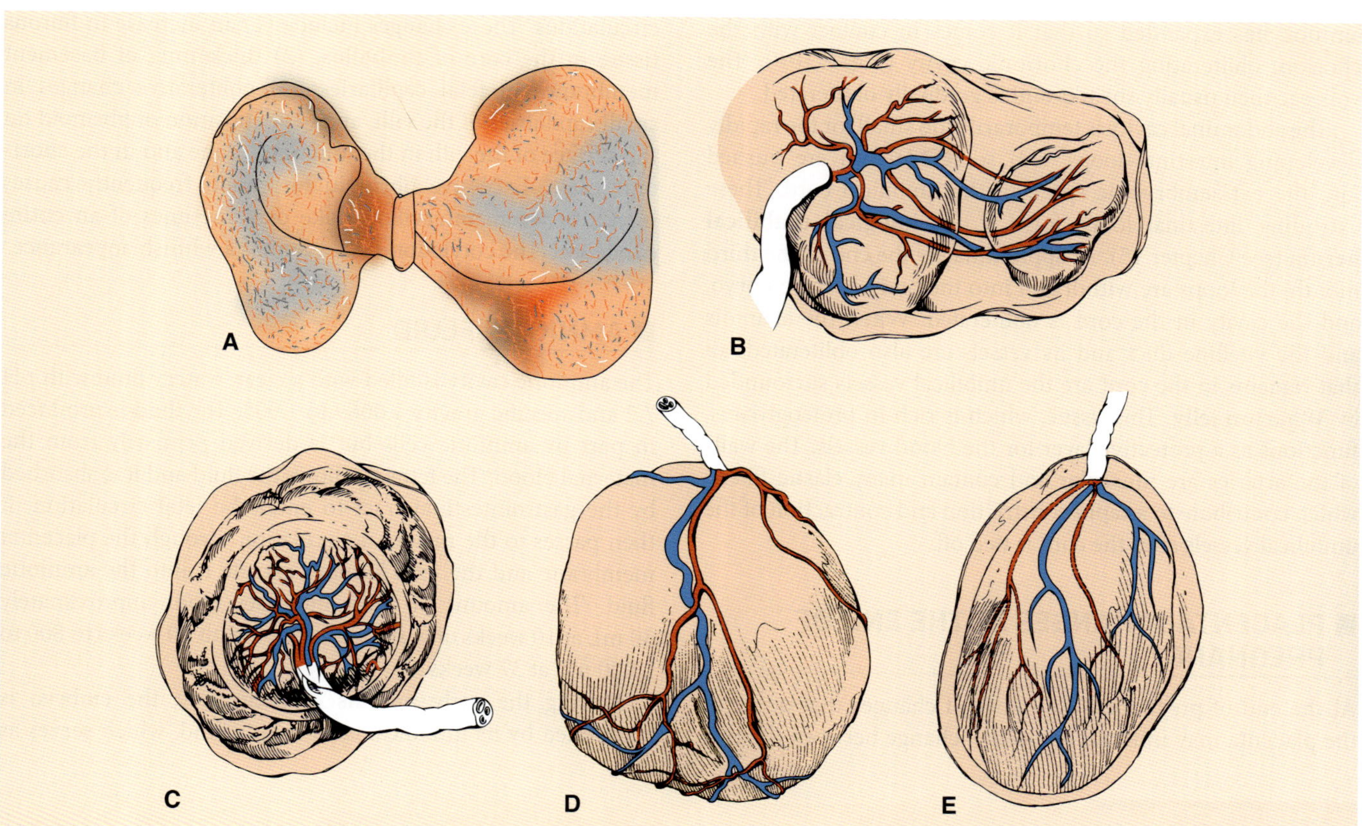


**FIGURE 8.18** **A.** Placenta bilobata. **B.** Placenta succenturiata. **C.** Placenta circumvallate. **D.** Velamentous placenta. **E.** Battledore placenta.

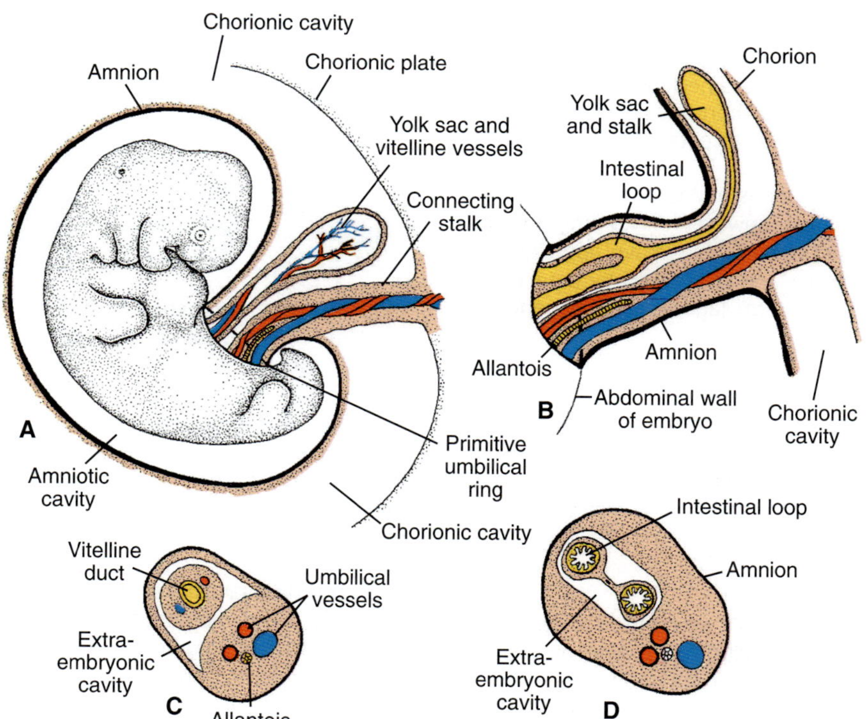


**FIGURE 8.19** **A.** A 5-week embryo showing structures passing through the primitive umbilical ring. **B.** The primitive umbilical cord of a 10-week embryo. **C.** Transverse section through the structures at the level of the umbilical ring. **D.** Transverse section through the primitive umbilical cord showing intestinal loops protruding in the cord.

amnion has expanded so that it comes in contact with the chorion, obliterating the chorionic cavity (Fig. 8.10*B*). The yolk sac then usually shrinks and is gradually obliterated.

The abdominal cavity is temporarily too small for the rapidly developing intestinal loops, and some of them are pushed into the extraembryonic space in the umbilical cord. These extruding intestinal loops form a **physiological umbilical hernia** (see Chapter 15). At approximately the end of the third month, the loops are withdrawn into the body of the embryo, and the cavity in the cord is obliterated. When the allantois and the vitelline duct and its vessels are also obliterated, all that remains in the cord are the umbilical vessels surrounded by **Wharton jelly**. This tissue, which is rich in proteoglycans, functions as a protective layer for the blood vessels. The walls of the arteries are muscular and contain many elastic fibers, which contribute to a rapid constriction and contraction of the umbilical vessels after the cord is tied off.

## PLACENTAL CHANGES AT THE END OF PREGNANCY

At the end of pregnancy, a number of changes that occur in the placenta may indicate reduced exchange between the two circulations. These changes include (1) an increase in fibrous tissue in the core of the villus, (2) thickening of basement membranes in fetal capillaries, (3) obliterative changes in small capillaries of the villi, and (4) deposition of fibrinoid on the surface of the villi in the junctional zone and in the chorionic plate. Excessive fibrinoid formation frequently causes infarction of an intervillous lake or sometimes of an entire cotyledon. The cotyledon then assumes a whitish appearance.

## AMNIOTIC FLUID

The amniotic cavity is filled with a clear, watery fluid with pH 7.2 and specific gravity 1.0069 to 1.008. The fluid is produced in part by amniotic cells but is derived primarily from the maternal blood. The fetus swallows the fluid and it is absorbed by the gastrointestinal tract to enter the fetal circulation. It then passes to the maternal circulation through the placental membrane and the fetal kidneys excrete it into the amniotic fluid. The amount of fluid increases from approximately 30 mL at 10 weeks of gestation to 450 mL at 20 weeks to 800 to 1,000 mL at 37 weeks.

During the early months of pregnancy, the embryo is suspended by its umbilical cord in this fluid, which serves as

### *Clinical Correlates*

#### Umbilical Cord Abnormalities

At birth, the umbilical cord is approximately 1 to 2 cm in diameter and 50 to 60 cm long. It is tortuous, causing **false knots**. Length of a cord reflects the amount of intrauterine movement of the fetus, and shortened cords have been observed in fetal movement disorders and with intrauterine constraint. An extremely long cord may encircle the neck of the fetus, usually without increased risk, whereas a short one may cause difficulties during delivery by pulling the placenta from its attachment in the uterus.

Normally, there are two arteries and one vein in the umbilical cord. In 1 in 200 newborns, however, only a **single umbilical artery** is present, and these babies have approximately 20% chance of having cardiac and other vascular defects. The missing artery either fails to form (agenesis) or degenerates early in development.

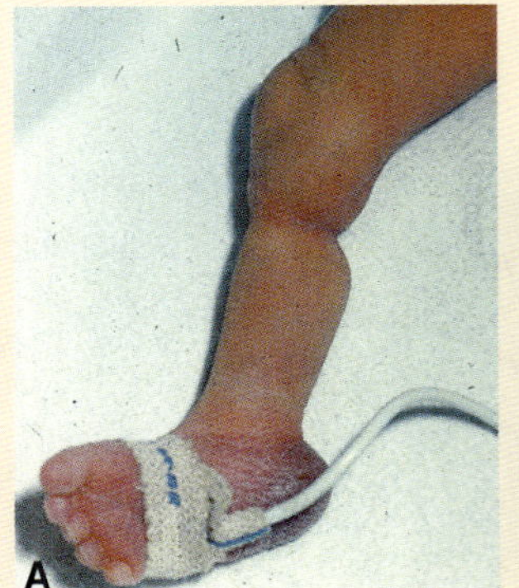


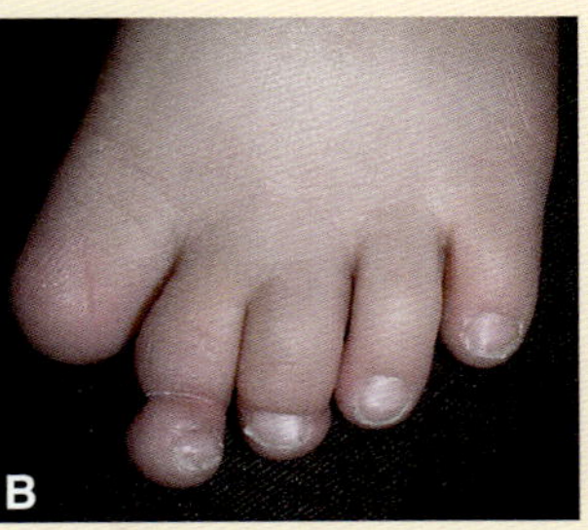


**FIGURE 8.20** Limb abnormalities caused by amniotic bands. **A.** Limb constriction ring. **B.** Digit amputation (big toe) and ring constriction (second toe).

#### Amniotic Bands

Occasionally, tears in the amnion result in **amniotic bands** that may encircle part of the fetus, particularly the limbs and digits. Amputations, **ring constrictions**, and other abnormalities, including craniofacial deformations, may result (Fig. 8.20). Origin of the bands is unknown.

#### Amniotic Fluid

**Hydramnios** or **polyhydramnios** is the term used to describe an excess of amniotic fluid (1,500 to 2,000 mL), whereas **oligohydramnios** refers to a decreased amount (<400 mL). Both conditions are associated with an increase in the incidence of birth defects. Primary causes of hydramnios include idiopathic causes (35%), maternal diabetes (25%), and congenital malformations, including central nervous system disorders (e.g., anencephaly) and gastrointestinal defects (atresias, e.g., esophageal) that prevent the infant from swallowing the fluid. Oligohydramnios is a rare occurrence that may result from renal agenesis. The lack of fluid in the amniotic cavity may constrict the fetus or there may be too little fluid for the fetus to "breathe" into its lungs resulting in lung hypoplasia.

**Premature rupture of the membranes (PROM)** refers to rupture of the membranes before uterine contractions begin and occurs in 10% of pregnancies. **Preterm** PROM occurs before 37 completed weeks of pregnancy, occurs in 3% of pregnancies, and is a common cause of preterm labor. Causes of preterm PROM are unknown, but risk factors include a previous pregnancy affected by prematurity or PROM, black race, smoking, infections, and severe polyhydramnios.

a protective cushion. The fluid (1) absorbs jolts, (2) prevents adherence of the embryo to the amnion, and (3) allows for fetal movements. The volume of amniotic fluid is replaced every 3 hours. From the beginning of the fifth month, the fetus swallows its own amniotic fluid, and it is estimated that it drinks about 400 mL a day, about half of the total amount. Fetal urine is added daily to the amniotic fluid in the fifth month, but this urine is mostly water because the placenta is functioning as an exchange for metabolic wastes. During childbirth, the amniochorionic membrane forms a hydrostatic wedge that helps to dilate the cervical canal.

## FETAL MEMBRANES IN TWINS

The frequency of multiple gestation (e.g., twins, triplets) has increased substantially in recent years and now accounts for over 3% of all live births in the United States. The rate of twin births has increased to a high of 32.6 per 1,000 births in 2008. The reasons for this increase are twofold: the increasing age of mothers at the time of their infants' birth and the increasing use of fertility treatments, including assisted reproductive technologies (ARTs).

### Dizygotic Twins

Approximately 90% of twins are **dizygotic**, or **fraternal**, and their incidence increases with maternal age (doubling at age 35 years) and with fertility procedures, including ART. They result from simultaneous shedding of two oocytes and fertilization by different spermatozoa. Because the two zygotes have different genetic constitutions, the twins have no more resemblance than any other brothers or sisters. They may or may not be of different sex. The zygotes implant individually in the uterus, and usually each develops its own placenta, amnion, and chorionic sac (Fig. 8.21*A*). Sometimes, however, the two placentas are so close together that they fuse. Similarly, the walls of the chorionic sacs may also come into close apposition and fuse (Fig. 8.21*B*). Occasionally, each dizygotic twin possesses red blood cells of two different types (**erythrocyte mosaicism**), indicating that fusion of the two placentas was so intimate that red cells were exchanged.

### Monozygotic Twins

The second type of twins, which develops from a single fertilized ovum, is **monozygotic**, or **identical**, twins. The rate for monozygotic twins is 3 to 4 per 1,000. They result from splitting of the zygote at various stages of development. The earliest separation is believed to occur at the two-cell stage, in which case two separate zygotes develop. The blastocysts implant separately, and each embryo has its own placenta and chorionic sac (Fig. 8.22*A*). Although the arrangement of the membranes of these twins resembles that of dizygotic twins, the two can be recognized as partners of a monozygotic pair by their strong resemblance in blood groups, fingerprints, sex, and external appearance, such as eye and hair color.

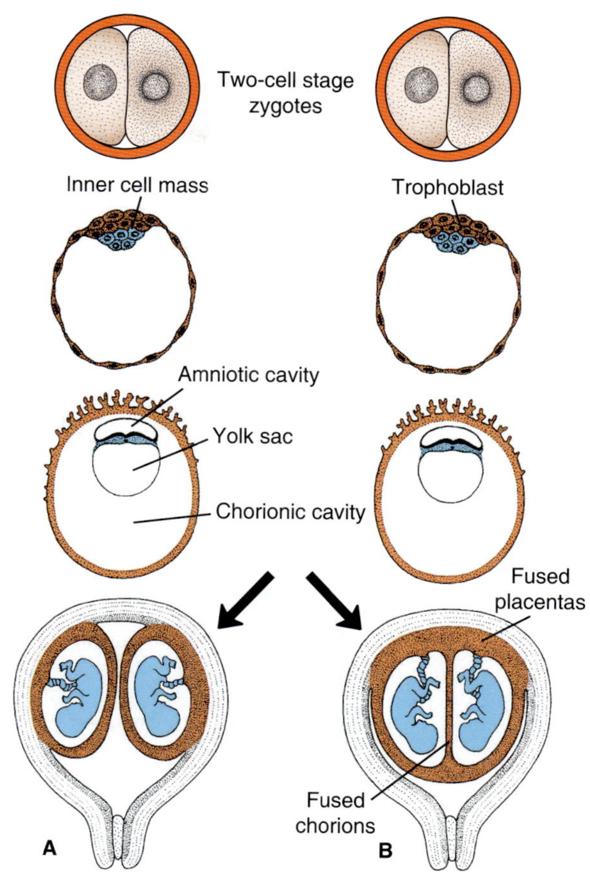


**FIGURE 8.21** Development of dizygotic twins. Normally, each embryo has its own amnion, chorion, and placenta **(A)**, but sometimes, the placentas are fused **(B)**. Each embryo usually receives the appropriate amount of blood, but on occasion, large anastomoses shunt more blood to one of the partners than to the other.

Splitting of the zygote usually occurs at the early blastocyst stage. The inner cell mass splits into two separate groups of cells within the same blastocyst cavity (Fig. 8.22*B*). The two embryos have a common placenta and a common chorionic cavity but separate amniotic cavities (Fig. 8.22*B*). In rare cases, the separation occurs at the bilaminar germ disc stage, just before the appearance of the primitive streak (Fig. 8.22*C*). This method of splitting results in formation of two partners with a single placenta and a common chorionic and amniotic sac. Although the twins have a common placenta, blood supply is usually well balanced.

Although triplets are rare (about 1 per 7,600 pregnancies), birth of quadruplets, quintuplets, and so forth is rarer. In recent years, multiple births have occurred more frequently in mothers given gonadotropins (fertility drugs) for ovulatory failure.

## PARTURITION (BIRTH)

For the first 34 to 38 weeks of gestation, the uterine myometrium does not respond to signals for **parturition (birth)**.

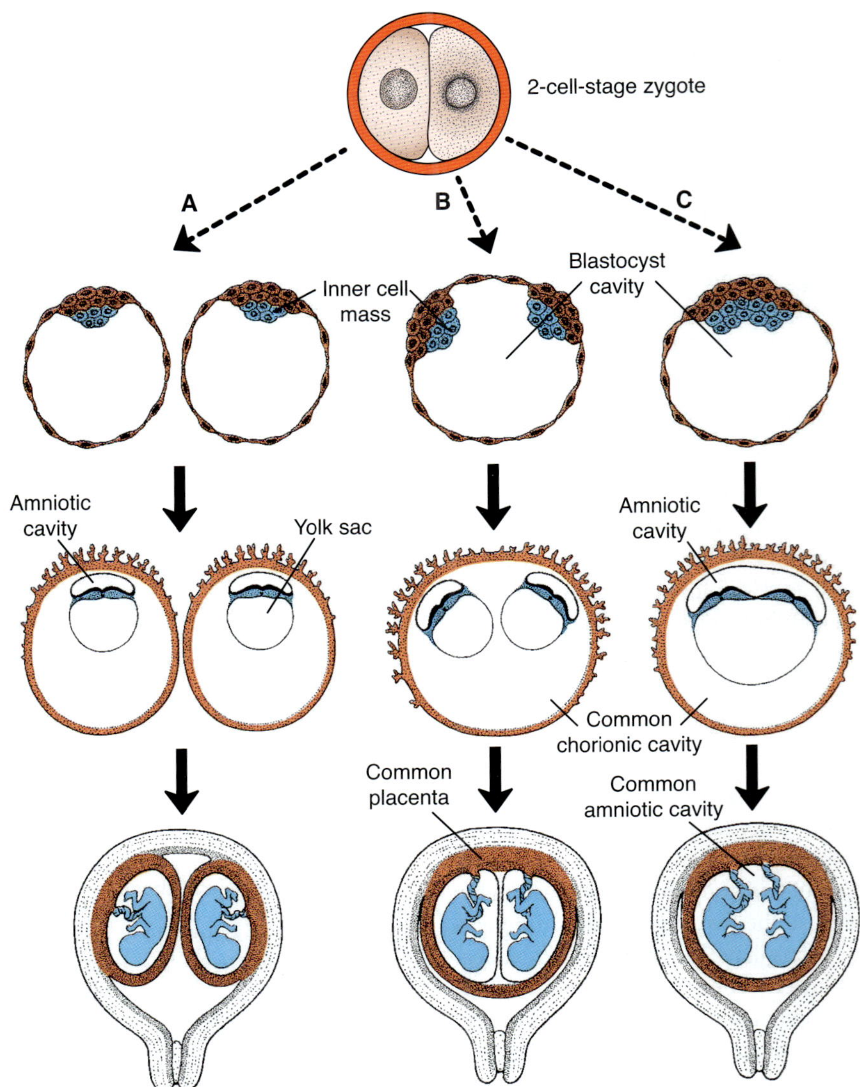


**FIGURE 8.22** Possible relations of fetal membranes in monozygotic twins. **A.** Splitting occurs at the two-cell stage, and each embryo has its own placenta, amniotic cavity, and chorionic cavity. **B.** Splitting of the inner cell mass into two completely separated groups. The two embryos have a common placenta and a common chorionic sac but separate amniotic cavities. **C.** Splitting of the inner cell mass at a late stage of development. The embryos have a common placenta, a common amniotic cavity, and a common chorionic cavity.

During the last 2 to 4 weeks of pregnancy, however, this tissue undergoes a transitional phase in preparation for the onset of **labor**. Ultimately, this phase ends with a thickening of the myometrium in the upper region of the uterus and a softening and thinning of the lower region and cervix.

Labor itself is divided into three stages: (1) **effacement** (thinning and shortening) and dilatation of the cervix (this stage ends when the cervix is fully dilated), (2) **delivery of the fetus**, and (3) **delivery of the placenta and fetal membranes. Stage 1** is produced by uterine contractions that force the amniotic sac against the cervical canal like a wedge, or if the membranes have ruptured, then pressure will be exerted by the presenting part of the fetus, usually the head. **Stage 2** is also assisted by uterine contractions, but the most important force is provided by increased intra-abdominal pressure from contraction of abdominal muscles. **Stage 3** requires uterine contractions and is aided by increasing intra-abdominal pressure.

As the uterus contracts, the upper part retracts, creating a smaller and smaller lumen, while the lower part expands, thereby producing direction to the force. Uterine contractions usually begin about 10 minutes apart; thereafter, during the second stage of labor, the contractions are more frequent in duration and are approximately 1 minute apart. These contractions are intense and can be of 30- to 90-second duration. Their occurrence in pulses is essential to fetal survival, as they are of sufficient force to compromise uteroplacental blood flow to the fetus.

## Clinical Correlates

### Abnormalities Associated with Twins

Twin pregnancies have a high incidence of perinatal mortality and morbidity and an increased risk for preterm delivery. Approximately 60% of twins are born preterm and also have a high incidence of being LBW. Both of these factors put twin pregnancies at great risk, and twin pregnancies have an infant mortality rate three times higher than that for singletons.

The incidence of twinning may be much higher than the number observed at birth because twins are conceived more often than they are born. Many twins die before birth, and some studies indicate that only 29% of women pregnant with twins actually give birth to two infants. The term **vanishing twin** refers to the death of one fetus. This disappearance, which occurs in the first trimester or the early second trimester, may result from resorption or formation of a fetus papyraceus (Fig. 8.23).

Another problem leading to increased mortality among twins is twin–twin transfusion syndrome, which occurs in 15% of monochorionic monozygotic pregnancies. In this condition, placental vascular anastomoses, which occur in a balanced arrangement in most monochorionic placentas, are formed, so that one twin receives most of the blood flow, and flow to the other is compromised. As a result, one twin is larger than the other (Fig. 8.24). The outcome is poor, with the death of both twins occurring in 50% to 70% of cases.

At later stages of development, partial splitting of the primitive node and streak may result in formation of conjoined twins. These twins are classified according to the nature and degree of their union (Figs. 8.25 and 8.26). Occasionally, monozygotic twins are connected only by a common skin bridge or by a common liver bridge. The type of twins formed depends on when and to what extent abnormalities of the node and streak occurred. Misexpression of genes, such as *GOOSECOID*, may also result in conjoined twins. Many conjoined twins have survived, including the most famous pair, Chang and Eng, who were joined at the abdomen and who traveled to England and the United States on exhibitions in the mid-1800s. Finally settling in North Carolina, they farmed and fathered 21 children with their two wives.

In brother–sister pairs of dizygotic twins, testosterone from the male twin can affect development of the female. Thus, females in such pairs tend to have square jaws, larger teeth, perform better on spatial ability tests and have better ball skills than most girls. They are 15% less likely to get married and they have fertility problems, producing 25% fewer children.

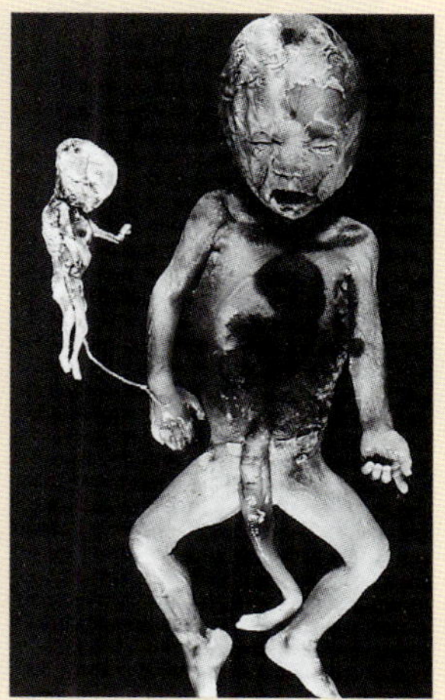

**FIGURE 8.23** Fetus papyraceus. One twin is larger, and the other has been compressed and mummified, hence, the term *papyraceus*.

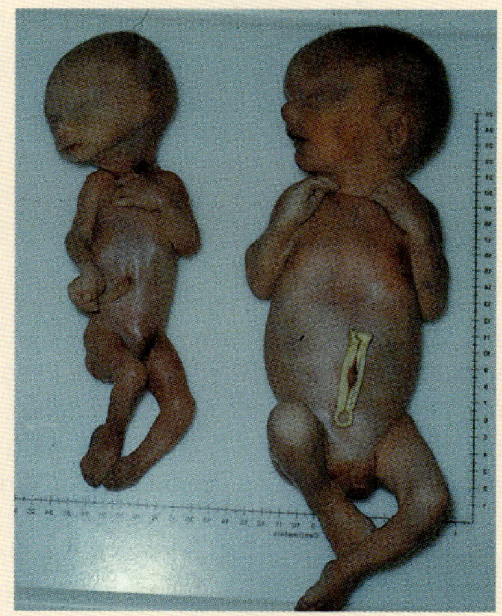

**FIGURE 8.24** Monozygotic twins with twin transfusion syndrome. Placental vascular anastomoses produced unbalanced blood flow to the two fetuses.

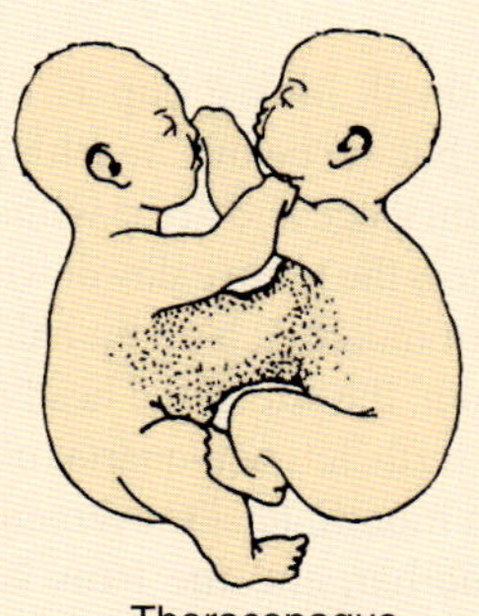

Thoracopagus

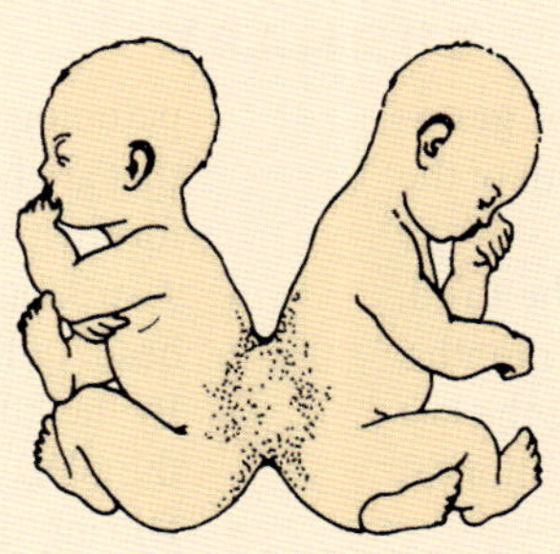

Pygopagus

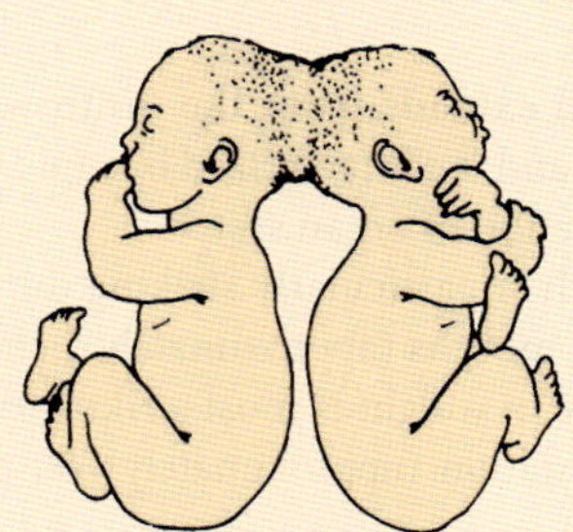

Craniopagus

**FIGURE 8.25** Thoracopagus, pygopagus, and craniopagus twins (*pagus*; fastened). Conjoined twins can be separated only if they have no vital parts in common.

(*Continued*)

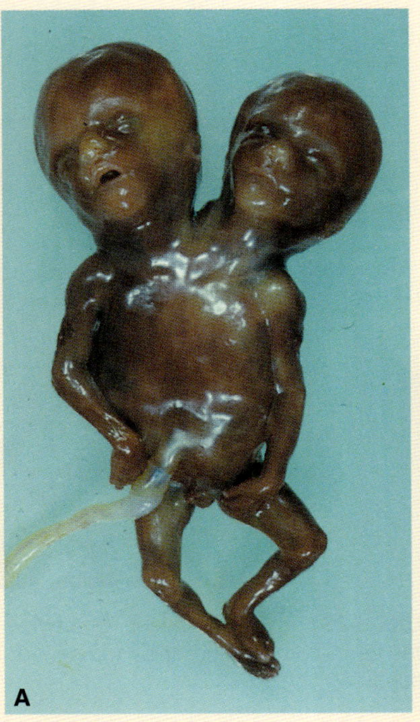

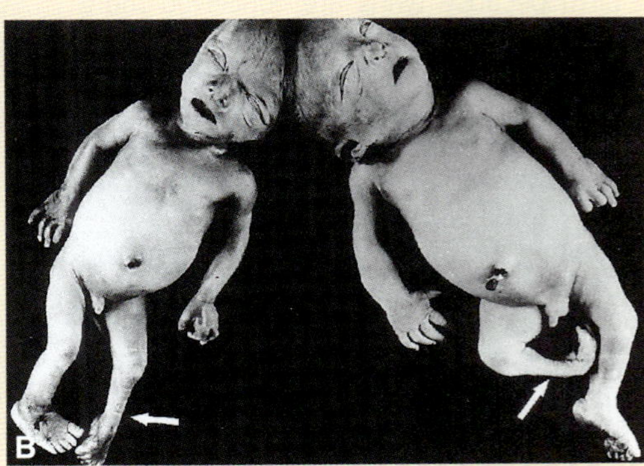

**FIGURE 8.26** Examples of conjoined twins. **A.** Dicephalus (two heads). **B.** Craniopagus (joined at the head).

## *Clinical Correlates*

### Preterm Birth

Factors initiating labor are not known and may involve "**retreat from maintenance of pregnancy**," in which pregnancy-supporting factors (e.g., hormones) are withdrawn, or **active induction** caused by stimulatory factors targeting the uterus. Probably, components of both phenomena are involved. Unfortunately, a lack of knowledge about these factors has restricted progress in preventing **preterm birth**. Preterm birth (delivery before 37 completed weeks) of **premature infants** occurs in approximately 12% of births in the United States and is a leading cause of infant mortality and also contributes significantly to morbidity. In India, among the total 27 million babies born annually, 3.6 million babies are born preterm, and over 300,000 of these preterm babies die each year due to associated complications. India has the highest number of preterm births and the highest number of preterm deaths worldwide, thus contributing to 25% of the overall global preterm-related deaths. It is caused by preterm PROM, premature onset of labor, or pregnancy complications requiring premature delivery. Risk factors include previous preterm birth; black race; multiple gestations; infections, such as periodontal disease and bacterial vaginosis; and low maternal body mass index.

## SUMMARY


- The **fetal period extends from the ninth week of gestation until birth** and is characterized by rapid growth of the body and maturation of organ systems.
- Growth in length is particularly striking during the third, fourth, and fifth months (approximately 5 cm per month), whereas increase in weight is most striking during the last 2 months of gestation (approximately 700 g per month) (Table 8.1, p. 87).
- Most babies weigh between 2,700 and 4,000 g (6 to 9 lb) at birth. Those babies weighing **<2,500 g (5 lb 8 oz)** are considered **low birth weight**; those below **1,500 g (3 lb 5 oz)** are considered **very low birth weight**.
- **IUGR** is a term applied to babies who do not achieve their genetically determined potential size and are pathologically small. This group is distinct from babies that are healthy but are below the 10th percentile in weight for their gestational age and are classified as **SGA**.
- A striking change is the relative slowdown in the growth of the head. In the third month, it is about half the size of the CRL. By the fifth month, the size of the head is about one-third of the CHL, and at birth, it is one-quarter of the CHL (Fig. 8.2).
- During the fifth month, fetal movements are clearly recognized by the mother, and the fetus is covered with fine, small hair.
- A fetus born during the sixth or the beginning of the seventh month has difficulty surviving, mainly because the respiratory and central nervous systems have not differentiated sufficiently.

- In general, the **length of pregnancy** for a full-term fetus is considered to be **280 days, or 40 weeks after onset of the last menstruation**, or, **more accurately, 266 days or 38 weeks after fertilization**.
- The **placenta** consists of two components:
  - A fetal portion, derived from the **chorion frondosum** or **villous chorion**
  - A maternal portion, derived from the **decidua basalis**.
- The space between the chorionic and decidual plates is filled with **intervillous lakes** of maternal blood.
- **Villous trees** (fetal tissue) grow into the maternal blood lakes and are bathed in them.
- The fetal circulation is at all times separated from the maternal circulation by (1) a syncytial membrane (a chorion derivative) and (2) endothelial cells from fetal capillaries. Hence, the human placenta is of the **hemochorial** type.
- Intervillous lakes of the fully grown placenta contain approximately 150 mL of maternal blood, which is renewed three or four times per minute. The villous area varies from 4 to 14 $m^2$, facilitating exchange between mother and child.
- Main functions of the placenta are (1) exchange of gases; (2) exchange of nutrients and electrolytes; (3) transmission of maternal antibodies, providing the fetus with passive immunity; (4) production of hormones, such as progesterone, estradiol, and estrogen (in addition, it produces hCG and somatomammotropin); and (5) detoxification of some drugs.
- The **amnion** is a large sac containing amniotic fluid in which the fetus is suspended by its umbilical cord. The fluid (1) absorbs jolts, (2) allows for fetal movements, and (3) prevents adherence of the embryo to the amnion.
- The fetus swallows amniotic fluid, which is absorbed through its gut and cleared by the placenta. The fetus adds urine to the amniotic fluid, but this is mostly water.
- An excessive amount of amniotic fluid (**hydramnios**) is associated with anencephaly and esophageal atresia, whereas an insufficient amount (**oligohydramnios**) is related to renal agenesis.
- The **umbilical cord**, surrounded by the amnion, contains (1) two umbilical arteries; (2) one umbilical vein; and (3) Wharton jelly, which serves as a protective cushion for the vessels.
- Fetal membranes in twins vary according to their origin and time of formation.
- Two-thirds of twins are **dizygotic**, or **fraternal**; they have two amnions, two chorions, and two placentas, which sometimes are fused.
- **Monozygotic twins** usually have two amnions, one chorion, and one placenta. In cases of **conjoined twins**, in which the fetuses are not entirely split from each other, there is one amnion, one chorion, and one placenta.
- Signals initiating **parturition** (birth) are not clear, but preparation for labor usually begins between 34 and 38 weeks.
- Labor itself consists of three stages: (1) effacement and dilatation of the cervix, (2) delivery of the fetus, and (3) delivery of the placenta and fetal membranes.

Part 1

## Self-Assessment

### Comprehensive Questions

1. Write a brief note on chorion.
2. Write a short note on placental barrier.
3. Describe the embryological basis of the formation of dizygotic/monozygotic twins.
4. Discuss the formation and functions of fetal membranes.

### Problem Solving Questions

1. A 26-year-old pregnant lady comes to the OPD for antenatal checkup. She has a regular 28-day monthly cycle. Her LMP was January 20, 2023. Calculate her expected date of delivery.
2. An ultrasound at 7 months' gestation shows too much space (fluid accumulation) in the amniotic cavity. What is this condition called, and what are its causes?
3. Later in her pregnancy, a woman realizes that she was probably exposed to toluene in the workplace during the third week of gestation but tells a fellow worker that she is not concerned about her baby because the placenta protects her infant from toxic factors by acting as a barrier. Is she correct?
4. A 22-year-old primigravida presented with 24 weeks of pregnancy for her regular antenatal check-up. On examination, her blood pressure was observed to be 160/100 mm Hg with pedal edema. Urine routine microscopic examination showed proteinuria. Her natal scan showed a single live fetus compatible with her gestational age. What is the probable diagnosis of this maternal condition?
5. A 29-year-old primigravida presented with onset of labor at 40 weeks of pregnancy. The antenatal ultrasound scans and growth of fetus were compatible with the gestational age throughout her pregnancy. She delivered a dead male fetus with the umbilical cord encircling the neck of the baby. On examination, the umbilical cord was observed to be more than double the normal length and the cord was looped as knot. What is the probable cause of fetal demise?
6. A 32-year-old primigravida was diagnosed with twin pregnancy with two gestational sacs observed in a 7-week ultrasound scan. She returned for her next antenatal visit to the obstetrics clinic at 16 weeks of pregnancy. On her routine check-up, only one fetal heart sound was heard with a Doppler. She was immediately scanned ultrasonographically and only a single live intrauterine fetus was observed. There was no sign of the second fetus. What is the probable diagnosis and what was the cause?

### Multiple Choice Questions

1. A 35-year-old woman came to the hospital for antenatal care. During the examination by ultrasonography, it was found that the implantation took place in the lower segment of the uterus. Which of the following is the name of the condition?
   (a) Discoid placenta
   (b) Placenta accreta
   (c) Placenta previa
   (d) Fused placenta

(Continued)

2. Human placenta is
   (a) Hemoendothelial
   (b) Hemoallantoic
   (c) Chorioallantoic
   (d) Hemochorial
3. Umbilical cord contains
   (a) Two arteries and one vein
   (b) Two veins and one artery
   (c) One vein and two arteries
   (d) One artery and one vein
4. Placental barrier at term is formed by
   (a) Syncytium and endothelium
   (b) Cytotrophoblast, syncytium endothelium
   (c) Syncytium, cytotrophoblast, extraembryonic mesoderm basement membrane, and endothelium
   (d) Cytotrophoblast and endothelium
5. Human placenta is formed by
   (a) Decidua capsularis and chorion laeve
   (b) Decidua basalis and chorion laeve
   (c) Decidua parietalis and chorion frondosum
   (d) Decidua basalis and chorion frondosum
6. The growth-promoting factor of a fetus in prenatal and postnatal periods is
   (a) β-Galactose
   (b) Vascular endothelial growth factor
   (c) Insulin-like growth factor
   (d) Growth hormone
7. Primary centers of ossification of long bones start at
   (a) 8 weeks
   (b) 10 weeks
   (c) 12 weeks
   (d) 20 weeks
8. The chorion consists of which of the following?
   (a) Cytotrophoblast, syncytiotrophoblast, and extraembryonic mesoderm
   (b) Cytotrophoblast and extraembryonic mesoderm
   (c) Cytotrophoblast, syncytiotrophoblast, and intraembryonic mesoderm
   (d) Amnion and extraembryonic mesoderm
9. Hormones secreted by the placenta are all of the following except
   (a) Progesterone and estrogen
   (b) hCG
   (c) Placental lactogen
   (d) Insulin
10. All of the following structures are present in the connecting stalk except
   (a) Allantois
   (b) Vitelline duct
   (c) Chorionic cavity
   (d) Umbilical vessels

**Answers**

1. (c) 2. (d) 3. (a) 4. (a) 5. (d) 6. (c) 7. (c) 8. (a) 9. (d) 10. (c)

CHAPTER

# 9 Birth Defects and Prenatal Diagnosis



**Specific Learning Objectives**

- Birth defects
  - Causes
  - Environmental
  - Genetic
  - Infection agents
- Types
  - Disruption
  - Malformation
  - Deformation
- Teratology
- Prenatal diagnosis

**Competencies Covered**

AN77.6 Describe teratogenic influences.
AN81.1 Describe various methods of prenatal diagnosis.
AN81.2 Describe indications, process, and disadvantages of amniocentesis.
AN81.3 Describe indications, process, and disadvantages of chorion villus biopsy.

## BIRTH DEFECTS

**Birth defect**, **congenital malformation**, and **congenital anomaly** are synonymous terms used to describe structural, behavioral, functional, and metabolic disorders present at birth. Terms used to describe the study of these disorders are **teratology** (Gr. *teratos*; monster) and **dysmorphology**. Major structural anomalies occur in approximately 3% of liveborn infants and birth defects are a leading cause of infant mortality, accounting for approximately 25% of infant deaths. They are the fifth leading cause of years of potential life lost prior to age 65 and a major contributor to disabilities. They are also nondiscriminatory; the frequencies of birth defects are the same for Asians, African Americans, Latin Americans, Whites, and Native Americans.

The causes of birth defects fall into three categories: those that are caused by environmental factors (15%), those caused by genetic factors (30%), and those caused by an interaction of the environment with a person's genetic susceptibility. Most birth defects fall into this last category (55%), and for most of these congenital malformations, details of their origin are unknown (Fig. 9.1).

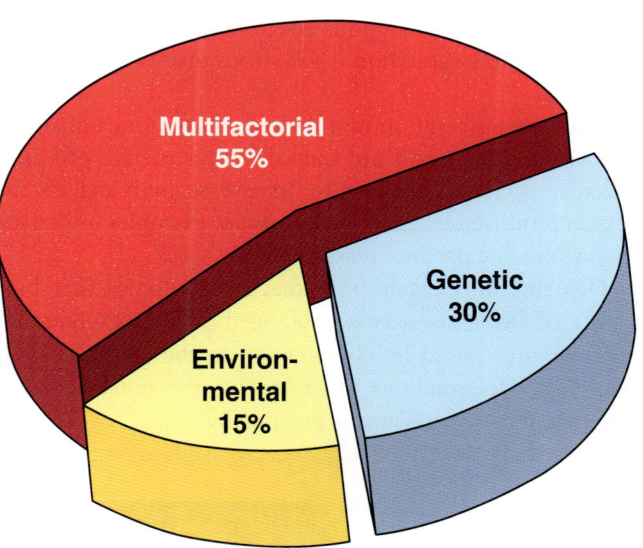


FIGURE 9.1 Pie chart showing the contributions of various factors to the causes of birth defects. Approximately 15% have purely environmental causes, such as drugs, environmental pollutants, infectious diseases, and maternal diseases, such as diabetes, phenylketonuria, obesity, etc.; 30% are purely genetic, including chromosomal abnormalities and single gene mutations; and 55% are multifactorial and will involve gene teratogen interactions. This latter group also includes birth defects of unknown origin.

**Minor anomalies** occur in approximately 15% of newborns. These structural abnormalities, such as microtia (small ears), pigmented spots, and short **palpebral fissures**, are not themselves detrimental to health but, in some cases, are associated with major defects. For example, infants with one minor anomaly have a 3% chance of having a major malformation; those with two minor anomalies have a 10% chance; and those with three or more minor anomalies have a 20% chance. Therefore, minor anomalies serve as clues for diagnosing more serious underlying defects. In particular, ear anomalies are easily recognizable indicators of other defects and are observed in virtually all children with syndromic malformations.

## Types of Abnormalities

Many **malformations** occur during formation of structures, for example, during the period of organogenesis that extends from the beginning of the **third to the end of the eighth week of gestation** (Fig. 9.2). They may result in complete or partial absence of a structure or in alterations of its normal configuration. Malformations are caused by environmental and/or genetic factors acting independently or in concert. Teratogenic insults prior to the third week were thought to follow the all or none rule: Either the embryo died and was spontaneously aborted, or its growth was slowed, but it recovered and showed no ill effects. Although this tenet holds true for many insults to normal development, it is important to note that **axis formation** begins late in the **first week** at the blastocyst stage (see Chapter 3, p. 36) and that a great variety of birth defects can be caused by disruptions in cell signaling during specification of the cranial-caudal and left-right axes (see Chapter 5, p. 49, and Chapter 13, p. 148). Therefore, the critical period for causing most structural birth defects extends from **fertilization through the eighth week of gestation** (Fig. 9.2). In the period following the eighth week until birth, structural defects do not often occur following a toxic insult because organ systems have formed and have passed the critical period. However, differentiation of organs, particularly the brain, remains sensitive throughout this period and can be affected. Thus, no time in gestation is safe from insults by teratogens (Fig. 9.2).

**Disruptions** result in morphological alterations of already formed structures and are caused by destructive processes. Vascular accidents leading to transverse limb defects and defects produced by amniotic bands are examples of destructive factors that produce disruptions (Fig. 9.3).

**Deformations** result from mechanical forces that mold a part of the fetus over a prolonged period. Clubfeet, for example, are caused by compression in the amniotic cavity (Fig. 9.4). Deformations often involve the musculoskeletal system and may be reversible postnatally.

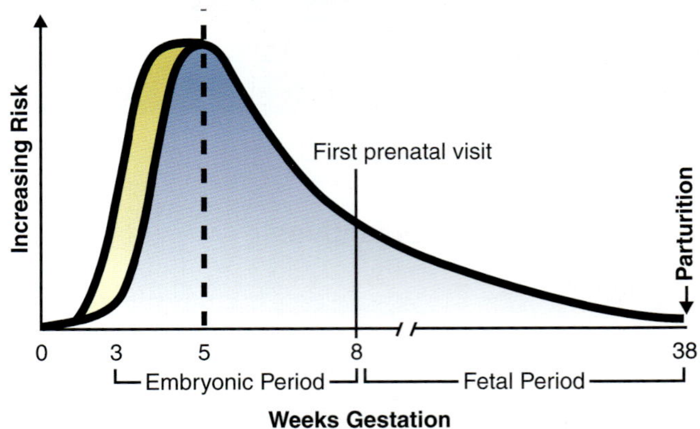


**FIGURE 9.2** Graph showing the times in gestation versus the risks of birth defects being induced. Many malformations are induced in the embryonic period (period of organogenesis) during the third to eighth weeks (*blue area*). However, embryos are also sensitive in the first 2 weeks when the cranial-caudal and left-right axes are established, and virtually any type of birth defect can be induced at this time (*yellow area*). After the eighth week, the fetal period begins and extends to term. During this time, the risk for gross structural defects being induced decreases, but organ systems may still be affected. For example, the brain continues to differentiate during the fetal period, such that toxic exposures may cause learning disabilities or intellectual disability. The fact that most birth defects occur prior to the eighth week makes it imperative to initiate birth defects prevention strategies prior to conception. Unfortunately, most women do not appear for their first prenatal visit until the eighth week, which is after the critical time for prevention of most birth defects.

A **syndrome** is a group of anomalies occurring together that have a specific common cause. This term indicates that a diagnosis has been made and that the risk of recurrence is known. In contrast, **association** is the nonrandom appearance of two or more anomalies that occur together more frequently than by chance alone, but the cause has not been determined. An example is the VACTERL association (*v*ertebral anomalies, *a*nal atresia, *c*ardiac defects, *t*racheo*e*sophageal fistula, *r*enal anomalies, and *l*imb defects).

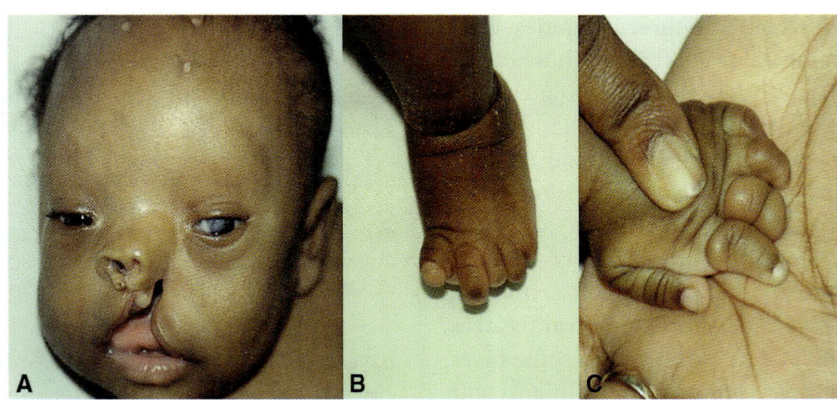


**FIGURE 9.3** Defects produced by amniotic bands as examples of disruptions. **A.** Cleft lip. **B.** Toe amputations. **C.** Finger amputations. Strands of amnion may be swallowed or become wrapped around structures causing various disruption-type defects. The origin of the bands of amniotic tissue is unknown.

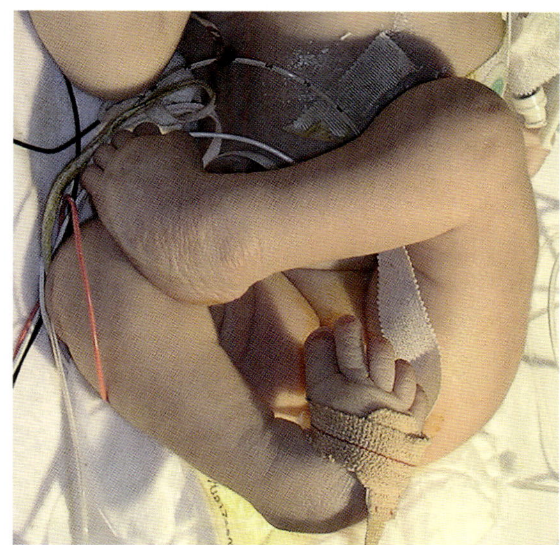

**FIGURE 9.4** Abnormal positioning of the lower limbs and clubfeet as examples of deformations. These defects are probably caused by oligohydramnios (too little amniotic fluid).

Although they do not constitute a diagnosis, associations are important because recognition of one or more of the components promotes the search for others in the group.

## Environmental Factors

Until the early 1940s, it was assumed that congenital defects were caused primarily by hereditary factors. With the discovery by N. Gregg that rubella (German measles) affecting a mother during early pregnancy caused abnormalities in the embryo, it suddenly became evident that congenital malformations in humans could also be caused by environmental factors. In 1961, observations by W. Lenz linked limb defects to the sedative **thalidomide** and made it clear that drugs could also cross the placenta and produce birth defects (Fig. 9.5). Since that time, many agents have been identified as **teratogens** (factors that cause birth defects) (Table 9.1, p. 108).

### *Principles of Teratology*

Factors determining the capacity of an agent to produce birth defects have been defined and set forth as the **principles of teratology**. They include the following:

1. Susceptibility to teratogenesis depends on the **genotype of the conceptus** and the manner in which this genetic composition interacts with the environment. The **maternal genome** is also important with respect to drug metabolism, resistance to infection, and other biochemical and molecular processes that affect the conceptus.
2. Susceptibility to teratogens varies with the **developmental stage at the time of exposure**. Many birth defects are induced during the **third to eighth weeks** of gestation, which is the period of **embryogenesis** (organogenesis). Organ systems are established and develop during this period, and each may have one or more stages of susceptibility. For example, cleft palate can be induced at the blastocyst stage (day 6), during gastrulation (day 14), at the early limb bud stage (fifth week), or when the palatal shelves are forming (seventh week). Also, it is important to note that not all defects are induced during the third to eighth weeks. Virtually any type of malformation can be induced during the period of axis formation that begins in the first week. Also, other defects can be caused after 8 weeks, especially those that affect the brain resulting in learning and motor disabilities (Fig. 9.2). Therefore, no stage of development is completely safe.
3. Manifestations of abnormal development depend **on dose and duration of exposure** to a teratogen.



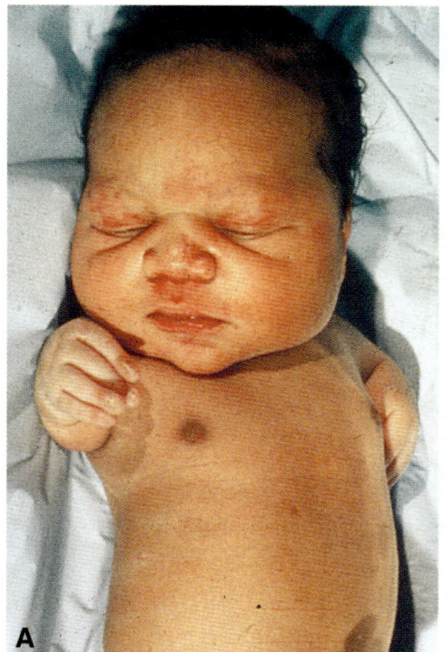

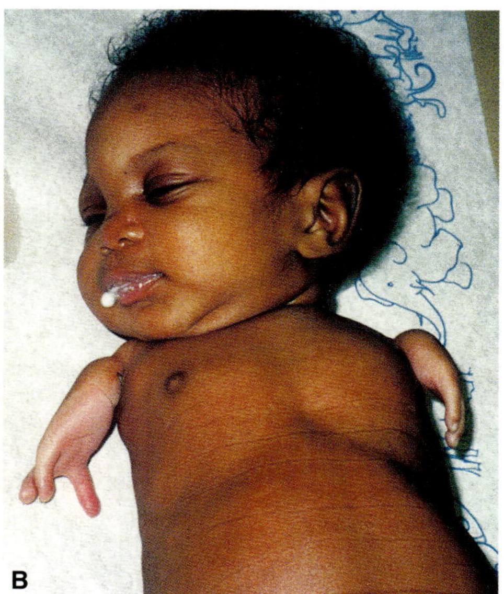

**FIGURE 9.5 A,B.** Examples of phocomelia. Limb defects characterized by loss of the long bones of the limb. These defects were commonly produced by the drug thalidomide.

Table 9.1 Teratogens Associated with Human Malformations

| Teratogen | Congenital Malformations |
|---|---|
| ***Infectious agents*** | |
| Rubella virus | Cataracts, glaucoma, heart defects, hearing loss, tooth abnormalities |
| Cytomegalovirus | Microcephaly, visual impairment, intellectual disability, fetal death |
| Herpes simplex virus | Microphthalmia, microcephaly, retinal dysplasia |
| Varicella virus | Skin scarring, limb hypoplasia, intellectual disability, muscle atrophy |
| Toxoplasmosis | Hydrocephalus, cerebral calcifications, microphthalmia |
| Syphilis | Intellectual disability, hearing loss |
| ***Physical agents*** | |
| X-rays | Microcephaly, spina bifida, cleft palate, limb defects |
| Hyperthermia | Anencephaly, spina bifida, intellectual disability |
| ***Chemical agents*** | |
| Thalidomide | Limb defects, heart malformations |
| Aminopterin | Anencephaly, hydrocephaly, cleft lip and palate |
| Diphenylhydantoin (phenytoin) | Fetal hydantoin syndrome: facial defects, intellectual disability |
| Valproic acid | Neural tube defects; heart, craniofacial, and limb anomalies |
| Trimethadione | Cleft palate, heart defects, urogenital and skeletal abnormalities |
| Topamax (topiramate) | Cleft lip and/or cleft palate |
| Lithium | Heart malformations |
| Selective serotonin reuptake inhibitors (SSRIs) | Heart malformations, neural tube defects, anal atresia, facial clefts, and many other defects |
| Ondansetron | Facial clefts, heart defects |
| Opioids (codeine, hydrocodone, oxycodone) | Neural tube defects, heart defects, gastroschisis |
| Amphetamines | Cleft lip and palate, heart defects |
| Warfarin | Skeletal abnormalities (nasal hypoplasia, stippled epiphyses) |
| ACE inhibitors | Growth retardation, fetal death |
| Mycophenolate mofetil | Cleft lip and palate, heart defects, microtia, microcephaly |
| Alcohol | FAS, short palpebral fissures, maxillary hypoplasia, heart defects, intellectual disability |
| Isotretinoin (vitamin A) | Isotretinoin embryopathy: small, abnormally shaped ears, mandibular hypoplasia, cleft palate, heart defects |
| Industrial solvents | Spontaneous abortion, prematurity, low birth weight, heart, craniofacial, and neural tube defects |
| Organic mercury | Neurological symptoms similar to those of cerebral palsy |
| Lead | Growth retardation, neurological disorders |
| ***Hormones*** | |
| Androgenic agents | Masculinization of female genitalia: fused labia, clitoral hypertrophy (ethisterone, norethisterone) |
| DES | Malformation of the uterus, uterine tubes, and upper vagina; vaginal cancer; malformed testes |
| Maternal diabetes | Various malformations; heart and neural tube defects most common |
| Maternal obesity | Neural tube defects, heart defects, omphalocele |

*ACE*, angiotensin-converting enzyme; *FAS*, fetal alcohol syndrome; *DES*, diethylstilbestrol.

4. Teratogens act in specific ways (**mechanisms**) on developing cells and tissues to initiate abnormal embryogenesis (**pathogenesis**). Mechanisms may involve inhibition of a specific biochemical or molecular process; pathogenesis may involve cell death, decreased cell proliferation, or other cellular phenomena.
5. Manifestations of abnormal development are death, malformation, growth retardation, and functional disorders.

### Infectious Agents

Infectious agents that cause birth defects (Table 9.1) include a number of viruses. Birth defects due to **rubella** (German measles) during pregnancy (congenital rubella syndrome) used to be a major problem, but development and widespread use of a vaccine have nearly eliminated congenital malformations from this cause.

**Cytomegalovirus** is a serious threat. Often, the mother has no symptoms, but the effects on the fetus can be devastating. The infection can cause serious illness at birth and is sometimes fatal. On the other hand, some infants are asymptomatic at birth but develop abnormalities later, including hearing loss, visual impairment, and intellectual disability.

**Herpes simplex virus** and **varicella virus** can cause birth defects. Herpes-induced abnormalities are rare, and usually, infection is transmitted to the child during delivery, causing severe illness and sometimes death. Intrauterine infection with varicella causes scarring of the skin, limb hypoplasia, and defects of the eyes and central nervous system. The occurrence of birth defects after prenatal infection with varicella is infrequent and depends on the timing of the infection. Among infants born to women infected before 13 weeks' gestation, 0.4% are malformed, whereas the risk increases to 2% among infants whose mothers are infected during 13 to 20 weeks of gestation.

**Zika virus** causes **congenital Zika syndrome (CZS)** following transmission of the virus from an infected mother to her unborn child. Infections late in the first trimester (7 to 12 weeks) are the most likely to harm the fetus, although abnormalities have been observed following infections up to 18 weeks. Approximately 30% of pregnancies in which the mothers test positive for the virus are adversely affected. Infection is spread primarily by mosquitoes, but cases of sexual transmission have been reported. Zika infection causes a unique pattern of birth defects in affected children including (1) **severe microcephaly** with overlapping cranial sutures, redundant scalp skin, and a prominent occipital bone (Fig. 9.6); (2) thinning of the cerebral cortex with abnormal gyri and subcortical calcifications; (3) microphthalmia and coloboma; (4) joint contractures (arthrogryposis); and (5) neurological sequelae, including motor and cognitive deficits. The cellular target for the virus is neural progenitor cells, which undergo decreased proliferation rates and increased cell necrosis following infection.

Zika virus was first discovered in 1947 in the Zika forest in Uganda, but few effects on humans were documented until 2007 when large numbers of cases of a mild febrile illness among people living in a number of South Pacific islands were shown to be caused by the virus. This outbreak was followed by another from 2013 to 2016 over a larger number of islands in this same region, and in these cases, some individuals developed Guillain-Barré syndrome. In 2015, the virus made its way to the Americas, reaching Brazil and subsequently the Southern United States. Once the virus reached Brazil, increasing numbers of infants with microcephaly were observed, and the connection between maternal Zika infection and this unique birth defect was established. Retrospectively, cases of microcephaly were identified in some of the South Pacific islands.

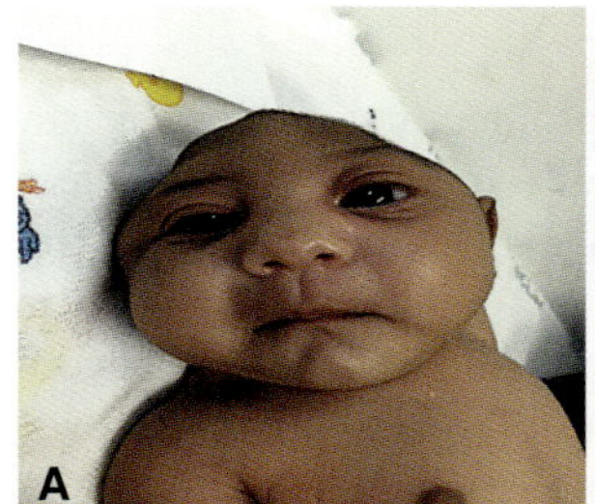

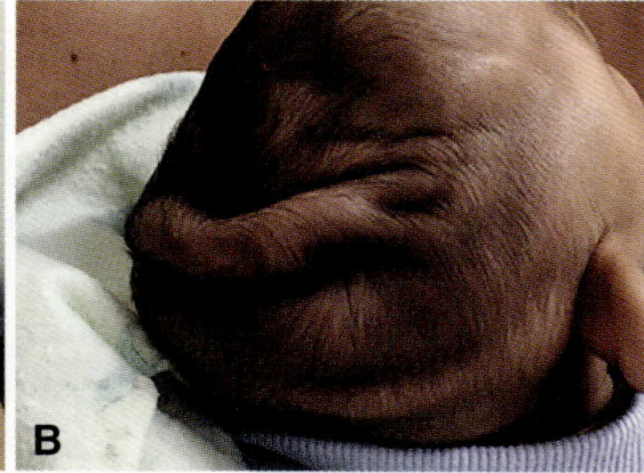


**FIGURE 9.6** Infants showing the effects of Zika virus infection early in gestation. **A.** Microcephaly. **B.** Redundant scalp folds due to the small size of the cranium.

### Other Viral Infections and Hyperthermia

Malformations apparently do not occur following maternal infection with measles, mumps, hepatitis, poliomyelitis, echovirus, coxsackie virus, and influenza, but some of these infections may cause spontaneous abortion or fetal death or may be transmitted to the fetus. For example, coxsackie B virus may cause an increase in spontaneous abortion, whereas measles and mumps may cause an increase in early and late fetal death and neonatal measles and mumps. Hepatitis B has a high rate of transmission to the fetus, causing fetal and neonatal hepatitis, whereas hepatitis A, C, and E are rarely transmitted transplacentally. Echoviruses seem to have no adverse effects on the fetus. Also, there is no evidence that immunizations against any of these diseases harm the fetus.

A complicating factor introduced by these and other infectious agents is that most are **pyrogenic** (cause fevers), and elevated body temperature (**hyperthermia**) caused by fevers or possibly by external sources, such as hot tubs and saunas, is teratogenic. Characteristically, neurulation is affected by elevated temperatures, and neural tube defects, such as anencephaly and spina bifida, are produced.

**Toxoplasmosis** can cause birth defects. Poorly cooked meat; feces of domestic animals, especially cats; and soil contaminated with feces can carry the protozoan parasite *Toxoplasmosis gondii*. A characteristic feature of fetal toxoplasmosis infection is cerebral calcifications. Other features that may be present at birth include microcephaly (small head), macrocephaly (large head), or hydrocephalus (an increase in cerebrospinal fluid in the brain). In a manner similar to cytomegalovirus, infants who appear normal at birth may later develop visual impairment, hearing loss, seizures, and intellectual disability.

### Radiation

**Ionizing radiation** kills rapidly proliferating cells, so it is a potent teratogen, producing virtually any type of birth defect depending on the dose and stage of development of the conceptus at the time of exposure. Radiation from nuclear explosions is also teratogenic. Among women survivors pregnant at the time of the atomic bomb explosions over Hiroshima and Nagasaki, 28% spontaneously aborted, 25% gave birth to children who died in their first year of life, and 25% gave birth to children who had severe birth defects involving the central nervous system. Similarly, the explosion of the nuclear reactor at Chernobyl, which released up to 400 times the amount of radiation as the nuclear bombs, has also resulted in an increase in birth defects throughout the region. Radiation is also a mutagenic agent and can lead to genetic alterations of germ cells and subsequent malformations.

### Pharmaceutical Drugs and Chemical Agents

The role of chemical agents and pharmaceutical drugs (medications) in the production of abnormalities in humans is difficult to assess for two reasons: (1) Most studies are retrospective, relying on the mother's memory for a history of exposure and (2) pregnant women take a large number of medications. A National Institutes of Health study discovered that pregnant women, on average, took four medications during pregnancy. Only 20% of pregnant women used no drugs during their pregnancy. Even with this widespread use of medications during pregnancy, insufficient information is available to judge the safety of approximately 90% of these drugs if taken during pregnancy.

On the other hand, relatively few of the many drugs used during pregnancy have been positively identified as being teratogenic. One example is **thalidomide**, an antinauseant and sleeping pill. In 1961, it was noted in West Germany that the frequency of **amelia** and **meromelia** (total or partial absence of the extremities), a rare abnormality that was usually inherited, had suddenly increased (Fig. 9.5). This observation led to examination of the prenatal histories of affected children and to the discovery that many mothers had taken thalidomide early in pregnancy. The causal relation between thalidomide and meromelia was discovered only because the drug produced such an unusual abnormality. If the defect had been a more common type, such as cleft lip or heart malformation, the association with the drug might easily have been overlooked.

The discovery that a drug like thalidomide could cross the placenta and cause birth defects was revolutionary and led directly to the science of teratology and founding of the Teratology Society. Today, thalidomide is still in use as an immunomodulatory agent in the treatment of people with AIDS and other immunopathological diseases such as leprosy, lupus erythematosus, and graft-versus-host disease. Limb defects still occur in babies exposed to the drug, but it is now clear that other malformations are produced as well. These abnormalities include heart malformations, orofacial clefts, intellectual disability, autism, and defects of the urogenital and gastrointestinal systems.

**Isotretinoin**, an analogue of **vitamin A**, has been shown to cause a characteristic pattern of malformations known as the **isotretinoin embryopathy**. The drug is prescribed for the treatment of cystic acne and other chronic dermatoses, but it is highly teratogenic and can produce virtually any type of malformation. Even topical retinoids, such as etretinate, may have the potential to cause abnormalities. Vitamin A itself may be teratogenic at high doses, based on animal studies and the fact that isotretinoin is a closely related compound. Precisely how much is potentially harmful (>10,000 or >25,000 IU) is controversial, but the amount of vitamin A typically contained in multivitamins (2,000 to 8,000 IU) is below these doses, unless an individual takes more than one multivitamin a day.

Other drugs with teratogenic potential include the **anticonvulsants diphenylhydantoin (phenytoin)**, **valproic acid**, and **trimethadione**, which are used by women who have seizure disorders. Specifically, trimethadione and diphenylhydantoin produce a broad spectrum of abnormalities that constitute distinct patterns of dysmorphogenesis known as the **trimethadione** and **fetal hydantoin syndromes**. Facial clefts are particularly common in these syndromes. The anticonvulsant **valproic acid** increases the risk for several defects, including atrial septal defects (ASD), cleft palate, hypospadias, polydactyly, and craniosynostosis, but the highest risk is for the neural tube defect, spina bifida. The anticonvulsant carbamazepine also has been associated with an increased risk for neural tube defects and possibly other types of malformations. Even newer anticonvulsant drugs like **topiramate** increase the risk for cleft lip and/or cleft palate. A confounding issue with these patients is the fact that they require these medications to prevent seizures. Because of their teratogenic potential, however, the type of drug employed and the dose should be considered to provide the best outcome for the mother and her child.

**Antipsychotic** and **antianxiety agents** (major and minor tranquilizers, respectively) are suspected producers of congenital malformations. The antipsychotics **phenothiazine** and **lithium** have been implicated as teratogens. Although evidence for the teratogenicity of phenothiazines is conflicting, an association between lithium and congenital heart defects, especially Ebstein anomaly (see Chapter 13, p. 163), is better documented, although the risk is small.

**Antidepressant drugs** that work as **selective serotonin reuptake inhibitors (SSRIs)** including fluoxetine, paroxetine, sertraline, citalopram, and escitalopram have been linked by epidemiological studies to multiple birth defects, presumably because of serotonin's role in establishing the left–right axis (laterality; see Chapter 5, p. 52). The heart is particularly sensitive because of its complex laterality, and many types of heart defects have been observed in infants born to mothers taking the drugs. Even malformations in the midline, such as neural tube defects, cleft palate, and anal atresia have been associated with exposure to these drugs, which animal studies have demonstrated may be due to disruption of coordinated signaling essential to establishing the cranial–caudal and left–right axes of the embryo (see Chapter 5, p. 49). Prenatal exposure to these types of drugs has also been associated with an increase in adolescent depression and anxiety.

**Ondansetron** was developed for prevention of the nausea and vomiting experienced following cancer therapy and surgery but has become a popular treatment, through off-label use, to prevent nausea and vomiting associated with pregnancy. Approximately 70% to 85% of pregnant women suffer from nausea and vomiting, and in some cases, the symptoms can become severe. Ondansetron is an effective treatment for these symptoms, but recent evidence suggests that the drug can cause facial clefts and heart defects when taken during the early weeks of pregnancy when nausea and vomiting usually occur.

**Opioid** medications such as **codeine**, **hydrocodone**, and **oxycodone** are used to treat severe pain, and both their use and abuse have been increasing in recent years. Epidemiology studies demonstrate an association with the use of these drugs and neural tube defects, heart defects, and gastroschisis (an abdominal wall defect).

**Mycophenolate mofetil (MMF)** is an immunosuppressant drug used to prevent rejection in organ transplant patients. Use of the drug in pregnancy has resulted in spontaneous abortions and birth defects, including cleft lip and palate, microtia (small ears), microcephaly, and heart defects.

The **anticoagulant warfarin** is teratogenic. Infants born to mothers with first trimester exposures typically have skeletal abnormalities, including nasal hypoplasia, abnormal epiphyses in their long bones, and limb hypoplasia. In contrast, the anticoagulant **heparin** does not appear to be teratogenic.

**Antihypertensive agents** that inhibit **angiotensin-converting enzyme (ACE) inhibitors** produce growth retardation, renal dysfunction, fetal death, and oligohydramnios if exposures occur during the second or third trimester. Effects of exposure to these compounds in the first trimester are less clear.

Caution has also been expressed regarding a number of other compounds that may damage the embryo or fetus. The most prominent among these are propylthiouracil and potassium iodide (goiter and intellectual disability), streptomycin (hearing loss), sulfonamides (kernicterus), the antidepressant imipramine (limb deformities), tetracyclines (bone and tooth anomalies), amphetamines (oral clefts and cardiovascular abnormalities), and quinine (hearing loss).

### *Illicit Drugs, Alcohol, and Cigarettes*

One of the problems in today's society is the effect of maternal use of social drugs, such as lysergic acid diethylamide (LSD), phencyclidine (PCP) or "angel dust," marijuana, cocaine, alcohol, and tobacco on embryonic and fetal development. In the case of LSD, limb abnormalities and malformations of the central nervous system have been reported. A comprehensive review of more than 100 publications, however, led to the conclusion that pure LSD used in moderate doses is not teratogenic and does not cause genetic damage. A similar lack of conclusive evidence for teratogenicity has been described for PCP. **Cocaine** use has been linked to premature labor, intrauterine growth retardation, and spontaneous abortion. Also, malformations of the heart, genitourinary system, and brain have been observed in babies whose mothers used cocaine, and there may be long-term effects on behavior. One difficulty in assessing the drug's effects is the fact that women who use cocaine often use other drugs as well, especially alcohol.

There is a well-documented association between maternal **alcohol** ingestion and congenital abnormalities, and because of its widespread use, there is a high incidence of alcohol-related birth defects. For example, the incidence of **fetal alcohol syndrome (FAS)** is estimated to be 2 to 9 infants per 1,000 births, whereas that of **fetal alcohol spectrum disorder (FASD)** is 24 to 48 infants per 1,000 births. Because alcohol may induce a broad spectrum of defects, ranging from intellectual disability to structural abnormalities of the brain (microcephaly, holoprosencephaly), face, and heart, the term **fetal alcohol spectrum disorder** is used to refer to any alcohol-related defects. **Fetal alcohol syndrome** represents the severe end of the spectrum. Necessary criteria for the diagnosis of FAS include decreased growth (<10th percentile), decreased head circumference (10th percentile), and two of three key facial features (short palpebral fissures, smooth philtrum, and thin upper lip). In addition, affected individuals always have some cognitive disorders and may have structural birth defects (Fig. 9.7). **Alcohol-related neurodevelopmental disorder (ARND)** refers to cases with evidence of involvement of the central nervous system that do not meet the diagnostic criteria for FAS. The incidence of FAS and ARND together has been estimated to be 1 in 100 live births. Furthermore, **alcohol is the leading cause of intellectual disability**. It is not clear how much alcohol is necessary to cause a developmental problem. The dose and timing during gestation are both critical, but there is probably no "safe" level. Even binge drinking (>5 drinks per sitting) at a critical stage of development appears to increase the risk for birth defects, including orofacial clefts.

Recent scientific evidence suggests that in some cases, alcohol acts as a teratogen by downregulating sonic hedgehog

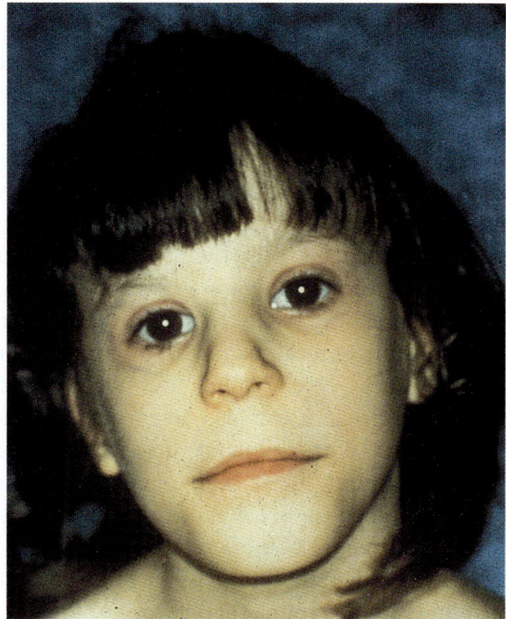

**FIGURE 9.7** Characteristic features of a child with fetal alcohol syndrome (FAS), including an indistinct philtrum, thin upper lip, depressed nasal bridge, short nose, and flat midface.

(SHH) signaling through interference with SHH binding to cholesterol. In turn, this downregulation results in abnormal brain development and the death of neural crest cells that are essential for normal craniofacial development.

**Marijuana** (tetrahydrocannabinol [THC]) has been linked to a number of adverse pregnancy outcomes whether it is smoked or ingested. Some studies have shown an association with an increase in the neural tube defect anencephaly if the drug is used during the first 4 weeks of pregnancy. Other studies have shown an association with marijuana use and an increase in neurodevelopmental deficiencies, such as attention-deficit/hyperactivity disorder (ADHD), learning disabilities, and memory impairment. The drug may also cause premature births and low birth weight.

**Cigarette smoking** has been linked to an increased risk for orofacial clefts (cleft lip and cleft palate) and is a moderate risk factor for heart defects, including transposition of the great arteries (TGA), ASD, pulmonary stenosis, and common truncus arteriosus. It also contributes to intrauterine growth restriction, premature delivery, spontaneous abortions, and stillbirths. Postnatally, there is an increased risk of low birth weight, sudden infant death syndrome (SIDS), asthma, and upper respiratory infections.



### Hormones

#### Androgenic Agents

In the past, synthetic progestins were frequently used during pregnancy to prevent abortion. The progestins ethisterone and norethisterone have considerable androgenic activity, and many cases of masculinization of the genitalia in female embryos have been reported. The abnormalities consist of an enlarged clitoris associated with varying degrees of fusion of the labioscrotal folds.

#### Endocrine Disrupters

**Endocrine disrupters** are exogenous agents that interfere with the normal regulatory actions of hormones controlling developmental processes. Most commonly, these agents interfere with the action of estrogen through its receptor to cause developmental abnormalities of the central nervous system and reproductive tract. For some time, it has been known that the synthetic estrogen **diethylstilbestrol (DES)**, which was used to prevent abortion, raised the incidence of carcinomas of the vagina and cervix in women exposed to the drug in utero. Furthermore, a high percentage of these women had reproductive dysfunction caused in part by congenital malformations of the uterus, uterine tubes, and upper vagina. Male embryos exposed in utero can also be affected, as evidenced by an increase in malformations of the testes and abnormal sperm analysis among these individuals. In contrast to women, however, men do not demonstrate an increased risk of developing carcinomas of the genital system.

Today, **environmental estrogens** are a concern, and numerous studies to determine their effects on the unborn are under way. Decreasing sperm counts and increasing incidences of testicular cancer, hypospadias, and other abnormalities of the reproductive tract in humans, together with documented central nervous system abnormalities (masculinization of female brains and feminization of male brains) in other species with high environmental exposures, have raised awareness of the possible harmful effects of these agents. Many are formed from chemicals used for industrial purposes and from pesticides.

#### Oral Contraceptives

**Birth control pills**, containing estrogens and progestogens, appear to have a low teratogenic potential. Because other hormones such as DES produce abnormalities, however, use of oral contraceptives should be discontinued if pregnancy is suspected.

#### Cortisone

Experimental work has repeatedly shown that cortisone injected into mice and rabbits at certain stages of pregnancy causes a high percentage of cleft palates in the offspring. Some recent epidemiological studies also suggest that women who take corticosteroids during pregnancy are at a modestly increased risk for having a child with an orofacial cleft.

### In Vitro Fertilization

Evidence from several studies indicates that **in vitro fertilization** techniques are associated with an increase in birth defects and that these rates are higher with **intracytoplasmic sperm injection (ICSI)** procedures. Furthermore, any treatment for infertility, whether chemical induction of ovulation or in vitro fertilization, is associated with an increased risk for stillbirths, low birth weight, and prematurity.

### Maternal Disease

#### Diabetes

Disturbances in carbohydrate metabolism during pregnancy in diabetic mothers cause a high incidence of stillbirths, neonatal deaths, abnormally large infants, and congenital malformations. The risk of congenital anomalies in children born to mothers with pregestational diabetes (diabetes diagnosed before pregnancy; both type 1 [insulin-dependent] and type 2 [non–insulin-dependent]) is three to four times that for offspring of nondiabetic mothers and has been reported to be as high as 80% in the offspring of diabetics with long-standing disease. The increased risk is for a wide variety of malformations, including neural tube defects and congenital heart defects. There is also a higher risk for caudal dysgenesis (sirenomelia; see Fig. 5.8, p. 54).

Factors responsible for these abnormalities have not been delineated, although evidence suggests that altered glucose levels play a role and that **insulin** is not teratogenic. In this respect, a significant correlation exists between the severity and duration of the mother's disease and the incidence of malformations. Also, strict control of maternal glucose levels beginning before conception and continuing throughout gestation reduces the occurrence of malformations to incidences approaching those in the general population.

The risk for birth defects associated with gestational diabetes (diabetes that is first diagnosed during pregnancy) is less clear, with some, but not all, studies showing a slightly increased risk. Given that the onset of gestational diabetes is believed to be after the critical period for inducing structural birth defects (3 to 8 weeks' gestation), some investigators have suggested that any observed increased risk may be due to the fact that some women diagnosed with gestational diabetes probably had diabetes before pregnancy, but it was not diagnosed.

#### PHENYLKETONURIA

Mothers with **phenylketonuria (PKU)**, in which the enzyme phenylalanine hydroxylase is deficient or reduced, resulting in increased serum concentrations of phenylalanine, are at risk for having infants with intellectual disability, microcephaly, and cardiac defects. Women with PKU who maintain their low-phenylalanine diet prior to conception and throughout pregnancy reduce the risk to their infants to that observed in the general population.

### *Nutritional Deficiencies*

Although many nutritional deficiencies, particularly vitamin deficiencies, have been proven to be teratogenic in laboratory animals, the evidence for specific cause and effects in humans is more difficult to document. One example is **endemic cretinism**, caused by **iodine deficiency** and characterized by stunted mental and physical growth. Recent evidence also indicates that methyl-deficient diets alter expression of imprinted genes and may result in birth defects and diseases, such as cancer postnatally. Finally, recent studies show that poor maternal nutrition prior to and during pregnancy contributes to low birth weight and birth defects and that severe starvation during pregnancy is associated with a two- to threefold increase in schizophrenia in the offspring.

### *Obesity*

Obesity has reached epidemic proportions in the United States and has nearly doubled in the past 15 years. **In 2007 to 2008, over one-third of women of reproductive age were obese (body mass index >30).**

Prepregnancy obesity is associated with a twofold increased risk for having a child with a neural tube defect. Causation has not been determined but may relate to maternal metabolic disturbances affecting glucose, insulin, or other factors. Prepregnancy obesity also increases the risk for having a baby with a heart defect, omphalocele, and multiple congenital anomalies.

### *Hypoxia*

Hypoxia induces congenital malformations in a great variety of experimental animals. Whether the same is valid for humans remains to be seen. Although children born at relatively high altitudes are usually lighter in weight and smaller than those born near or at sea level, no increase in the incidence of congenital malformations has been noted. In addition, women with cyanotic cardiovascular disease often give birth to small infants but usually without gross congenital malformations.

### *Heavy Metals*

Several years ago, researchers in Japan noted that a number of mothers with diets consisting mainly of fish had given birth to children with multiple neurological symptoms resembling cerebral palsy. Further examination revealed that the fish contained an abnormally high level of **organic mercury**, which was spewed into Minamata Bay and other coastal waters of Japan by large industries. Many of the mothers did not show any symptoms themselves, indicating that the fetus was more sensitive to mercury than the mother. In the United States, similar observations were made when seed corn sprayed with a mercury-containing fungicide was fed to hogs and the meat was subsequently eaten by pregnant women. Likewise, in Iraq, several thousand babies were affected after mothers ate grain treated with mercury-containing fungicides.

**Lead** has been associated with increased abortions, growth retardation, and neurological disorders.

## Male-Mediated Teratogenesis

A number of studies have indicated that exposures to chemicals and other agents, such as ethylnitrosourea and radiation, can cause mutations in male germ cells. Epidemiological investigations have linked paternal occupational and environmental exposures to mercury, lead, solvents, alcohol, cigarette smoking, and other compounds to spontaneous abortion, low birth weight, and birth defects. **Advanced paternal age** is a factor for an increased risk for some types of structural birth defects, Down syndrome, and new autosomal dominant mutations. With respect to mutations, men transmit a higher number of mutations to their children than women, and the age of the father is the dominant factor in determining how many de novo mutations appear in the child. Thus, the age at which

### *Clinical Correlates*

#### Prevention of Birth Defects

Many birth defects can be prevented. For example, supplementation of salt with iodine eliminates intellectual disability and bone deformities resulting from **cretinism**. Placing women with diabetes or PKU under strict metabolic control prior to conception reduces the incidence of birth defects in their offspring. **Folate supplementation** lowers the incidence of neural tube defects, such as spina bifida and anencephaly, and also reduces the risk for hyperthermia-induced abnormalities. Avoidance of alcohol during **all** stages of pregnancy reduces the incidence of birth defects. An essential component of all prevention strategies is to initiate interventions **prior to conception**.

It is important for physicians prescribing medications to women of childbearing age to consider the possibility of pregnancy and the potential teratogenicity of the compounds. Hundreds of children have been born with severe birth defects produced by **retinoids (isotretinoin embryopathy)**, compounds used for the treatment of cystic acne (isotretinoin). Because patients with acne are usually young and may be sexually active, these agents must be used cautiously.

males reproduce can dramatically affect the rate of genomic change in a population such that the older males are when they produce children the more mutations occur in their offspring. Even transmission of paternally mediated toxicity is possible through seminal fluid and from household contamination from chemicals brought home on work clothes by the father.

## ■ PRENATAL DIAGNOSIS

The perinatologist has several approaches for assessing growth and development of the fetus in utero, including **ultrasound**, **maternal serum screening**, **amniocentesis**, and **chorionic villus sampling (CVS)**. In combination, these techniques are designed to detect malformations, genetic abnormalities, overall fetal growth, and complications of pregnancy, such as placental or uterine abnormalities. The overall goal of these tests is to provide women who are at risk with information that gives them the opportunity to make informed choices about their pregnancy. Thus, the use and development of in utero therapies have heralded a new concept in which the fetus is now a patient.

### Ultrasonography

**Ultrasonography** is a relatively noninvasive technique that uses high-frequency sound waves reflected from tissues to create images. The approach may be transabdominal or transvaginal, with the latter producing images with higher resolution (Fig. 9.8). In fact, the technique, which was first developed in the 1950s, has advanced to a degree whereby detection of blood flow in major vessels, movement of heart valves, and flow of fluid in the trachea and bronchi are possible. The technique is safe and commonly used, with approximately 80% of pregnant women in the United States receiving at least one scan.

Important parameters revealed by ultrasound include characteristics of fetal age and growth; presence or absence of congenital anomalies; status of the uterine environment, including the amount of amniotic fluid (Fig. 9.9*A*); placental position and umbilical blood flow; and whether multiple gestations are present (Fig. 9.9*B*). All of these factors are then used to determine proper approaches for management of the pregnancy.

Determination of fetal age and growth is crucial in planning pregnancy management, especially for low-birth-weight infants. In fact, studies show that ultrasound-screened and managed pregnancies with low-birth-weight babies reduced the mortality rate by 60% compared with an unscreened group. Fetal age and growth are assessed by **crown-rump length** during the 5th to the 10th weeks of gestation. After that, a combination of measurements—including the **biparietal diameter (BPD)** of the skull, **femur length**, and **abdominal circumference**—are used (Fig. 9.10). Multiple measurements of these parameters over time improve the ability to determine the extent of fetal growth.

Congenital malformations that can be determined by ultrasound include the neural tube defects anencephaly and spina bifida (see Chapter 18); abdominal wall defects, such as omphalocele and gastroschisis (see Chapter 15); and heart (see Chapter 13) and facial defects, including cleft lip and palate (see Chapter 17).

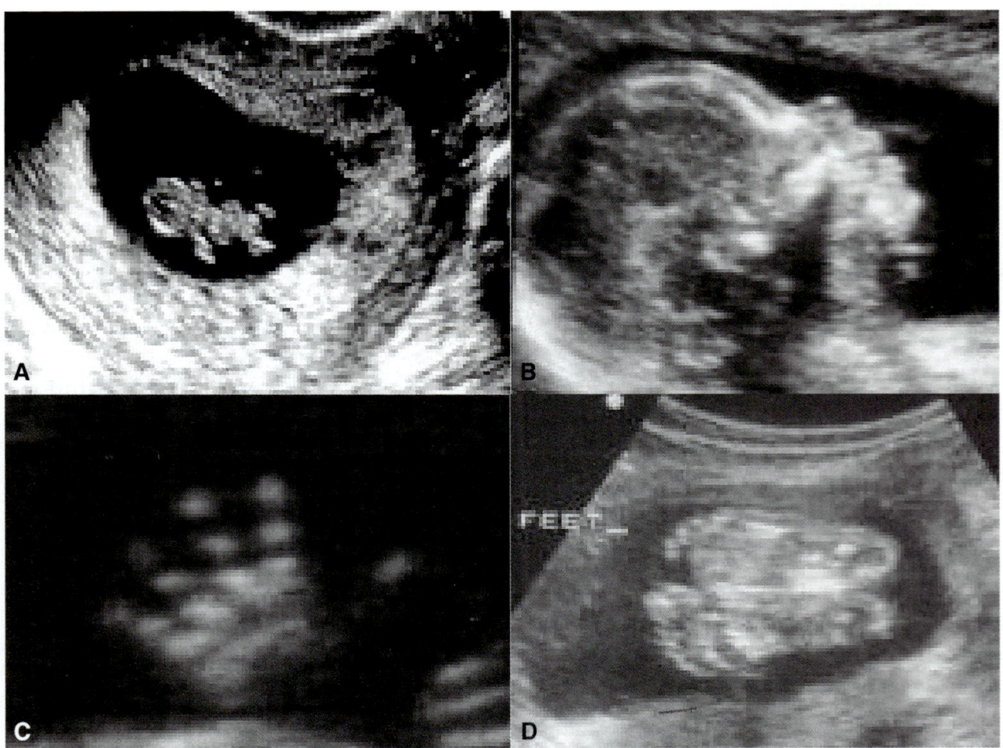


**FIGURE 9.8** Examples of the effectiveness of ultrasound in imaging the embryo and fetus. **A.** A 6-week embryo. **B.** Lateral view of the fetal face. **C.** Hand. **D.** Feet.

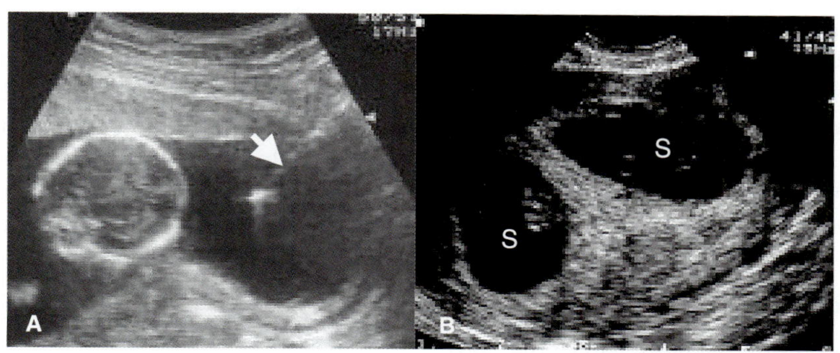


**FIGURE 9.9** **A.** Ultrasound image showing position of the fetal skull and placement of the needle into the amniotic cavity (*arrow*) during amniocentesis. **B.** Twins. Ultrasound showing the presence of two gestational sacs (*S*).

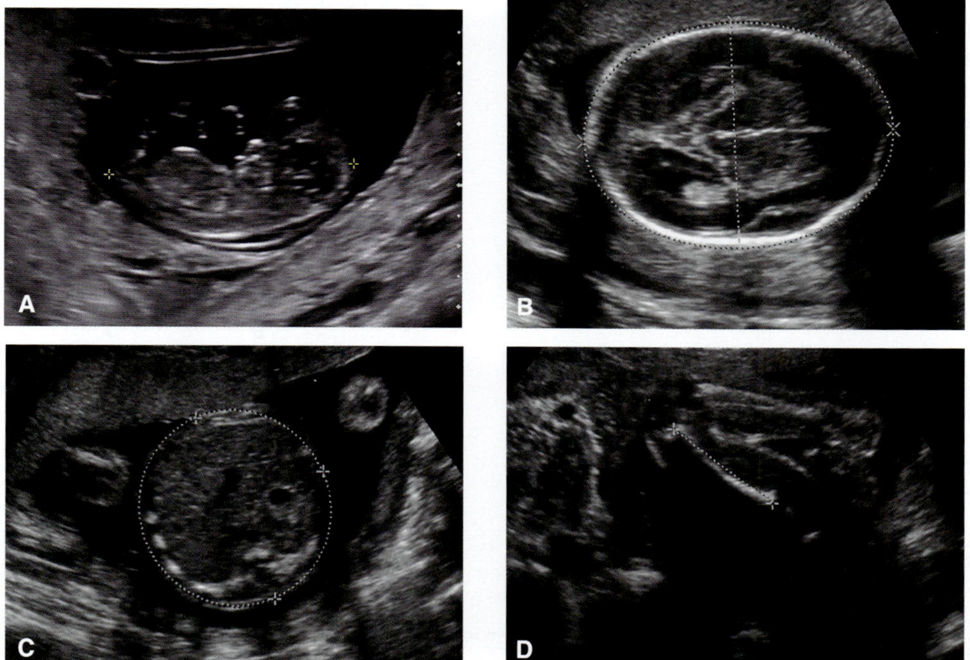


**FIGURE 9.10** Ultrasounds showing measures used to assess embryonic and fetal growth. **A.** Crown-rump length in a 10-week, 6-day fetus. **B.** Head circumference and biparietal diameter of the skull (20 weeks). **C.** Abdominal circumference (20 weeks). **D.** Femur length (20 weeks).

Ultrasound can also be used to screen for Down syndrome and some other chromosome-related abnormalities through a test called **nuchal translucency**. This test involves measurement of the translucent space at the posterior of the baby's neck, where fluid accumulates when Down syndrome and some other abnormalities, especially heart defects are present. The test is performed at 11 to 14 weeks of pregnancy. Information from this test, combined with maternal serum screening test results and the mother's age, can be combined to provide a risk estimate for Down syndrome. Then, based on this risk assessment, a woman can decide whether she wants invasive testing, such as amniocentesis, which would provide a definitive diagnosis.

## Amniocentesis

During amniocentesis, a needle is inserted transabdominally into the amniotic cavity (identified by ultrasound; Fig. 9.9*A*), and approximately 20 to 30 mL of fluid is withdrawn. Because of the amount of fluid required, the procedure is not usually performed before 14 weeks' gestation, when sufficient quantities are available without endangering the fetus. Recent studies suggest that the risk of fetal loss related to the procedure is as low as 1 in 300 to 500 but may be even less for individuals and centers highly skilled in the technique.

The fluid itself is analyzed for biochemical factors, such as AFP and acetylcholinesterase. In addition, fetal cells, sloughed into the amniotic fluid, can be recovered and used for metaphase karyotyping and other genetic analyses (see Chapter 2). Unfortunately, the harvested cells are not rapidly dividing, and therefore, cell cultures containing mitogens must be established to provide sufficient metaphase cells for analysis. Thus, results are available 1 to 2 weeks after the procedure. Once chromosomes are obtained, major chromosomal alterations, such as translocations, breaks, trisomies, and monosomies, can be identified. With special stains (Giemsa) and high-resolution techniques, chromosome-banding patterns can be determined. Furthermore, with recent advances in molecular biology, more sophisticated molecular analyses using polymerase chain reaction (PCR) and genotyping assays have increased the level of detection for genetic abnormalities.

### Chorionic Villus Sampling

**CVS** involves inserting a needle transabdominally or transvaginally into the placental mass and aspirating approximately 5 to 30 mg of villus tissue. Cells may be analyzed immediately, but accuracy of results is problematic because of the high frequency of chromosomal errors in the normal placenta. Therefore, cells from the mesenchymal core are isolated by trypsinization of the external trophoblast and cultured. Because of the large number of cells obtained, only 2 to 3 days in culture are necessary to permit genetic analysis. Thus, the time for genetic characterization of the fetus is reduced compared with amniocentesis. The risk of procedure-related pregnancy loss from CVS when performed by experienced individuals appears to approach that of amniocentesis. However, there have been indications that the procedure carries an increased risk for limb reduction defects, especially of the digits.

### Cordocentesis or Percutaneous Umbilical Blood Sampling

**Cordocentesis, or percutaneous umbilical blood sampling (PUBS)**, is the preferred method for obtaining fetal blood. The technique can be employed in the 14th week and is accomplished by using ultrasound guidance to insert a needle into the umbilical cord. Blood samples provide cells for rapid cytogenetic analysis and are used for diagnosis of hematological diseases. The technique has a slightly higher incidence of fetal loss than amniocentesis.

Invasive prenatal diagnostic tests such as amniocentesis, chorionic villus biopsy, and PUBS are reserved for use in high-risk pregnancies. Factors that place women at higher risk include the following:

- Advanced maternal age (35 years and older)
- Previous family history of a genetic problem, such as the parents having had a child with Down syndrome or a neural tube defect
- The presence of maternal disease, such as diabetes
- An abnormal ultrasound or serum screening test

### Maternal Serum Screening

A search for biochemical markers of fetal status led to development of **maternal serum screening tests**. One of the first of these tests assessed serum **α-fetoprotein (AFP)** concentrations. AFP is produced normally by the fetal liver, peaks at approximately 14 weeks, and "leaks" into the maternal circulation (maternal serum α-fetoprotein [MSAFP]) via the placenta. Thus, AFP concentrations increase in maternal serum during the second trimester and then begin a steady decline after 30 weeks of gestation. In cases of neural tube defects and several other abnormalities, including omphalocele, gastroschisis, bladder exstrophy, amniotic band syndrome, sacrococcygeal teratoma, and intestinal atresia, AFP levels increase in amniotic fluid and maternal serum. In other instances, AFP concentrations decrease, as, for example, in Down syndrome, trisomy 18, sex chromosome abnormalities, and triploidy. AFP screening, combined with testing other second trimester markers (e.g., human chorionic gonadotropin [hCG], unconjugated estriol, and inhibin A) can increase the detection rate for birth defects using these serum screening studies. Because these studies are "screening" studies and are not definitive for a diagnosis, positive results require additional confirmation by invasive techniques, such as amniocentesis.

### Noninvasive Prenatal Screening

It is now possible to isolate fetal cells and DNA from maternal blood to screen for genetic abnormalities. Fetal cells cross the placental barrier beginning at 4 to 6 weeks after conception and can be analyzed by fluorescent in situ hybridization (FISH) and PCR techniques. However, isolating sufficient numbers of these cells from the mother's blood has been difficult. More recently, investigators have focused on circulating fragments of cell-free DNA (cfDNA) originating from placental trophoblasts undergoing apoptosis. This cfDNA comprises 5% to 50% of all cfDNA in maternal plasma and can be isolated and sequenced resulting in full fetal genome sequences. Consequently, the test has greater specificity and predictive value for detection of aneuploidy (trisomy 13, 18, 21) than standard screening. Currently, the test is only used for screening, such that a positive result is then confirmed by either CVS or amniocentesis. However, many investigators believe that the test will ultimately replace these invasive procedures.

## ■ FETAL THERAPY

### Fetal Transfusion

In cases of fetal anemia produced by maternal antibodies or other causes, blood transfusions for the fetus can be performed. Ultrasound is used to guide insertion of a needle into the umbilical cord vein, and blood is transfused directly into the fetus.

### Fetal Medical Treatment

Treatment for infections, fetal cardiac arrhythmias, compromised thyroid function, and other medical problems is usually provided to the mother and reaches the fetal compartment after crossing the placenta. In some cases, however, agents may be administered to the fetus directly by intramuscular injection into the gluteal region or via the umbilical vein.

### Fetal Surgery

Because of advances in ultrasound and surgical procedures, operating on fetuses has become possible. Because of risks

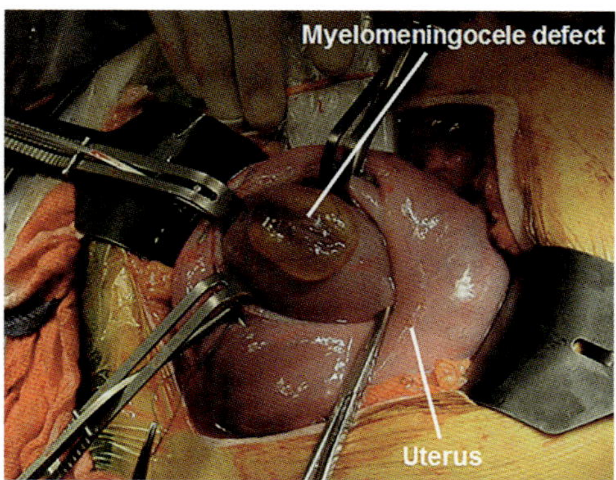


**FIGURE 9.11** Open fetal surgery in a fetus with spina bifida. The uterus has been excised and the fetus exposed directly to the surgical procedure.

to the mother, infant, and subsequent pregnancies, however, procedures are only performed in centers with well-trained teams and only when there are no reasonable alternatives. There are two types of fetal surgeries: **open fetal surgery**, whereby the uterus is exposed and opened to operate directly on the fetus; and **fetoscopic surgery**, using small incisions through the mother's abdominal wall and the uterus. Open surgery is conducted between 18 and 30 weeks of gestation and is employed to repair neural tube defects, heart abnormalities, diaphragmatic hernias, and other conditions. Surgical intervention with neural tube defects (Fig. 9.11) has resulted in a lower incidence of dependence on ventriculoperitoneal shunts and Chiari malformation (herniation of the cerebellum into the foramen magnum) and an improvement in motor skills and the ability to walk. The largest risk factor regarding such surgeries is premature labor and delivery. The overall mortality rate is 6%. Fetoscopy is utilized to place shunts in cases of urinary tract obstruction; to relieve problems caused by amniotic bands; to remove abnormal vessels, such as those that occur in twin transfusion syndrome; and to repair diaphragmatic hernias. Because the technique is less invasive than open surgery, the attendant risks are fewer.

## Stem Cell Transplantation and Gene Therapy

Because the fetus does not develop any immunocompetence before 18 weeks' gestation, it may be possible to transplant tissues or cells before this time without rejection. Research in this field is focusing on hematopoietic stem cells for treatment of immunodeficiency and hematologic disorders. Gene therapy for inherited metabolic diseases, such as Tay-Sachs and cystic fibrosis, is also being investigated.

Part 1

## SUMMARY

- Various agents (Table 9.1, p. 108) and genetic factors are known to cause congenital malformations and **approximately 3% of all live-born infants will have a birth defect**.
- Factors that cause birth defects include the following:
  - Viruses, such as rubella, Zika, and cytomegalovirus
  - Radiation
  - Drugs, such as thalidomide, aminopterin, anticonvulsants, antipsychotics, and antidepressant compounds
  - Substance abuse and social drugs, such as cigarettes, marijuana, and alcohol
  - Hormones, such as DES
  - Maternal diabetes
- Effects of teratogens depend on the **maternal and fetal genotype**, the **stage of development** when exposure occurs, and the **dose and duration of exposure** of the agent.
- Many major malformations are produced during the **period of embryogenesis (teratogenic period; third to eighth weeks).**
- A wide spectrum of birth defects can also be induced during the period of **axis formation** in the first and second weeks (Fig. 9.2). Even after 8 weeks, the fetus remains susceptible so that no period of gestation is completely free of risk.
- **Prevention** of many birth defects is possible, but it depends on beginning preventative measures **before conception** and increasing physicians' and women's awareness of the risks.
- Many techniques are available to assess the growth and developmental status of the fetus.
- **Ultrasound** can accurately determine fetal age and growth parameters, and can detect many malformations.
- **Maternal serum screening** for **α-fetoprotein (AFP)** and other markers can indicate the presence of a neural tube defect or other abnormalities.
- Combinations of maternal serum screening and ultrasound to detect **nuchal translucency** can be used for detecting Down syndrome and some other chromosome-related abnormalities.
- Screening maternal serum is considered a **noninvasive prenatal screening (NIPS) technique** that can also be used to isolate fragments of cell-free fetal DNA (cfDNA) derived from dying placental trophoblast cells. These fragments can be sequenced to detect genetic abnormalities. Currently, NIPS is only a screening technique, meaning that a positive result is followed by a more invasive procedure to confirm or negate a diagnosis.
- **Amniocentesis** is an invasive procedure in which a needle is placed into the amniotic cavity and a fluid sample is withdrawn. This fluid can be analyzed biochemically and also provides cells for culture and genetic analysis.
- **Chorionic villus sampling (CVS)** involves aspirating a tissue sample directly from the placenta to obtain cells for genetic analysis.
- **Cordocentesis (percutaneous umbilical blood sampling [PUBS])** is another invasive test in which a needle is used to draw blood from the umbilical cord in utero. Blood cells obtained in this way can be used for cytogenetic analysis and to diagnose hematological diseases.
- **Invasive procedures** such as amniocentesis, CVS, and PUBS are offered to women at a high risk for having a child with an abnormality. These risks include (1) advanced maternal age (35 years and older); (2) a family history of genetic

(Continued)

abnormalities; (3) maternal disease, such as diabetes; and (4) an abnormal ultrasound or serum screening test.

- **Fetal medicine:** Modern medicine has also made the fetus a patient who can receive treatment, such as transfusions and medications for disease.
- **Fetal surgery and gene therapy:** Fetal surgery can be accomplished in two ways—**open fetal surgery** techniques, in which the uterus is incised and repairs are made for neural tube defects, heart malformations, diaphragmatic hernias, and other defects; and **fetoscopy**, which is less invasive than open surgery with fewer risks and employs an endoscope to place shunts, sever amniotic bands, and repair less severe diaphragmatic hernias.



## Self-Assessment

### Comprehensive Questions

1. Differentiate between amniocentesis and chorionic villous sampling.
2. List the indications of stem cell therapy.
3. Write briefly on multifactorial birth defects.

### Problem Solving Questions

1. Amniocentesis reveals an elevated AFP level. What should be included in a differential diagnosis, and how would a definitive one be made?
2. A 40-year-old woman is approximately 8 weeks pregnant. What tests are available to determine whether her unborn child has Down syndrome? What are the risks and advantages of each technique?
3. Why is it important to determine the status of an infant prenatally? What maternal or family factors might raise your concern about the well-being of an unborn infant?
4. What factors influence the action of a teratogen?
5. A young woman in only the third week of her pregnancy develops a fever of 104°F but refuses to take any medication because she is afraid that drugs will harm her baby. Is she correct?
6. A young woman who is planning a family seeks advice about folic acid and other vitamins. Should she take such a supplement, and if so, when and how much?
7. A young insulin-dependent diabetic woman who is planning a family is concerned about the possible harmful effects of her disease on her unborn child. Are her concerns valid, and what would you recommend?
8. A 26-year-old woman on anticonvulsant therapy with valproic acid gets pregnant. Should she continue with the pregnancy?
9. A 30-year-old multigravida female with one child presented in an obstetrics clinic with 18 weeks of pregnancy. Her antenatal ultrasound revealed generalized subcutaneous edema with severe bilateral pleural effusion and pericardial effusion. Her blood investigations showed Rh negative blood group and her husband was found to be Rh positive. In view of these findings, she was advised medical termination of pregnancy. What is the probable diagnosis in this case?

### Multiple Choice Questions

1. Features of fetal alcohol syndrome are all of the following except
   (a) Flat nose
   (b) Bridge of the nose is indistinct
   (c) Wide midface
   (d) Thin upper lip and flat philtrum
2. Antenatal vaccinations are usually not done against which of the following infections?
   (a) Tetanus
   (b) Toxoplasmosis
   (c) Hepatitis
   (d) Rubella
3. α-Fetoprotein in maternal serum is an indicator of
   (a) GIT abnormalities
   (b) Defect in the mesonephric duct
   (c) Neural tube defect
   (d) Septal defects of the heart
4. Neural tube defects can be prevented by maternal intake of
   (a) Iron
   (b) Vitamin B
   (c) Calcium
   (d) Folic acid
5. Iodine deficiency causes
   (a) Cretinism
   (b) Thyrotoxicosis
   (c) Neural tube defects
   (d) Malabsorption syndrome
6. In ultrasound, nuchal translucency is seen in
   (a) Down syndrome
   (b) Cretinism
   (c) Anencephaly
   (d) Turner syndrome
7. Disruption is
   (a) A group of anomalies occurring together
   (b) Genetic disorder causing a birth defect
   (c) Insult of the fetus due to substance abuse
   (d) Morphological disruptions of normally formed structures
8. Example of a congenital disruption is
   (a) Clubfoot
   (b) Skeletal dysplasia
   (c) Amniotic band causing amputation of a limb
   (d) Fetal alcohol syndrome

### Answers

1. (c) 2. (c) 3. (c) 4. (d) 5. (a) 6. (a) 7. (d) 8. (c)

# Part 2

# Systems-Based Embryology

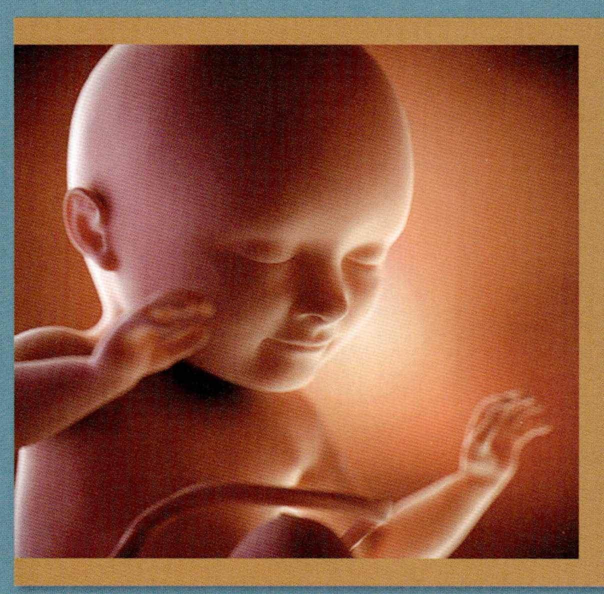

# The Axial Skeleton

## Specific Learning Objectives

- Development of skull
  - Neurocranium
  - Viscerocranium
  - Craniofacial defects
- Development of vertebrae and vertebral column
  - Vertebral defects
- Ribs and sternum

## Competencies Covered

AN79.5 Explain the embryological basis of nucleus pulposus and the embryological basis of vertebral defects.
AN26.1 Explain the concept of bone ossification.



The axial skeleton includes the skull, vertebral column, ribs, and sternum. In general, the skeletal system develops from **paraxial** and **lateral plate (parietal layer) mesoderm** and from **neural crest**. Paraxial mesoderm forms a **segmented** series of tissue blocks on each side of the neural tube, known as **somitomeres** in the head region and **somites** from the occipital region caudally. Somites differentiate into a ventromedial part, the **sclerotome**, and a dorsolateral part, the **dermomyotome**. At the end of the fourth week, sclerotome cells become polymorphous and form loosely organized tissue, called **mesenchyme**, or embryonic connective tissue (Fig. 10.1). It is characteristic for mesenchymal cells to migrate and to differentiate in many ways. They may become fibroblasts, chondroblasts, or **osteoblasts (bone-forming cells)**.

The bone-forming capacity of mesenchyme is not restricted to cells of the sclerotome but occurs also in the parietal layer of the lateral plate mesoderm of the body wall. This layer of mesoderm forms bones of the pelvic and shoulder girdles, limbs, and sternum. Neural crest cells in the head region also differentiate into mesenchyme and participate in formation of bones of the face and skull. The remainder of the skull is derived from occipital somites and somitomeres. In some bones, such as the flat bones of the skull, mesenchyme in the dermis differentiates directly into bone, a process known as **intramembranous ossification** (Fig. 10.2). In most bones, however, including the base of the skull and the limbs, mesenchymal cells first give rise to **hyaline cartilage models**, which in turn become ossified by **endochondral ossification** (Fig. 10.3). The following paragraphs discuss development

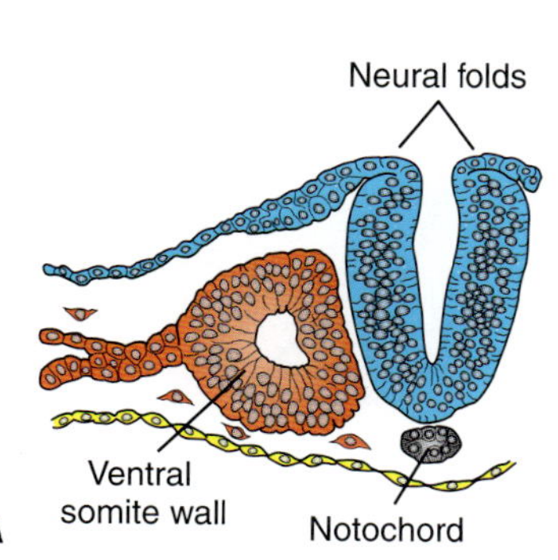


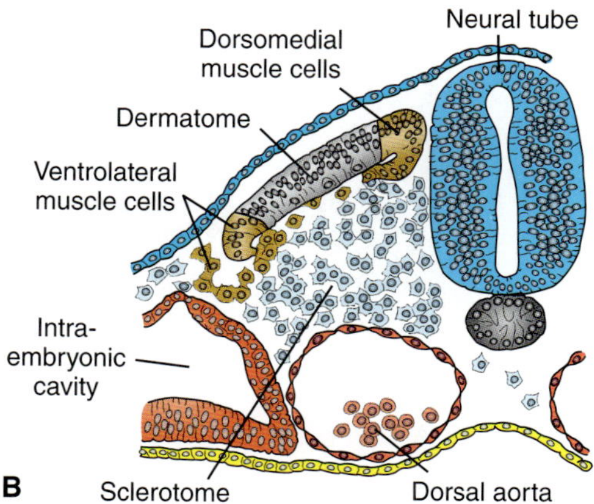


**FIGURE 10.1** Development of the somite. **A.** Paraxial mesoderm cells are arranged around a small cavity. **B.** As a result of further differentiation, cells in the ventromedial wall lose their epithelial arrangement and become mesenchymal. Collectively, they are called the *sclerotome*. Cells in the ventrolateral and dorsomedial regions form muscle cells and also migrate beneath the remaining dorsal epithelium (the dermatome) to form the myotome.

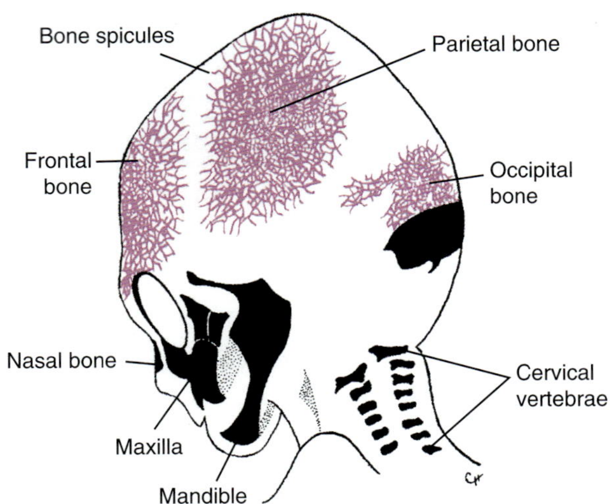


**FIGURE 10.2** Skull bones of a 3-month-old fetus show the spread of bone spicules from primary ossification centers in the flat bones of the skull.

of the most important bony structures and some of their abnormalities.

## SKULL

The skull can be divided into two parts: the **neurocranium**, which forms a protective case around the brain, and the **viscerocranium**, which forms the skeleton of the face.

### Neurocranium

The neurocranium is most conveniently divided into two portions: (1) the membranous part, consisting of **flat bones**, which surround the brain as a vault, and (2) the **cartilaginous part**, or **chondrocranium**, which forms bones of the base of the skull.

#### *Membranous Neurocranium*

The membranous portion of the skull is derived from neural crest cells and paraxial mesoderm as indicated in Figure 10.4. Mesenchyme from these two sources invests the brain and undergoes **intramembranous ossification**. The result is formation of a number of flat, membranous bones that are characterized by the presence of needle-like **bone spicules**. These spicules progressively radiate from primary ossification centers toward the periphery (Fig. 10.2). With further growth during fetal and postnatal life, membranous bones enlarge by apposition of new layers on the outer surface and by simultaneous osteoclastic resorption from the inside.

### Newborn Skull

At birth, the flat bones of the skull are separated from each other by narrow seams of connective tissue, the **sutures**. At points where more than two bones meet, sutures are wide and are called **fontanelles** (Fig. 10.5). The most prominent of these is the **anterior fontanelle**, which is found where the two parietal and two frontal bones meet. Sutures and fontanelles



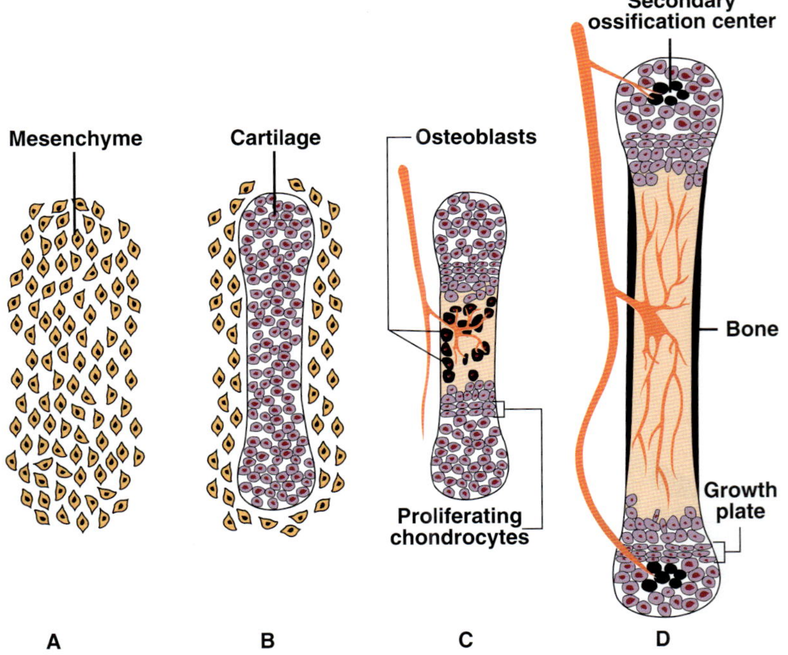


**FIGURE 10.3** Endochondral bone formation. **A.** Mesenchyme cells begin to condense and differentiate into chondrocytes. **B.** Chondrocytes form a cartilaginous model of the prospective bone. **C,D.** Blood vessels invade the center of the cartilaginous model, bringing osteoblasts (*black* cells) and restricting proliferating chondrocytic cells to the ends (epiphyses) of the bones. Chondrocytes toward the shaft side (diaphysis) undergo hypertrophy and apoptosis as they mineralize the surrounding matrix. Osteoblasts bind to the mineralized matrix and deposit bone matrices. Later, as blood vessels invade the epiphyses, secondary ossification centers form. Growth of the bones is maintained by proliferation of chondrocytes in the growth plates.

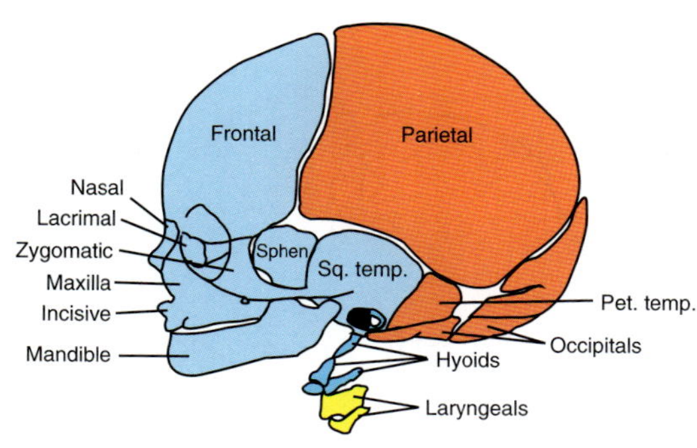


**FIGURE 10.4** Skeletal structures of the head and face. Mesenchyme for these structures is derived from neural crest (*blue*), paraxial mesoderm (somites and somitomeres) (*red*), and lateral plate mesoderm (*yellow*).

allow the bones of the skull to overlap (**molding**) during birth. Soon after birth, membranous bones move back to their original positions, and the skull appears large and round. In fact, the size of the vault is large compared with the small facial region (Fig. 10.5*B*).

Several sutures and fontanelles remain membranous for a considerable time after birth, which allows bones of the vault to continue to grow after birth to accommodate postnatal growth of the brain. Although a 5- to 7-year-old child has nearly all of his or her cranial capacity, some sutures remain open until adulthood. In the first few years after birth, palpation of the anterior fontanelle may give valuable information as to whether ossification of the skull is proceeding normally and whether intracranial pressure is normal. In most cases, the anterior fontanelle closes by 18 months of age, and the posterior fontanelle closes by 1 to 2 months of age.

### *Cartilaginous Neurocranium or Chondrocranium*

The cartilaginous neurocranium or chondrocranium of the skull initially consists of a number of separate cartilages. Those that lie in front of the rostral limit of the notochord, which ends at the level of the pituitary gland in the center of the sella turcica, are derived from neural crest cells. They form the **prechordal chondrocranium**. Those that lie posterior to this limit arise from occipital sclerotomes formed by paraxial mesoderm and form the **chordal chondrocranium**. The base of the skull is formed when these cartilages fuse and ossify by endochondral ossification (Figs. 10.3 and 10.6).

## Viscerocranium

The viscerocranium, which consists of the bones of the face, is formed mainly from the first two pharyngeal arches (see Chapter 17). The first arch gives rise to a dorsal portion, the **maxillary process**, which extends forward beneath the region of the eye and gives rise to the **maxilla**, the **zygomatic bone**, and **part of the temporal bone** (Fig. 10.7). The ventral portion, the **mandibular process**, contains the **Meckel cartilage**. Mesenchyme around the Meckel cartilage condenses and ossifies by intramembranous ossification to give rise to the **mandible**. The Meckel cartilage disappears except in the **sphenomandibular** ligament. The dorsal tip of the mandibular process, along with that of the second pharyngeal arch, later gives rise to the **incus**, the **malleus**, and the **stapes** (Fig. 10.7). Ossification of the three ossicles begins in the fourth month, making these the first bones to become fully ossified. Mesenchyme for formation of the bones of the face is derived from neural crest cells, including the nasal and lacrimal bones (Fig. 10.4).

At first, the face is small in comparison with the neurocranium. This appearance is caused by (1) virtual absence of the paranasal air sinuses and (2) the small size of the bones, particularly the jaws. With the appearance of teeth and development of the air sinuses, the face loses its babyish characteristics.



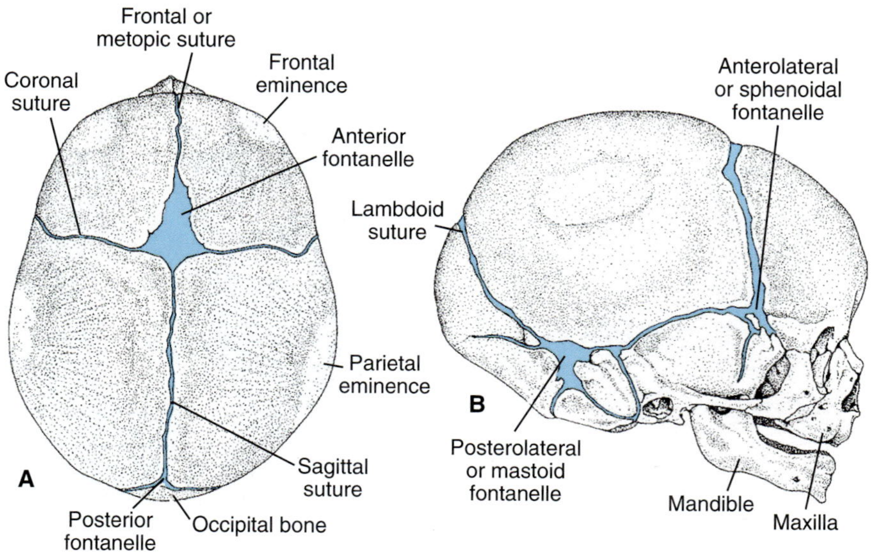


**FIGURE 10.5** Skull of a newborn, seen from above **(A)** and the right side **(B)**. Note the anterior and posterior fontanelles and sutures. The posterior fontanelle closes about 3 months after birth; the anterior fontanelle closes around the middle of the second year. Many of the sutures disappear during adult life.

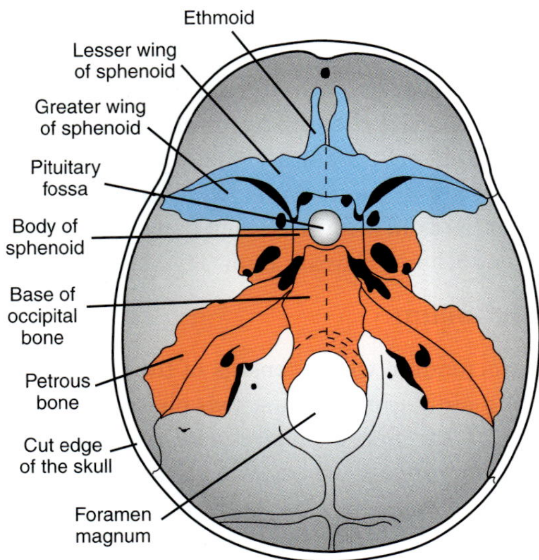


**FIGURE 10.6** Dorsal view of the chondrocranium, or base of the skull, in the adult showing bones formed by endochondral ossification. Bones that form rostral to the rostral half of the sella turcica arise from neural crest and constitute the prechordal (in front of the notochord) chondrocranium (*blue*). Those forming posterior to this landmark arise from paraxial mesoderm (chordal chondrocranium) (*red*).

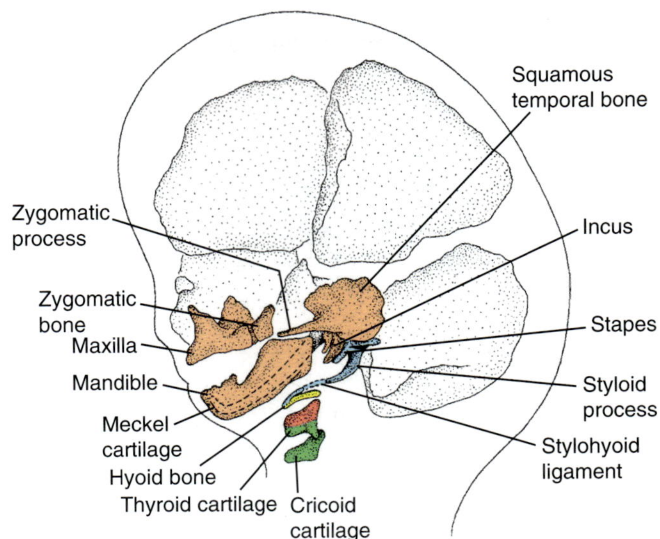


**FIGURE 10.7** Lateral view of the head and neck region of an older fetus, showing derivatives of the arch cartilages participating in formation of bones of the face.

Part 2

## *Clinical Correlates*

### Craniofacial Defects and Skeletal Dysplasias

#### *Neural Crest Cells*

Neural crest cells originating in the neuroectoderm form the facial skeleton and part of the skull. These cells also constitute a vulnerable population as they leave the neuroectoderm; they are often a target for teratogens. Therefore, it is not surprising that craniofacial abnormalities are common birth defects (see Chapter 17).

#### *Cranioschisis*

In some cases, the cranial vault fails to form (**cranioschisis**), and brain tissue exposed to amniotic fluid degenerates, resulting in **anencephaly**. Cranioschisis is caused by failure of the cranial neuropore to close (Fig. 10.8*A*). Children with such severe skull and brain defects cannot survive. Children with relatively small defects in the skull through which meninges and/or brain tissue herniate (**cranial meningocele** and **meningoencephalocele**,

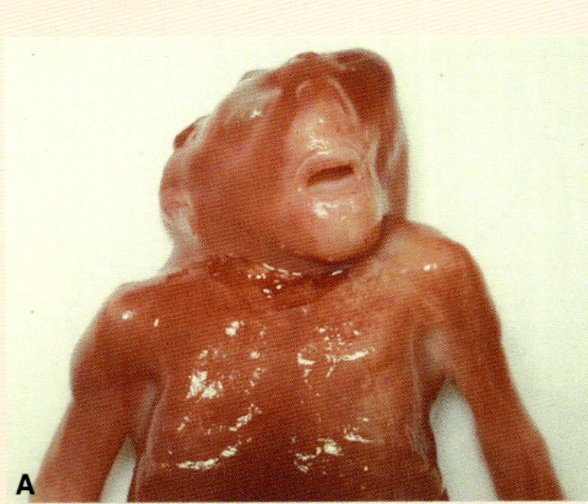


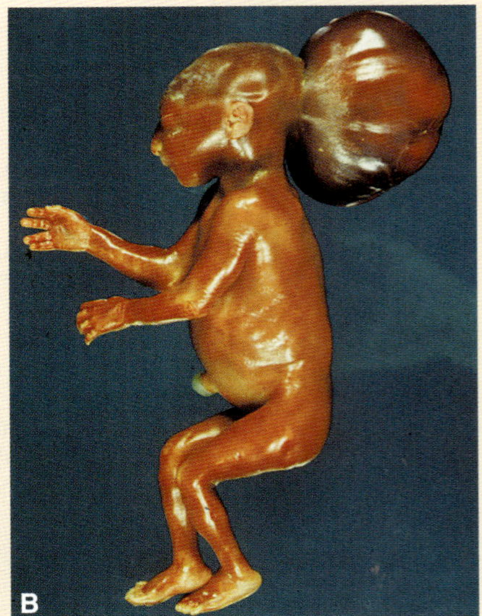


**FIGURE 10.8** **A.** Child with anencephaly. Cranial neural folds fail to elevate and fuse, leaving the cranial neuropore open. The skull never forms, and brain tissue degenerates. **B.** Patient with meningocele. This rather common abnormality may be successfully repaired.

respectively) (Fig. 10.8*B*) may be treated successfully. In such cases, the extent of neurological deficits depends on the amount of damage to brain tissue.

### *Craniosynostosis*

Another important category of cranial abnormalities is caused by premature closure of one or more sutures. These abnormalities are collectively known as **craniosynostosis**, which occurs in 1 in 2,500 births and is **a feature of more than 100 genetic syndromes**. Regulation of suture growth and closure is not well understood but may involve interactions between neural crest–mesoderm cell boundaries. For example, crest cells form the frontal bones, whereas paraxial mesoderm forms the parietal bones and the loose mesenchyme in the coronal sutures. Also, crest cells migrate between the parietal bones and form the first part of the sagittal suture. Molecular signaling at these boundaries regulates cell proliferation and differentiation. For example, *EFNB1* encodes ephrin-B1, a ligand for EphB receptors that causes cells to repel each other, a kind of antiadhesive activity and important for preventing premature suture closure. Loss of function mutations in *EFNB1* causes **craniofrontonasal syndrome**, characterized by coronal suture synostosis and hypertelorism. Proliferation of neural crest cells in the frontal bones is regulated in part by the transcription factors *MSX2* and *TWIST1* that act cooperatively in parallel pathways. Mutations in *MSX2* cause **Boston-type craniosynostosis** that can affect a number of sutures, whereas mutations in *TWIST1* cause **Saethre–Chotzen syndrome**, characterized by coronal suture synostosis and polydactyly.

**Fibroblast growth factors (FGFs)** and **fibroblast growth factor receptors (FGFRs)** play important roles in most of skeletal development. There are many members of the FGF family and their receptors. Together, they regulate cellular events, including proliferation, differentiation, and migration. Signaling is mediated by the receptors, which are **transmembrane tyrosine kinase receptors**, each of which has three extracellular immunoglobulin domains, a transmembrane segment, and a cytoplasmic tyrosine kinase domain. FGFR1 and FGFR2 are coexpressed in prebone and precartilage regions, including craniofacial structures; FGFR3 is expressed in the cartilage growth plates of long bones and in the occipital region. In general, FGFR2 increases proliferation, and FGFR1 promotes osteogenic differentiation, whereas the role of FGFR3 is unclear. Mutations in these receptors, which often involve only a single amino acid substitution, have been linked to specific types of **craniosynostosis** (FGFR1, FGFR2, and FGFR3) and several forms of **skeletal dysplasia** (FGFR3) (Table 10.1).

**Table 10.1 Genes Associated with Skeletal Defects**

| Gene | Chromosome | Abnormality | Phenotype |
|---|---|---|---|
| *FGFR1* | 8p12 | Pfeiffer syndrome | Craniosynostosis, broad great toes and thumbs, cloverleaf skull (severe craniosynostosis), underdeveloped face |
| *FGFR2* | 10q26 | Pfeiffer syndrome | Same |
| | | Apert syndrome | Craniosynostosis, underdeveloped face, symmetric syndactyly of hands and feet |
| | | Jackson–Weiss syndrome | Craniosynostosis, underdeveloped face, foot anomalies, hands usually spared |
| | | Crouzon syndrome | Craniosynostosis, underdeveloped face, no foot or hand defects |
| *FGFR3* | 4p16 | Achondroplasia (ACH) | Short-limb dwarfism, underdeveloped face |
| | | Thanatophoric dysplasia (type I) | Curved short femurs, with or without cloverleaf skull |
| | | Thanatophoric dysplasia (type II) | Relatively long femurs, severe cloverleaf skull |
| | | Hypochondroplasia | Milder form of ACH with normal craniofacial features |
| *MSX2* | 5q35 | Boston-type craniosynostosis | Craniosynostosis |
| *TWIST* | 7p21 | Saethre–Chotzen syndrome | Craniosynostosis, midfacial hypoplasia, cleft palate, vertebral anomalies, hand and foot abnormalities |
| *HOXA13* | 7p15 | Hand-foot-genital syndrome | Small, short digits, divided uterus, hypospadias |
| *HOXD13* | 2q31 | Synpolydactyly | Fused, multiple digits |
| *TBX5* | 12q24.1 | Upper limb and heart defects | Digit defects, absent radius, limb bone hypoplasia, atrial and ventricular septal defects, conduction abnormalities |
| *COLIA1* and *COLIA2* | 17q21 and 7q21 | Limb defects, blue sclera | Shortening, bowing, and hypomineralization of the long bones, blue sclera |
| *Fibrillin (FBNI)* | 15q15-21 | Marfan syndrome | Long limbs and face, sternal defects (pectus excavatum and carinatum), dilation and dissection of the ascending aorta, lens dislocation |

*(Continued)*

The shape of the skull depends on which of the sutures closes prematurely. Early closure of the sagittal suture (57% of cases) results in frontal and occipital expansion, and the skull becomes long and narrow (**scaphocephaly**) (Fig. 10.9). Premature closure of the coronal sutures (20% to 25% of cases) results in a short skull called **brachycephaly** (Fig. 10.10*A*). If the coronal sutures close prematurely on one side only, then the result is an asymmetric flattening of the skull called **plagiocephaly** (Fig. 10.10*B*,*C*).

By far, the most common causes of craniosynostosis are genetic (Table 10.1). Other causes include, vitamin D deficiency; exposure to teratogens, including, diphenylhydantoin, retinoids, valproic acid, methotrexate, and cyclophosphamide; and intrauterine factors that constrain the fetus, such as oligohydramnios and multiple birth pregnancies.

### *Skeletal Dysplasias*

**Achondroplasia (ACH)**, the most common form of skeletal dysplasia (1/20,000 live births), primarily affects the long bones (Fig. 10.11*A*). Other skeletal defects include a large skull (**megalocephaly**) with a small midface (Fig. 10.11*B*), short fingers, and accentuated spinal curvature. ACH is inherited as an autosomal dominant, and 90% of cases appear sporadically due to new mutations.

**Thanatophoric dysplasia** is the most common neonatal lethal form of skeletal dysplasia (1/40,000 live births). There are two types; both are autosomal dominant. Type I is characterized by short, curved femurs with or without cloverleaf skull; type II individuals have straight, relatively long femurs and severe cloverleaf skull caused by craniosynostosis (Fig. 10.12). Another term for cloverleaf skull is **kleeblattschädel**. It occurs when all of the sutures close prematurely, resulting in the brain growing through the anterior and sphenoid fontanelles.

**Hypochondroplasia**, another autosomal dominant form of skeletal dysplasia, appears to be a milder type of ACH. Common to all of these forms of skeletal dysplasias are mutations in *FGFR3* causing abnormal endochondral bone formation so that growth of the long bones and the base of the skull are adversely affected.

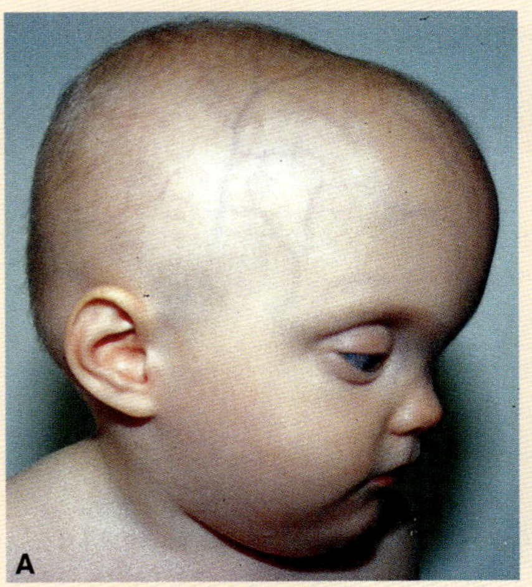

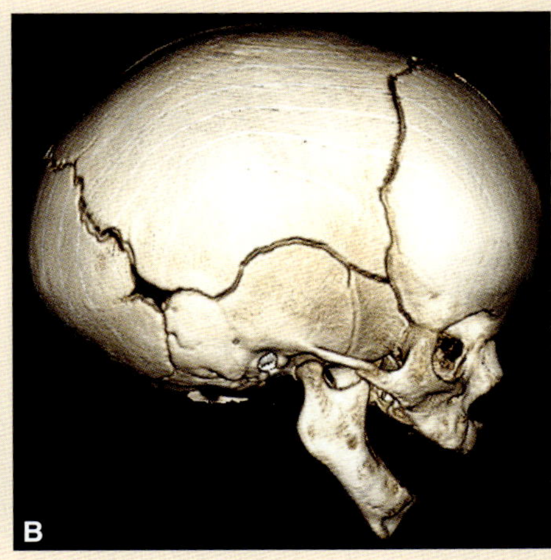

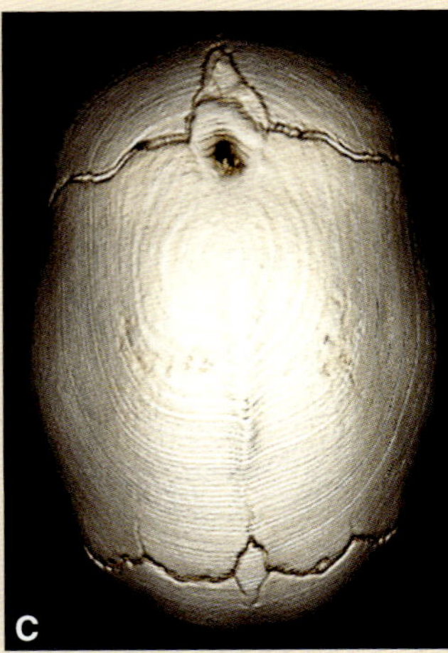


**FIGURE 10.9** Craniosynostosis involving the sagittal suture. **A.** Child with scaphocephaly caused by early closure of the sagittal suture. Note the long narrow shape of the head with prominent frontal and occipital regions. **B,C.** Computed tomography (CT) scans of the skull showing the long narrow shape of the head with bossing of the frontal and occipital regions **(B)** caused by premature closure of the sagittal suture **(C)**.

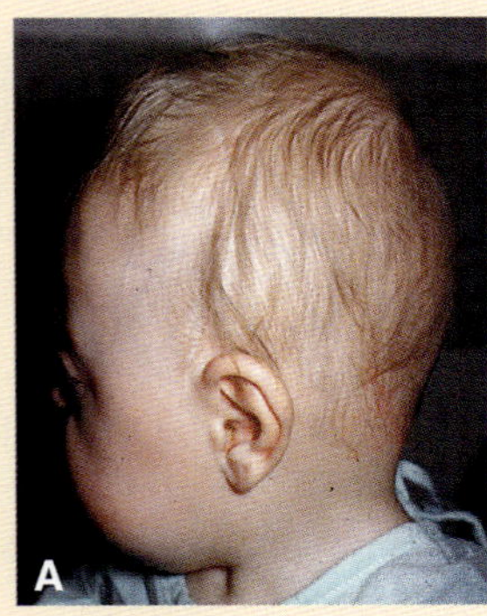

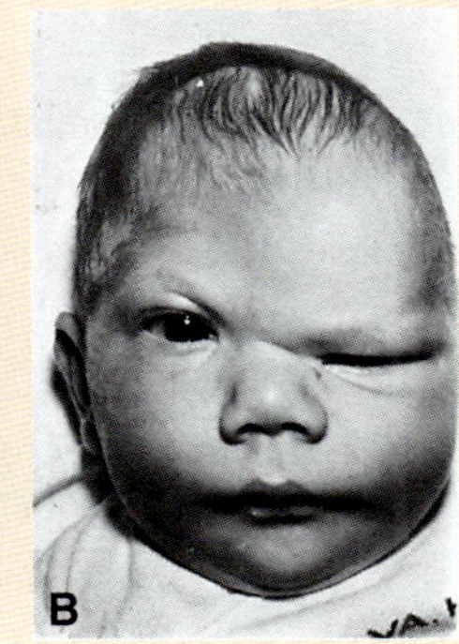

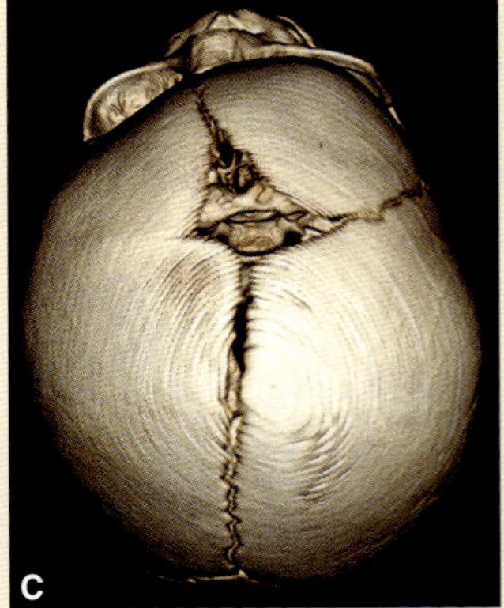


**FIGURE 10.10** Craniosynostosis involving the coronal sutures. **A.** Child with brachycephaly caused by early closure of both coronal sutures. Note the tall shape of the skull with flattened frontal and occipital regions. **B.** Child with plagiocephaly resulting from premature closure of the coronal suture on one side of the skull. **C.** Computed tomography (CT) scan of the skull showing plagiocephaly resulting from premature closure of the coronal suture on one side.

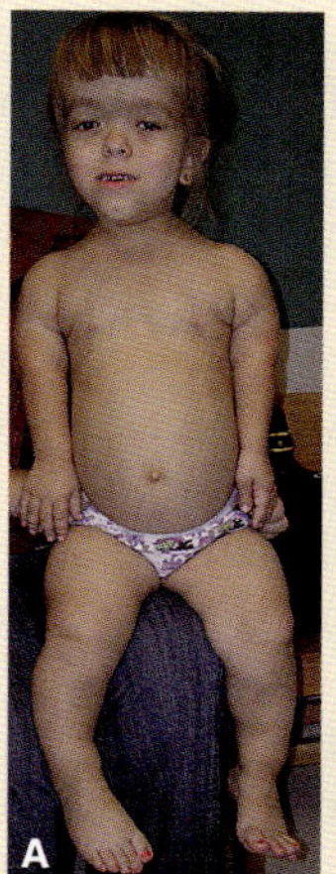


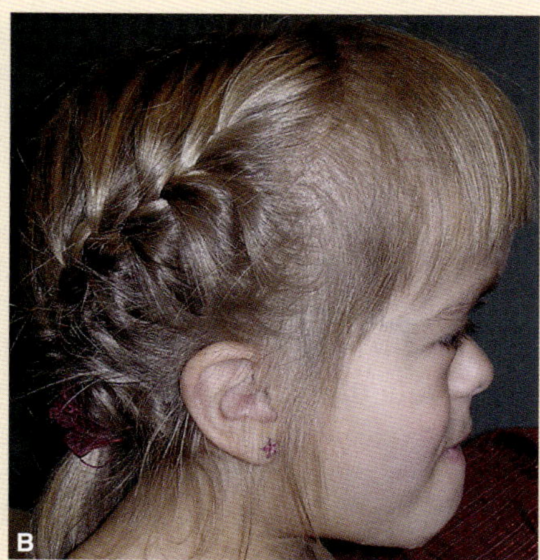


**FIGURE 10.11 A.** Nine-year-old child with achondroplasia (ACH) showing a large head, short extremities, short fingers, and protruding abdomen. **B.** Lateral view of the patient's head showing a prominent forehead and midfacial hypoplasia.

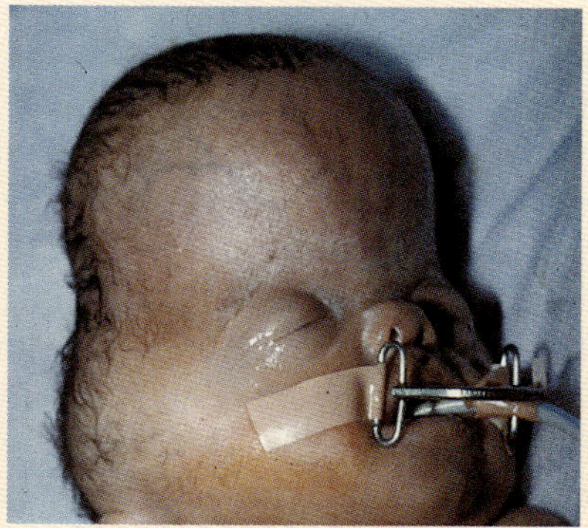

**FIGURE 10.12** Patient with cloverleaf skull characteristic of thanatophoric dwarfism type II. The shape of the skull results from abnormal growth of the cranial base, caused by a mutation in *FGFR3*, followed by craniosynostosis. The sagittal, coronal, and lambdoid sutures are commonly involved.

### *Generalized Skeletal Dysplasia*

**Cleidocranial dysostosis** is an example of a generalized dysplasia of osseus and dental tissues that is characterized by late closure of the fontanelles and decreased mineralization of the cranial sutures resulting in bossing (enlargement) of the frontal, parietal, and occipital bones (Fig. 10.13). Other parts of the skeleton are affected as well, and oftentimes, the **clavicles are underdeveloped or missing**.

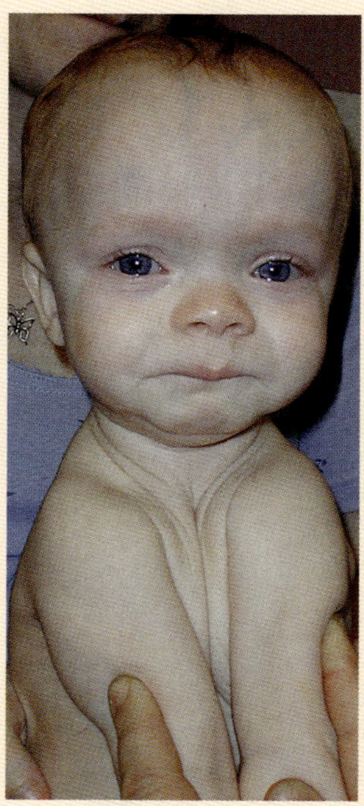

**FIGURE 10.13** Child with cleidocranial dysostosis with generalized skeletal dysplasias. One characteristic of the condition is delayed closure of the fontanelles and decreased mineralization of the cranial sutures, such that the head appears larger due to bossing of the frontal, parietal, and occipital bones. Other parts of the skeleton are affected as well, and often, the clavicles are underdeveloped or missing, as in this case.

### *Acromegaly*

**Acromegaly** is caused by congenital hyperpituitarism and excessive production of growth hormone. It is characterized by disproportional enlargement of the face, hands, and feet. Sometimes, it causes more symmetrical excessive growth and gigantism.

### *Microcephaly*

**Microcephaly** is usually an abnormality in which the brain fails to grow and, as a result, the skull fails to expand (Fig. 10.14). Many children with microcephaly are severely intellectually disabled.

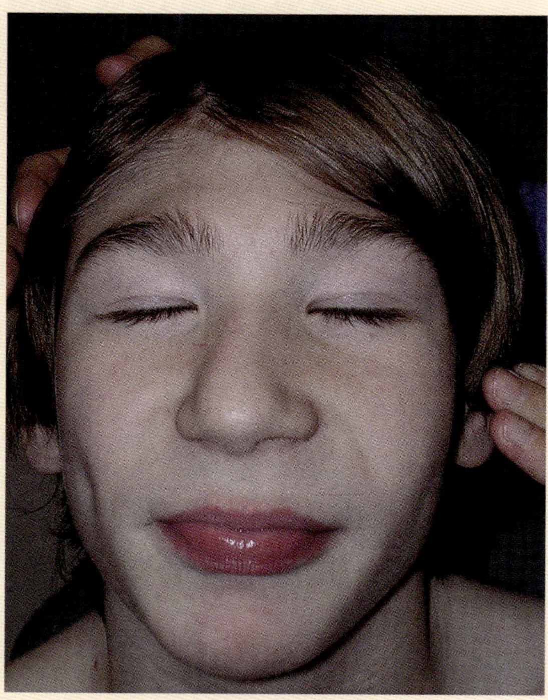

**FIGURE 10.14** Child with microcephaly showing a small head due to the fact that the brain failed to grow to its normal size. One cause for this abnormality is exposure to alcohol in utero. In most cases, microcephaly is associated with significant intellectual disabilities.

(*Continued*)

## VERTEBRAE AND THE VERTEBRAL COLUMN

Vertebrae form from the sclerotome portions of the somites, which are derived from paraxial mesoderm (Fig. 10.15*A*). A typical vertebra consists of a **vertebral arch** and **foramen** (through which the spinal cord passes), a **body**, **transverse processes**, and usually a **spinous process** (Fig. 10.15*B*). During the fourth week, sclerotome cells migrate around the neural tube and notochord to merge with cells from the opposing somite on the other side of the neural tube (Fig. 10.15*A*). As development continues, the sclerotome portion of each somite also undergoes a process called **resegmentation**. Resegmentation occurs when the caudal half of each sclerotome grows into and fuses with the cephalic half of each subjacent sclerotome (*arrows* in Fig. 10.16*A,B*). Thus, each vertebra is formed from the combination of the caudal half of one somite and the cranial half of its neighbor. As a result of this process, muscles derived from the myotome region of each sclerotomes become attached to two adjacent sclerotomes across the intervertebral discs and can therefore move the vertebral column. Patterning of the shapes of the different vertebrae is regulated by *HOX* genes.

Mesenchymal cells between cephalic and caudal parts of the original sclerotome segment do not proliferate but fill the space between two precartilaginous vertebral bodies. In this way, they contribute to formation of the **intervertebral disc** (Fig. 10.16*B*). Although the notochord regresses entirely in the region of the vertebral bodies, it persists and enlarges in the region of the intervertebral disc. Here, it contributes to the **nucleus pulposus**, which is later surrounded by circular fibers of the **annulus fibrosus**. Combined, these two structures form the **intervertebral disc** (Fig. 10.16*C*).

Resegmentation of sclerotomes into definitive vertebrae causes the myotomes to bridge the intervertebral discs, and this alteration gives them the capacity to move the spine (Figs. 10.16*C* and 10.17). For the same reason, intersegmental arteries, at first lying between the sclerotomes, now pass midway over the vertebral bodies. Spinal nerves, however, come to lie near the intervertebral discs and leave the vertebral column through the intervertebral foramina.

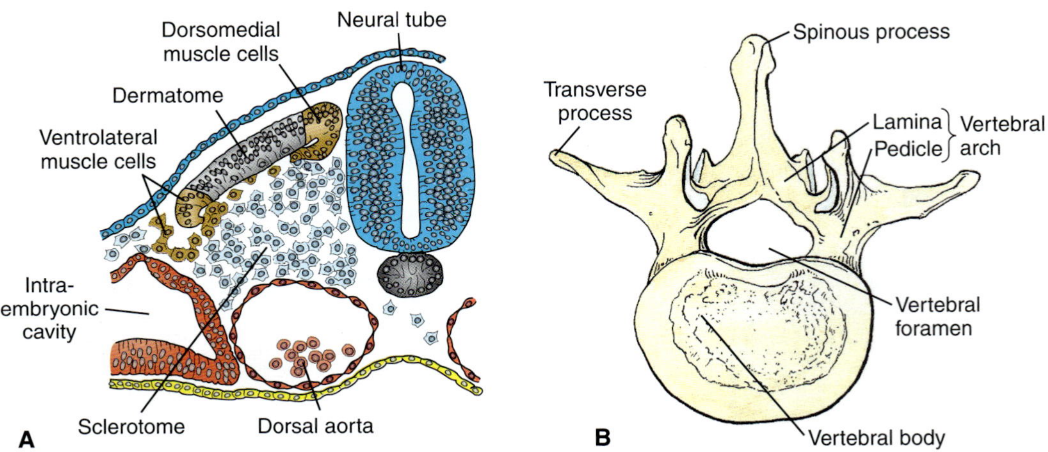


**FIGURE 10.15** **A.** Cross section showing the developing regions of a somite. Sclerotome cells are dispersing to migrate around the neural tube and notochord to contribute to vertebral formation. **B.** Example of a typical vertebra showing its various components.

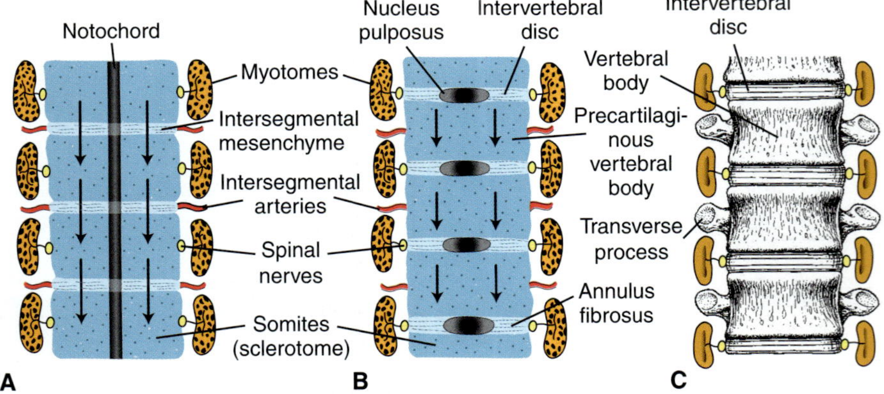


**FIGURE 10.16** Formation of the vertebral column at various stages of development. **A.** At the fourth week of development, sclerotomic segments are separated by less dense intersegmental tissue. Note the position of the myotomes, intersegmental arteries, and segmental nerves. **B.** Proliferation of the caudal half of one sclerotome proceeds into the intersegmental mesenchyme and cranial half of the subjacent sclerotome [*arrows*]. Note the appearance of the intervertebral discs. **C.** Vertebrae are formed by the upper and lower halves of two successive sclerotomes and the intersegmental tissue. Myotomes bridge the intervertebral discs and, therefore, can move the vertebral column.

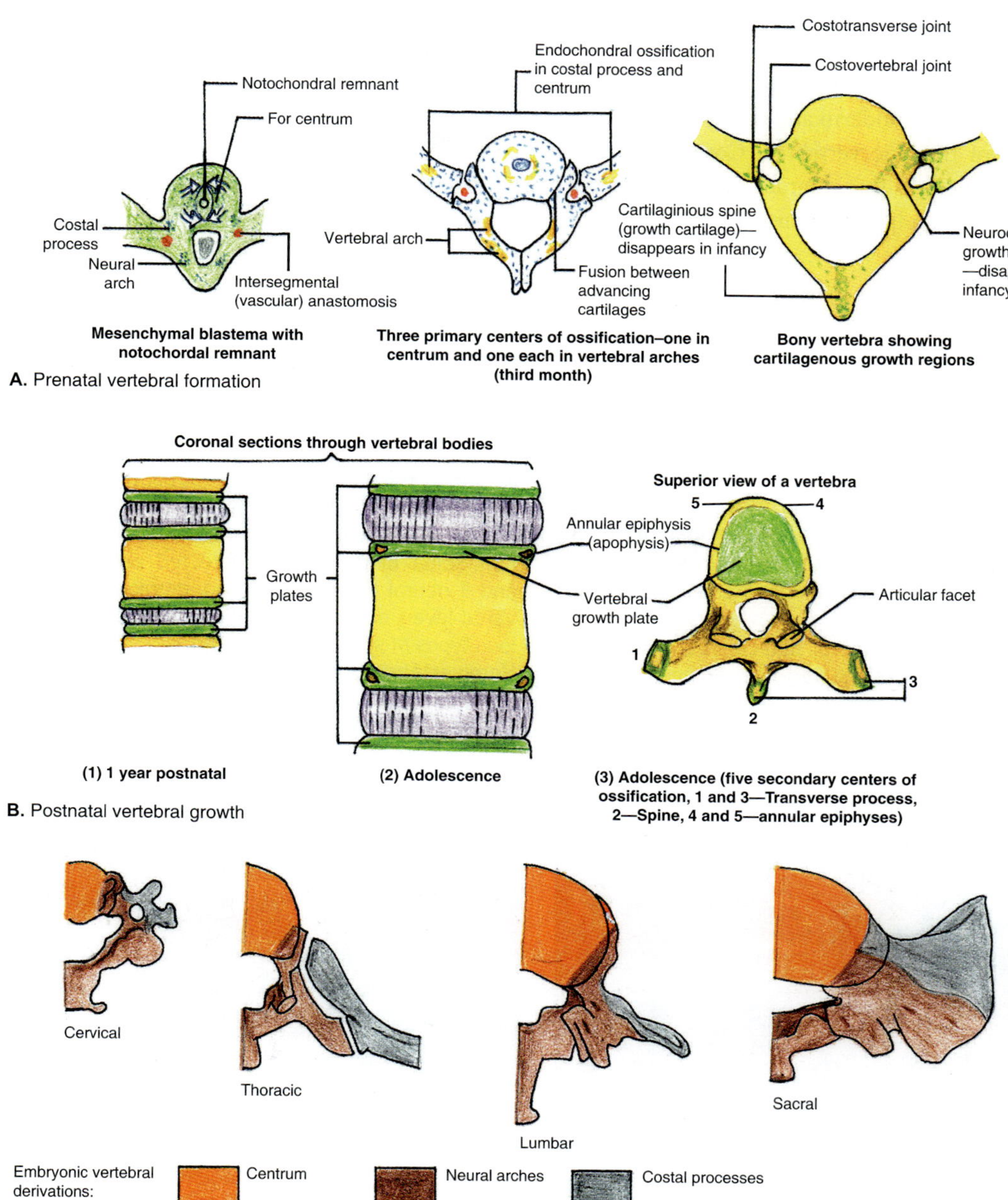


**FIGURE 10.17 A, B.** Development of vertebra showing different stages of growth: blasternal, cartilaginous, and pre- and postnatal. **C.** Morphological parts of an adult vertebra showing principal derivations.

## Formation of Vertebra

The centers of ossification of a vertebra are as follows:

- During the sixth week of gestation, chondrification centers appear in each mesenchymal vertebra.
- Two for each centrum and neural arch simultaneously develop.
- The centers in neural arches fuse with each other and also with the centrum.
- The spinous in the midline and transverse processes laterally develop from extension of centers from the neural arch.
- At birth, each vertebra consists of three bony parts connected by cartilage.
- The vertebral arch articulates with centrum neurocentral joints which permits the vertebral arches to grow and accommodate the developing spinal cord.
- Patterning of the shapes of the different vertebrae is regulated by *HOX* genes. They also determine their cranial caudal orientation.
- As the vertebrae form, two **primary curves** of the spine are established: the **thoracic** and **sacral curvatures**. Later, two secondary curves are established: the **cervical curvature**, as the child learns to hold up its head, and the **lumbar curvature**, which forms when the child learns to walk.

## RIBS AND STERNUM

The bony portion of each rib is derived from sclerotome cells that remain in the paraxial mesoderm and that grow out from the costal processes of thoracic vertebrae. Costal cartilages are formed by sclerotome cells that migrate across the **lateral somitic frontier** into the adjacent lateral plate mesoderm (see Chapter 11 for a description of the lateral somitic frontier). The sternum develops independently in the parietal layer of lateral plate mesoderm in the ventral body wall. Two sternal bands are formed in the parietal (somatic) layer of lateral plate mesoderm on either side of the midline, and these later fuse to form cartilaginous models of the manubrium, sternebrae, and xiphoid process.

### Clinical Correlates

#### Vertebral Defects

The process of formation and rearrangement of segmental sclerotomes into definitive vertebrae is complicated, and it is fairly common to have two successive vertebrae fuse asymmetrically or have half a vertebra missing, a cause of **scoliosis (lateral curving of the spine)**. Also, the number of vertebrae is frequently more or less than the norm. In **Klippel-Feil sequence**, the cervical vertebrae are fused causing reduced mobility and a short neck.

One of the most serious vertebral defects is the result of imperfect fusion or nonunion of the vertebral arches. Such an abnormality, known as **cleft vertebra (spina bifida)**, may involve only the bony vertebral arches, leaving the spinal cord intact. In these cases, the bony defect is covered by skin, and no neurological deficits occur (**spina bifida occulta**). A more severe abnormality is **spina bifida cystica**, in which the neural tube fails to close, vertebral arches fail to form, and neural tissue is exposed. Any neurological deficits depend on the level and extent of the lesion (Fig. 10.18). This defect, which occurs in 1 per 2,500 births, may be prevented, in many cases, by providing mothers with folic acid prior to conception (see Chapter 6, p. 65). Spina bifida can be detected prenatally by ultrasound, and if neural tissue is exposed, amniocentesis can detect elevated levels of $\alpha$-fetoprotein in the amniotic fluid. (For the various types of spina bifida, see Fig. 6.7, p. 65.)

**Hemivertebra:** Suppression of one of the epiphyses of the centrum forms a cuneiform vertebra (hemivertebra) which is one of the causes for congenital scoliosis (lateral bending of the vertebral column).

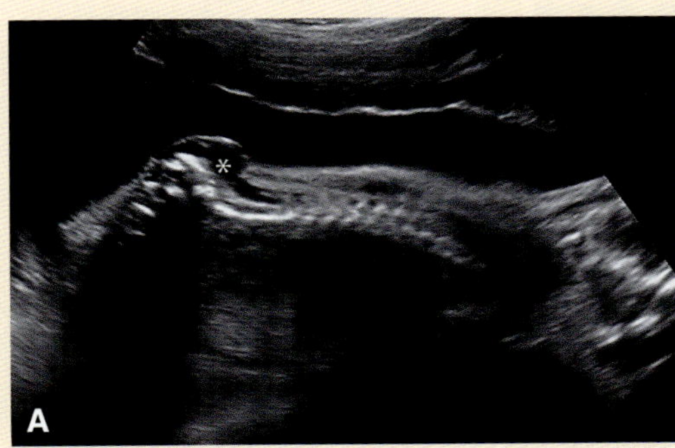


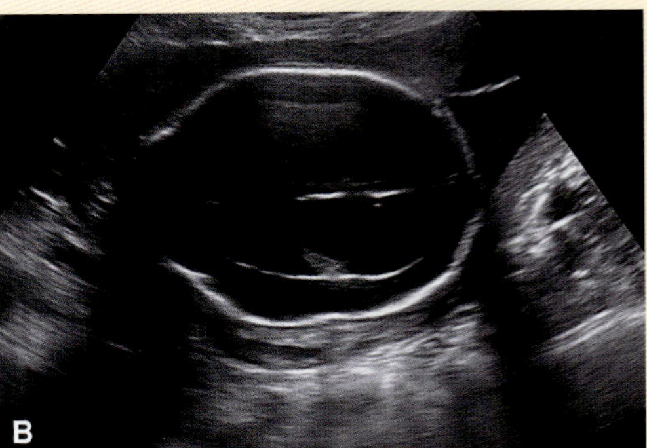


**FIGURE 10.18** **A.** Ultrasound scan of a 26-week-old fetus with spina bifida in the lumbosacral region (*asterisk*). **B.** Ultrasound scan showing the skull of a 26-week-old fetus with spina bifida. Because of the shape of the skull, the image is called the "lemon sign," which occurs in some of these cases and is due to the brain being pulled caudally, changing the shape of the head (see Arnold–Chiari malformation, p. 263).

### Clinical Correlates

#### Rib Defects

Occasionally, extra ribs are formed, usually in the lumbar or cervical regions. **Cervical ribs** occur in approximately 1% of the population and are usually attached to the seventh cervical vertebra. Because of its location, this type of rib may impinge on the brachial plexus or the subclavian artery, resulting in varying degrees of anesthesia in the limb.

#### Defects of the Sternum

**Cleft sternum** is a very rare defect and may be complete or located at either end of the sternum. Thoracic organs are covered only by skin and soft tissue. The defect arises when the sternal bands fail to grow together in the midline. **Hypoplastic ossification centers** and **premature fusion of sternal segments** also occur particularly in infants with congenital heart defects (20% to 50%). Multiple manubrial ossification centers occur in 6% to 20% of all children but are especially common in those with Down syndrome.

**Pectus excavatum** is the term for a depressed sternum that is sunken posteriorly. **Pectus carinatum** refers to a flattening of the chest bilaterally with an anteriorly projecting sternum. The projection of the sternum resembles the keel of a boat. Both defects may result from abnormalities of ventral body wall closure or formation of the costal cartilages and sternum.

Part 2

## SUMMARY


- The skeletal system develops from mesenchyme, which is derived from the mesodermal germ layer and from the neural crest.
- Some bones, such as the flat bones of the skull, undergo **intramembranous ossification**; that is, mesenchyme cells are directly transformed into osteoblasts (Fig. 10.2).
- In most bones, such as the long bones of the limbs, mesenchyme condenses and forms hyaline cartilage models of bones (Fig. 10.3).
- Ossification centers appear in these cartilage models, and the bone gradually ossifies by **endochondral ossification**.
- The skull consists of the **neurocranium** and the **viscerocranium** (face).
- The neurocranium includes a **membranous portion**, which forms the cranial vault, and a cartilaginous portion, the **chondrocranium**, which forms the base of the skull.
- Neural crest cells form the face, part of the cranial vault, and the prechordal part of the chondrocranium (the part that lies rostral to the pituitary gland). Paraxial mesoderm forms the remainder of the skull.
- The **vertebral column** and **ribs** develop from the **sclerotome** compartments of the **somites**, and the **sternum is derived from mesoderm in the ventral body wall.**
- A definitive vertebra is formed by condensation of the caudal half of one sclerotome and fusion with the cranial half of the subjacent sclerotome (Fig. 10.16).
- Abnormalities of the skeletal system include vertebral (**spina bifida**), cranial (**cranioschisis** and **craniosynostosis**), and facial (**cleft palate**) defects.
- Major malformations of the limbs are rare, but defects of the radius and digits are often associated with other abnormalities (**syndromes**).


## Self-Assessment

### Comprehensive Questions

1. Write about the craniofacial defects.
2. Discuss about the development of the vertebral column.

### Problem Solving Questions

1. Why are cranial sutures important? Are they involved in any abnormalities?
2. Explain the origin of scoliosis as a vertebral anomaly. What genes might be involved in this abnormality?
3. A 42-year-old male dwarf had a large head but an underdeveloped face with short limbs. He has normal intelligence. Explain this disorder. Which gene is usually affected in this disorder? What kind of inheritance is usually seen in this disorder?
4. A full-term aborted fetus was received for fetal autopsy, which demonstrated enlargement of frontal, parietal, and occipital bone with missing clavicle. Explain this anomaly.
5. A 5-year-old male child has a lateral bending of his vertebral column. What is the probable cause?
6. What is the embryological basis of spina bifida?

### Multiple Choice Questions

1. All of the following are derived from neural crest cells except
   (a) Frontal
   (b) Greater wing of sphenoid
   (c) Lesser wing of sphenoid
   (d) Petrous part of temporal bone
2. Membranous neurocranium is derived from all of the following except
   (a) Neural crest cells
   (b) Paraxial mesoderm
   (c) Somitomeres
   (d) Intermediate mesoderm
3. Which of the following is the most common type of skeletal dysplasia?
   (a) Achondroplasia
   (b) Thanatophoric dysplasia (type 1)
   (c) Thanatophoric dysplasia (type 2)
   (d) Hypochondroplasia
4. Patterning of the shapes of the different vertebrae is regulated by
   *(a) HOX* gene
   (b) FGFR1
   (c) FGFR3
   (d) FGFR2
5. All of the following muscles take origin from primaxial precursors except
   (a) Scalene
   (b) Geniohyoid
   (c) Intercostals
   (d) External obliques

### Answers

1. (d) 2. (d) 3. (a) 4. (a) 5. (d)

Part 2

CHAPTER

# 11 Muscular System

**Specific Learning Objectives**

- Development of skeletal muscle
- Innervation of skeletal muscle
- Skeletal muscles and tendons
- Molecular regulations and patterning of muscles
- Head and limb muscle development
- Cardiac muscle
- Smooth muscle

**Competency Covered**

AN79.4 Describe the development of somites.

Part 2

With the exception of some smooth muscle tissue (see p. 135), the muscular system develops from the mesodermal germ layer and consists of **skeletal**, **smooth**, and **cardiac muscle**.

Skeletal muscle is derived from **paraxial mesoderm**, which forms somites from the occipital to the sacral regions and somitomeres in the head.

Smooth muscle differentiates from **visceral (splanchnic) mesoderm** surrounding the gut and its derivatives and from ectoderm (pupillary, mammary gland, and sweat gland muscles).

Cardiac muscle is derived from **visceral (splanchnic) mesoderm** surrounding the heart tube.

## STRIATED SKELETAL MUSCULATURE

Head musculature (see Chapter 17) is derived from seven **somitomeres**, which are partially segmented whorls of mesenchymal cells derived from paraxial mesoderm (see Chapter 6, p. 66). Musculature of the axial skeleton, body wall, and limbs is derived from **somites**, which initially form as somitomeres and extend from the occipital region to the tail bud. Immediately after segmentation, these somitomeres undergo a process of **epithelization** and form a "ball" of epithelial cells with a small cavity in the center (Fig. 11.1*A*). The ventral region of each somite then becomes mesenchymal again and forms the **sclerotome** (Fig. 11.1*B–D*), the bone-forming cells for the vertebrae and ribs. Cells in the upper region of the somite form the dermatome and two muscle-forming areas at the ventrolateral (VLL) and dorsomedial (DML) lips (or edges), respectively (Fig. 11.1*B*). Cells from these two areas migrate and proliferate to form progenitor muscle cells ventral to the **dermatome**, thereby forming the **dermomyotome** (Fig. 11.1*B,C*; Fig. 11.2). Some cells from the VLL region also migrate into the adjacent parietal layer of the lateral plate mesoderm (Fig. 11.1*B*). Here, they form **infrahyoid**, **abdominal wall** (rectus abdominis, internal and external oblique, and transversus abdominis), and **limb muscles**. The remaining cells in the myotome form **muscles of the back**, **shoulder girdle**, and **intercostal muscles** (Table 11.1).

Initially, there is a well-defined border between each somite and the parietal layer of lateral plate mesoderm called the **lateral somitic frontier** (Fig. 11.1*B*). This frontier separates two mesodermal domains in the embryo:

1. The **primaxial domain** that comprises the region around the neural tube and contains only somite-derived (paraxial mesoderm) cells
2. The **abaxial domain** that consists of the parietal layer of lateral plate mesoderm together with somite cells that have migrated across the lateral somitic frontier

**Table 11.1 Origins of Muscles from Abaxial and Primaxial Precursors**

| | Primaxial | Abaxial |
|---|---|---|
| **Cervical region** | Scalenes<br>Geniohyoid<br>Prevertebral | Infrahyoid |
| **Thoracoabdominal region** | Intercostals | Pectoralis major and minor<br>External oblique<br>Internal oblique<br>Transversus abdominis<br>Sternalis<br>Rectus abdominis<br>Pelvic diaphragm |
| **Upper limb** | Rhomboids<br>Levator scapulae<br>Latissimus dorsi | Distal limb muscles |
| **Lower limb**[a] | | All lower limb muscles |

[a]The precise origin of muscles in the pelvic region and lower limb has not been determined, but most, if not all, are abaxial in origin.

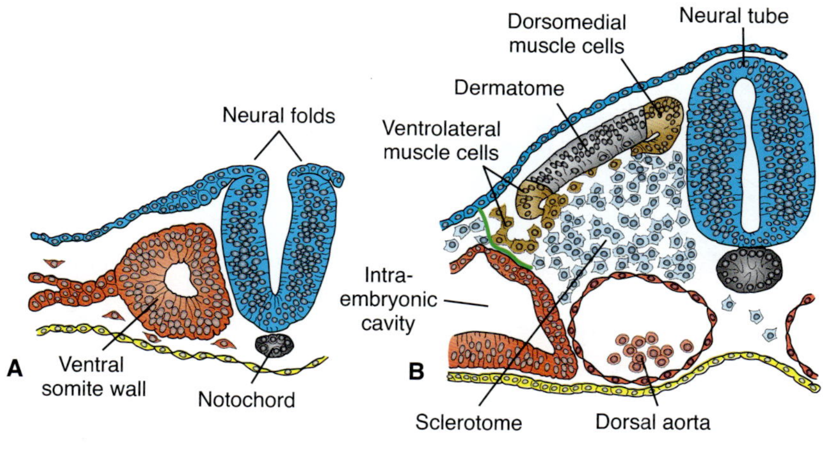


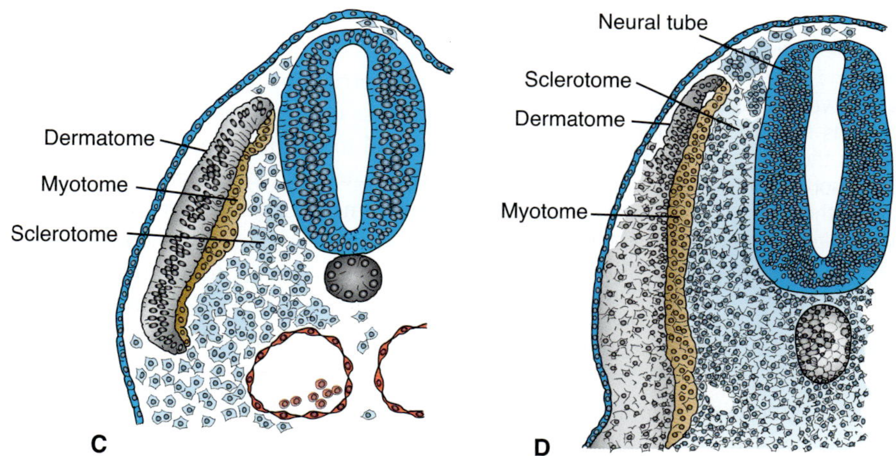




**FIGURE 11.1** Cross-sectional drawings showing the stages of development in a somite. **A.** Mesoderm cells become epithelial and are arranged around a small lumen. **B.** Cells in the ventral and medial walls of the somite lose their epithelial characteristics and migrate around the neural tube and notochord, and some move into the parietal layer of lateral plate mesoderm. Collectively, these cells constitute the sclerotome. Cells at the dorsomedial (DML) and ventrolateral (VLL) regions of the somite form muscle cell precursors. Cells from both regions migrate ventral to the dermatome to form the dermomyotome. VLL cells also migrate into the parietal layer of lateral plate mesoderm across the lateral somitic frontier (*green line*). In combination, somitic cells and lateral plate mesoderm cells constitute the abaxial mesodermal domain, whereas the primaxial mesodermal domain only contains somitic cells (paraxial mesoderm). **C.** Together, dermatome cells and the muscle cells that associate with them form the dermomyotome. **D.** The dermomyotome begins to differentiate: Myotome cells contribute to primaxial muscles, and dermatome cells form the dermis of the back.

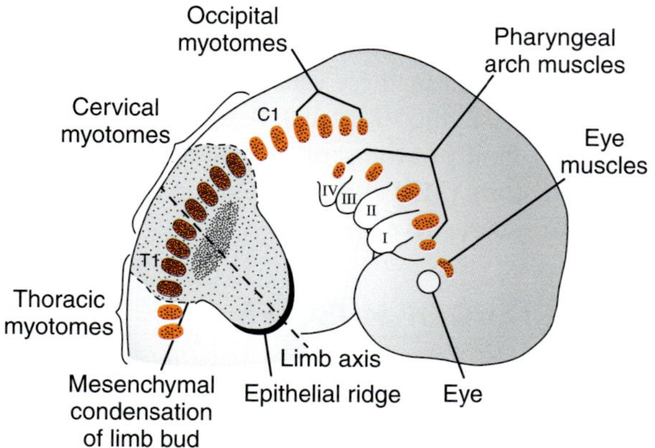


**FIGURE 11.2** Drawing showing musculature in the head and neck derived from somitomeres and myotomes that form from the occipital region caudally in a 7-week embryo.

Muscle cells that cross this frontier (those from the VLL edge of the myotome) and enter the lateral plate mesoderm comprise the **abaxial** muscle cell precursors and receive many of their signals for differentiation from lateral plate mesoderm (Fig. 11.3); those that remain in the paraxial mesoderm and do not cross the frontier (the remaining VLL cells and all of the DML cells) comprise the **primaxial** muscle cell precursors and receive many of their developmental signals from the neural tube and notochord (Fig. 11.3). Regardless of their domain, **each myotome receives its innervation from spinal nerves derived from the same segment as the muscle cells.**

The lateral somitic frontier also defines the border between dermis derived from dermatomes in the back and dermis derived from lateral plate mesoderm in the body wall. It also defines a border for rib development, such that the bony components of each rib are derived from primaxial

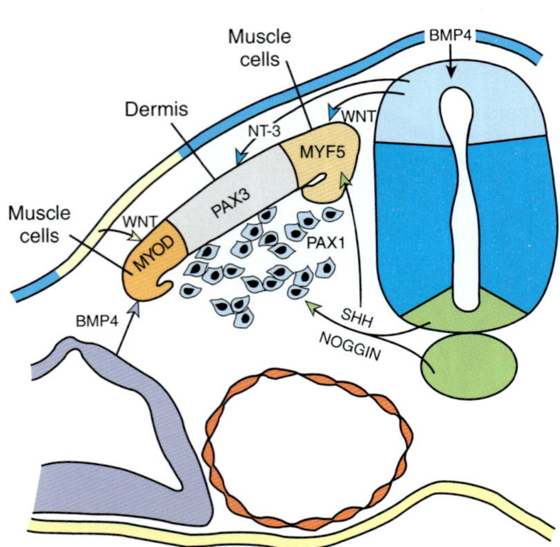


**FIGURE 11.3** Expression patterns of genes that regulate somite differentiation. Sonic hedgehog (SHH) and noggin, secreted by the notochord and floor plate of the neural tube, cause the ventral part of the somite to form sclerotome and to express *PAX1*, which in turn controls chondrogenesis and vertebral formation. WNT and low concentrations of SHH proteins from the dorsal neural tube activate *PAX3*, which demarcates the dermatome. WNT proteins also direct the dorsomedial (DML) portion of the somite to form muscle precursor cells and to express the muscle-specific gene *MYF5*. The dermatome portion of the somite is directed to become dermis by neurotrophin 3 (NT-3) secreted by the dorsal neural tube. The combined influence of activating WNT proteins and inhibitory bone morphogenetic protein 4 (BMP4) protein activates *MyoD* expression in the VLL region to create a second group of muscle cell precursors.

sclerotome cells and the cartilaginous parts of those ribs that attach to the sternum are derived from sclerotome cells that migrate across the lateral somitic frontier (abaxial cells).

## INNERVATION OF AXIAL SKELETAL MUSCLES

The **new description** of muscle development characterized by primaxial and abaxial domains differs from the old concept of epimeres (back muscles) and hypomeres (limb and body wall muscles), which was based on a functional definition of innervation: Epimeric muscles were innervated by dorsal primary rami, and hypomeric muscles by ventral primary rami. The new description is based on the actual **embryological origin** of muscle cells from two different populations of muscle cell precursors, the abaxial and primaxial cells, and not their innervation. The description does not preclude the fact that **epaxial (above the axis) muscles (back muscles) are innervated by dorsal primary rami**, whereas **hypaxial (below the axis) muscles (body wall and limb muscles) are innervated by ventral primary rami** (Fig. 11.4).

## SKELETAL MUSCLE AND TENDONS

During differentiation, precursor cells, the **myoblasts**, fuse and form long, multinucleated muscle fibers. Myofibrils soon appear in the cytoplasm, and by the end of the third month,

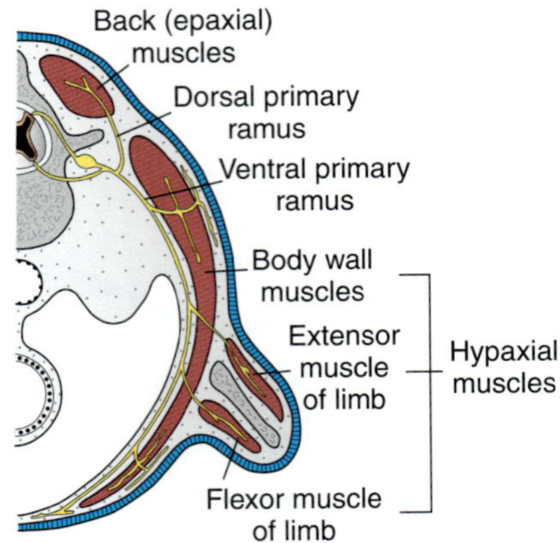


**FIGURE 11.4** Cross section through half the embryo showing innervation to developing musculature. Epaxial (true back muscles) are innervated by dorsal (posterior) primary rami. Hypaxial muscles (limb and body wall) are innervated by ventral (anterior) primary rami.

cross-striations, typical of skeletal muscle, appear. A similar process occurs in the seven somitomeres in the head region rostral to the occipital somites. However, somitomeres never segregate into recognizable regions of sclerotome and dermomyotome segments prior to differentiation. **Tendons** for the attachment of muscles to bones are derived from sclerotome cells lying adjacent to myotomes at the anterior and posterior borders of somites. The transcription factor ***SCLERAXIS*** regulates development of tendons.

## MOLECULAR REGULATION OF MUSCLE DEVELOPMENT

Genes regulating muscle development have recently been identified. Bone morphogenetic protein 4 (BMP4) and probably fibroblast growth factors from lateral plate mesoderm, together with WNT proteins from adjacent ectoderm, signal VLL cells of the dermomyotome to express the muscle-specific gene *MyoD* (Fig. 11.3). BMP4, secreted by ectoderm cells, induces production of WNT proteins by the dorsal neural tube at the same time that low concentrations of sonic hedgehog (SHH) proteins, secreted by the notochord and floor plate of the neural tube, reach the DML cells of the dermomyotome. Together, these proteins induce expression of *MYF5* and *MyoD* in these cells (note that SHH does not play a role in specifying VLL cells). Both *MyoD* and *MYF5* are members of a family of transcription factors called **myogenic regulatory factors (MRFs)**, and this group of genes activates pathways for muscle development.

## PATTERNING OF MUSCLES

Patterns of muscle formation are controlled by connective tissue into which myoblasts migrate. In the head region, these connective tissues are derived from **neural crest cells**; in cervical and occipital regions, they differentiate from **somitic mesoderm**; and in the body wall and limbs, they originate from the **parietal layer of lateral plate mesoderm**.

**Table 11.2 Origins of the Craniofacial Muscles**

| Mesodermal Origin | Muscles | Innervation |
|---|---|---|
| Somitomeres 1 and 2 | Superior, medial, inferior recti | Oculomotor (III) |
| Somitomere 3 | Superior oblique | Trochlear (IV) |
| Somitomere 4 | Jaw closing | Trigeminal (V) |
| Somitomere 5 | Lateral rectus | Abducens (VI) |
| Somitomere 6 | Jaw opening, other second arch | Facial (VII) |
| Somitomere 7 | Stylopharyngeus | Glossopharyngeal (IX) |
| Somites 1 and 2 | Intrinsic laryngeals | Vagus (X) |
| Somites 2–5[a] | Tongue | Hypoglossal (XII) |

[a]Somites 2 to 5 constitute the occipital group (somite 1 degenerates for the most part).

## HEAD MUSCULATURE

All voluntary muscles of the head region are derived from paraxial mesoderm (somitomeres and somites), including musculature of the tongue, eye (except that of the iris, which is derived from optic cup ectoderm), and that associated with the pharyngeal (visceral) arches (Table 11.2 and Fig. 11.2). Patterns of muscle formation in the head are directed by connective tissue elements derived from neural crest cells.

## LIMB MUSCULATURE

The first indication of limb musculature is observed in the seventh week of development as a condensation of mesenchyme near the base of the limb buds (Fig. 11.2). The mesenchyme is derived from muscle cell precursors from somites that migrate into the limb bud to form the muscles. As in other regions, connective tissue dictates the pattern of muscle formation, and this tissue is derived from the parietal layer of lateral plate mesoderm, which also gives rise to the bones of the limb (see Chapter 12).

## CARDIAC MUSCLE

Cardiac muscle develops from visceral mesoderm surrounding the endothelial heart tube. Myoblasts adhere to one another by special attachments that later develop into **intercalated discs**. Myofibrils develop as in skeletal muscle, but myoblasts do not fuse. During later development, a few special bundles of muscle cells with irregularly distributed myofibrils become visible. These bundles, **Purkinje fibers**, form the conducting system of the heart.

## SMOOTH MUSCLE

Smooth muscle for the dorsal aorta and large arteries is derived from lateral plate mesoderm and neural crest cells. In the coronary arteries, smooth muscle originates from proepicardial cells (see Chapter 13) and neural crest cells (proximal segments). Smooth muscle in the wall of the gut and gut derivatives is derived from the visceral layer of lateral plate mesoderm that surrounds these structures. Only the sphincter and dilator muscles of the pupil and muscle tissue in the mammary and sweat glands are derived from ectoderm.

**Serum response factor (SRF)** is a transcription factor responsible for smooth muscle cell differentiation. This factor is upregulated by growth factors through kinase phosphorylation pathways. **Myocardin** and ***myocardin-related transcription factors (MRTFs)*** then act as coactivators to enhance the activity of SRF, thereby initiating the genetic cascade responsible for smooth muscle development.

Part 2

### *Clinical Correlates*

Partial or complete absence of a muscle is common and usually not debilitating. Examples include partial or complete absence of the palmaris longus, serratus anterior, or quadratus femoris muscles. A more serious defect is called **Poland sequence** that occurs in 1 per 20,000 individuals and is characterized by absence of the pectoralis minor and partial loss of the pectoralis major (usually the sternal head) muscles (Fig. 11.5). The nipple and areola are absent or displaced, and there are often digital defects (syndactyly [fused digits] and brachydactyly [short digits]) on the affected side. The disfiguring nature of the defects can be problematic, especially in females because of breast development.

Partial or complete absence of abdominal musculature is called **prune belly syndrome** (Fig. 11.6). Usually, the abdominal wall is so thin that organs are visible and easily palpated. This defect is sometimes associated with malformations of the urinary tract and bladder, including urethral obstruction. These defects cause an accumulation of fluid that distends the abdomen, resulting in atrophy of the abdominal muscles.

**Muscular dystrophy** is the term for a group of inherited muscle diseases that cause progressive muscular wasting and weakness. There are a large number of these types of diseases of which **Duchenne muscular dystrophy (DMD)** is the most common (1 per 4,000 male births). The disease is inherited

*(Continued)*

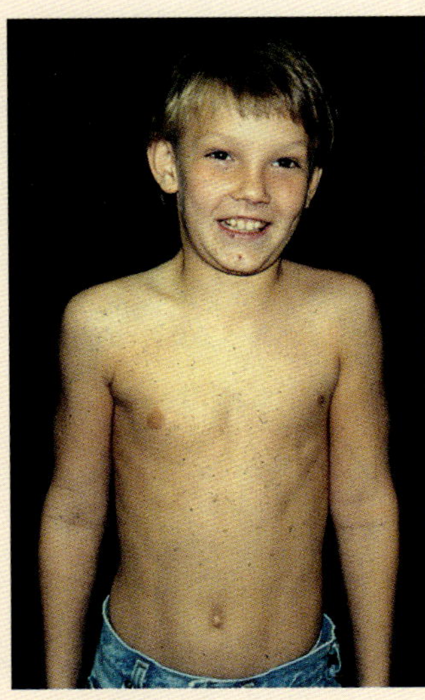

**FIGURE 11.5** Poland sequence. The pectoralis minor and part of the pectoralis major muscles are missing on the patient's left side. Note displacement of the nipple and areola.

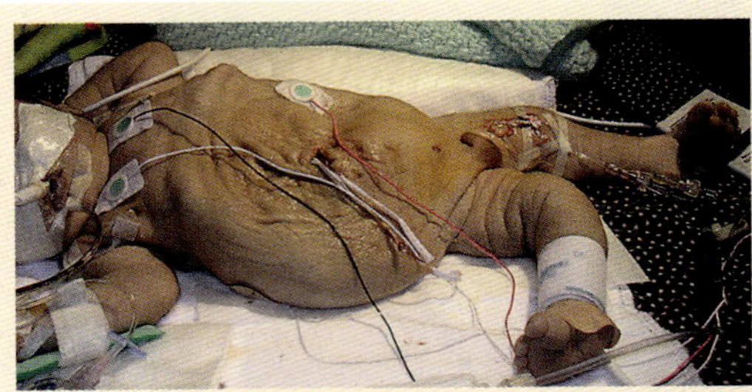

**FIGURE 11.6** Prune belly syndrome: a distended abdomen from atrophy of abdominal wall musculature.

as **X-linked recessive** such that males are much more often affected than females. Both DMD and **Becker muscular dystrophy (BMD)** are caused by mutations in the gene for **dystrophin** on the X chromosome. However, in DMD, no functional dystrophin is made, and the disease is much more severe with an earlier onset [<5 years of age versus 8 to 25 years of age in BMD]. Dystrophin is a cytoplasmic protein that forms a dystrophin-associated protein complex linking the cytoskeleton to the extracellular matrix.



## SUMMARY

- **Most muscles** arise from the **mesoderm**.
- Skeletal muscles are derived from paraxial mesoderm, including (1) **somites**, which give rise to muscles of the axial skeleton, body wall, and limbs, and (2) **somitomeres**, which give rise to muscles of the head.
- Progenitor cells for muscle tissues are derived from the ventrolateral (VLL) and dorsomedial (DML) edges (lips) of the prospective dermomyotome. Cells from both regions contribute to formation of the myotome. Some cells from the VLL also migrate across the **lateral somitic frontier** into the parietal layer of the lateral plate mesoderm.
- This frontier or border separates two mesodermal domains in the embryo:
  - The **primaxial domain** that surrounds the neural tube and contains only somite-derived cells (paraxial mesoderm)
  - The **abaxial domain** that consists of the parietal layer of lateral plate mesoderm in combination with somite-derived cells that migrate across the frontier into this region (Fig. 11.1).
- Abaxial muscle precursor cells differentiate into **infrahyoid, abdominal wall (rectus abdominis, external and internal obliques, transversus abdominis), and limb muscles.**
- Primaxial muscle precursor cells form **muscles of the back, some muscles of the shoulder girdle, and intercostal muscles** (Table 11.1, p. 132).
- Muscles of the back (**epaxial muscles**) are innervated by **dorsal primary rami**; muscles of the limbs and body wall (**hypaxial muscles**) are innervated by **ventral primary rami.**
- Molecular signals for muscle cell induction arise from tissues adjacent to prospective muscle cells. Thus, signals from lateral plate mesoderm (**BMPs**) and overlying ectoderm (**WNTs**) induce VLL cells, whereas signals from the neural tube and notochord (**SHH** and **WNTs**) induce DML cells.
- **Connective tissue** derived from somites, parietal mesoderm, and neural crest (head region) provides a template for establishment of muscle patterns. **Most smooth muscles** and **cardiac muscle fibers** are derived from **visceral mesoderm.** Smooth muscles of the pupil, mammary gland, and sweat glands differentiate from ectoderm.

## Self-Assessment

### Comprehensive Questions

1. Discuss the development of skeletal muscles of the back with nerve supply.
2. Muscle cells are derived from what two regions of the somite? Which region contributes to the abaxial mesodermal domain? What muscles form from the abaxial and primaxial domains?

### Problem Solving Questions

1. In examining a newborn female infant, you note that her right nipple is displaced toward the axilla and that the right anterior axillary fold is nearly absent. What is your diagnosis?
2. How do you explain the fact that the phrenic nerve, which originates from cervical segments 3, 4, and 5, innervates the diaphragm in the thoracic region?

3. An 8-year-old male child comes to pediatrics OPD with muscle weakness and since 2 days is not able to stand. His elder brother is also affected by a similar condition and is bedridden. However, his sister is in good health. What is this condition and its cause? How will you counsel the parents?

## Multiple Choice Questions

1. All voluntary muscles of the back are derived from
   (a) Paraxial mesoderm
   (b) Lateral plate mesoderm
   (c) Intermediate mesoderm
   (d) Cardiogenic area
2. Skeletal muscles are formed by differentiation and fusion of
   (a) Myofibrils
   (b) Myoblasts
   (c) Fascicles
   (d) Mesoderm
3. Patterning of muscle formation are controlled by
   (a) Somites
   (b) Neural crest cell
   (c) Abaxial and primaxial cells
   (d) Connective tissue into which muscle cells migrate
4. Smooth muscle of gut is derived from
   (a) Paramesoderm
   (b) Intermediate mesoderm
   (c) Parietal layer of lateral plate mesoderm
   (d) Visceral layer of lateral plate mesoderm
5. Hypaxial muscles are
   (a) Muscles of the back
   (b) Muscles of the head and neck
   (c) Muscles of the body wall and limbs
   (d) Muscles of the viscera
6. Epaxial muscles are supplied by
   (a) Cranial nerves
   (b) Sympathetic plexus
   (c) Dorsal primary rami
   (d) Ventral primary rami

### Answers

1. (a) 2. (b) 3. (d) 4. (d) 5. (c) 6. (c)

Part 2

CHAPTER

# 12 Limbs

## Specific Learning Objectives

- Limb growth and development
- Limb musculature
- Molecular regulations
- Clinical correlations
- Bone age
- Limb defects

## Competencies Covered

AN13.8 Describe the development of the upper limb.
AN20.10 Describe the basic concept of the development of the lower limb.

Part 2

## LIMB GROWTH AND DEVELOPMENT

The limbs, including the shoulder and pelvic girdles, comprise the appendicular skeleton. At the end of the fourth week of development, limb buds become visible as outpocketings that form ridges on the lateral body wall (Fig. 12.1*A*). The forelimb appears first followed by the hind limb 1 to 2 days later. By the fifth week, limbs have attained the bud stage (Fig. 12.1*B*). Initially, the limb buds consist of a mesenchymal core derived from the parietal (somatic) layer of lateral plate mesoderm that will form the bones and connective tissues of the limb, covered by a layer of cuboidal ectoderm. Ectoderm at the distal border of the limb thickens and forms the **apical ectodermal ridge (AER)** (Fig. 12.2; see also Fig. 12.9*A*). This ridge exerts an inductive influence on adjacent mesenchyme, causing it to remain as a population of undifferentiated, rapidly proliferating cells, the **undifferentiated zone**. As the limb grows, cells farther from the influence of the AER begin to differentiate into cartilage and muscle. In this manner, development of each limb proceeds proximodistally into its three components: **stylopod** (humerus and femur), **zeugopod** (radius/ulna and tibia/fibula), and **autopod** (carpels, metacarpals, digits/tarsals, digits/metatarsals).

In 6-week-old embryos, the terminal portion of the limb buds becomes flattened to form the **hand-** and **footplates** and is separated from the proximal segment by a circular constriction (Fig. 12.1*C*). Later, a second constriction divides the proximal portion into two segments, and the main parts of the extremities can be recognized (Fig. 12.1*D*). Fingers and toes are formed when **cell death** in the AER separates this ridge into five parts (Fig. 12.3*A*). Further formation of the digits depends on their continued outgrowth under the influence of the five segments of ridge ectoderm, condensation of the mesenchyme to form cartilaginous digital rays, and the death of intervening tissue between the rays (Fig. 12.3*B*,*C*).

Development of the upper and lower limbs is similar except that morphogenesis of the lower limb is approximately 1 to

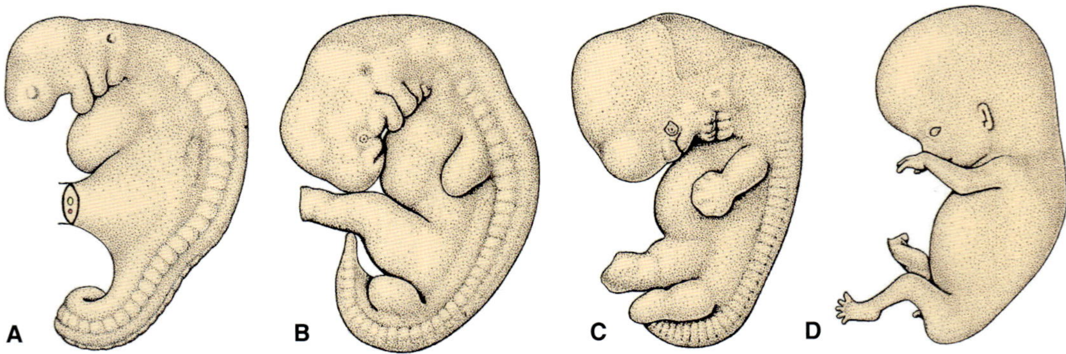


**FIGURE 12.1** Development of the limb buds in human embryos. **A.** At 4 weeks, outpocketings along the lateral body wall form ridges. **B.** At 5 weeks, the limb bud stage is attained. **C.** At 6 weeks, hand- and footplates are formed. **D.** By 8 weeks, fingers and toes are present. Hind limb development lags behind forelimb development by 1 to 2 days.

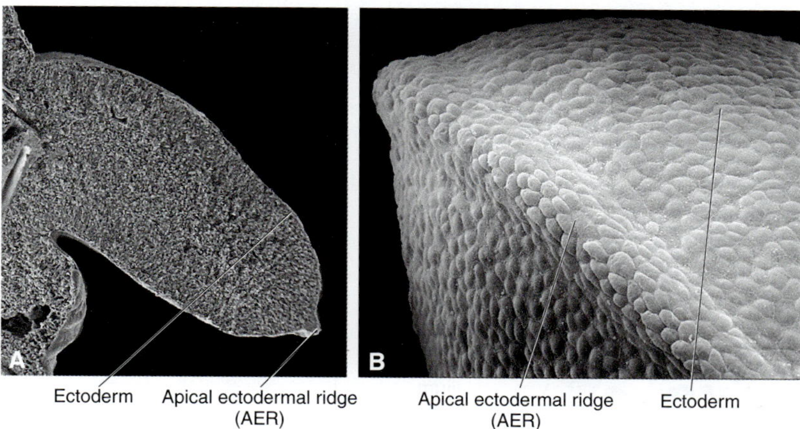


**FIGURE 12.2** **A.** Longitudinal section through the limb bud of a chick embryo, showing a core of mesenchyme covered by a layer of ectoderm that thickens at the distal border of the limb to form the apical ectodermal ridge (AER). In humans, this occurs during the fifth week of development. **B.** External view of a chick limb at high magnification showing the ectoderm and the specialized region at the tip of the limb called the AER.

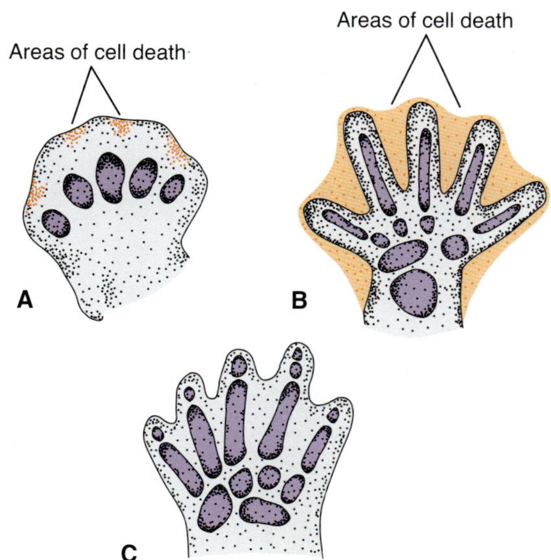


**FIGURE 12.3** Schematic of human hands. **A.** At 48 days, cell death in the apical ectodermal ridge (AER) creates a separate ridge for each digit. **B.** At 51 days, cell death in the interdigital spaces produces separation of the digits. **C.** At 56 days, digit separation is complete.

2 days behind that of the upper limb. Also, during the seventh week of gestation, the limbs rotate in opposite directions. **The upper limb rotates 90° laterally** so that the extensor muscles lie on the lateral and posterior surface, and the thumbs lie laterally, whereas **the lower limb rotates approximately 90° medially**, placing the extensor muscles on the anterior surface and the big toe medially.

While the external shape is being established, mesenchyme in the buds begins to condense, and these cells differentiate into chondrocytes (Fig. 12.4). By the sixth week of development, the first **hyaline cartilage models**, foreshadowing the bones of the extremities, are formed by these chondrocytes (Figs. 12.4 and 12.5). Joints are formed in the cartilaginous condensations when chondrogenesis is arrested, and a joint **interzone** is induced. Cells in this region increase in number and density, and then a joint cavity is formed by cell death. Surrounding cells differentiate into a joint capsule. Factors regulating the positioning of joints are not clear, but the secreted molecule **WNT14** appears to be the inductive signal.

Ossification of the bones of the extremities, **endochondral ossification**, begins by the end of the embryonic period. Primary **ossification centers** are present in all long bones of the limbs by the 12th week of development. From the primary center in the shaft or **diaphysis** of the bone, endochondral ossification gradually progresses toward the ends of the cartilaginous model (Fig. 12.5).

At birth, the diaphysis of the bone is usually completely ossified, but the two ends, the **epiphyses**, are still cartilaginous. Shortly thereafter, however, ossification centers arise in the epiphyses. Temporarily, a cartilage plate remains between the diaphyseal and epiphyseal ossification centers. This plate, the **epiphyseal plate**, plays an important role in growth in the length of the bones. Endochondral ossification proceeds on both sides of the plate (Fig. 12.5). When the bone has acquired its full length, the epiphyseal plates disappear, and the epiphyses unite with the shaft of the bone.

In long bones, an epiphyseal plate is found on each extremity; in smaller bones, such as the phalanges, it is found only at one extremity; and in irregular bones, such as the vertebrae, one or more primary centers of ossification and usually several secondary centers are present.

**Synovial joints** between bones begin to form at the same time that mesenchymal condensations initiate the process of forming cartilage. Thus, in the region between two chondrifying bone primordia, called the **interzone** (e.g., between the tibia and femur at the knee joint), the condensed mesenchyme differentiates into dense fibrous tissue. This fibrous tissue then forms **articular cartilage**, covering the ends of the two adjacent bones; the **synovial membranes**; and the **menisci and ligaments within the joint capsule** (e.g., the anterior and posterior cruciate ligaments in the knee). The **joint capsule** itself is derived from mesenchyme

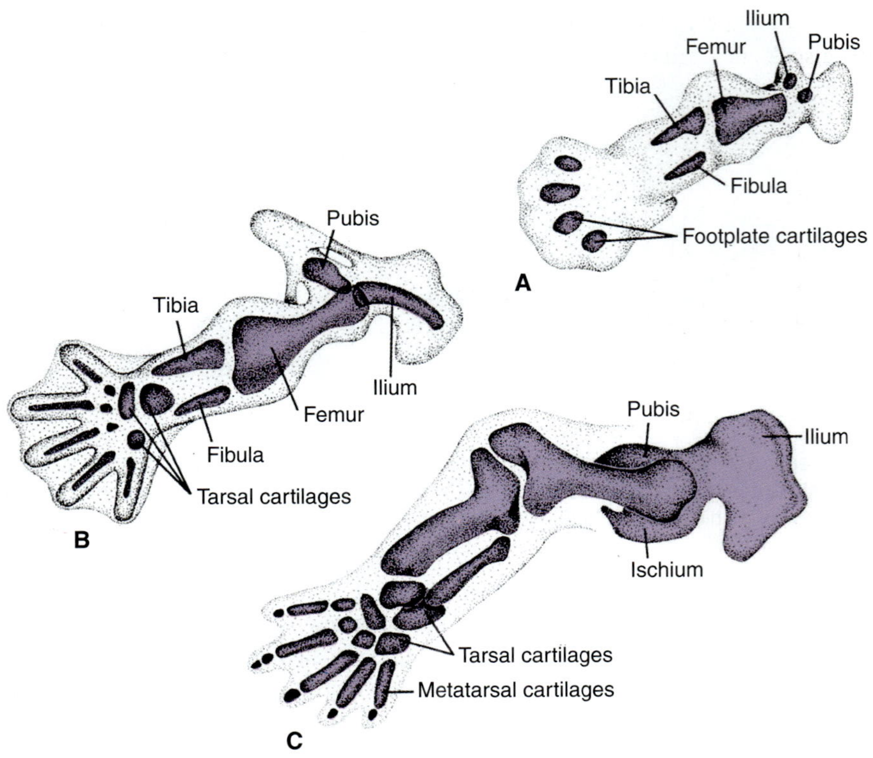


**FIGURE 12.4** **A.** Lower extremity of an early 6-week embryo, illustrating the first hyaline cartilage models. **B,C.** Complete set of cartilage models at the end of the sixth week and the beginning of the eighth week, respectively.



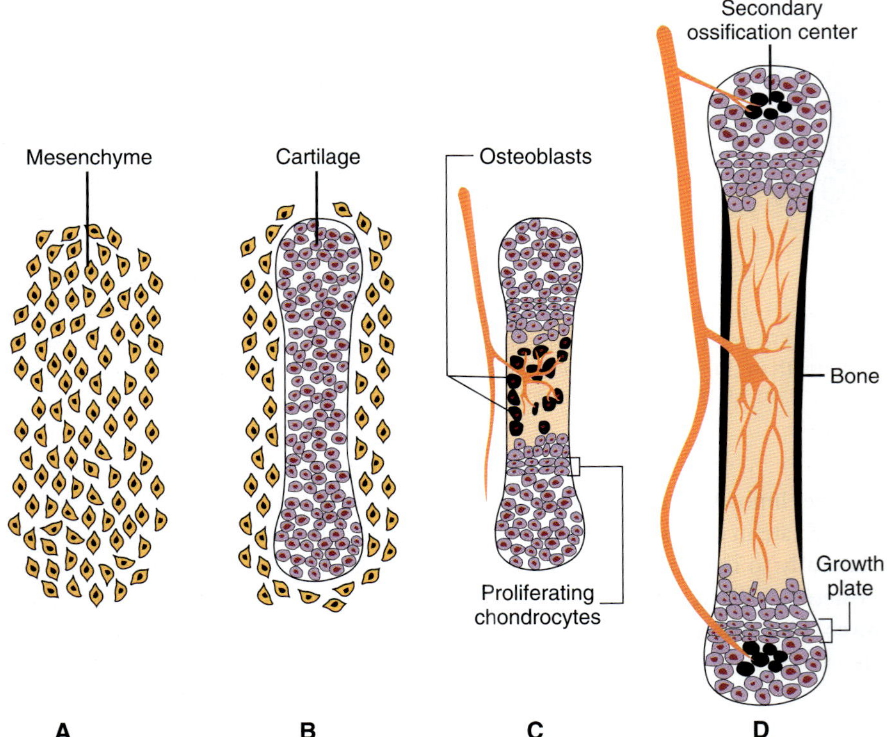


**FIGURE 12.5** Endochondral bone formation. **A.** Mesenchyme cells begin to condense and differentiate into chondrocytes. **B.** Chondrocytes form a cartilaginous model of the prospective bone. **C,D.** Blood vessels invade the center of the cartilaginous model, bringing osteoblasts (black cells) and restricting proliferating chondrocytic cells to the ends (epiphyses) of the bones. Chondrocytes toward the shaft side (diaphysis) undergo hypertrophy and apoptosis as they mineralize the surrounding matrix. Osteoblasts bind to the mineralized matrix and deposit bone matrices. Later, as blood vessels invade the epiphyses, secondary ossification centers form. Growth of the bones is maintained by proliferation of chondrocytes in the growth plates.

cells surrounding the interzone region. **Fibrous joints** (e.g., the sutures in the skull) also form from interzone regions, but, in this case, the interzone remains as a dense fibrous structure.

## ■ LIMB MUSCULATURE

Limb musculature is derived from ventrolateral cells of the somites that migrate into the limb to form muscles, and initially, these muscle components are segmented according to the somites from which they are derived (Fig. 12.6). However, with elongation of the limb buds, the muscle tissue first splits into flexor and extensor components (Fig. 12.7) and then additional splittings and fusions occur, such that a single muscle may be formed from more than one original segment. The resulting complex pattern of muscles is determined by connective tissue derived from lateral plate mesoderm.

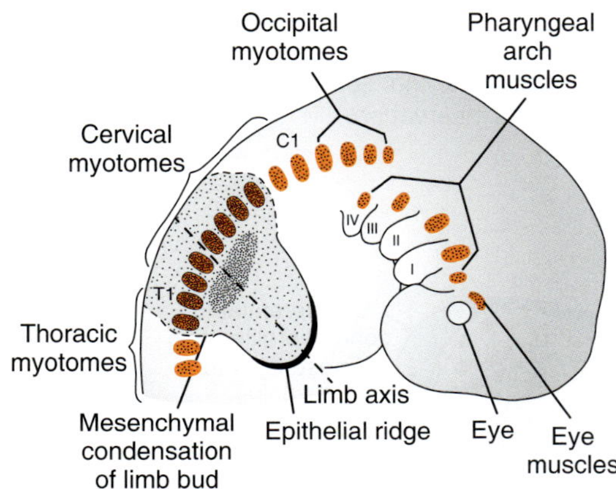


**FIGURE 12.6** Muscle cells for the limbs are derived from somites at specific segmental levels. For the upper limb, these segments are C5–T2; for the hind limb, they are L2–S2. Ultimately, muscles are derived from more than one segment and so the initial segmentation pattern is lost.

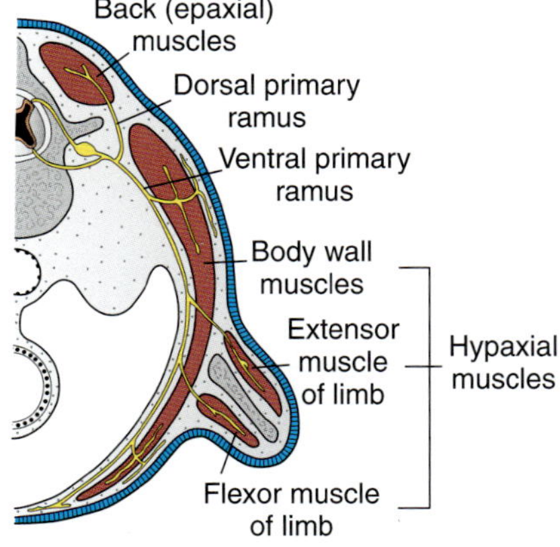


**FIGURE 12.7** As muscle cells move into the limb, they split into dorsal (extensor) and ventral (flexor) compartments. Muscles are innervated by ventral primary rami that initially divide to form dorsal and ventral branches to these compartments. Ultimately, branches from their respective dorsal and ventral divisions unite into large dorsal and ventral nerves.

Upper limb buds lie opposite the lower five cervical and upper two thoracic segments (Fig. 12.6), and the lower limb buds lie opposite the lower four lumbar and upper two sacral segments. As soon as the buds form, ventral primary rami from the appropriate spinal nerves penetrate into the mesenchyme. At first, each ventral ramus enters with dorsal and ventral branches derived from its specific spinal segment but soon branches in their respective divisions begin to unite to form large dorsal and ventral nerves (Fig. 12.7). Thus, the **radial nerve**, which supplies the extensor musculature, is formed by a combination of the dorsal segmental branches, whereas the **ulnar** and **median nerves**, which supply the flexor musculature, are formed by a combination of the ventral branches. Immediately after the nerves have entered the limb buds, they establish an intimate contact with the differentiating mesodermal condensations, and the early contact between the nerve and muscle cells is a prerequisite for their complete functional differentiation.

Spinal nerves not only play an important role in differentiation and motor innervation of the limb musculature but also provide **sensory innervation** for the **dermatomes**. Although the original dermatomal pattern changes with growth and rotation of the extremities, an orderly sequence can still be recognized in the adult (Fig. 12.8).

### Molecular Regulation of Limb Development

Positioning of the limbs along the craniocaudal axis in the flank regions of the embryo is regulated by the ***HOX* genes** expressed along this axis. These **homeobox** genes are expressed in overlapping patterns from head to tail (see Chapter 6, p. 75), with some having more cranial limits than others. For example, the cranial limit of expression of ***HOXB8*** is at the cranial border of the forelimb, and misexpression of this gene alters the position of these limbs. Specification of the forelimb is regulated by the transcription factor ***TBX5***; specification of the hind limb is regulated by ***TBX4***.

Once positioning along the craniocaudal axis is determined, growth must be regulated along the proximodistal, anteroposterior, and dorsoventral axes (Fig. 12.9). Limb outgrowth is initiated by fibroblast growth factor (FGF) 10 secreted by lateral plate mesoderm cells (Fig. 12.9*A*). Once outgrowth is initiated, bone morphogenetic proteins (BMPs), expressed in ventral ectoderm, induce formation of the AER by signaling through the homeobox gene *MSX2*. Expression of ***RADICAL FRINGE***, a homologue of *Drosophila fringe*, in the dorsal half of the limb ectoderm, restricts the location of the AER to the distal tip of the limbs. This gene induces expression of ***SER2***, a homologue of *Drosophila serrate*, at the border between cells that are expressing *RADICAL FRINGE* and those that are not. It is at this border that the AER is established. Formation of the border itself is assisted by expression of ***ENGRAILED-1*** in ventral ectoderm cells, because this gene represses expression of *RADICAL FRINGE* (Fig. 12.9*A*). After the ridge is established, it expresses **FGF4** and **FGF8**, which maintain the **undifferentiated zone**, the rapidly proliferating population of mesenchyme cells adjacent to the

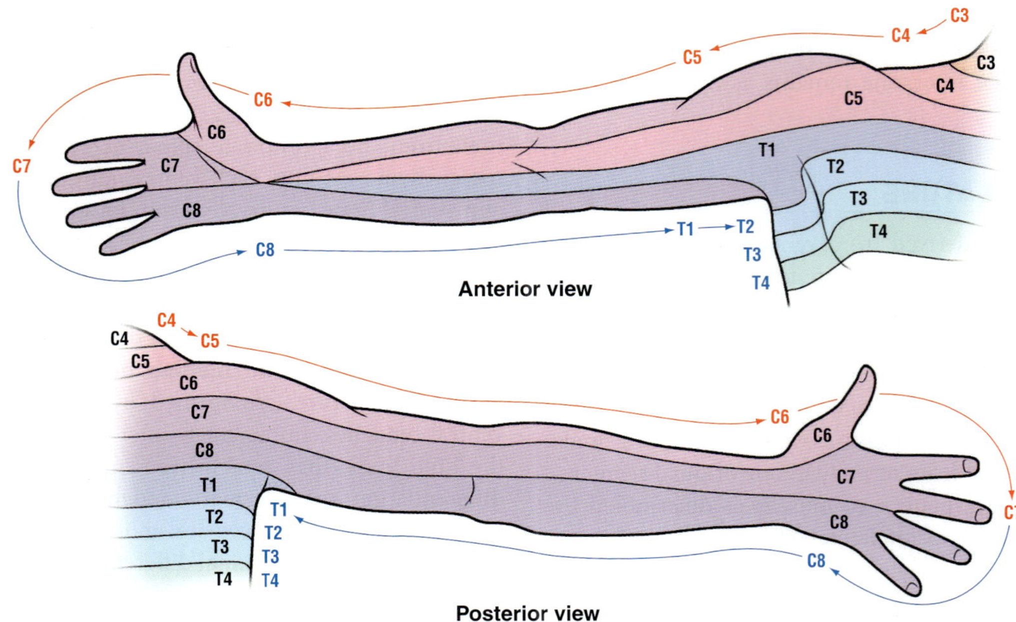


**FIGURE 12.8** Forelimbs with their sensory innervation to the dermatomes represented. Note that sensory innervation to the limb maintains a segmental pattern reflecting the embryological origin of each dermatome and its innervation.



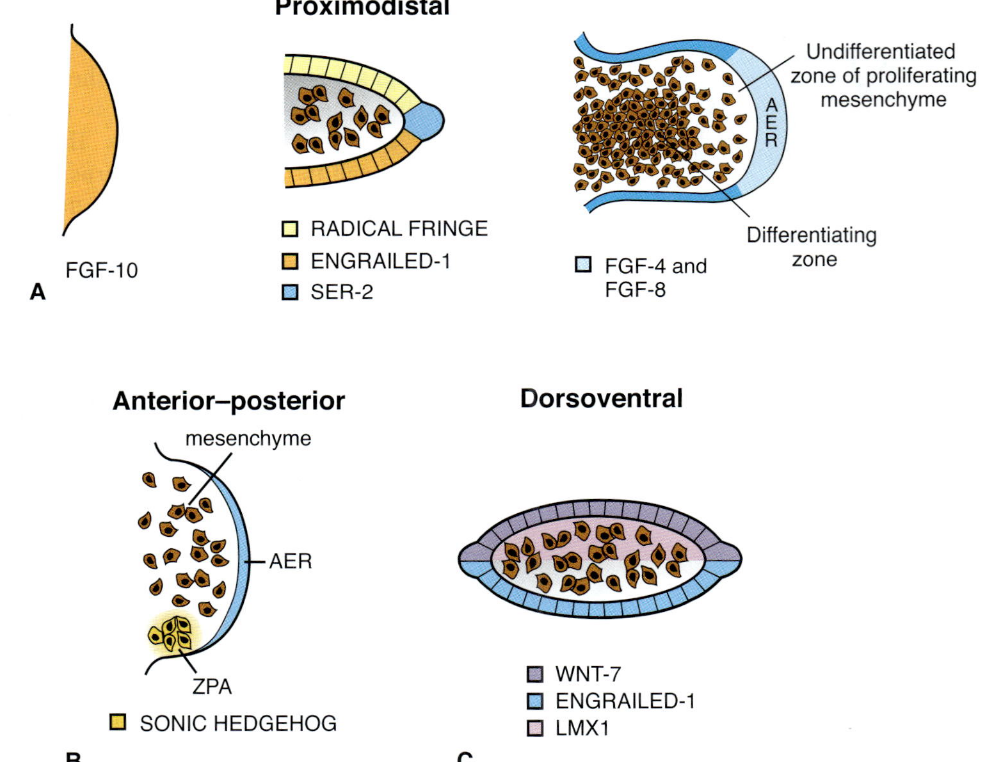


**FIGURE 12.9** Molecular regulation of patterning and growth in the limb. **A.** Limb outgrowth is initiated by fibroblast growth factor (FGF) 10 secreted by lateral plate mesoderm in the limb-forming regions. Once outgrowth is initiated, the apical ectodermal ridge (AER) is induced by bone morphogenetic proteins (BMPs) and restricted in its location by the gene *RADICAL FRINGE* expressed in dorsal ectoderm. In turn, this expression induces that of *SER2* in cells destined to form the AER. After the ridge is established, it expresses FGF4 and FGF8 to maintain the **progress zone**, the rapidly proliferating mesenchyme cells adjacent to the ridge. **B.** Anteroposterior patterning of the limb is controlled by cells in the zone of polarizing activity (ZPA) at the posterior border. These cells produce retinoic acid (vitamin A), which initiates expression of *SHH*, regulating patterning. **C.** The dorsoventral limb axis is directed by *WNT7a*, which is expressed in the dorsal ectoderm. This gene induces expression of the transcription factor *LMX1* in the dorsal mesenchyme, specifying these cells as dorsal.

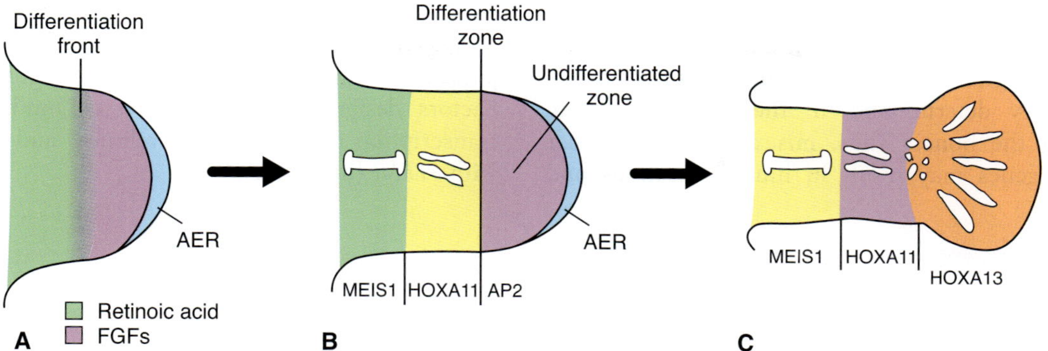


**FIGURE 12.10** Drawing showing limb patterning along the proximodistal axis. **A.** During early stages of limb outgrowth, cells beneath the apical ectodermal ridge (AER) are maintained in a highly proliferative undifferentiated state (the undifferentiated zone) by exposure to fibroblast growth factors (FGFs) secreted by the AER. Meanwhile, cells that are farther away from the AER are exposed to retinoic acid secreted by flank mesenchyme cells. These two cell populations meet at the differentiation front. **B.** As continued growth occurs, proximal cells under the influence of retinoic acid and a genetic cascade differentiate into the stylopod. As this process occurs, the differentiation front moves distally and, under the influence of *SHH* and other genes, the zeugopod differentiates. **C.** Finally, secretion of FGFs by the AER is terminated and the autopod differentiates. While the AER is active, the marker gene for the undifferentiated zone is the transcription factor *AP2* **(B)**, which may play a role in maintaining FGF secretion by the AER. Marker genes for the three differentiated limb regions **(C)** include *MEIS1* (stylopod), *HOXA11* (zeugopod), and *HOXA13* (autopod).

ridge (Fig. 12.9*A*). Distal growth of the limb is then effected by these rapidly proliferating cells under the influence of the FGFs. As growth occurs, mesenchymal cells at the proximal end of the undifferentiated zone are no longer influenced by signals from FGFs and, instead, begin to differentiate under the control of other signaling molecules (Fig. 12.10). For example, **retinoic acid**, made in flank mesenchyme cells, acts as a morphogen to initiate a genetic cascade to specify and cause differentiation of the stylopod. A marker gene for this region is the transcription factor *MEIS1* that may participate in this process. Differentiation of the zeugopod and autopod regions involves other genes, including *SONIC HEDGEHOG* (*SHH*). Marker genes for these regions are *HOXA11* for the zeugopod and *HOXA13* for the autopod (Fig. 12.10*C*). It is not clear whether or not these markers play a role in the differentiation process, but *HOX* genes in general play a critical role in patterning the bones of the limbs.

Patterning of the anteroposterior axis of the limb is regulated by the **zone of polarizing activity (ZPA)**, a cluster of mesenchymal cells at the posterior border of the limb near the AER (Fig. 12.9*B*). These cells produce the secreted factor **SHH**, a morphogen that contributes to specification of the anteroposterior axis. For example, digits appear in the proper order, with the thumb on the radial (anterior) side. As the limb grows, the ZPA moves distalward to remain in proximity to the posterior border of the AER. Misexpression of *SHH* in the anterior margin of a limb containing a normally expressing ZPA in the posterior border results in a mirror image duplication of limb structures (Fig. 12.11).

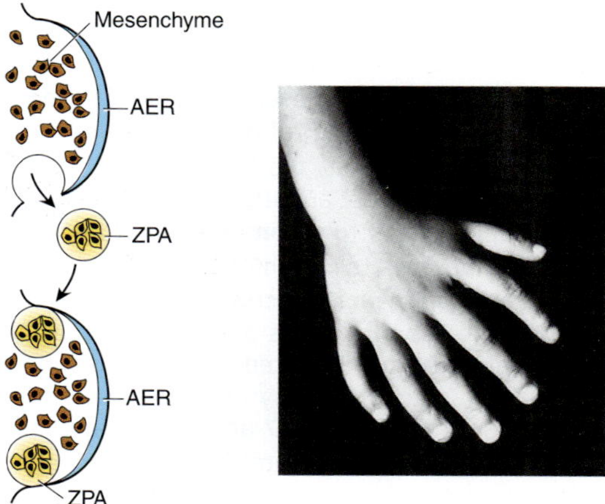


**FIGURE 12.11** Experimental procedure for grafting a new zone of polarizing activity (ZPA) from one limb bud into another using chick embryos. The result is the production of a limb with mirror image duplication of the digits much like that shown in the adjacent figure, indicating the role of the ZPA in regulating anteroposterior patterning of the limb. *SHH* protein is the molecule secreted by the ZPA responsible for this regulation.

The dorsoventral axis is also regulated by BMPs in the ventral ectoderm, which induce expression of the transcription factor *EN1*. In turn, *EN1* represses *WNT7a* expression, restricting it to the dorsal limb ectoderm. WNT7a is a secreted factor that induces expression of *LMX1*, a transcription factor containing a homeodomain, in the dorsal mesenchyme (Fig. 12.9*C*). *LMX1* specifies cells to be dorsal, establishing the dorsoventral components. In addition, *WNT7a* maintains *SHH* expression in the ZPA and therefore indirectly affects anteroposterior patterning as well. These two genes are also intimately linked in signaling pathways in *Drosophila*, and this interaction is conserved in vertebrates. In fact, all of the patterning genes in the limb have feedback loops. Thus, FGFs in the AER activate *SHH* in the ZPA, whereas *WNT7a* maintains the SHH signal, which in turn can upregulate *FGF* expression in the AER.

Although patterning genes for the limb axes have been determined, it is the *HOX* genes that regulate the types and shapes of the bones of the limb. This *HOX* gene expression is dependent on the combinatorial (involving combinations) expression of *FGF*, *SHH*, and *WNT7a* genes that cause *HOX* expression in three phases in the limb that correspond to the proximal (stylopod: humerus and femur), middle (zeugopod: radius/ulna; tibia/fibula), and distal (autopod: hand and foot) regions. Genes of the *HOXA* and *D* clusters are the primary determinants in the limb accounting for patterning the bones. Thus, misexpression of either of these two genes may result in limb truncations and anterior–posterior duplications. Just as in the craniocaudal axis of the embryo, *HOX* genes are nested in overlapping patterns of expression that somehow regulate patterning. Factors designating forelimb versus hind limb are the transcription factors *TBX5* (forelimbs) and *TBX4* together with *PITX1* (hind limbs).

## Clinical Correlates

### Bone Age

Radiologists use the appearance of various ossification centers to determine whether a child has reached his or her proper maturation age. Useful information about **bone age** is obtained from ossification studies in the hands and wrists of children. Prenatal analysis of fetal bones by ultrasonography provides information about fetal growth and gestational age.

### Limb Defects

Limb malformations occur in approximately 6 per 10,000 live births, with 3.4 per 10,000 affecting the upper limb and 1.1 per 10,000 affecting the lower. These defects are often associated with other birth defects involving the craniofacial, cardiac, and genitourinary systems. Abnormalities of the limbs vary greatly, and they may be represented by partial (**meromelia**) or complete absence (**amelia**) of one or more of the extremities (Fig. 12.12*A*). Sometimes, the long bones are absent, and rudimentary hands and feet are attached to the trunk by small, irregularly shaped bones (**phocomelia**, a form of meromelia) (Fig. 12.12*B*). Sometimes, all segments of the extremities are present but abnormally short (**micromelia**).

Although these abnormalities are rare and mainly hereditary, cases of teratogen-induced limb defects have been documented. For example, many children with limb malformations were born between 1957 and 1962. Many mothers of these infants had taken **thalidomide**, a drug widely used as a sleeping pill and antinauseant. It was subsequently established that thalidomide causes a characteristic syndrome of malformations consisting of absence or gross deformities of the long bones, intestinal atresia, and cardiac anomalies. Studies indicate that the fourth and the fifth weeks of gestation are the most sensitive period for induction of the limb defects. Because the drug is now being used to treat AIDS and cancer patients, distribution of thalidomide is carefully regulated to avoid its use by pregnant women.

A different category of limb defects involves the digits. Sometimes, the digits are shortened (**brachydactyly**; Fig. 12.13*A*). If two or more fingers or toes are fused, it is called **syndactyly** (Fig. 12.13*B*). Normally, mesenchyme between prospective digits in hand- and footplates is removed by cell death (apoptosis). In 1 per 2,000 births, this process fails, and the result is fusion between two or more digits. The presence of extra fingers or toes is called **polydactyly** (Fig. 12.13*C*). The extra digits frequently lack proper muscle connections. Abnormalities involving polydactyly are usually bilateral, whereas absence of a digit (**ectrodactyly**), such as a thumb, usually occurs unilaterally.

**Cleft hand and foot** consists of an abnormal cleft between the second and fourth metacarpal bones and soft tissues. The third metacarpal and phalangeal bones are almost always absent, and the thumb and index finger and the fourth and fifth fingers may be fused (Fig. 12.13*D*). The two parts of the hand are somewhat opposed to each other.

A number of gene mutations have been identified that affect the limbs and sometimes other structures (see Table 10.1, p. 125). The role of the *HOX* genes in limb development is

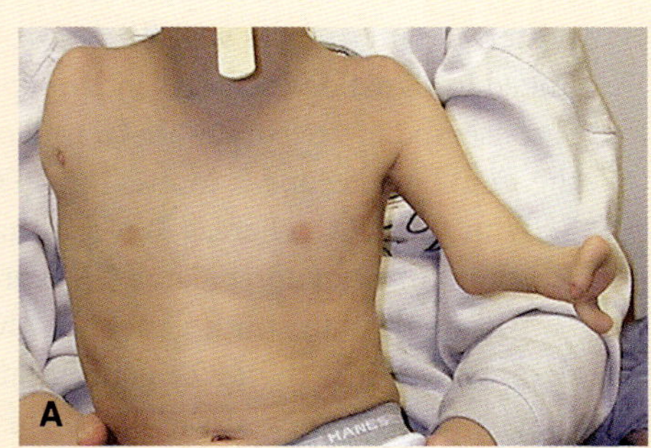


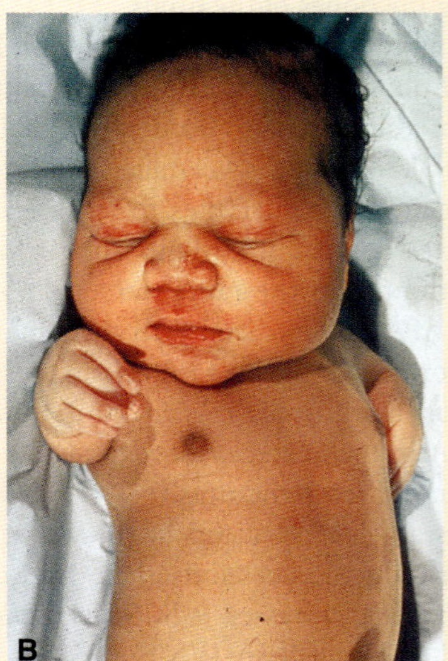


**FIGURE 12.12** **A.** Child with unilateral amelia and multiple defects of the left upper limb. **B.** Patient with a form of meromelia called *phocomelia*. The hands are attached to the trunk by irregularly shaped bones.

Part 2

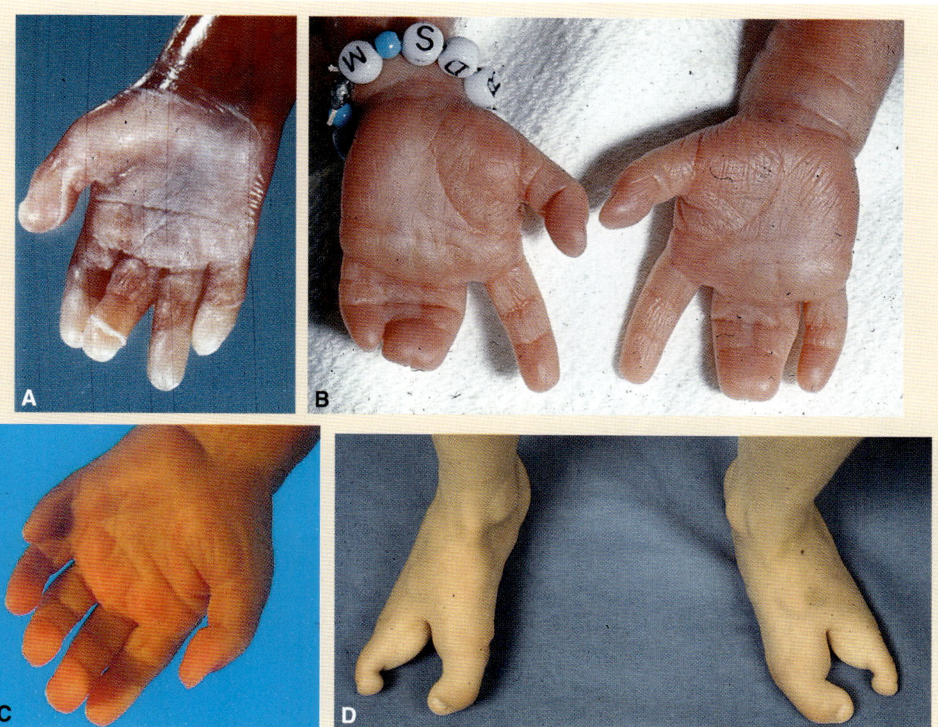

**FIGURE 12.13** Digital defects. **A.** Brachydactyly, short digits. **B.** Syndactyly, fused digits. **C.** Polydactyly, extra digits. **D.** Cleft foot. Any of these defects may involve either the hands or feet or both.

illustrated by two abnormal phenotypes produced by mutations in this family of genes: Mutations in ***HOXA13*** result in **hand–foot–genital syndrome**, characterized by fusion of the carpal bones and small short digits. Affected females often have a partially (bicornuate) or a completely (didelphic) divided uterus and abnormal positioning of the urethral orifice. Affected males may have hypospadias. The genital defects are due to the fact that *HOXA13* plays an important role in development of the cloaca into the urogenital sinus and anal canal (see Chapter 16). Mutations in ***HOXD13*** result in a combination of syndactyly and polydactyly (**synpolydactyly**).

***TBX5*** mutations (chromosome 12q24.1) result in **Holt-Oram syndrome**, characterized by upper limb abnormalities and heart defects consistent with a role for this gene in upper limb and heart development. Virtually all types of limb defects affecting the upper limb have been observed, including absent digits, polydactyly, syndactyly, absent radius, and hypoplasia of any of the limb bones. Heart defects include atrial and ventricular septal defects and conduction abnormalities.

**Osteogenesis imperfecta** is characterized by shortening, bowing, and hypomineralization of the long bones of the limbs that can result in fractures and blue sclera (Fig. 12.14). Several types of osteogenesis imperfecta occur, ranging from persons with a mildly increased frequency of fractures to a severe form that is lethal in the neonatal period. In most cases, dominant mutations in the ***COL1A1*** or ***COL1A2*** genes that are involved in production of **type I collagen** cause the abnormalities.

**Marfan syndrome** is caused by mutations in the ***FIBRILLIN* (*FBN1*)** gene located on chromosome 15q21.1. Affected individuals are usually tall and slender with long thin limbs and a long thin face. Other characteristics include sternal defects (pectus excavatum or carinatum), joint hyperflexibility, dilatation and/or dissection of the ascending aorta, and dislocation of the lens of the eye.

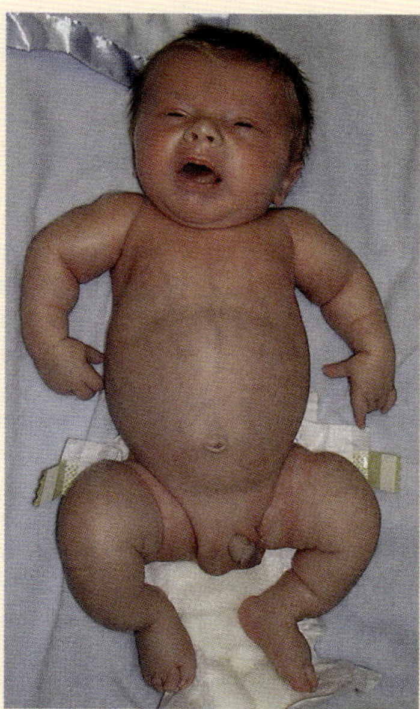

**FIGURE 12.14** Newborn with osteogenesis imperfecta. Note the shortness and bowing of the limbs.

**Arthrogryposis (congenital joint contractures)** (Fig. 12.15) usually involves more than one joint and may be caused by neurological defects (motor horn cell deficiency, meningomyelocele), muscular abnormalities (myopathies, muscle agenesis), and joint and contiguous tissue problems (synostosis, abnormal development). **Clubfoot** may be caused by arthrogryposis but

(*Continued*)

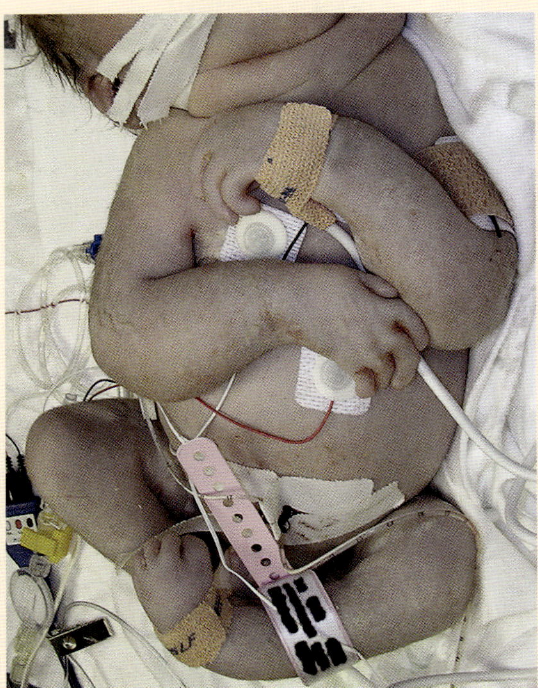

**FIGURE 12.15** Infant with arthrogryposis (congenital joint contractures).

is more commonly considered to be idiopathic in origin. The fact that 25% of cases are familial and that prevalence varies across ethnic populations suggests that many cases occur from genetic causes. In this regard, recent studies have linked clubfoot with mutations and microdeletions involving *PITX1*, a transcription factor important for hind limb development. Other causes include abnormal cartilage and bone formation.

**Congenital absence or deficiency of the radius** is usually a genetic abnormality observed with malformations in other structures, such as **craniosynostosis–radial aplasia syndrome** (Baller-Gerold syndrome). These individuals have synostosis in one or more cranial sutures, absence of the radius, and other defects.

**Amniotic bands** may cause ring constrictions and amputations of the limbs or digits (Fig. 12.16; see also Fig. 8.18, p. 97). The origin of the bands is not clear, but they may represent adhesions between the amnion and affected structures in the fetus. Other investigators believe that bands originate from tears in the amnion that detach and surround part of the fetus.

**Transverse limb deficiencies** are limb defects in which proximal structures are intact, but structures distal to a transverse plane are partially or completely absent (Fig. 12.17). The defects may be due to disruption of the AER or its signaling or to vascular abnormalities, such as thromboses or vasoconstriction.

**Congenital hip dislocation** consists of underdevelopment of the acetabulum and head of the femur. It is rather common and occurs mostly in female newborns. Although dislocation usually occurs after birth, the abnormality of the bones develops prenatally. Because many babies with congenital hip dislocation are breech deliveries, it has been thought that breech posture may interfere with development of the hip joint. It is frequently associated with laxity of the joint capsule.

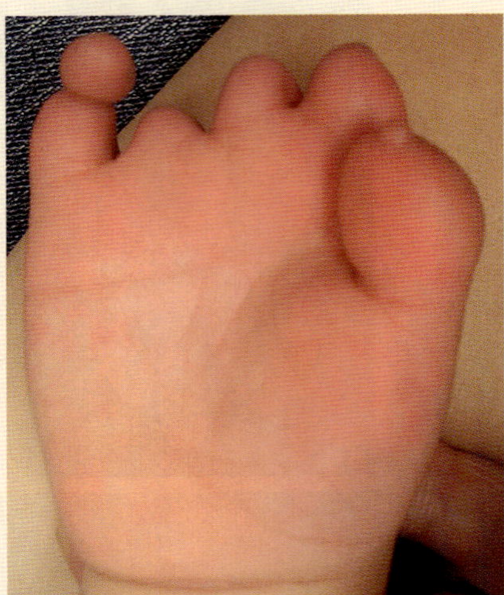

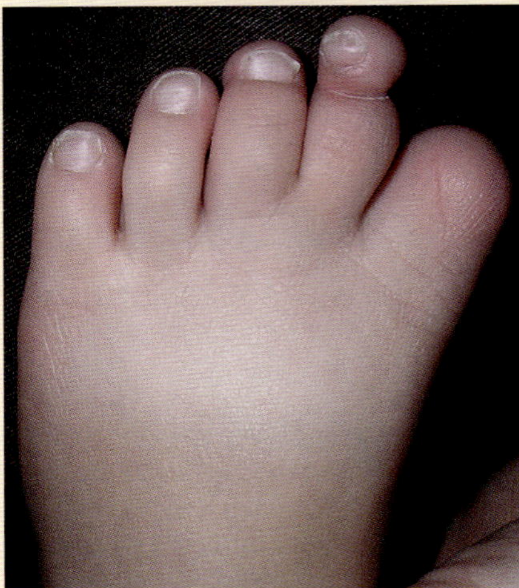

**FIGURE 12.16** Digit amputations resulting from amniotic bands.

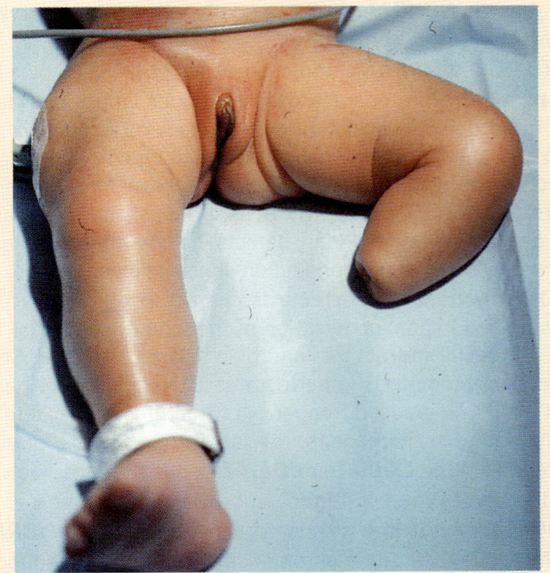

**FIGURE 12.17** Transverse limb deficiency, which may be caused by disruptions to the AER or to vascular abnormalities.

## SUMMARY

- Limbs form at the end of the fourth week as buds along the body wall adjacent to specific spinal segments determined by ***HOX genes*** (upper limb, C5–T2; lower limb, L2–S2).
- The **apical ectodermal ridge (AER)** at the distal border of the limb regulates proximodistal limb outgrowth by secreting **FGFs** that maintain a region of rapidly dividing cells immediately adjacent to the ridge called the **undifferentiated zone**.
- As the limb grows, cells near the flank are exposed to **retinoic acid** that causes them to differentiate into the **stylopod** (humerus/femur).
- Next to differentiate is the **zeugopod** (radius/ulna and tibia/fibula) and then the **autopod** (wrist and fingers, ankle and toes).
- The **zone of polarizing activity (ZPA)** located at the posterior border of the limb secretes **SHH** and controls anterior–posterior patterning (thumb to little finger).
- Bones of the limb form by **endochondral ossification** and are derived from the parietal layer of lateral plate mesoderm.
- Muscle cells migrate from somites in a segmental fashion and segregate into dorsal and ventral muscle groups. Later fusion and splitting of these groups into different muscles distorts the original segmental pattern.
- Muscles are innervated by **ventral primary rami** that split into dorsal and ventral branches.
- The dorsal and ventral branches eventually unite into dorsal and ventral nerves to innervate the dorsal (extensor) and ventral (flexor) compartments, respectively.
- Digits form when apoptosis (programmed cell death) occurs in the AER to separate this structure into five separate ridges.
- Final separation of the digits is achieved by additional apoptosis in the interdigital spaces.
- Many digital defects occur that are related to these patterns of cell death, including polydactyly, syndactyly, and clefts (Fig. 12.13).

## Self-Assessment

### Comprehensive Questions

1. Explain the rotation of the upper limb and lower limb.
2. Draw labeled diagrams to show the dermatome of the upper/lower limb.

### Problem Solving Questions

1. If you observe congenital absence of the radius or digital defects, such as absent thumb or polydactyly, would you consider examining the infant for other malformations? Why?
2. A young boy has a thin, long face. He is very tall with slender, long arms. What is this anomaly called? What is the cause of this condition?

### Multiple Choice Questions

1. During limb development, rotation takes place in which
   (a) The upper limb rotates laterally and the lower limb rotates medially.
   (b) The lower limb rotates laterally and the upper limb rotates medially.
   (c) Both the upper and lower limbs rotate medially.
   (d) Both the upper and lower limbs rotate laterally.
2. Limb buds of both the upper and lower limbs are initially visible on ultrasound at which week of gestation?
   (a) 3 weeks
   (b) 4 weeks
   (c) 5 weeks
   (d) 6 weeks
3. Induction of limb buds is by
   (a) Apical ectodermal ridges
   (b) Somites
   (c) Ventral rami of nerves
   (d) Neural crest cells
4. Patterning of limb buds is regulated by
   (a) *PAX* genes
   (b) *SHH*
   (c) *HOX* genes
   (d) *BMP4*

### Answers

1. (a) 2. (c) 3. (a) 4. (c)

Part 2

CHAPTER

# 13 Cardiovascular System

## Specific Learning Objectives

- Development of heart
  - Formation of heart tube
  - Folding of heart tube: Formation of cardiac loop
  - Development of atrial and ventricular chambers
  - Formation of interatrial septum
  - Formation of interventricular septum
  - Development of sinus venosus
  - Molecular regulation of heart development and establishment of laterality
- Development of the vascular system
  - Arterial system: Aortic arches and their derivatives
  - Venous system: Development of SVC, IVC, coronary sinus, and portal vein
- Congenital anomalies/defects of the cardiovascular system
  - Heart defects: Dextrocardia, atrial septal defect, ventricular septal defect, and Fallot's tetralogy
- Arterial system defects: Transposition of great vessels, patent ductus arteriosus, and coarctation of aorta
- Fetal circulation and changes occurring at birth



## Competencies Covered

**AN25.2** Describe the development of the heart.

**AN25.3** Describe fetal circulation and changes occurring at birth.

**AN25.4** Describe embryological basis of the following: (1) atrial septal defect, (2) ventricular septal defect, and (3) Fallot's tetralogy

**AN25.5** Describe the developmental basis of congenital anomalies, transposition of great vessels, dextrocardia, patent ductus arteriosus, and coarctation of the aorta.

**AN25.6** Mention the development of aortic arch arteries, SVC, IVC, and coronary sinus.

## ESTABLISHMENT AND PATTERNING OF THE PRIMARY HEART FIELD

The vascular system appears in the middle of the third week, when the embryo is no longer able to satisfy its nutritional requirements by diffusion alone. **Progenitor heart cells** lie in the epiblast, immediately adjacent to the cranial end of the primitive streak. From there, they migrate through the streak and into the visceral layer of lateral plate mesoderm where some form a horseshoe-shaped cluster of cells called the **primary heart field (PHF)** cranial to the neural folds (Fig. 13.1). The cells of the primary heart field form portions of the atria and the entire left ventricle. The right ventricle and outflow tract (conus cordis and truncus arteriosus) are derived from the **secondary heart field (SHF)**, which also contributes cells to formation of the atria at the caudal end of the heart (Fig. 13.2). This secondary field of cells resides in visceral (splanchnic) mesoderm ventral to the pharynx (Fig. 13.2).

As progenitor heart cells migrate through the primitive streak on approximately day 16 of gestation, they are specified on both sides from lateral to medial to become the different parts of the heart (Fig. 13.1*A*). Patterning of these cells occurs about the same time that laterality (left–right sidedness) is being established for the entire embryo, and this process and the signaling pathway it is dependent upon (Fig. 13.3) are essential for normal heart development.

Cells in the SHF also exhibit laterality such that those on the right side contribute to the left of the outflow tract region and those on the left contribute to the right. This laterality is determined by the same signaling pathway that establishes laterality for the entire embryo (Fig. 13.3) and explains the spiraling nature of the pulmonary artery and aorta and ensures that the aorta exits from the left ventricle and the pulmonary artery from the right ventricle.

Once cells establish the PHF, they are induced by the underlying pharyngeal endoderm to form cardiac myoblasts and blood islands that will form blood cells and vessels by the process of vasculogenesis. With time, the islands unite and form a **horseshoe-shaped** endothelial-lined tube surrounded by myoblasts. This region is known as the **cardiogenic region**; the intraembryonic (primitive body) cavity over it later develops into the **pericardial cavity** (Fig. 13.1*B,C*).

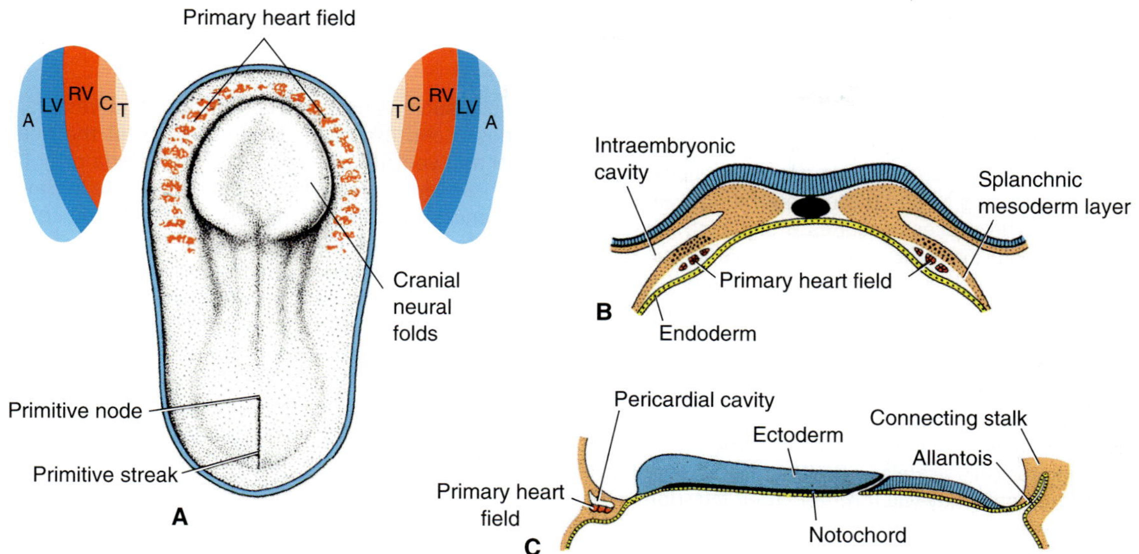


**FIGURE 13.1** **A.** Dorsal view of a late presomite embryo (approximately 18 days) after removal of the amnion. Progenitor heart cells have migrated and formed the horseshoe-shaped PHF located in the splanchnic layer of lateral plate mesoderm. As they migrate, PHF cells are specified to develop the left and right sides of the heart, including the left ventricle (LV) and parts of both atria (A). The right ventricle (RV), outflow tract (conus cordis [C] and truncus arteriosus [T]), and remainder of both atria also exhibit left-right patterning and are formed by the SHF. **B.** Transverse section through a similar-staged embryo to show the position of PHF cells in the visceral mesoderm layer. **C.** Cephalocaudal section through a similar-staged embryo showing the position of the pericardial cavity and PHF. *C*, conus arteriosus; *T*, truncus arteriosus.

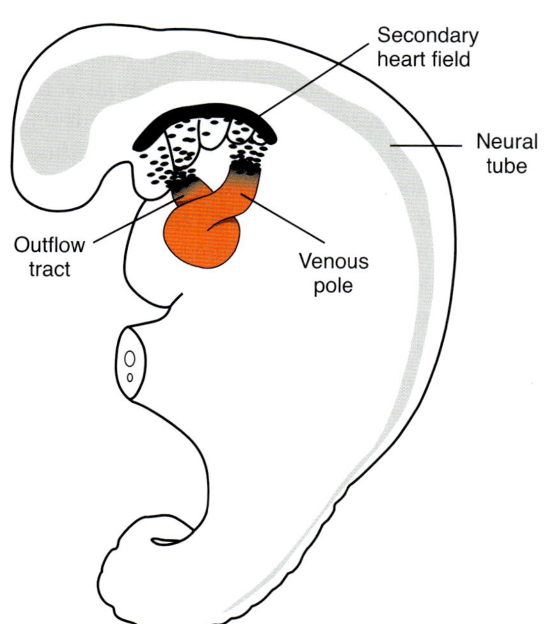


**FIGURE 13.2** Drawing showing the SHF that lies in visceral mesoderm at the posterior of the pharynx. The SHF provides cells that lengthen the arterial and venous poles of the heart, which includes the right ventricle and the outflow tract (conus cordis and truncus arteriosus) and atria and sinus venosus, respectively. Disruption of the SHF causes shortening of the outflow tract region, resulting in outflow tract defects.

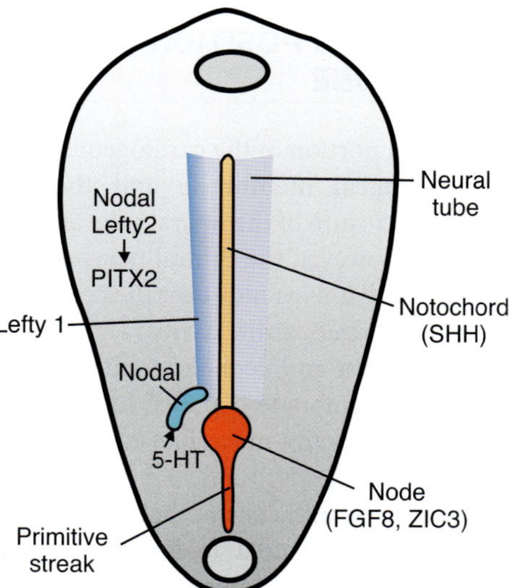


**FIGURE 13.3** Dorsal view of a drawing of a 16-day embryo showing the laterality pathway. The pathway is expressed in lateral plate mesoderm on the left side and involves a number of signaling molecules, including serotonin (5-HT), which result in expression of the transcription factor *PITX2*, the master gene for left sidedness. This pathway specifies the left side of the body and also programs heart cells in the primary and SHFs. The right side is specified as well, but genes responsible for this patterning have not been completely determined. Disruption of the pathway on the left results in laterality abnormalities, including many heart defects (see Chapter 5, p. 54).

Part 2

## Clinical Correlates

### Laterality and Heart Defects

Establishing laterality during gastrulation (see Chapter 5, p. 48) is essential for normal heart development because it specifies cells contributing to and patterning the right and left sides of the heart. The process requires a signaling cascade that includes serotonin (5-HT) as a key molecule in initiating the pathway (Fig. 13.3). 5-HT is concentrated on the left side of the embryo and, by signaling through the transcription factor *MAD3*, restricts *Nodal* expression to the left where this gene initiates a signaling cascade culminating in expression of *PITX2*, the master gene for left sidedness (see Chapter 5, p. 52; Fig. 13.3). The right side is also specified, but signals responsible for this event have not been as well established.

Cardiac progenitor cells are also specified at this time both for the parts of the heart they will form and their left-right sidedness by the laterality pathway. Thus, this period (days 16 to 18) is critical for heart development and individuals with laterality defects, such as heterotaxy, often have many different types of heart defects, including dextrocardia (right-sided heart), ventricular septal defects (VSDs), atrial septal defects (ASDs), double outlet right ventricle (DORV; both the aorta and pulmonary artery exit the right ventricle), and outflow tract defects, such as transposition of the great vessels, pulmonary stenosis, and others. Laterality defects of the heart, such as atrial and ventricular isomerisms (both atria or both ventricles have similar characteristics instead of the normal left-right differences) and inversions (the characteristics of the atria or ventricles are reversed), also occur because of disruptions in specifying left and right sidedness in the progenitor heart cells. Even for individuals with isolated heart defects, the cause can be due to abnormalities in establishing laterality. There is also a strong genetic component to the defects as illustrated by the fact that heterotaxy can be familial and individuals within such families often have heart defects whether or not they exhibit other laterality abnormalities. Similarly, individuals with situs inversus (complete reversal of left-right asymmetry in all organs) have a slightly higher risk of having a heart defect, but the risk for their offspring is greatly increased.

The importance of laterality in normal heart development explains the teratogenic effects of antidepressants of the selective serotonin reuptake inhibitor (SSRI) class that have been linked by epidemiology studies to an increase in heart defects. The mechanism for this effect appears to be a disruption of 5-HT signaling important in the laterality pathway (see Chapter 5, p. 57).

In addition to the cardiogenic region, other blood islands appear bilaterally, parallel, and close to the midline of the embryonic shield. These islands form a pair of longitudinal vessels, the **dorsal aortae**.

## FORMATION AND POSITION OF THE HEART TUBE

Initially, the central portion of the cardiogenic area is anterior to the **oropharyngeal membrane** and the neural plate (Fig. 13.4*A*). With closure of the neural tube and formation of the brain vesicles, however, the central nervous system grows cranially so rapidly that it extends over the central cardiogenic region and the future pericardial cavity (Fig. 13.4). As a result of growth of the brain and cephalic folding of the embryo, the oropharyngeal membrane is pulled forward, whereas the heart and pericardial cavity move first to the cervical region and finally to the thorax (Fig. 13.4).

Under the inductive influence of the pharyngeal endoderm and due to the cephalocaudal folding of the embryo, the horseshoe-shaped cardiogenic area fuses in the center to form a single heart tube. The progression of fusion of the heart tubes begins at the cranial end of the developing heart tube and extends caudally. This single heart tube has a cranial end which is the arterial end (outflow channel of ventricles) and is connected to the aortic sac and thereafter to the dorsal aorta. The caudal end of the developing heart tube is the venous end (inflow channel to atria) which is embedded in the septum transversum. The venous end receives three veins on both the sides as umbilical, vitelline, and common cardinal veins.

Three constrictions appear in the developing heart tube from the craniocaudal direction as bulboventricular groove, atrioventricular groove, and sinoatrial groove. The straightened heart tube is thus divided into four distinct regions by these constrictions craniocaudally as bulbus cordis, ventricles, atria, and sinus venosus. The bulbus cordis is divided into truncus arteriosus (distal part), conus cordis (middle part) and portion adjacent to the ventricle (proximal part of the conus cordis).

As the embryo grows and bends cephalocaudally, it also folds laterally (Fig. 13.5). As a result, the caudal regions of the paired cardiac tube merge except at their caudalmost ends (Fig. 13.6). Simultaneously, the central part of the horseshoe-shaped tube expands to form the future outflow tract and ventricular regions. Thus, the heart becomes a continuous expanded tube consisting of an inner endothelial lining and an outer myocardial layer (Fig. 13.5*C*). It receives venous drainage at its caudal pole and begins to pump blood out of the first aortic arch into the dorsal aorta at its cranial pole (Figs. 13.6 and 13.7).

The developing heart tube bulges more and more into the pericardial cavity. Initially, however, the tube remains attached to the dorsal side of the pericardial cavity by a fold of mesodermal tissue, the **dorsal mesocardium** that is derived from the SHF (Fig. 13.5*C*; see Fig. 13.16*A*, p. 157). No ventral mesocardium is ever formed. With further development, the middle section of the dorsal mesocardium disappears, creating the **transverse pericardial sinus**, which connects both sides of the pericardial cavity. The heart is now suspended in the cavity by blood vessels at its cranial and caudal poles (Fig. 13.7*D*).

During these events, the myocardium thickens and secretes a layer of extracellular matrix, rich in hyaluronic acid called *cardiac jelly*, which separates it from the endothelium (Fig. 13.5*C*; see Fig. 13.15, p. 156). In addition, formation of the **proepicardial organ** occurs in mesenchymal cells located at the caudal border of the dorsal mesocardium. Cells from this structure proliferate

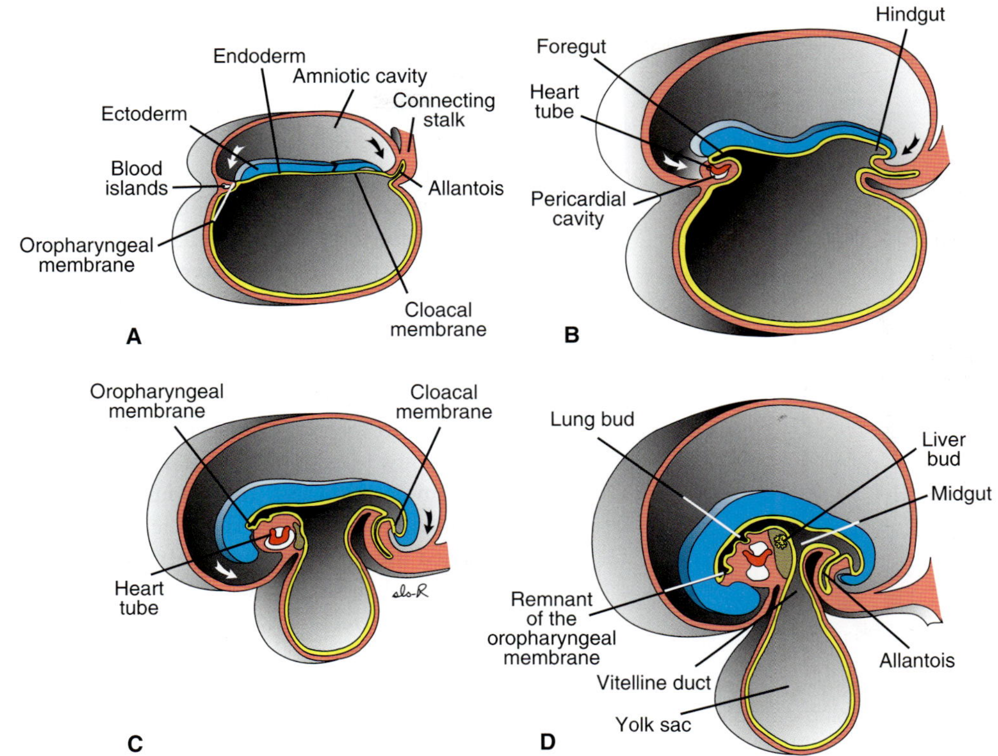


**FIGURE 13.4** Figures showing effects of the rapid growth of the brain on positioning of the heart. Initially, the cardiogenic area and the pericardial cavity are in front of the oropharyngeal membrane. **A.** 18 days. **B.** 20 days. **C.** 21 days. **D.** 22 days.

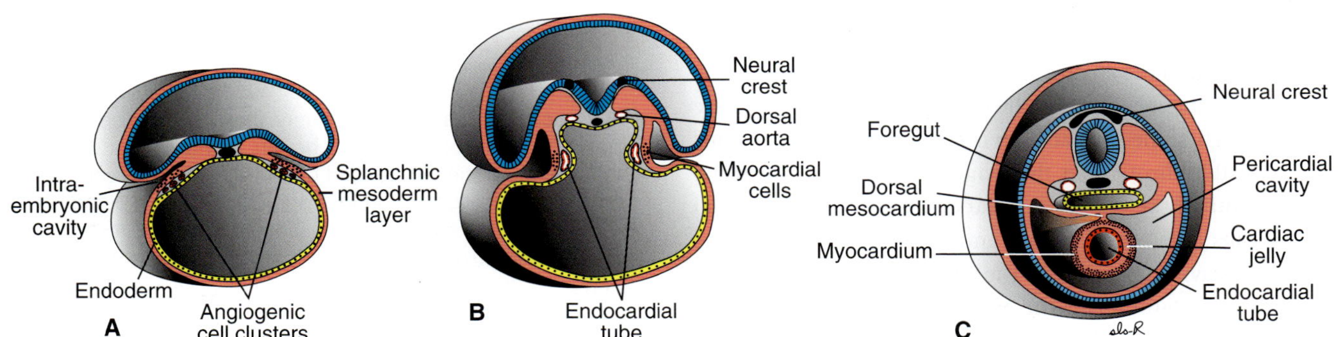


**FIGURE 13.5** Cross sections through embryos at different stages of development, showing formation of a single heart tube from paired primordia. **A.** Early presomite embryo (17 days). **B.** Late presomite embryo (18 days). **C.** Eight-somite stage (22 days). Fusion occurs only in the caudal region of the horseshoe-shaped tube. The outflow tract and most of the ventricular region form by expansion and growth of the crescent portion of the horseshoe.

and migrate over the surface of the myocardium to form the epicardial layer (**epicardium**) of the heart. Thus, the heart tube consists of three layers: (1) the **endocardium**, forming the internal endothelial lining of the heart; (2) the **myocardium**, forming the muscular wall; and (3) the **epicardium** or **visceral pericardium**, covering the outside of the tube. This outer layer is responsible for formation of the coronary arteries, including their endothelial lining and smooth muscle.

## ■ FORMATION OF THE CARDIAC LOOP

The heart tube continues to elongate as cells are added from the SHF to its cranial end (Fig. 13.2). This lengthening process is essential for normal formation of the right ventricle and the outflow tract region (conus cordis and truncus arteriosus that form part of the aorta and pulmonary artery) and for the looping process. If this lengthening is inhibited, then a variety of outflow tract defects occur, including DORV (both the aorta and pulmonary artery arise from the right ventricle), VSDs, tetralogy of Fallot (see Fig. 13.34), pulmonary atresia (see Fig. 13.36*B*), and pulmonary stenosis.

As the outflow tract lengthens, the cardiac tube begins to bend on day 23. The cephalic portion of the tube (bulboventricular tube) bends ventrally, caudally, and to the right (Fig. 13.7); and the atrial (caudal) portion shifts dorsocranially and to the left (Figs. 13.7 and 13.8*A*). Bending or looping of the heart tube leads to a shift of the atrium dorsocranially in respect to the ventricle and also leads to a shift of the sinus

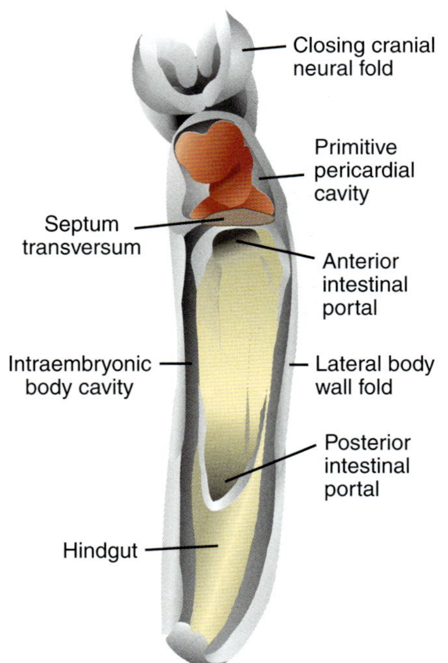


**FIGURE 13.6** Frontal view of an embryo showing the heart in the pericardial cavity and the developing gut tube with the anterior and posterior intestinal portals. The original paired tubes of the heart primordia have fused into a single tube except at their caudal ends, which remain separate. These caudal ends of the heart tube are embedded in the septum transversum, whereas the outflow tract leads to the aortic sac and aortic arches.

venosus caudal to the atrium. This bending, which may be due to cell shape changes, creates the **cardiac loop**. It is complete by day 28. While the cardiac loop is forming, local expansions become visible throughout the length of the tube. The **atrial portion**, initially a paired structure outside the pericardial cavity, forms a common atrium and is incorporated into the pericardial cavity (Fig. 13.7). The **atrioventricular junction** remains narrow and forms the **atrioventricular canal**, which connects the common atrium and the early embryonic ventricle (Fig. 13.9). The **bulbus cordis** is narrow except for its proximal third. This portion will form the **trabeculated part of the right ventricle** (Figs. 13.7 and 13.9). The midportion, the **conus cordis**, will form the outflow tracts of both ventricles. The distal part of the bulbus, the **truncus arteriosus**, will form the roots and proximal portion of the aorta and pulmonary artery (Fig. 13.9). The junction between the ventricle and the bulbus cordis, externally indicated by the **bulboventricular sulcus** (Fig. 13.7*C*), remains narrow. It is called the **primary interventricular foramen** (Fig. 13.9). Thus, the cardiac tube is organized by regions along its craniocaudal axis from the conotruncus to the right ventricle to the left ventricle to the atrial region, respectively (Fig. 13.7*A–C*). When **looping** is completed, the smooth-walled heart tube begins to form primitive trabeculae in two sharply defined areas just proximal and distal to the primary interventricular foramen (Fig. 13.9). The bulbus temporarily remains smooth-walled. The primitive ventricle, which is now trabeculated, is called the **primitive left ventricle**. Likewise, the trabeculated proximal third of the bulbus cordis is called the **primitive right ventricle** (Fig. 13.9).

The conotruncal portion of the heart tube, initially on the right side of the pericardial cavity, shifts gradually to a more medial position. This change in position is the result of formation of two transverse dilations of the atrium, bulging on each side of the bulbus cordis (Figs. 13.8*B* and 13.9).

## *Clinical Correlates*

### Abnormalities of Cardiac Looping

**Dextrocardia** is a condition where the heart lies on the right side of the thorax instead of the left and it occurs when the heart loops to the left instead of the right. The defect may be induced during gastrulation, when laterality is established, or slightly later when cardiac looping occurs. Dextrocardia occurs with **situs inversus**, a complete reversal of asymmetry in all organs, or may be associated with **laterality sequences (heterotaxy)** in which only some organ positions are reversed (see Chapter 5, p. 54).

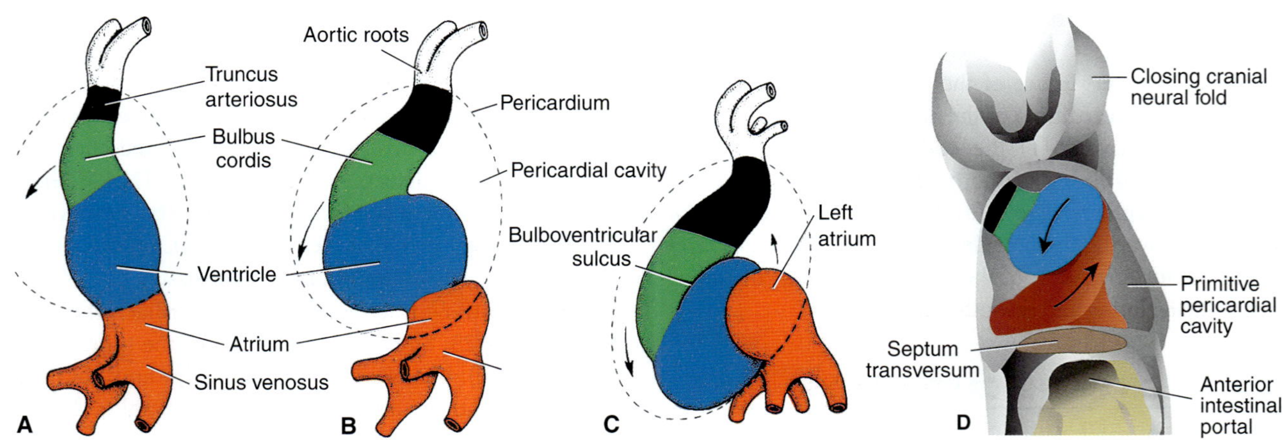


**FIGURE 13.7** Formation of the cardiac loop. **A.** 22 days. **B.** 23 days. **C.** 24 days. **D.** Frontal view of the heart tube undergoing looping in the pericardial cavity. The primitive ventricle is moving ventrally and to the right, whereas the atrial region is moving dorsally and to the left (*arrows*).

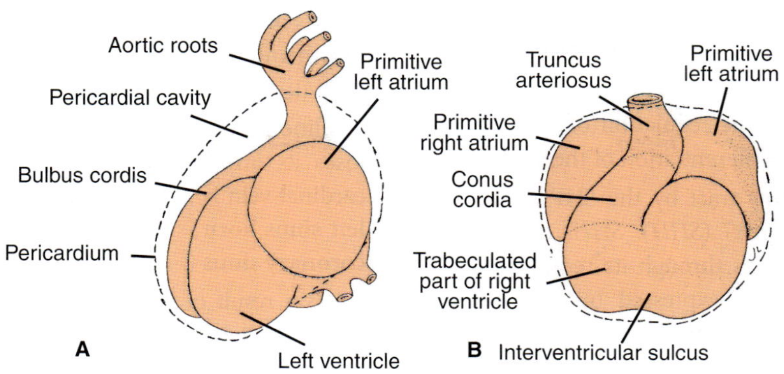


**FIGURE 13.8** Heart of a 5-mm embryo (28 days). **A.** Viewed from the left. **B.** Frontal view. The bulbus cordis is divided into the truncus arteriosus, conus cordis, and trabeculated part of the right ventricle. *Broken line*, pericardium.

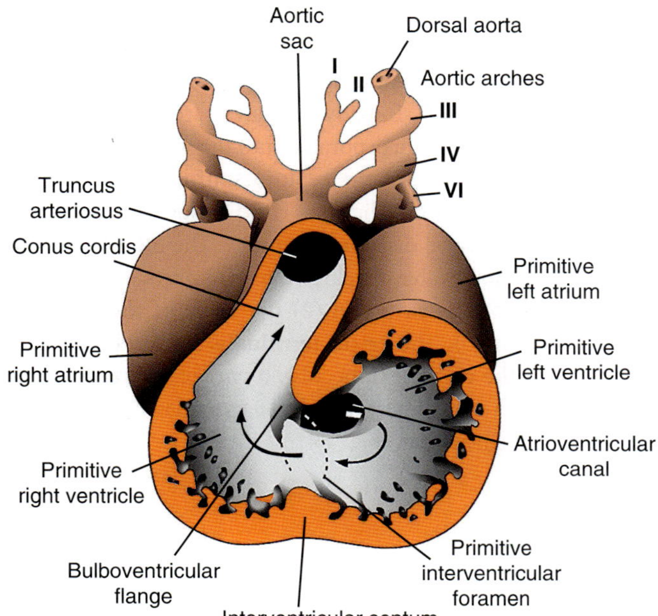


**FIGURE 13.9** Frontal section through the heart of a 30-day embryo showing the primary interventricular foramen and entrance of the atrium into the primitive left ventricle. Note the bulboventricular flange. *Arrows*, direction of blood flow.

## ■ MOLECULAR REGULATION OF CARDIAC DEVELOPMENT

Signals from anterior (cranial) endoderm induce a heart-forming region in overlying visceral mesoderm by inducing the transcription factor ***NKX2.5***. The signals require secretion of bone morphogenetic proteins (**BMPs**) **2** and **4** secreted by the endoderm and lateral plate mesoderm. Concomitantly, the activity of **WNT proteins** (3a and 8), secreted by the neural tube, must be blocked because they normally inhibit heart development. Inhibitors (CRESCENT and CERBERUS) of the WNT proteins are produced by endoderm cells immediately adjacent to heart-forming mesoderm in the anterior half of the embryo. The combination of BMP activity and WNT inhibition by CRESCENT and CERBERUS causes expression of *NKX2.5*, the master gene for heart development (Figs. 13.1 and 13.10). *BMP* expression also upregulates expression of

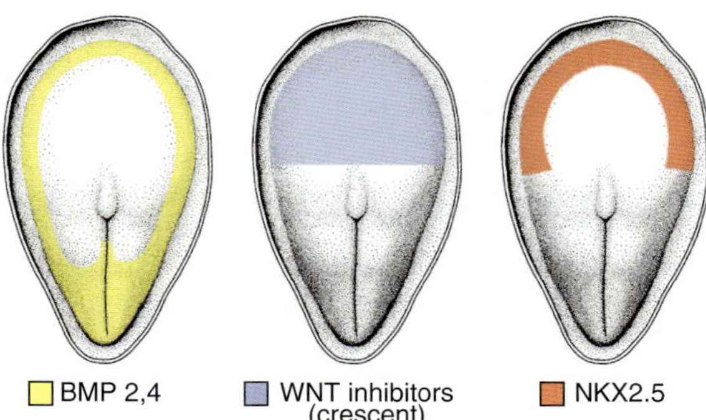


**FIGURE 13.10** Heart induction. BMPs secreted by the endoderm and lateral plate mesoderm in combination with inhibition of *WNT* expression by CRESCENT in the anterior half of the embryo induce expression of *NKX2.5* in the heart-forming region of the lateral plate mesoderm (visceral layer). *NKX2.5* is then responsible for heart induction.

fibroblast growth factor 8 (***FGF8***) that is important for the expression of cardiac-specific proteins.

Once the cardiac tube is formed, the venous portion is specified by **retinoic acid (RA)** produced by mesoderm adjacent to the presumptive sinus venosus and atria. Following this initial exposure to RA, these structures express the gene for retinaldehyde dehydrogenase, which allows them to make their own RA and commits them to becoming caudal cardiac structures. Lower concentrations of RA in more anterior cardiac regions (ventricles and outflow tract) contribute to specification of these structures. The importance of RA in cardiac signaling explains why the compound can produce a variety of cardiac defects.

*NKX2.5* contains a homeodomain and is a homologue of the gene ***tinman*** that regulates heart development in *Drosophila*. ***TBX5*** is another transcription factor that contains a DNA-binding motif known as the *T-box*. Expressed later than *NKX2.5*, it plays an important role in septation.

Cardiac looping is dependent upon several factors, including the laterality pathway and expression of the transcription factor ***PITX2*** in lateral plate mesoderm on the left side. *PITX2* may play a role in the deposition and function of extracellular matrix molecules that assist in looping. In addition, *NKX2.5* upregulates expression of ***HAND1*** and ***HAND2***, transcription factors that are expressed in the

Part 2

primitive heart tube and that later become restricted to the future left and right ventricles, respectively. Downstream effectors of these genes participate in the looping phenomenon. *HAND1* and *HAND2*, under the regulation of *NKX2.5*, also contribute to expansion and differentiation of the ventricles.

Lengthening of the outflow tract by the SHF is regulated in part by *SONIC HEDGEHOG* (*SHH*). *SHH*, expressed by pharyngeal arch endoderm, acts through its receptor patched (PTC; see Chapter 1, p. 313), expressed by SHF cells, to stimulate proliferation of cells in the SHF. Meanwhile, *NOTCH* signaling through its ligand *JAG1* (see Chapter 1, p. 314) is responsible for upregulation of FGFs in the SHF that in turn regulate migration and differentiation of neural crest cells essential for outflow tract septation (see p. 163) and for development and patterning of the aortic arches (see p. 169). Mutations in *SHH*, *NOTCH*, and *JAG1* are responsible for some outflow tract, aortic arch, and cardiac defects.

## ■ DEVELOPMENT OF THE SINUS VENOSUS

In the middle of the fourth week, the **sinus venosus** receives venous blood from the **right** and **left sinus horns** (Fig. 13.11*A*). Each horn receives blood from three important veins: (1) the **vitelline** or the **omphalomesenteric vein**, (2) the **umbilical vein**, and (3) the **common cardinal vein**. At first, communication between the sinus and the atrium is wide. Soon, however, the entrance of the sinus shifts to the right (Fig. 13.11*B*). This shift is caused primarily by left-to-right shunts of blood, which occur in the venous system during the fourth and fifth weeks of development.

With obliteration of the right umbilical vein and the left vitelline vein during the fifth week, the left sinus horn rapidly loses its importance (Fig. 13.11*B*). When the left common cardinal vein is obliterated at 10 weeks, all that remains of the **left sinus horn** is the **oblique vein of the left atrium** and the **coronary sinus** (Fig. 13.12).

As a result of left-to-right shunts of blood, the right sinus horn and veins enlarge greatly. The **right sinus horn**, which now forms the only communication between the original sinus venosus and the atrium, is incorporated into the right atrium to form the smooth-walled part of the right atrium **(sinus venarum)** (Fig. 13.13). Its entrance, the **sinoatrial orifice**, is flanked on each side by a valvular fold, the **right** and **left venous valves** (Fig. 13.13*A*). Dorsocranially, both the **right** and the **left venous** valves fuse, forming a ridge known as the **septum spurium** (Fig. 13.13*A*). Initially the valves are large, but when the right sinus horn is incorporated into the wall of the atrium, the left venous valve and the septum spurium fuse with the developing atrial septum (Fig. 13.13*B*). The superior portion of the right venous valve disappears entirely. The inferior portion of the right venous valve develops into two parts: (1) the **valve of the inferior vena cava** and (2) the **valve of the coronary sinus** (Fig. 13.13*B*). The **crista terminalis** forms the dividing line between the original trabeculated part of the right atrium and the smooth-walled part (**sinus venarum**), which originates from the right sinus horn (Fig. 13.13*B*).

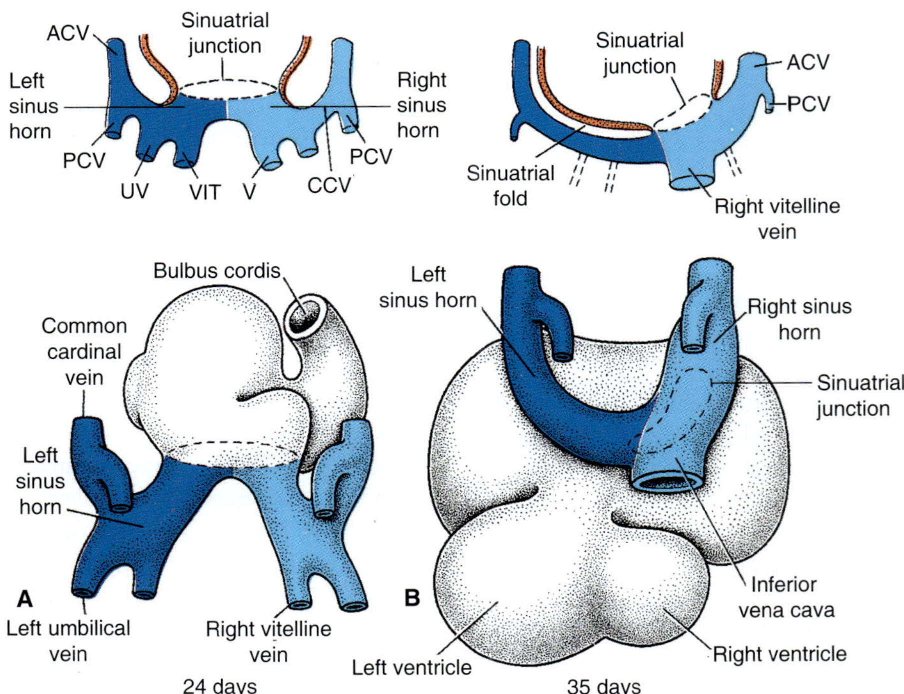


**FIGURE 13.11** Dorsal view of two stages in the development of the sinus venosus at approximately 24 days **(A)** and 35 days **(B)**. *Broken line*, Sinoatrial junction: the entrance of the sinus venosus into the atrial cavity. Each drawing is accompanied by a scheme to show in transverse section the great veins and their relation to the atrial cavity. *ACV*, anterior cardinal vein; *PCV*, posterior cardinal vein; *UV*, umbilical vein; *VIT V*, vitelline vein; *CCV*, common cardinal vein.

Part 2

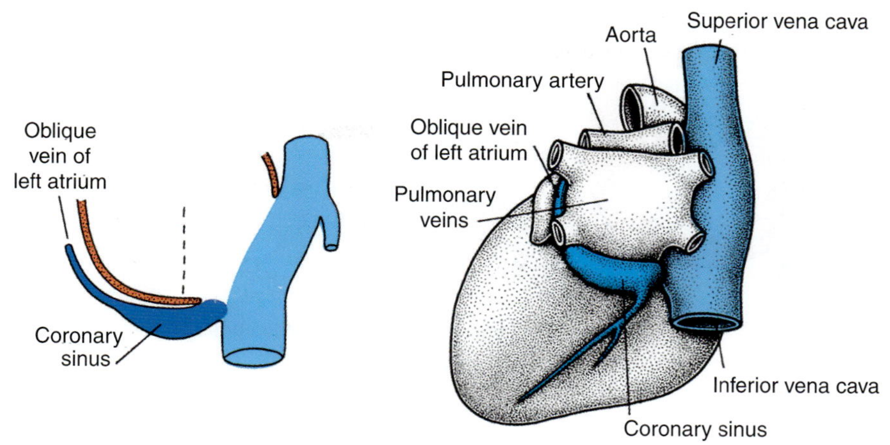


**FIGURE 13.12** Final stage in development of the sinus venosus and great veins.

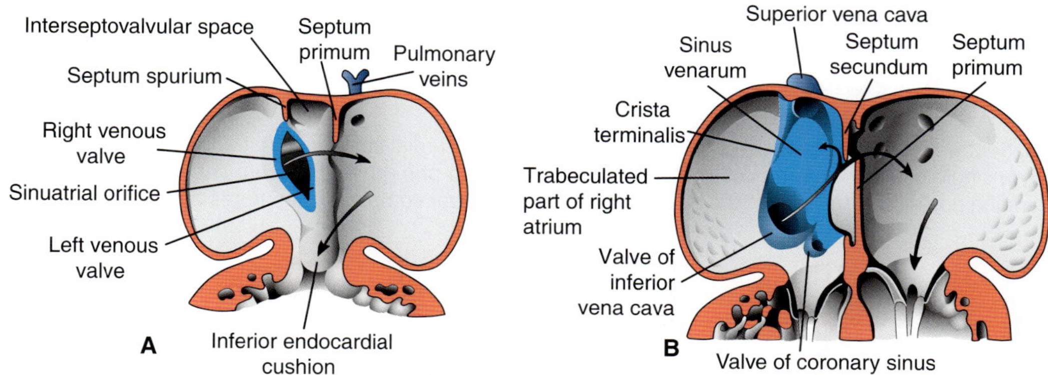


**FIGURE 13.13** Ventral view of coronal sections through the heart at the level of the atrioventricular canal to show development of the venous valves. **A.** 5 weeks. **B.** Fetal stage. The sinus venarum (*blue*) is smooth-walled; it derives from the right sinus horn. *Arrows*, blood flow.

## FORMATION OF THE CARDIAC SEPTA

The major septa of the heart are formed between the 27th and 37th days of development, when the embryo grows in length from 5 mm to approximately 16 to 17 mm. The formation of the cardiac septum involves two theories.

One method by which a septum may be formed involves two actively growing masses of tissue that approach each other until they fuse, dividing the lumen into two separate canals (Fig. 13.14*A,B*). Such a septum may also be formed by active growth of a single tissue mass that continues to expand until it reaches the opposite side of the lumen (Fig. 13.14*C*). Formation of such tissue masses, called **endocardial cushions**, depends on synthesis and deposition of extracellular matrices and cell migration and proliferation. Thus, in regions where such cushions form, there is increased synthesis of extracellular matrix that produces endocardial cell covered protrusions into the lumen (Fig. 13.15*A,B*).

These endocardial cushion protrusions develop in the (1) **atrioventricular** and (2) **conotruncal** regions, and in these locations, they assist in formation of the **atrial and ventricular (membranous portion) septa**, the **atrioventricular canals and valves** (Fig. 13.16), and the **aortic and pulmonary channels** (see Fig. 13.20). Eventually, cushions are populated by cells migrating and proliferating into the matrix:

- In **atrioventricular cushions,** the cells are derived from overlying endocardial cells that detach from their neighbors and move into the matrix (Fig. 13.15C).
- In **conotruncal cushions,** the cells are derived from neural crest cells migrating from the cranial neural folds to the outflow tract region (see p. 163 and Fig. 13.30, p. 165).

Because of their key location, abnormalities in endocardial cushion formation may cause cardiac malformations, including **ASDs** and **VSDs** and defects involving the **great vessels** (i.e., **transposition of the great vessels, common truncus arteriosus,** and **tetralogy of Fallot**).

The second way in which a septum is formed does not involve endocardial cushions. If, for example, a narrow strip of tissue in the wall of the atrium or ventricle should fail to grow while areas on each side of it expand rapidly, a narrow ridge forms between the two expanding portions (Fig. 13.14*D,E*). When growth of the expanding portions continues on either side of the narrow portion, the two walls approach each other and eventually merge, forming a septum (Fig. 13.14*F*). Such a septum never completely divides the original lumen but leaves a narrow communicating canal between the two expanded sections. It is usually closed secondarily by tissue contributed by neighboring proliferating tissues. Such a septum partially divides the atria and ventricles.

Part 2

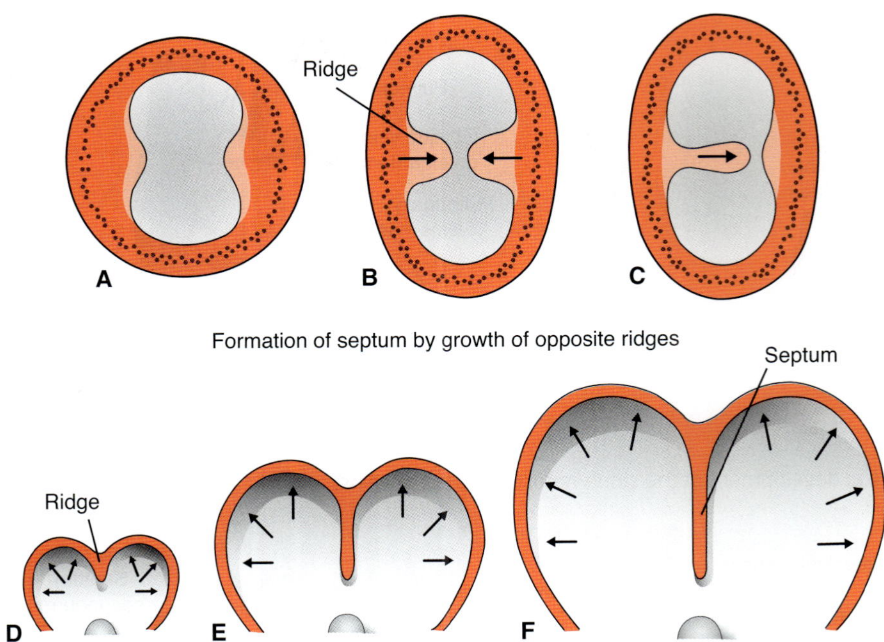


**FIGURE 13.14** **A,B.** Septum formation by two actively growing ridges (endocardial cushions) that approach each other until they fuse. **C.** Septum formed by a single actively growing cell mass, such as the septum primum and septum secundum. **D–F.** Septum formation by merging two expanding portions of the wall of the heart. Such a septum never completely separates two cavities.

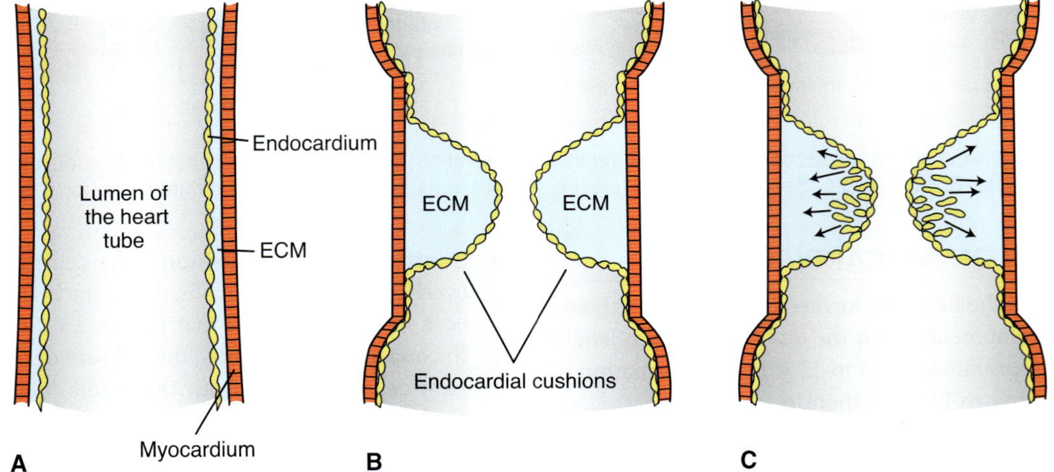


**FIGURE 13.15** Drawings showing development of endocardial cushions. **A.** Initially, the heart tube consists of the myocardium and endocardium separated by a layer of extracellular matrix (*ECM*). **B.** Endocardial cushions form in the atrioventricular canal and in the outflow tract as expansions of the ECM. **C.** Cells migrate into the cushions and proliferate: In the atrioventricular canal, these cells are derived from the endocardium; in the outflow tract, they are derived from neural crest cells (see p. 163).

## Septum Formation in the Common Atrium

At the end of the fourth week, a sickle-shaped crest grows from the roof of the common atrium into the lumen. This crest is the first portion of the septum primum (Figs. 13.13*A* and 13.16*A*,*B*). The two limbs of this septum extend toward the endocardial cushions in the atrioventricular canal. The opening between the lower rim of the septum primum and the endocardial cushions is the **ostium primum** (Fig. 13.16*A*,*B*). With further development, extensions of the superior and inferior endocardial cushions grow along the edge of the septum primum, closing the ostium primum (Fig. 13.16*C*,*D*). Before closure is complete, however, **programmed cell death (apoptosis)** produces perforations in the upper portion of the septum primum. Coalescence of these perforations forms the **ostium secundum**, ensuring free blood flow from the right to the left primitive atrium (Fig. 13.16*B*,*D*).

When the lumen of the right atrium expands as a result of incorporation of the sinus horn, a new crescent-shaped fold appears. This new fold, the **septum secundum** (Fig. 13.16*C*,*D*), never forms a complete partition in the atrial cavity (Fig. 13.16*F*,*G*). Its anterior limb extends downward to the septum in the atrioventricular canal. When the left

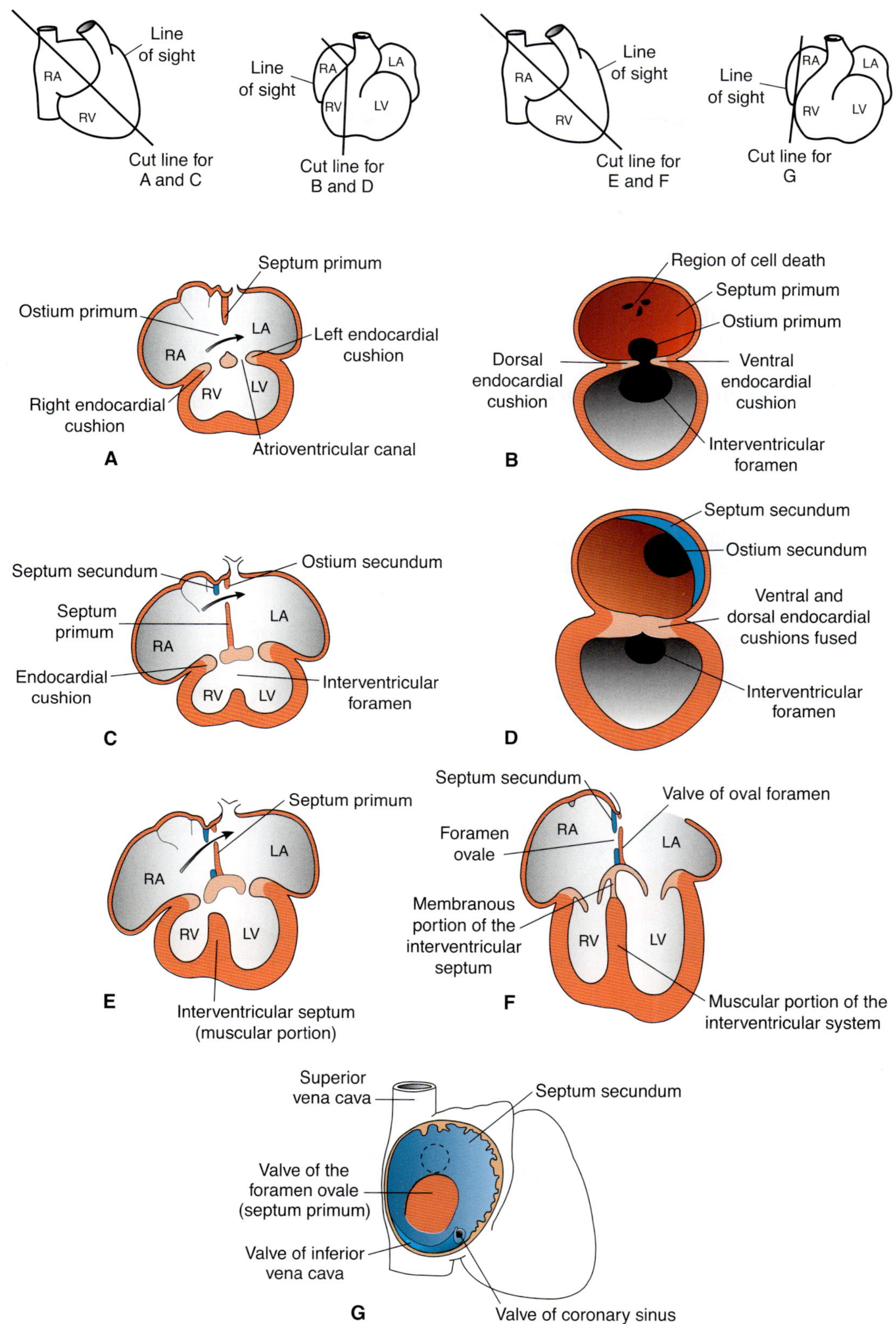


**FIGURE 13.16** Atrial septa at various stages of development. **A.** 30 days (6 mm). **B.** Same stage as **(A)**, viewed from the right. **C.** 33 days (9 mm). **D.** Same stage as **(C)**, viewed from the right. **E.** 37 days (14 mm). **F.** Newborn. **G.** The atrial septum from the right; same stage as **(F)**, *RA*, right atrium; *RV*, right ventricle; *LA*, left atrium; *LV*, left ventricle.

venous valve and the septum spurium fuse with the right side of the septum secundum, the free concave edge of the septum secundum begins to overlap the ostium secundum (Fig. 13.16*E*,*F*). The opening left by the septum secundum is called the **oval foramen (foramen ovale)**. When the upper part of the septum primum gradually disappears, the remaining part becomes the **valve of the oval foramen**. The passage between the two atrial cavities consists of an obliquely elongated cleft (Fig. 13.16*E–G*) through which blood from the right atrium flows to the left side (arrows in Figs. 13.13*B* and 13.16*E*).

After birth, when lung circulation begins and pressure in the left atrium increases, the valve of the oval foramen is pressed against the septum secundum, obliterating the oval foramen and separating the right and left atria. In about 20% of cases, fusion of the septum primum and septum secundum is incomplete, and a narrow oblique cleft remains between the two atria. This condition is called **probe patency** of the oval foramen; it does not allow intracardiac shunting of blood.

### Formation of the Left Atrium and Pulmonary Vein

While the primitive right atrium enlarges by incorporation of the right sinus horn, the primitive left atrium is likewise expanding. Meanwhile, mesenchyme at the caudal end of the dorsal mesocardium that suspends the heart tube in the pericardial cavity (Fig. 13.17*A*) begins to proliferate. Then, as the septum primum grows downward from the roof of the common atrium, this proliferating mesenchyme forms the **dorsal mesenchymal protrusion (DMP)**, and this tissue grows with the septum primum toward the atrioventricular canal (Fig. 13.17*B,C*). Within the DMP is the developing **pulmonary vein** that is positioned in the left atrium by the growth and movement of the DMP (Fig. 13.17*C*). Eventually, the remaining portion of the DMP at the tip of the septum primum contributes to endocardial cushion formation in the atrioventricular canal (Fig. 13.17*D*). The main stem of the pulmonary vein that opens into the left atrium sends two branches to each lung. Then, as expansion of the left atrium continues, the main stem is incorporated into the posterior wall until the point where branching of the vessel occurs, resulting in four separate openings for pulmonary veins into the atrial chamber (Figs. 13.17*D* and 13.18).

Thus, each atrium develops by expansion (Fig. 13.14*D–F*) and by incorporation of vascular structures: the sinus venosus in the right atrium and the stem of the pulmonary vein in the left (Fig. 13.18). In the fully developed heart, the original embryonic right atrium becomes the trabeculated **right atrial appendage** containing the pectinate muscles, whereas the smooth-walled **sinus venarum** originates from

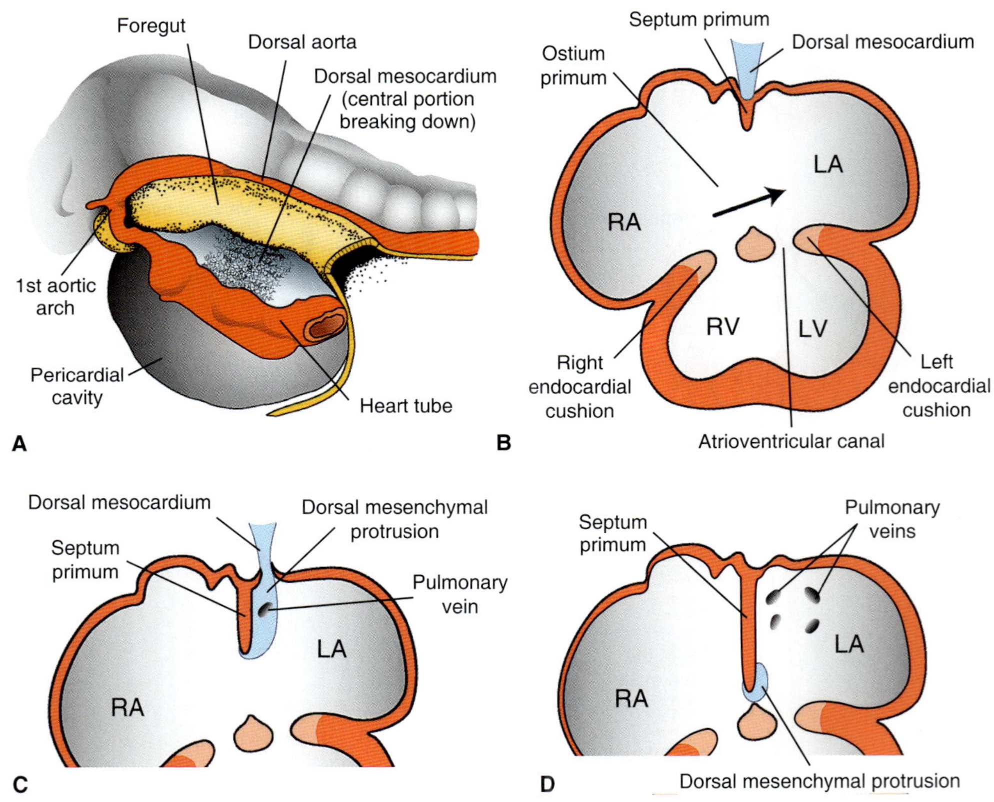


**FIGURE 13.17 A.** Drawing showing the heart tube suspended into the pericardial cavity by the dorsal mesocardium, a mesentery attached to mesoderm surrounding the gut tube, that is derived from the SHF (see Fig 13.5*C*). At this stage, the central portion of the mesocardium breaks down such that only the two ends of the heart tube remain attached. **B,C.** At the atrial pole, a portion of the dorsal mesocardium proliferates to form the dorsal mesenchymal protrusion (DMP) that penetrates the atrial wall to the left of the septum primum. The pulmonary vein forms within the mesenchyme of the DMP and becomes positioned in the posterior wall of the left atrium as the DMP grows downward with the septum primum. **D.** Initially, only the main stem of the pulmonary vein enters the left atrium, but, as the atrial walls expand, this stem is incorporated into the left atrium to the point where its four branches diverge to go to the lungs. Consequently, once the process of atrial expansion is complete, there are four openings for pulmonary veins into the left atrium. The remaining portion of the DMP remains at the tip of the septum primum and contributes to endocardial cushion formation around the atrioventricular canal. *RA*, right atrium; *RV*, right ventricle; *LA*, left atrium; *LV*, left ventricle.

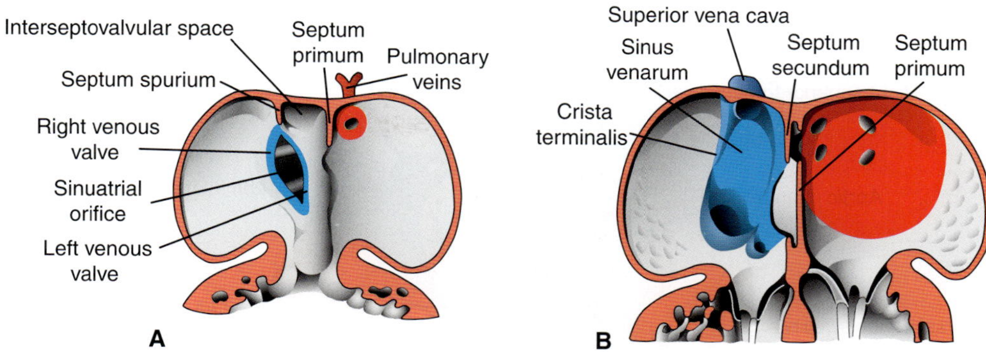


**FIGURE 13.18** Coronal sections through the heart to show development of the smooth-walled portions of the right and left atria. Both the wall of the right sinus horn (*blue*) and the pulmonary vein (*red*) are incorporated into the heart to form the smooth-walled parts of the atria.

### Clinical Correlates

Until recently, the pulmonary vein was thought to originate as an outgrowth of the left atrium, and this concept made it difficult to determine the etiology of a rare birth defect where the pulmonary veins drain into other vessels or directly into the right atrium, a condition called **total anomalous pulmonary venous return (TAPVR)**. However, understanding that the vein arises in the dorsal mesocardium as part of the DMP provides a rationale for how the defect can occur simply by abnormal positioning of the DMP. For example, deviation of the DMP to the right places the pulmonary vein in the right atrium instead of the left (20% of cases) or if deviation to the right is more pronounced, the vein can enter the superior vena cava or the brachiocephalic vein (50% of cases). Because the dorsal mesocardium is normally a midline structure, it is not surprising that TAPVR often occurs in individuals with heterotaxy.

the right horn of the sinus venosus (Fig. 13.18*A*). The original embryonic left atrium is represented by little more than the **trabeculated atrial appendage**, whereas the smooth-walled part originates from the pulmonary vein (Fig. 13.18*B*).

## Septum Formation in the Atrioventricular Canal

At the end of the fourth week, four **atrioventricular endocardial cushions** appear: one on each side plus one at the dorsal (superior) and one at the ventral (inferior) border of the atrioventricular canal (Figs. 13.19 and 13.20). Initially, the atrioventricular canal gives access only to the primitive left ventricle and is separated from the bulbus cordis by the **bulbo (cono) ventricular flange** (Fig. 13.9). Near the end of the fifth week, however, the posterior extremity of the flange terminates almost midway along the base of the dorsal endocardial cushion and is much less prominent than before (Fig. 13.20). Because the atrioventricular canal enlarges to the right, blood passing through the atrioventricular orifice now has direct access to the primitive left as well as the primitive right ventricle.

In addition to the dorsal and ventral endocardial cushions, two **lateral atrioventricular cushions** appear on the right and left borders of the canal (Figs. 13.19 and 13.20). The dorsal and ventral cushions, in the meantime, project further into the lumen and fuse, resulting in a complete division of the canal into right and left atrioventricular orifices by the end of the fifth week (Figs. 13.16*B,D* and 13.19).

### Atrioventricular Valves

After the atrioventricular endocardial cushions fuse, each atrioventricular orifice is surrounded by local proliferations of mesenchymal tissue derived from the endocardial cushions (Fig. 13.21*A*). When the bloodstream hollows out and thins tissue on the ventricular surface of these proliferations, the mesenchymal tissue becomes fibrous and forms the atrioventricular valves, which remain attached to the ventricular wall by muscular cords (Fig. 13.21*B,C*). Finally, muscular tissue in the cords degenerates and is replaced by dense connective tissue. The valves then consist of connective tissue covered by endocardium. They are connected to thick muscular trabeculae in the wall of the ventricle, the **papillary muscles**, by means



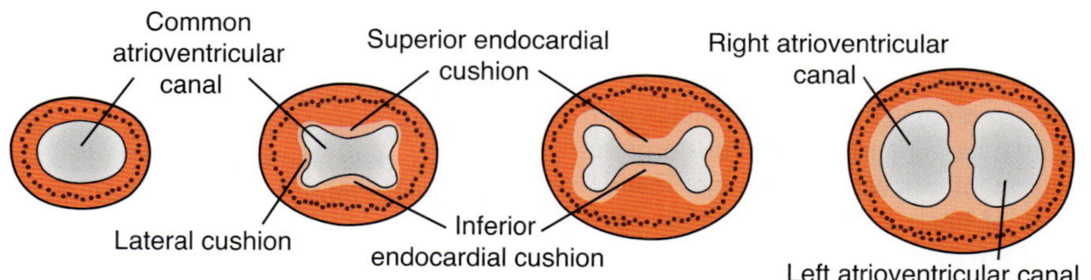


**FIGURE 13.19** Formation of the septum in the atrioventricular canal. From left to right, days 23, 26, 31, and 35. The initial circular opening widens transversely.

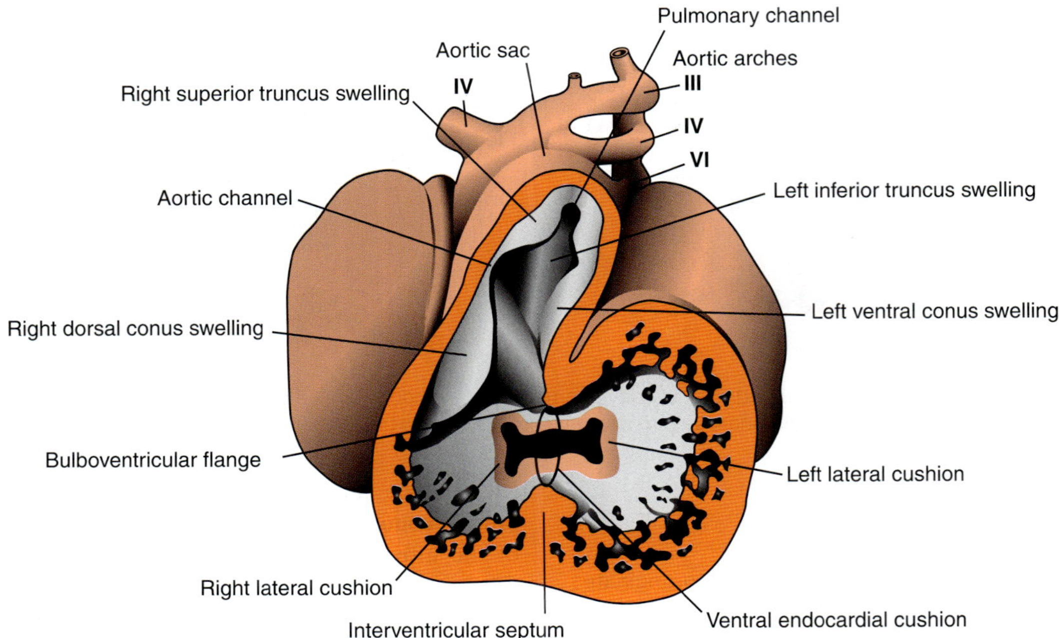


**FIGURE 13.20** Frontal section through the heart of a day-35 embryo. At this stage of development, blood from the atrial cavity enters the primitive left ventricle as well as the primitive right ventricle. Note development of the cushions in the atrioventricular canal. Cushions in the truncus and conus are also visible. *Ring*, primitive interventricular foramen.

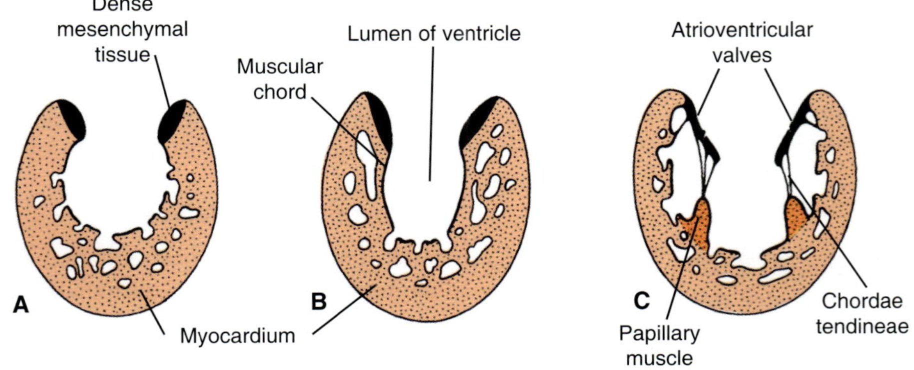


**FIGURE 13.21** Formation of the atrioventricular valves and chordae tendineae. The valves are hollowed out from the ventricular side but remain attached to the ventricular wall by the chordae tendineae.

## *Clinical Correlates*

### Heart Defects

Heart and vascular abnormalities make up the largest category of human birth defects and are present in **1%** of live born infants. The incidence among stillborns is 10 times as high. It is estimated that 12% of babies with heart defects have a chromosomal abnormality and, conversely, that 33% of babies with a chromosomal abnormality have a heart defect. Furthermore, 30% of heart defects occur in infants with other major malformations. Approximately 2% of heart defects are due to environmental agents, but most are caused by a complex interplay between genetic and environmental influences (**multifactorial** causes). Classic examples of cardiovascular teratogens include **rubella virus** and **thalidomide**. Others include **RA (Accutane)**, **alcohol**, and many other compounds. Maternal diseases, such as insulin-dependent **diabetes**, have also been linked to cardiac defects.

Targets for genetic or teratogen-induced heart defects include heart progenitor cells from the PHF and SHF, neural crest cells, endocardial cushions, and other cell types important for heart development (Table 13.1, p. 168). The fact that the same malformation can result from disrupting different targets (e.g., transposition of the great arteries can result from disruption of the SHF or neural crest cells) means that heart defects are heterogeneous in origin and difficult to classify epidemiologically.

Genes regulating cardiac development are being identified and mapped, and mutations that result in heart defects are being discovered. For example, mutations in the heart-specifying gene *NKX2.5*, on chromosome 5q35, can produce ASDs (secundum type), tetralogy of Fallot, and atrioventricular conduction delays in an autosomal dominant fashion. Mutations in the ***TBX5*** gene result in **Holt-Oram syndrome**, characterized by preaxial (radial) limb abnormalities and ASDs. Defects in the muscular portion of the interventricular septum may also occur. Holt-Oram syndrome is one of a group of **heart–hand syndromes** illustrating that the same genes may participate in multiple developmental processes. For example, *TBX5* regulates forelimb development and plays a role in septation of the heart. Holt-Oram syndrome is inherited as an autosomal dominant trait with a frequency of 1/100,000 live births.

Mutations in a number of genes regulating production of sarcomere proteins cause **hypertrophic cardiomyopathy** that may result in sudden death in athletes and the general population. The disease is inherited as an autosomal dominant, and most mutations (45%) target the β-myosin heavy-chain gene (14q11.2). The result is cardiac **hypertrophy** due to disruption in the organization of cardiac muscle cells (**myocardial disarray**), which may adversely affect cardiac output and/or conduction.

**Ventricular inversion** is a defect in which the morphologic left ventricle is on the right and connects to the right atrium through a mitral valve. The morphologic right ventricle is on the left side and connects to the left atrium through the tricuspid valve. The defect is sometimes called **L-transposition of the great arteries** because the pulmonary artery exits the morphologic left ventricle and the aorta exits the morphologic right ventricle. However, the arteries are in their normal positions, but the ventricles are reversed. The abnormality arises during the establishment of laterality and specification of the left and right sides of the heart by the laterality pathway.

**Hypoplastic right heart syndrome (HRHS)** and **hypoplastic left heart syndrome** (**HLHS**; Fig. 13.22) are rare defects that cause an underdevelopment of the right or left sides of the heart, respectively. On the right, the ventricle is very small, the pulmonary artery is affected and may be atretic or stenosed, and the atrium may be small; on the left, the ventricle is very small, the aorta may be atretic or stenotic, and the atrium may be reduced in size. The laterality associated with these defects suggests an adverse effect on specification of the left and right cardiac progenitor cells at an early stage of cardiac morphogenesis. The defects can also arise when the helix-loop-helix transcription factors *Hand1* (left ventricle) and *Hand2* (left ventricle) that regulate ventricular growth are misexpressed.

**ASD** is a congenital heart abnormality with an incidence of 6.4/10,000 births and with a 2:1 prevalence in female to male infants. One of the most significant defects is the **ostium secundum** defect, characterized by a large opening between the left and right atria. It may be caused by excessive cell death and resorption of the septum primum (Fig. 13.23*B,C*) or by inadequate development of the septum secundum (Fig. 13.23*D,E*). Depending on the size of the opening, considerable intracardiac shunting may occur from left to right.

The most serious abnormality in this group is complete absence of the atrial septum (Fig. 13.23*F*). This condition, known as common atrium or **cor triloculare biventriculare**, is always associated with serious defects elsewhere in the heart.

Occasionally, the oval foramen closes during prenatal life. This abnormality, **premature closure of the oval foramen**, leads to massive hypertrophy of the right atrium and ventricle and underdevelopment of the left side of the heart. Death usually occurs shortly after birth.

**Endocardial cushions** of the atrioventricular canal not only divide this canal into a right and left orifice but also participate in formation of the membranous portion of the interventricular septum and in closure of the ostium primum (Fig. 13.16). This region has the appearance of a cross, with the atrial and ventricular septa forming the post, and the atrioventricular cushions the crossbar (Fig. 13.16*E*). The integrity of this cross is an important sign in ultrasound scans of the heart. Whenever the atrioventricular cushions fail to fuse, the result is a **persistent atrioventricular canal**, combined with a defect in the cardiac septum (Fig. 13.24*A*). This septal defect has an atrial and a

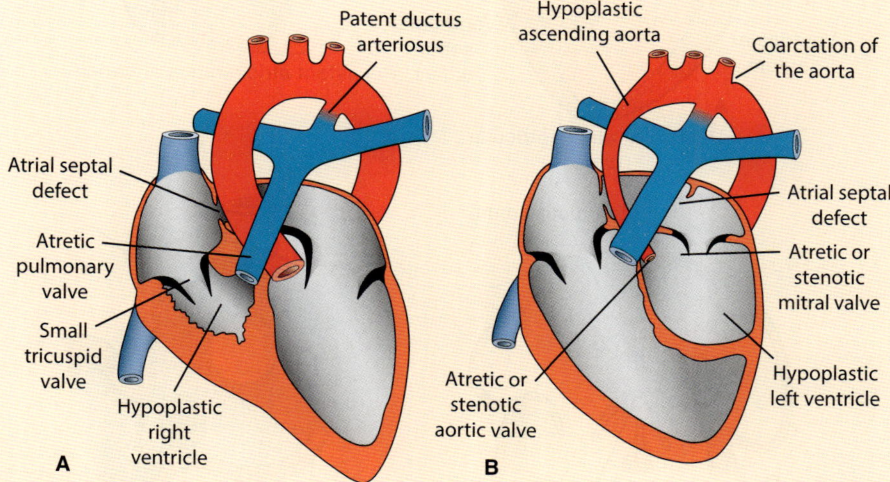


**FIGURE 13.22 A.** Hypoplastic right heart syndrome. **B.** Hypoplastic left heart syndrome. These are rare defects that cause an underdevelopment of the right or left sides of the heart, respectively. On the right, the ventricle is very small, the pulmonary artery is affected and may be atretic or stenosed and the atrium may be small; on the left, the ventricle is very small, the aorta may be atretic or stenotic, and the atrium may be reduced in size. The laterality associated with these defects suggests an adverse effect on specification of the left and right cardiac progenitor cells at an early stage of cardiac morphogenesis.

(*Continued*)

Part 2

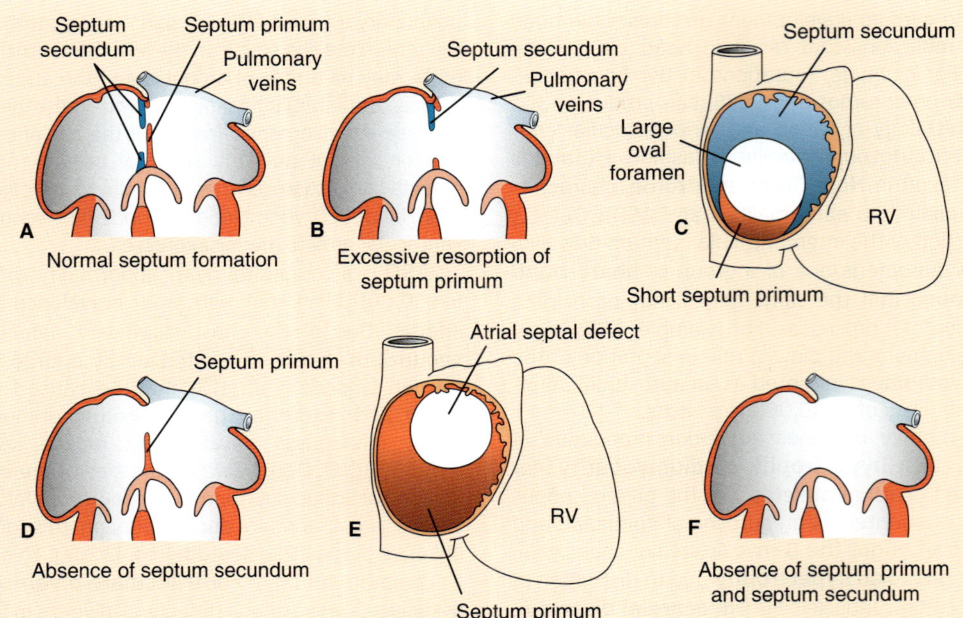


**FIGURE 13.23 A.** Normal atrial septum formation. **B,C.** Ostium secundum defect caused by excessive resorption of the septum primum. **D,E.** Similar defect caused by failure of development of the septum secundum. **F.** Common atrium, or cor triloculare biventriculare, resulting from complete failure of the septum primum and septum secundum to form. *RV*, right ventricle.

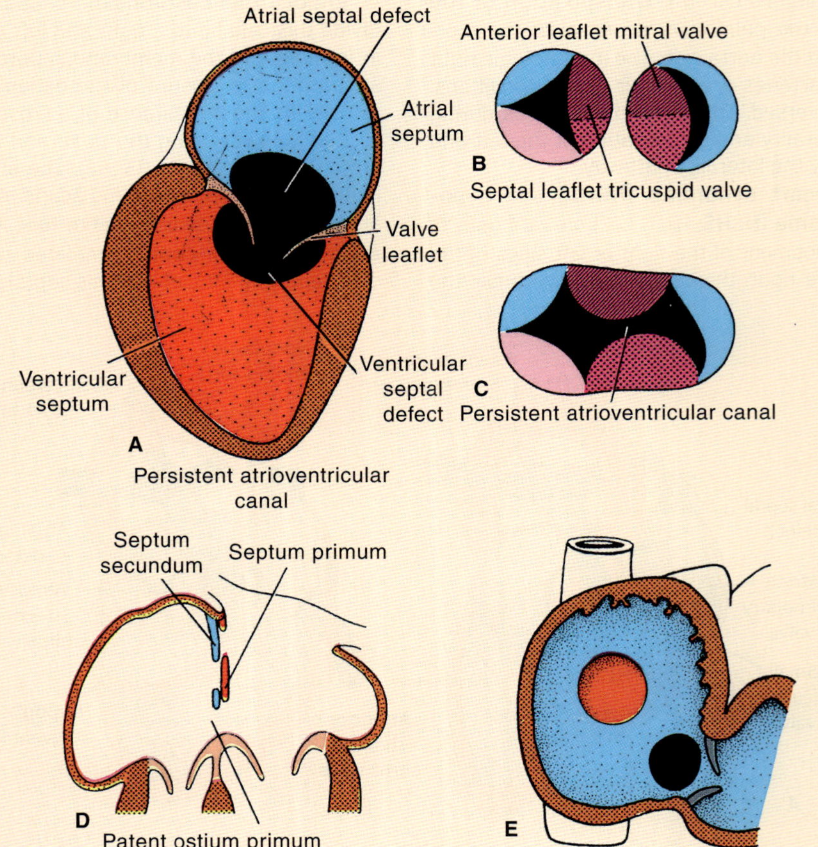


**FIGURE 13.24 A.** Persistent common atrioventricular canal. This abnormality is always accompanied by a septum defect in the atrial as well as in the ventricular portion of the cardiac partitions. **B.** Valves in the atrioventricular orifices under normal conditions. **C.** Split valves in a persistent atrioventricular canal. **D,E.** Ostium primum defect caused by incomplete fusion of the atrioventricular endocardial cushions.

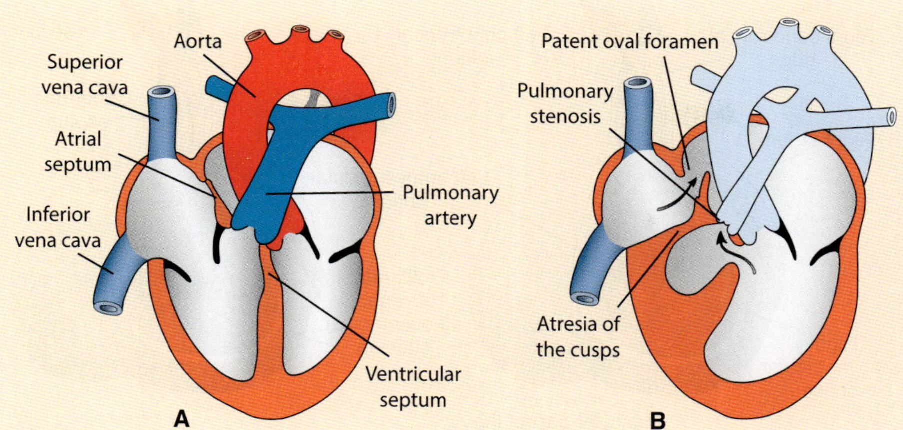


**FIGURE 13.25** **A.** Normal heart. **B.** Tricuspid atresia. Note the small right ventricle and the large left ventricle.

ventricular component, separated by abnormal valve leaflets in the single atrioventricular orifice (Fig. 13.24*B,C*).

Occasionally, endocardial cushions in the atrioventricular canal partially fuse. The result is a defect in the atrial septum, but the interventricular septum is closed (Fig. 13.24*D,E*). This defect, the **ostium primum defect**, is usually combined with a cleft in the anterior leaflet of the tricuspid valve (Fig. 13.24*C*).

**Tricuspid atresia**, which involves obliteration of the right atrioventricular orifice (Fig. 13.25), is characterized by the absence or fusion of the tricuspid valves. Tricuspid atresia is always associated with (1) patency of the oval foramen, (2) VSD, (3) underdevelopment of the right ventricle, and (4) hypertrophy of the left ventricle.

**Ebstein anomaly** is a condition where the tricuspid valve is displaced toward the apex of the right ventricle, and as a result, there is an expanded right atrium and a small right ventricle (Fig. 13.26). The valve leaflets are abnormally positioned, and the anterior one is usually enlarged.

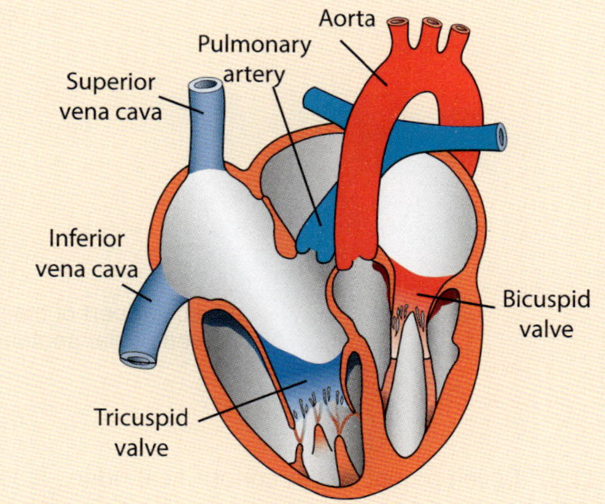


**FIGURE 13.26** Ebstein anomaly. The tricuspid valve leaflets are displaced toward the apex of the right ventricle, and there is expansion of the right atrial region.

of **chordae tendineae** (Fig. 13.21*C*). In this manner, two valve leaflets, constituting the **bicuspid** (or **mitral**) **valve**, form in the left atrioventricular canal, and three, constituting the **tricuspid valve**, form on the right side.

## Septum Formation in the Truncus Arteriosus and Conus Cordis

During the fifth week, pairs of opposing ridges appear in the truncus. These ridges, the **truncus swellings**, or **cushions**, lie on the right superior wall (**right superior truncus swelling**) and on the left inferior wall (**left inferior truncus swelling**) (Fig. 13.20). The right superior truncus swelling grows distally and to the left, and the left inferior truncus swelling grows distally and to the right. Hence, while growing toward the aortic sac, the swellings twist around each other, foreshadowing the spiral course of the future septum (Fig. 13.27). After complete fusion, the ridges form the **aorticopulmonary septum**, dividing the truncus into an **aortic** and a **pulmonary channel**.

When the truncus swellings appear, similar swellings (cushions) develop along the right dorsal and left ventral walls of the **conus cordis** (Figs. 13.20 and 13.27). The conus swellings grow toward each other and distally to unite with the truncus septum. When the two conus swellings have fused, the septum divides the conus into an anterolateral portion (the outflow tract of the right ventricle) (Fig. 13.28) and a posteromedial portion (the outflow tract of the left ventricle) (Fig. 13.29).

**Cardiac neural crest cells**, originating in the edges of the neural folds in the hindbrain region, migrate through pharyngeal arches 3, 4, and 6 to the outflow region of the heart, which they invade (Fig. 13.30). In this location, they contribute to endocardial cushion formation in both the conus cordis and truncus arteriosus. Migration and proliferation of cardiac neural crest cells is regulated by the SHF through the *NOTCH* signaling pathway (see p. 314). Therefore, outflow tract defects may occur by insults to the SHF or insults to cardiac neural crest cells that disrupt formation of the conotruncal septum. Heart defects caused by these mechanisms include tetralogy of Fallot (Fig. 13.34), pulmonary stenoses, persistent (common) truncus arteriosus (Fig. 13.35), and transposition of the great vessels (Fig. 13.36). **Because neural crest cells also contribute to craniofacial development, it is not**

Part 2

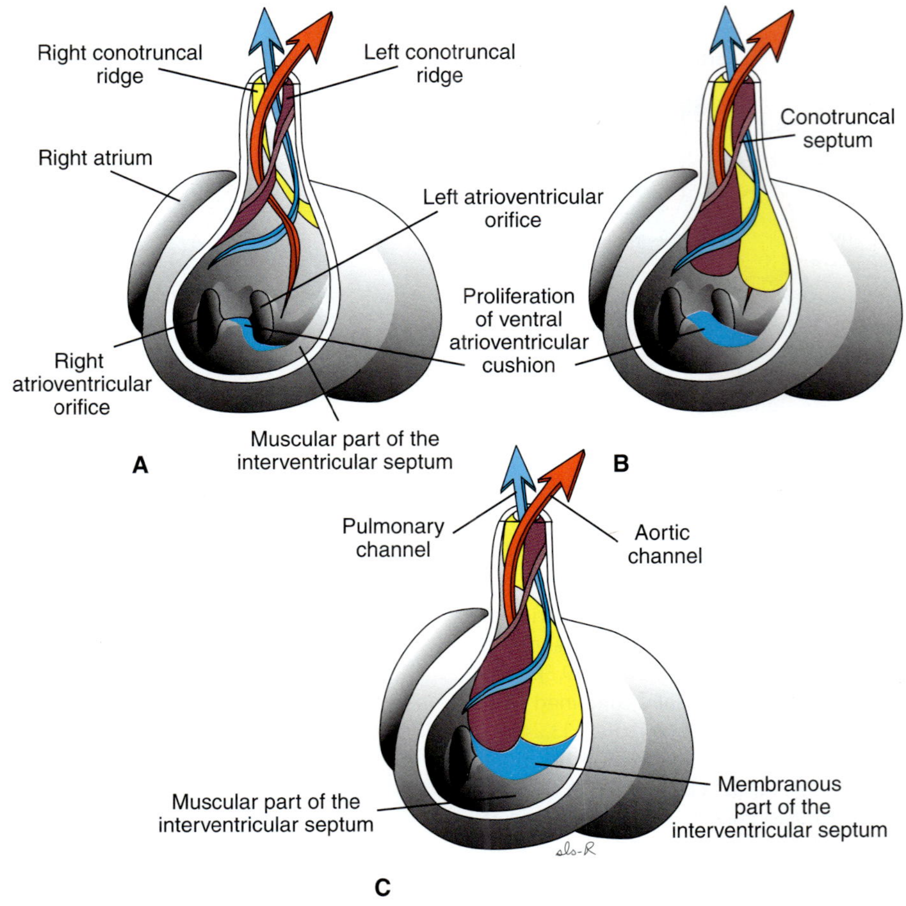


**FIGURE 13.27** Development of the conotruncal ridges (cushions) and closure of the interventricular foramen. Proliferations of the right and left conus cushions, combined with proliferation of the anterior endocardial cushion, close the interventricular foramen and form the membranous portion of the interventricular septum. **A.** 6 weeks (12 mm). **B.** Beginning of the seventh week (14.5 mm). **C.** End of the seventh week (20 mm).

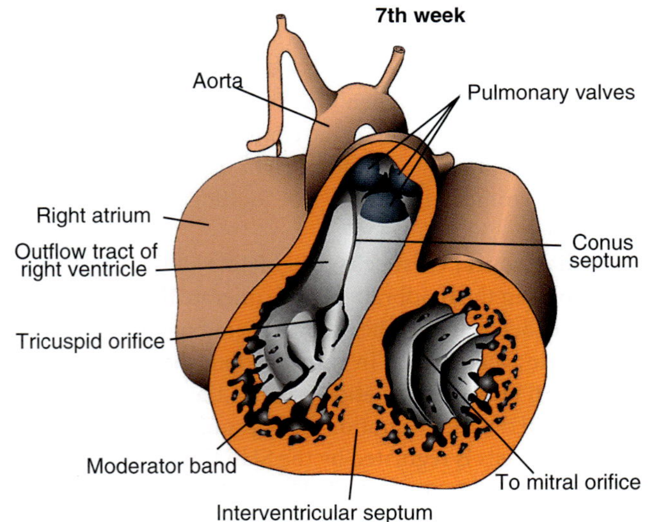


**FIGURE 13.28** Frontal section through the heart of a 7-week embryo. Note the conus septum and position of the pulmonary valves.

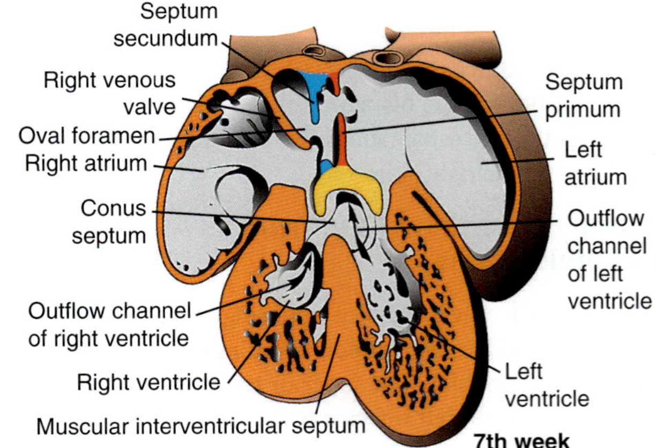


**FIGURE 13.29** Frontal section through the heart of an embryo at the end of the seventh week. The conus septum is complete, and blood from the left ventricle enters the aorta. Note the septum in the atrial region.

**uncommon to see facial and cardiac abnormalities in the same individual** (see Chapter 17, p. 235).

## Septum Formation in the Ventricles

By the end of the fourth week, the two primitive ventricles begin to expand. This is accomplished by continuous growth of the

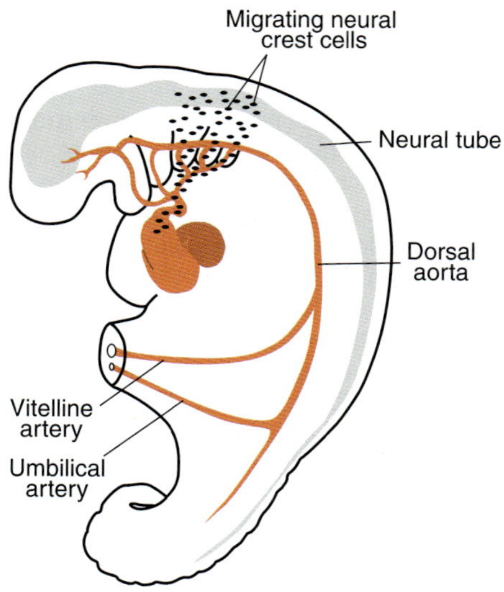


**FIGURE 13.30** Drawing showing the origin of neural crest cells in the hindbrain and their migration through pharyngeal arches 3, 4, and 6 to the outflow tract of the heart. In this location, they contribute to septation of the conus cordis and truncus arteriosus.

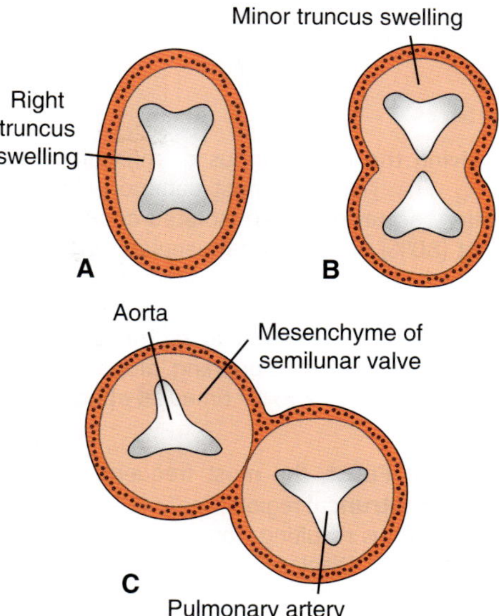


**FIGURE 13.31** Transverse sections through the truncus arteriosus at the level of the semilunar valves at weeks 5 **(A)**, 6 **(B)**, and 7 **(C)** of development.

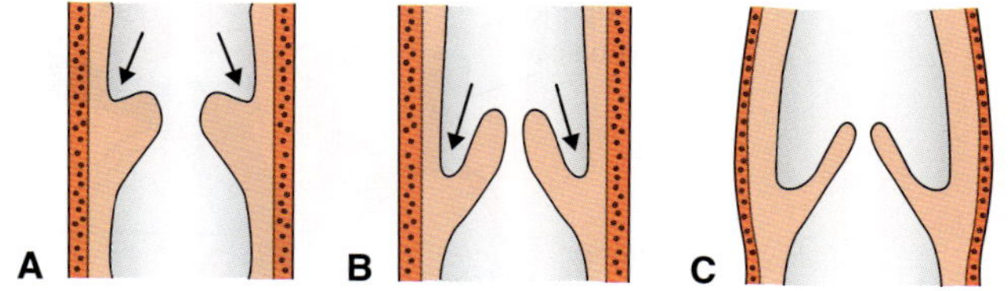


**FIGURE 13.32** Longitudinal sections through the semilunar valves at weeks 6 **(A)**, 7 **(B)**, and 9 **(C)** of development. The upper surface is hollowed (*arrows*) to form the valves.

myocardium on the outside and continuous diverticulation and trabecula formation on the inside (Figs. 13.20 and 13.29).

The medial walls of the expanding ventricles become apposed and gradually merge, forming the **muscular interventricular septum** (Fig. 13.29). Sometimes, the two walls do not merge completely, and a more or less deep apical cleft between the two ventricles appears. The space between the free rim of the muscular ventricular septum and the fused endocardial cushions permits communication between the two ventricles.

The **interventricular foramen**, above the muscular portion of the interventricular septum, shrinks on completion of the **conus septum** (Fig. 13.27). During further development, outgrowth of tissue from the anterior (inferior) endocardial cushion along the top of the muscular interventricular septum closes the foramen (Fig. 13.16*E,F*). This tissue fuses with the abutting parts of the conus septum. Complete closure of the interventricular foramen forms **the membranous part of the interventricular septum** (Fig. 13.16*F*).

### Semilunar Valves

When partitioning of the truncus is almost complete, primordia of the semilunar valves become visible as small tubercles found on the main truncus swellings. One of each pair is assigned to the pulmonary and aortic channels, respectively (Fig. 13.31). A third tubercle appears in both channels opposite the fused truncus swellings. Gradually, the tubercles hollow out at their upper surface, forming the **semilunar valves** (Fig. 13.32). Recent evidence shows that neural crest cells contribute to formation of these valves.

## FORMATION OF THE CONDUCTING SYSTEM OF THE HEART

Initially, all myocardial cells in the heart tube have pacemaker activity and the heart begins to beat at approximately 21 days of gestation. Soon, the **pacemaker** for the heart is restricted to the caudal part of the left side of the cardiac tube. Later, the sinus venosus assumes this function, and as the sinus is incorporated into the right atrium, pacemaker tissue lies near the opening of the superior vena cava. Thus, the **sinoatrial node (SAN)** is formed.

The **atrioventricular node (AVN)** begins as a collection of cells located around the atrioventricular canal that coalesce to form the AVN. Impulses from the AVN pass to the **atrioventricular bundle** and **left and right bundle branches** and finally to the **Purkinje fiber network** surrounding and activating the ventricles. With the exception of sympathetic and parasympathetic nerve fibers that terminate on the SAN to regulate heart rate, all of the cells for the heart's conduction system are derived from primary cardiac myocytes that differentiate into nodes, bundle branches, and Purkinje fibers. Expression of the transcription factor *TBX3* inhibits differentiation of these primary myocytes into ventricular muscle cells and allows them instead to differentiate into the conducting system.

## VASCULAR DEVELOPMENT

Blood vessel development occurs by two mechanisms: (1) **vasculogenesis** in which vessels arise by coalescence of **angioblasts** and (2) **angiogenesis** whereby vessels sprout

Part 2

## Clinical Correlates

### Heart Defects

**VSDs** involving the membranous or muscular portion of the septum (Fig. 13.33) are the most common congenital cardiac malformation, occurring as an isolated condition in 12/10,000 births. Most (80%) occur in the muscular region of the septum and resolve as the child grows. Membranous VSDs usually represent a more serious defect and are often associated with abnormalities in partitioning of the conotruncal region. Depending on the size of the opening, blood carried by the pulmonary artery may be 1.2 to 1.7 times as abundant as that carried by the aorta.

**Tetralogy of Fallot**, the most frequently occurring abnormality of the **conotruncal** region (Fig. 13.34), is due to an unequal division of the conus resulting from anterior displacement of the conotruncal septum. Displacement of the septum produces four cardiovascular alterations: (1) a narrow right ventricular outflow region, **pulmonary infundibular stenosis**; (2) a large defect of the interventricular septum; (3) an overriding aorta that arises directly above the septal defect; and (4) hypertrophy of the right ventricular wall because of higher pressure on the right side. Tetralogy of Fallot occurs in 9.6/10,000 births but occurs as a common feature in individuals with **Alagille syndrome**. In addition to the heart defect, these people have abnormalities in other organs, including the liver, and a characteristic face with a broad prominent forehead, deep set eyes, and a small pointed chin. In 90% of cases, there is a mutation in ***JAG1***, the ligand for ***NOTCH*** signaling that regulates neural crest cells forming the conotruncal (outflow tract) septum (see Chapter 1, p. 314).

**Persistent (common) truncus arteriosus** results when the conotruncal ridges fail to form such that no division of the outflow tract occurs (Fig. 13.35). In such a case, which occurs in 0.8/10,000 births, the pulmonary artery arises some distance above the origin of the undivided truncus. Because the ridges also participate in formation of the interventricular septum, the persistent truncus is always accompanied by a defective interventricular septum. The undivided truncus thus overrides both ventricles and receives blood from both sides.

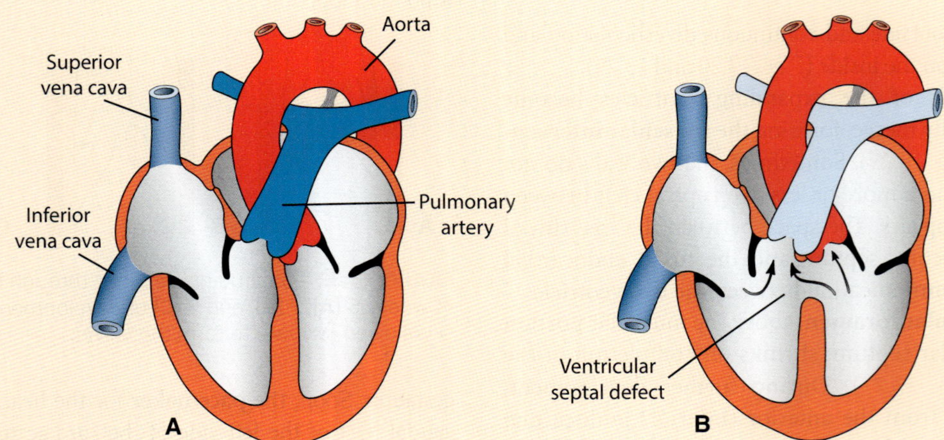


**FIGURE 13.33** **A.** Normal heart. **B.** Isolated defect in the membranous portion of the interventricular septum. Blood from the left ventricle flows to the right through the interventricular foramen (*arrows*).

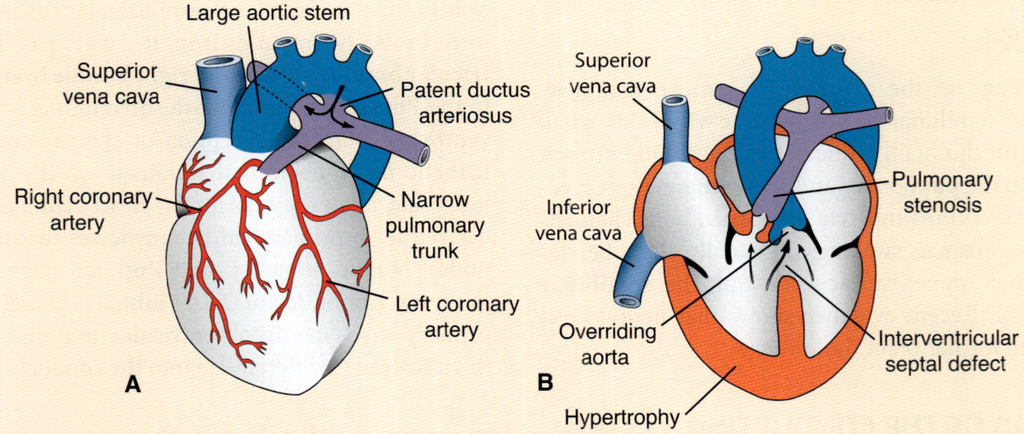


**FIGURE 13.34** Tetralogy of Fallot. **A.** Surface view. **B.** The four components of the defect: pulmonary stenosis, overriding aorta, interventricular septal defect, and hypertrophy of the right ventricle.

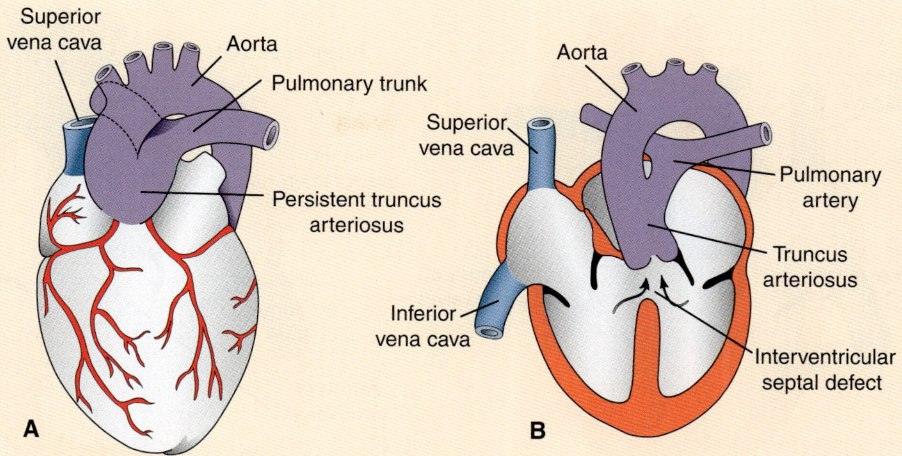


**FIGURE 13.35** Persistent truncus arteriosus. The pulmonary artery originates from a common truncus. **A.** The septum in the truncus and conus has failed to form. **B.** This abnormality is always accompanied by an interventricular septal defect.

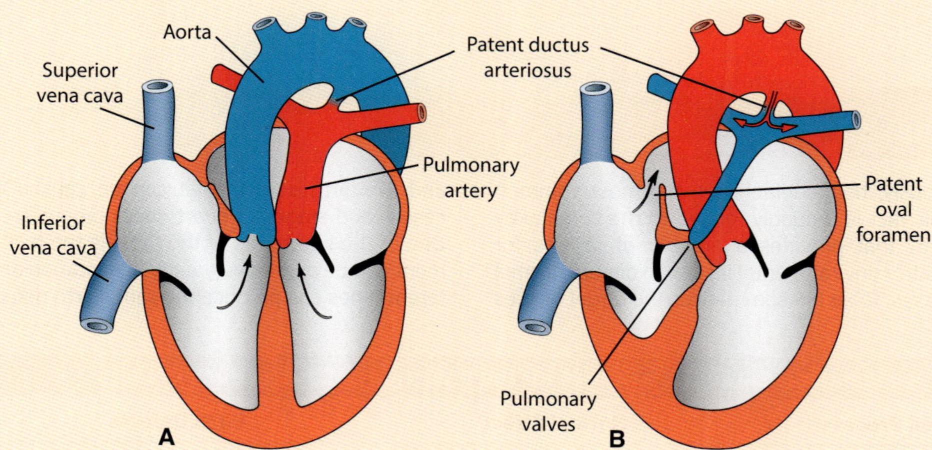


**FIGURE 13.36** **A.** Transposition of the great vessels. **B.** HRHS with pulmonary valvular atresia and a normal aortic root. The only access route to the lungs is by reverse blood flow through a PDA.

**Transposition of the great vessels** occurs when the conotruncal septum fails to follow its normal spiral course and runs straight down (Fig. 13.36*A*). As a consequence, the aorta originates from the right ventricle, and the pulmonary artery originates from the left ventricle. This condition, which occurs in 4.8/10,000 births, sometimes is associated with a defect in the membranous part of the interventricular septum. It is usually accompanied by an open ductus arteriosus. Because the SHF and neural crest cells contribute to the formation and septation of the outflow tract, respectively, insults to these cells contribute to cardiac defects involving the outflow tract.

**DiGeorge sequence** is an example of the 22q11 deletion syndrome (see Chapter 17, p. 243) characterized by a pattern of malformations that have their origin in abnormal neural crest development. These children have facial defects, thymic hypoplasia, parathyroid dysfunction, and cardiac abnormalities involving the outflow tract, such as persistent truncus arteriosus and tetralogy of Fallot. Craniofacial malformations are often associated with heart defects because neural crest cells play important roles in the development of both the face and heart.

**Valvular stenosis** of the pulmonary artery or aorta occurs when the semilunar valves are fused for a variable distance. The incidence of the abnormality is similar for both regions, being approximately 3 to 4/10,000 births. In the case of a **valvular stenosis of the pulmonary artery**, the trunk of the pulmonary artery is narrow or even atretic (Fig. 13.36*B*). The patent oval foramen then forms the only outlet for blood from the right side of the heart. The ductus arteriosus, always patent, is the only access route to the pulmonary circulation.

In **aortic valvular stenosis** (Fig. 13.37*A*), fusion of the thickened valves may be so complete that only a pinhole opening remains. The size of the aorta itself is usually normal.

When fusion of the semilunar aortic valves is complete—**aortic valvular atresia** (Fig. 13.37*B*)—the aorta, left ventricle, and left atrium are markedly underdeveloped. The abnormality is usually accompanied by an open ductus arteriosus, which delivers blood into the aorta.

**Ectopia cordis** is a rare anomaly in which the heart lies on the surface of the chest. It is caused by failure of the embryo to close the ventral body wall (see Chapter 7, p. 81).

(*Continued*)

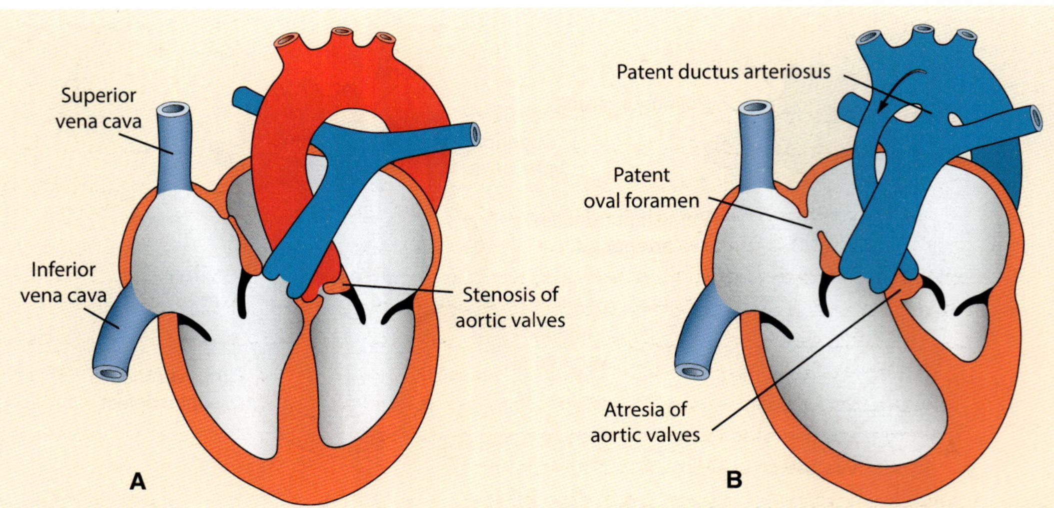


**FIGURE 13.37 A.** Aortic valvular stenosis. **B.** HLHS with aortic valvular atresia. *Arrow* in the arch of the aorta indicates direction of blood flow. The coronary arteries are supplied by this reverse blood flow. Note the small left ventricle and the large right ventricle.



## *Clinical Correlates*

As mentioned previously, heart defects are the most common birth defects, and this fact is probably related to the complexity of heart development that provides a number of targets for genetic mutations and/or environmental insults to disrupt normal embryological processes. Table 13.1 summarizes the target tissues and the birth defects that can be caused when different processes and stages of heart development are adversely affected. One of the key points of the table is the fact that heart development can be altered very early in gestation and that insults at different times can produce the same birth defects.

**Table 13.1 Heart Development: Susceptible Stages for the Induction of Cardiac Birth Defects**

| Target Tissue | Cell Process | Normal Effect | Birth Defects |
|---|---|---|---|
| PHF (days 16–18) | Establishment of laterality and patterning | Formation of the four chambered heart | DORV, TGA, l-TGA, ASD, VSD, atrial isomerism, ventricular inversion, dextrocardia |
| Heart tube (days 22–28) | Genetic signaling cascade for normal looping | Looping | Dextrocardia |
| AVC endocardial cushions (days 26–35) | Cushion formation: cell proliferation and migration | Division of the AVC into left and right channels; formation of the mitral and tricuspid valves and the IVS | VSD, mitral and tricuspid valve defects (mitral insufficiency, tricuspid atresia); positioning and leaflet defects |
| SHF (days 22–28) | Visceral mesoderm ventral to the pharynx and signaling from neural crest cells | Lengthening and partitioning the outflow tract into aortic and pulmonary channels | Tetralogy of Fallot, TGA, pulmonary atresia and stenosis |
| Outflow tract (conotruncus) (days 36–49) | Neural crest cell migration, proliferation and viability | Formation of the conotruncal cushions for division of the outflow tract | Common truncus arteriosus and other outflow tract defects |
| Aortic arches (days 22–42) | Neural crest cell migration, proliferation and viability | Patterning the arches into the great arteries | Anomalous right pulmonary artery; IAA type B |

Days give an approximate estimation of periods of vulnerability and are calculated from the time of fertilization.
*PHF*, primary heart field; *DORV*, double outlet right ventricle; *TGA*, transposition of the great arteries; *l-TGA*, left transposition of the great arteries; *ASD*, atrial septal defect; *VSD*, ventricular septal defect; *AVC*, atrioventricular canal; *IVS*, interventricular septum; *SHF*, secondary heart field; *IAA*, interrupted aortic arch.

from existing vessels. The major vessels, including the dorsal aorta and cardinal veins, are formed by vasculogenesis. The remainder of the vascular system then forms by angiogenesis. The entire system is patterned by guidance cues involving **vascular endothelial growth factor (VEGF)** and other growth factors (see Chapter 6, p. 70).

## Arterial System

### *Aortic Arches*

When pharyngeal arches form during the fourth and fifth weeks of development, each arch receives its own cranial nerve and its own artery (see Chapter 17). These arteries, the **aortic arches**, arise from the **aortic sac**, the most distal part of the truncus arteriosus (Figs. 13.9 and 13.38). The aortic arches are embedded in mesenchyme of the pharyngeal arches and terminate in the right and left dorsal aortae. (In the region of the arches, the dorsal aortae remain paired, but caudal to this region, they fuse to form a single vessel.) The pharyngeal arches and their vessels appear in a cranial-to-caudal sequence, so that they are not all present simultaneously. The aortic sac contributes a branch to each new arch as it forms, giving rise to a total of five pairs of arteries. (The fifth arch either never forms or forms incompletely and then regresses. Consequently, the five arches are numbered I, II, III, IV, and VI [Figs. 13.39 and 13.40*A*].) During further development, this arterial pattern becomes modified, and some vessels regress completely.

**Neural crest cells** in each pharyngeal arch contribute the coverings (smooth muscle and connective tissue) of the arch vessels and also regulate patterning of these vessels. Signals from endoderm and ectoderm lining the arches provide interactive signals to crest cells to regulate the patterning process. For example, FGF8 signaling in arch ectoderm is important for fourth arch development. Because patterning also involves left–right decisions, *PITX2*, the master gene for sidedness, expressed in the aortic sac, SHF, and arch mesoderm, regulates laterality during restructuring of the original aortic arch pattern.

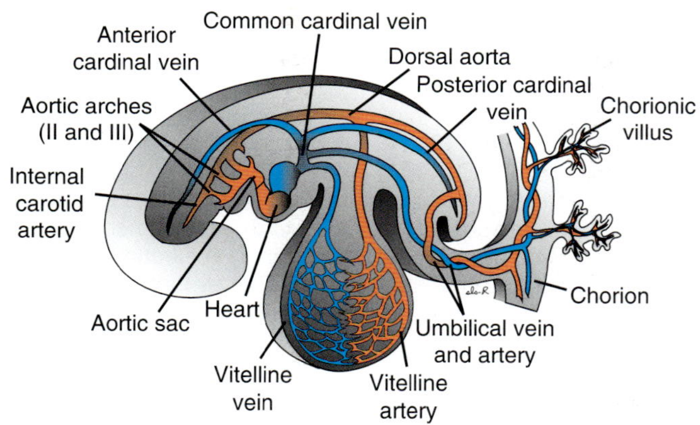


**FIGURE 13.38** Main intraembryonic and extraembryonic arteries (*red*) and veins (*blue*) in a 4-mm embryo (end of the fourth week). Only the vessels on the left side of the embryo are shown.

Division of the truncus arteriosus by the aorticopulmonary septum divides the outflow channel of the heart into the **ventral aorta** and the **pulmonary trunk**. The aortic sac then forms right and left horns, which subsequently give rise to the **brachiocephalic artery** and the proximal segment of the **aortic arch**, respectively (Fig. 13.40*B,C*).

By day 27, most of the **first aortic arch** has disappeared (Fig. 13.39), although a small portion persists to form the **maxillary artery**. Similarly, the **second aortic arch** soon disappears. The remaining portions of this arch are the **hyoid** and **stapedial arteries**. The third arch is large; the fourth and sixth arches are in the process of formation. Even though the sixth arch is not completed, the **primitive pulmonary artery** is already present as a major branch (Fig. 13.39*A*).

In the 29-day embryo, the first and second aortic arches have disappeared (Fig. 13.39*B*). The third, fourth, and sixth arches are large. The conotruncal region has divided so that the sixth arches are now continuous with the pulmonary trunk.

With further development, the aortic arch system loses its original symmetrical form, as shown in Figure 13.40*A* and establishes the definitive pattern illustrated in Figure 13.40*B,C*. This representation may clarify the transformation from the embryonic to the adult arterial system. The following changes occur:

The **third aortic arch** forms the **common carotid artery** and the first part of the **internal carotid artery**. The remainder of the internal carotid is formed by the cranial portion of the dorsal aorta. The **external carotid artery** is a sprout of the third aortic arch.

The **fourth aortic arch** persists on both sides, but its ultimate fate is different on the right and left sides. On the left,

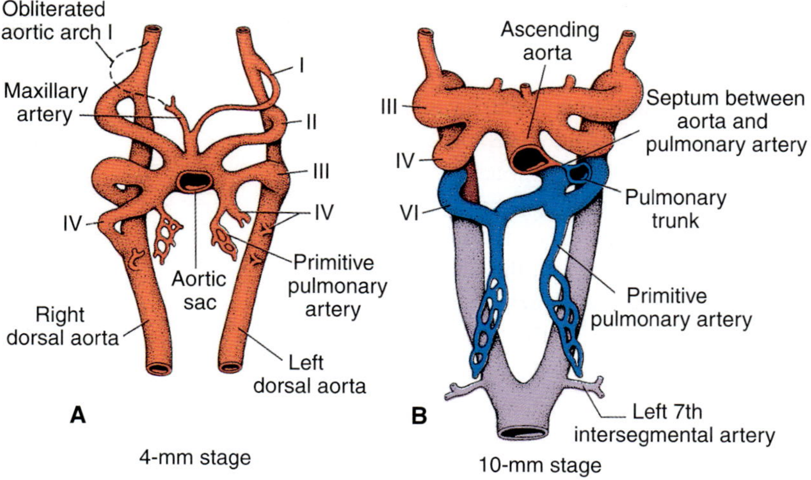


**FIGURE 13.39 A.** Aortic arches at the end of the fourth week. The first arch is obliterated before the sixth is formed. **B.** Aortic arch system at the beginning of the sixth week. Note the aorticopulmonary septum and the large pulmonary arteries.

Part 2

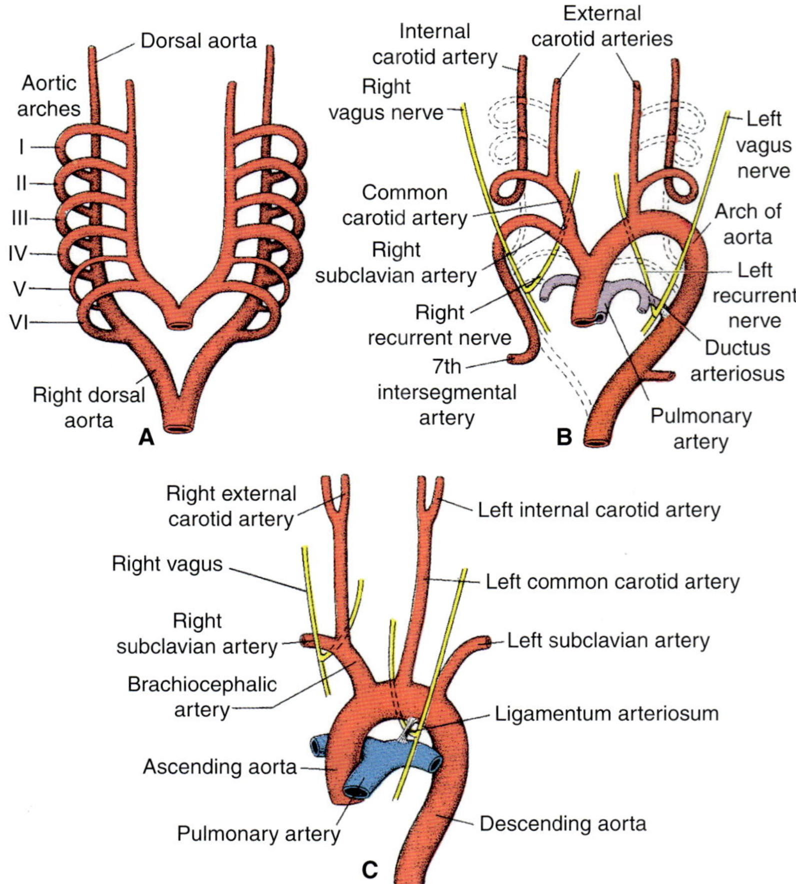


**FIGURE 13.40** **A.** Aortic arches and dorsal aortae before transformation into the definitive vascular pattern. **B.** Aortic arches and dorsal aortae after the transformation. *Broken lines*, obliterated components. Note the PDA and position of the seventh intersegmental artery on the left. **C.** The great arteries in the adult. Compare the distance between the place of origin of the left common carotid artery and the left subclavian in **(B)** and **(C)**. After disappearance of the distal part of the sixth aortic arch (the fifth arches never form completely), the right recurrent laryngeal nerve hooks around the right subclavian artery. On the left, the nerve remains in place and hooks around the ligamentum arteriosum.

Part 2

it forms part of the arch of the aorta, between the left common carotid and the left subclavian arteries. On the right, it forms the most proximal segment of the right subclavian artery, the distal part of which is formed by a portion of the right dorsal aorta and the seventh intersegmental artery (Fig. 13.40*B*).

The **fifth aortic arch** either never forms or forms incompletely and then regresses.

The **sixth aortic arch**, also known as the **pulmonary arch**, gives off an important branch that grows toward the developing lung bud (Fig. 13.40*B*). On the right side, the proximal part becomes the proximal segment of the right pulmonary artery. The distal portion of this arch loses its connection with the dorsal aorta and disappears. On the left, the distal part persists during intrauterine life as the **ductus arteriosus**. Table 13.2 summarizes the changes and derivatives of the aortic arch system.

A number of other changes occur along with alterations in the aortic arch system: (1) The dorsal aorta between the entrance of the third and fourth arches, known as the **carotid duct**, is obliterated (Fig. 13.41); (2) the right dorsal aorta disappears between the origin of the seventh intersegmental artery and the junction with the left dorsal aorta (Fig. 13.41); and (3) cephalic folding, growth of the forebrain, and elongation of the neck push the heart into the thoracic cavity. Hence,

**Table 13.2 Derivatives of the Aortic Arches**

| Arch | Arterial Derivative |
|---|---|
| 1 | Maxillary arteries |
| 2 | Hyoid and stapedial arteries |
| 3 | Common carotid and first part of the internal carotid arteries[a] |
| 4 left side | Arch of the aorta from the left common carotid to the left subclavian arteries[b] |
| Right side | Right subclavian artery (proximal portion)[c] |
| 6 left side | Left pulmonary artery and ductus arteriosus |
| Right side | Right pulmonary artery |

[a]Remainder of the internal carotid arteries are derived from the dorsal aorta; the external carotid arteries sprout from the third aortic arch.
[b]The proximal portion of the aortic arch is derived from the left horn of the aortic sac; the right horn of this sac forms the brachiocephalic artery.
[c]The distal portion of the right subclavian artery as well as the left subclavian artery form from the seventh intersegmental arteries on their respective sides.

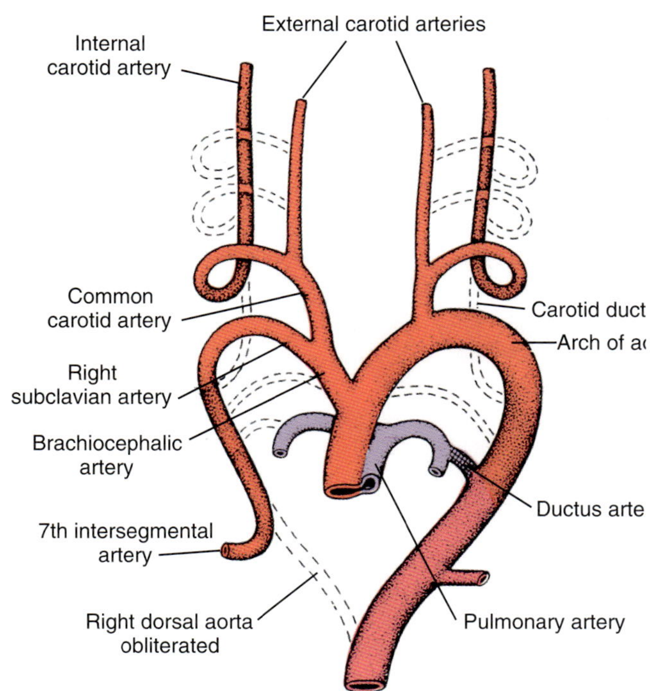


**FIGURE 13.41** Changes from the original aortic arch system.

the carotid and brachiocephalic arteries elongate considerably (Fig. 13.40*C*). As a further result of this caudal shift, the left subclavian artery, distally fixed in the arm bud, shifts its point of origin from the aorta at the level of the seventh intersegmental artery (Fig. 13.40*B*) to an increasingly higher point until it comes close to the origin of the left common carotid artery (Fig. 13.40*C*); and (4) as a result of the caudal shift of the heart and the disappearance of various portions of the aortic arches, the course of the **recurrent laryngeal nerves** becomes different on the right and left sides. Initially, these nerves, branches of the vagus, supply the sixth pharyngeal arches. When the heart descends, they hook around the sixth aortic arches and ascend again to the larynx, which accounts for their recurrent course. On the right, when the distal part of the sixth aortic arch and the fifth aortic arch disappear, the recurrent laryngeal nerve moves up and hooks around the right subclavian artery. On the left, the nerve does not move up because the distal part of the sixth aortic arch persists as the **ductus arteriosus**, which later forms the **ligamentum arteriosum** (Fig. 13.40).

### *Vitelline and Umbilical Arteries*

The **vitelline arteries**, initially a number of paired vessels supplying the yolk sac (Fig. 13.38), gradually fuse and form the arteries in the dorsal mesentery of the gut. In the adult, they are represented by the **celiac and superior mesenteric arteries. The inferior mesenteric arteries are derived from the umbilical arteries**. These three vessels supply derivatives of the **foregut**, **midgut**, and **hindgut**, respectively.

The **umbilical arteries**, initially paired ventral branches of the dorsal aorta, course to the placenta in close association with the allantois (Fig. 13.38). During the fourth week, however, each artery acquires a secondary connection with the dorsal branch of the aorta, the **common iliac artery**, and loses its earliest origin. After birth, the proximal portions of the umbilical arteries persist as the **internal iliac** and **superior vesical arteries**, and the distal parts are obliterated to form the **medial umbilical ligaments**.

### *Coronary Arteries*

**Coronary arteries** are derived from the **epicardium**, which differentiated from the **proepicardial organ** located in the caudal portion of the dorsal mesocardium, a derivative of the SHF. Some epicardial cells undergo an epithelial-to-mesenchymal transition induced by the underlying myocardium. The newly formed mesenchymal cells then contribute to endothelial and smooth muscle cells of the coronary arteries. Neural crest cells also may contribute smooth muscle cells along the proximal segments of these arteries and may direct connection of the coronary arteries to the aorta. Connection occurs by ingrowth of arterial endothelial cells from the arteries into the aorta causing the coronary arteries to "invade" the aorta.

Part 2

## *Clinical Correlates*

### Arterial System Defects

Under normal conditions, the **ductus arteriosus** is functionally closed through contraction of its muscular wall shortly after birth to form the **ligamentum arteriosum**. Anatomical closure by means of intima proliferation takes 1 to 3 months. A **patent ductus arteriosus (PDA)**, one of the most frequently occurring abnormalities of the great vessels (8/10,000 births), especially in premature infants, either may be an isolated abnormality or may accompany other heart defects (Figs. 13.34*A* and 13.36). In particular, defects that cause large differences between aortic and pulmonary pressures may cause increased blood flow through the ductus, preventing its normal closure.

In **coarctation of the aorta** (Fig. 13.42*A,B*), which occurs in 3.2/10,000 births, the aortic lumen below the origin of the left subclavian artery is significantly narrowed. Because the constriction may be above or below the entrance of the ductus arteriosus, two types (**preductal** and **postductal**) may be distinguished. The cause of aortic narrowing is primarily an abnormality in the media of the aorta, followed by intima proliferations. In the preductal type, the ductus arteriosus persists, whereas in the postductal type, which is more common, this channel is usually obliterated. In the latter case, collateral circulation between the proximal and distal parts of the aorta is established by way of large intercostal and internal thoracic arteries. In this manner, the lower part of the body is supplied with blood. Classic clinical signs associated with this condition include hypertension in the right arm concomitant with lowered blood pressure in the legs.

*(Continued)*

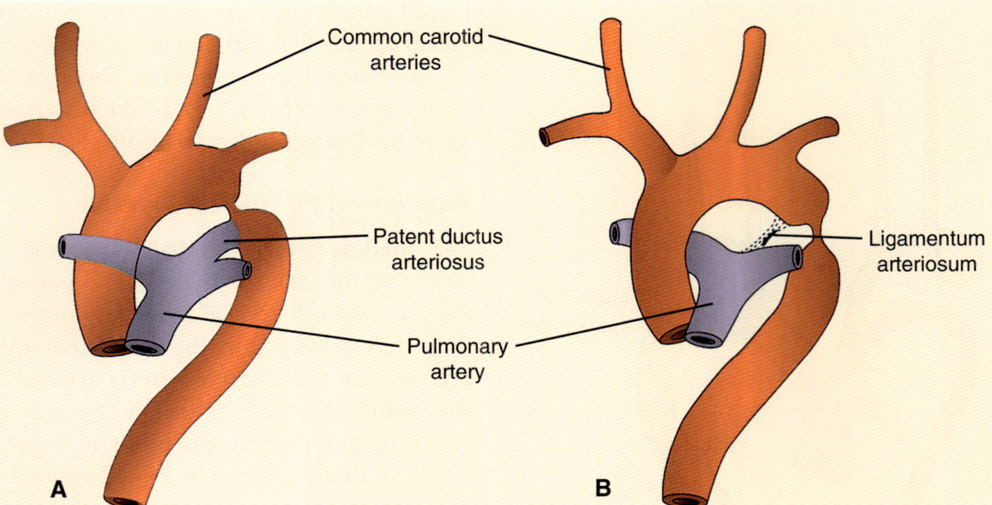


**FIGURE 13.42** Coarctation of the aorta. **A.** Preductal type. **B.** Postductal type. The caudal part of the body is supplied by large hypertrophied intercostal and internal thoracic arteries.

**Abnormal origin of the right subclavian artery** (Fig. 13.43*A,B*) occurs when the artery is formed by the distal portion of the right dorsal aorta and the seventh intersegmental artery. The right fourth aortic arch and the proximal part of the right dorsal aorta are obliterated. With shortening of the aorta between the left common carotid and left subclavian arteries, the origin of the abnormal right subclavian artery finally settles just below that of the left subclavian artery. Because its stem is derived from the right dorsal aorta, it must cross the midline behind the esophagus to reach the right arm. This location does not usually cause problems with swallowing or breathing because neither the esophagus nor the trachea is severely compressed.

With a **double aortic arch**, the right dorsal aorta persists between the origin of the seventh intersegmental artery and its junction with the left dorsal aorta (Fig. 13.44). A **vascular ring**

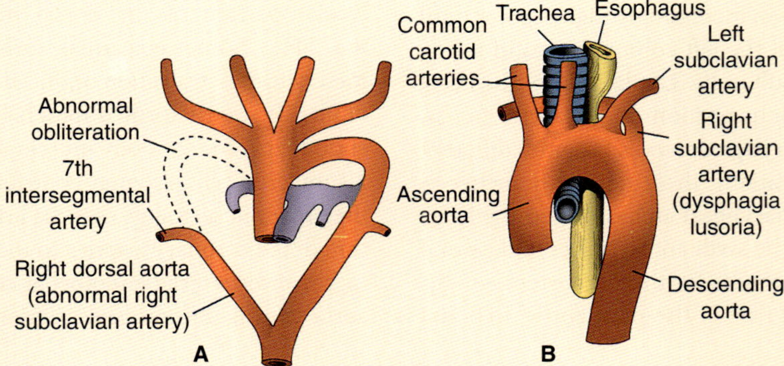


**FIGURE 13.43** Abnormal origin of the right subclavian artery. **A.** Obliteration of the right fourth aortic arch and the proximal portion of the right dorsal aorta with persistence of the distal portion of the right dorsal aorta. **B.** The abnormal right subclavian artery crosses the midline behind the esophagus and may compress it.

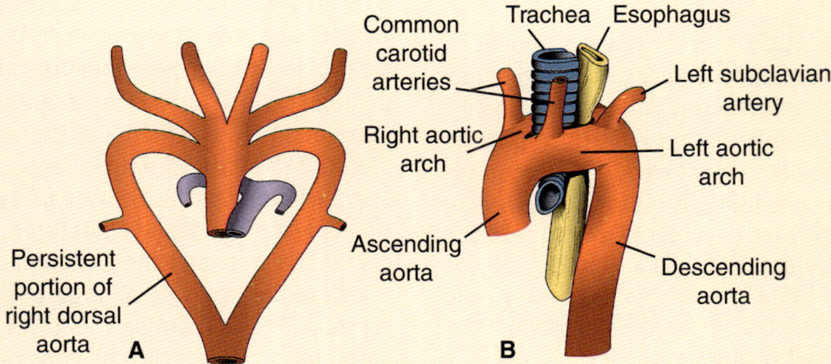


**FIGURE 13.44** Double aortic arch. **A.** Persistence of the distal portion of the right dorsal aorta. **B.** The double aortic arch forms a vascular ring around the trachea and esophagus.

surrounds the trachea and esophagus and commonly compresses these structures, causing difficulties in breathing and swallowing.

In a **right aortic arch**, the left fourth arch and left dorsal aorta are obliterated and replaced by the corresponding vessels on the right side. Occasionally, when the ligamentum arteriosum lies on the left side and passes behind the esophagus, it causes complaints with swallowing.

An **interrupted aortic arch (IAA)** is a very rare defect (3/1,000,000 live births) caused by abnormal regression patterns in the right and left fourth aortic arches (Fig. 13.45*A*). The result is an interruption between the aortic arch and descending aorta, and there are three types depending on where the break occurs: type A (3% to 40%), between the left subclavian artery and descending aorta (Fig. 13.45*B*); type B (50% to 60%), between the left common carotid and left subclavian arteries (Fig. 13.45*C*); and type C (4%), between the right and left common carotid arteries (Fig. 13.45*D*). The defect is accompanied by a VSD and a PDA that allows blood to reach the lower part of the body. Although rare, the defect occurs in 50% of children with DiGeorge syndrome, part of the 22q11 deletion syndrome complex (see Chapter 17, p. 243).

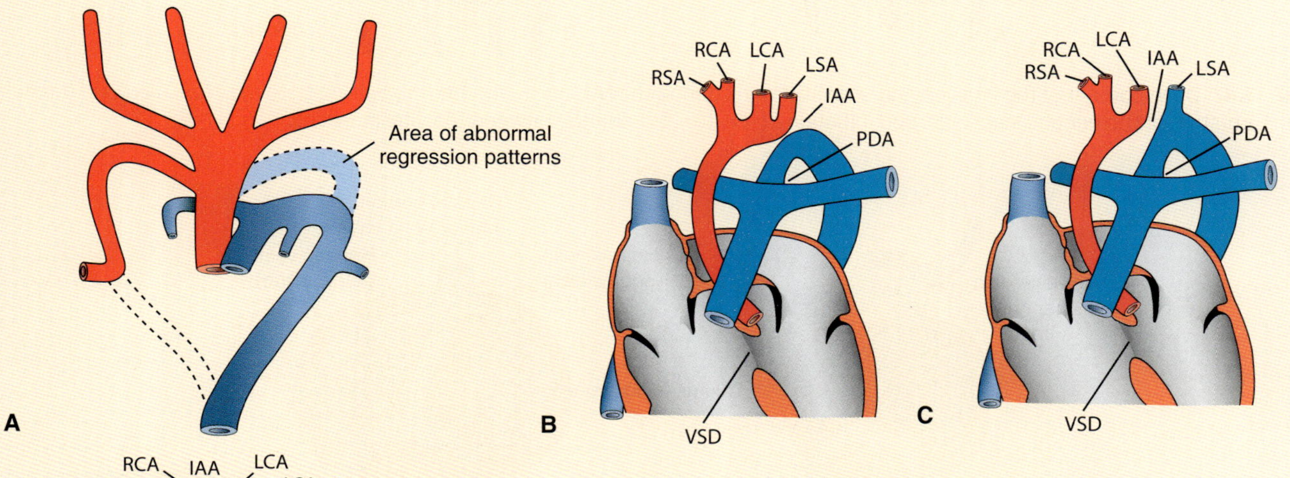


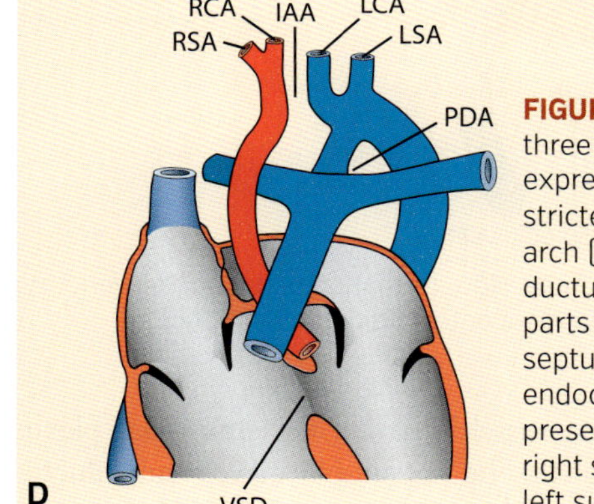


**FIGURE 13.45 A.** Abnormal regression patterns in the fourth aortic arch on the left result in three different types of interrupted aortic arch (*IAA*). These interruptions represent the ultimate expression of coarctation of the aorta where the vessel is split in two instead of simply constricted. **B.** Type A interrupted aortic arch (30% to 40% of cases). **C.** Type B interrupted aortic arch (40% to 50% of cases). **D.** Type C interrupted aortic arch (4% of cases). Note that a patent ductus arteriosus (*PDA*) is present to allow blood to reach the descending aorta to the lower parts of the body. A ventricular septal defect (*VSD*) is also present because the conotruncal septum responsible for septating the outflow tract fails to extend and fuse with the ventral endocardial cushion in the atrioventricular canal (see Fig. 13.27, p. 164). Type B IAA is often present in children with DiGeorge syndrome, part of the 22q11 deletion syndrome complex. *RSA*, right subclavian artery; *RCA*, right common carotid artery; *LCA*, left common carotid artery; *LSA*, left subclavian artery.



## Venous System

In the fifth week, three pairs of major veins can be distinguished: (1) the **vitelline veins**, or **omphalomesenteric veins**, carrying blood from the yolk sac to the sinus venosus; (2) the **umbilical veins**, originating in the chorionic villi and carrying oxygenated blood to the embryo; and (3) the **cardinal veins**, draining the body of the embryo proper (Fig. 13.46).

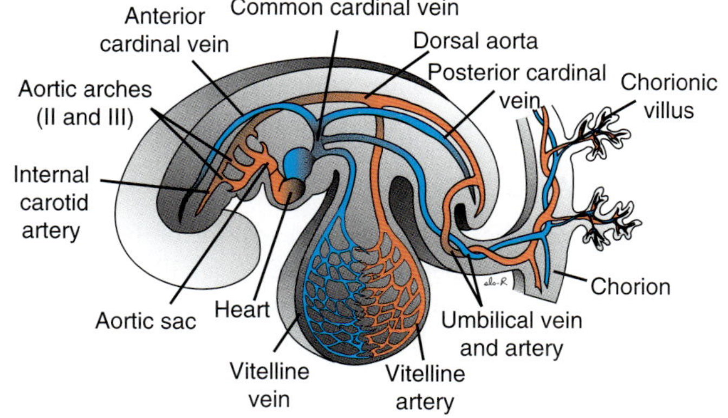


**FIGURE 13.46** Main components of the venous and arterial systems in a 4-mm embryo (end of the fourth week).

### *Vitelline Veins*

Before entering the sinus venosus, the vitelline veins form a plexus around the duodenum and pass through the septum transversum. The liver cords growing into the septum interrupt the course of the veins, and an extensive vascular network, the **hepatic sinusoids**, forms (Fig. 13.47).

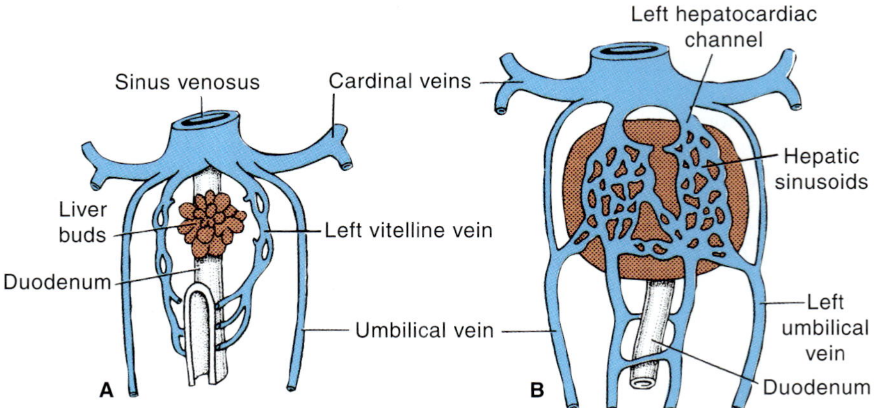


**FIGURE 13.47** Development of the vitelline and umbilical veins during the **(A)** fourth and **(B)** fifth weeks. Note the plexus around the duodenum, formation of the hepatic sinusoids, and initiation of left-to-right shunts between the vitelline veins.

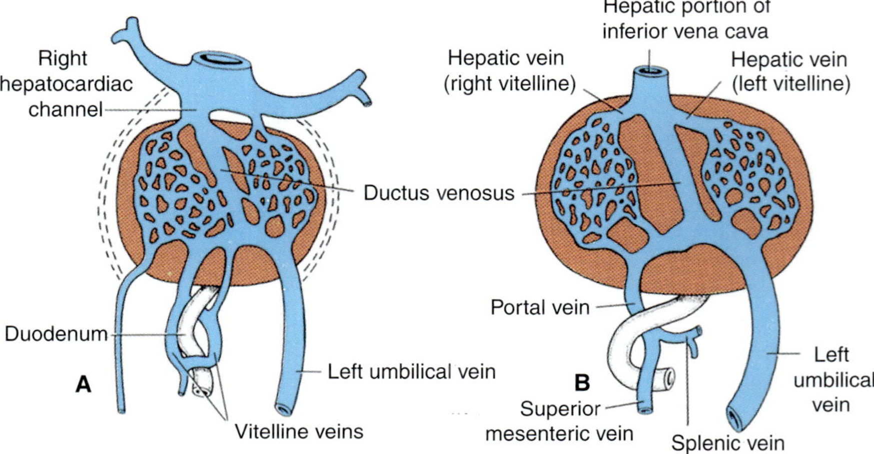


**FIGURE 13.48** Development of vitelline and umbilical veins in the **(A)** second and **(B)** third months. Note formation of the ductus venosus, portal vein, and hepatic portion of the inferior vena cava. The splenic and superior mesenteric veins enter the portal vein.

With reduction of the left sinus horn, blood from the left side of the liver is rechanneled toward the right, resulting in an enlargement of the right vitelline vein (right hepatocardiac channel). Ultimately, the right hepatocardiac channel forms the **hepatocardiac portion of the inferior vena cava**. The proximal part of the left vitelline vein disappears (Fig. 13.48*A,B*). The anastomotic network around the duodenum develops into a single vessel, the **portal vein** (Fig. 13.48*B*). The **superior** mesenteric vein, which drains the primary intestinal loop, derives from the right vitelline vein. The distal portion of the left vitelline vein also disappears (Fig. 13.48*A,B*).

### Umbilical Veins

Initially, the umbilical veins pass on each side of the liver, but some connect to the hepatic sinusoids (Fig. 13.47*A,B*). The proximal part of both umbilical veins and the remainder of the right umbilical vein then disappear, so that the left vein is the only one to carry blood from the placenta to the liver (Fig. 13.48). With the increase of the placental circulation, a direct communication forms between the left umbilical vein and the right hepatocardiac channel, the **ductus venosus** (Fig. 13.48*A,B*). This vessel bypasses the sinusoidal plexus of the liver. After birth, the left umbilical vein and ductus venosus are obliterated and form the **ligamentum teres hepatis** and **ligamentum venosum**, respectively.

### Cardinal Veins

Initially, the cardinal veins form the main venous drainage system of the embryo. This system consists of the **anterior cardinal veins**, which drain the cephalic part of the embryo, and the **posterior cardinal veins**, which drain the rest of the embryo. The anterior and posterior veins join before entering the sinus horn and form the short **common cardinal veins**. During the fourth week, the cardinal veins form a symmetrical system (Fig. 13.46).

During the fifth to the seventh weeks, a number of additional veins are formed: (1) the **subcardinal veins**, which mainly drain the kidneys; (2) the **sacrocardinal veins**, which drain the lower extremities; and (3) the **supracardinal veins**, which drain the body wall by way of the intercostal veins, taking over the functions of the posterior cardinal veins (Fig. 13.49).

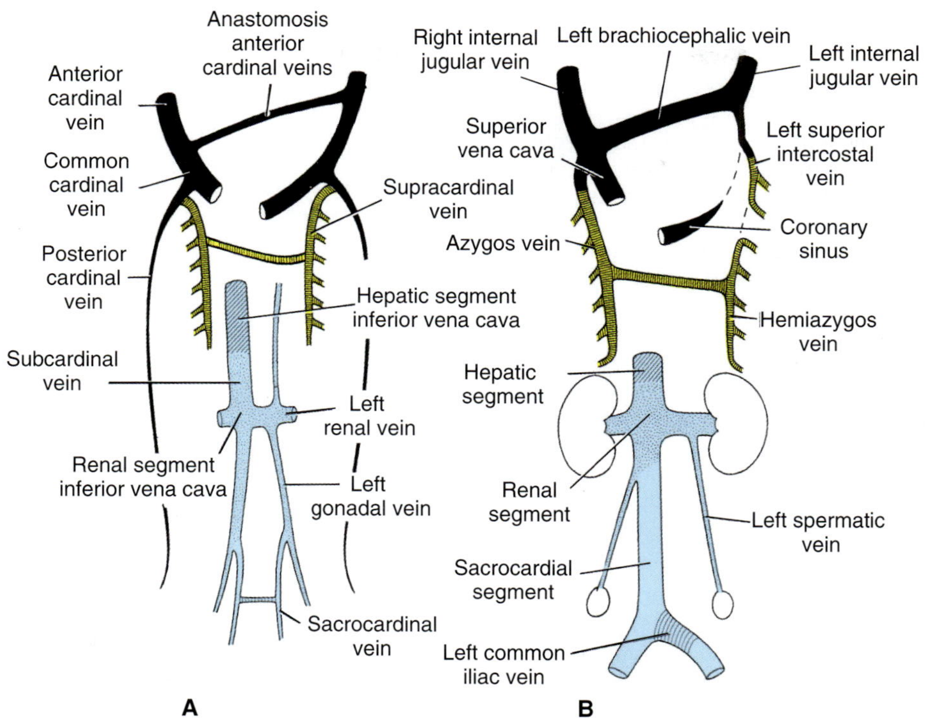


**FIGURE 13.49** Development of the inferior vena cava, azygos vein, and superior vena cava. **A.** Seventh week. The anastomosis lies between the subcardinals, supracardinals, sacrocardinals, and anterior cardinals. **B.** The venous system at birth showing the three components of the inferior vena cava.

Formation of the vena cava system is characterized by the appearance of anastomoses between left and right subcardinal, sacrocardinal, and supracardinal veins in such a manner that the blood from the left is channeled to the right side.

The **anastomosis between the anterior cardinal veins** develops into the **left brachiocephalic vein** (Fig. 13.49*A,B*). Most of the blood from the left side of the head and the left upper extremity is then channeled to the right. The terminal portion of the left posterior cardinal vein entering into the left brachiocephalic vein is retained as a small vessel, the **left superior intercostal vein** (Fig. 13.49*B*). This vessel receives blood from the second and third intercostal spaces. The **superior vena cava** is formed by the right common cardinal vein and the proximal portion of the right anterior cardinal vein. The anterior cardinal veins provide the primary venous drainage of the head during the fourth week of development and ultimately form the **internal jugular veins** (Fig. 13.49). **External jugular veins** are derived from a plexus of venous vessels in the face and drain the face and side of the head to the subclavian veins.

The **anastomosis between the subcardinal veins** forms the **left renal vein**. When this communication has been established, the left subcardinal vein disappears, and only its distal portion remains as the **left gonadal vein**. Hence, the right subcardinal vein becomes the main drainage channel and develops into the **renal segment of the inferior vena cava** (Fig. 13.49*B*).

The **anastomosis between the sacrocardinal veins** forms the **left common iliac vein** (Fig. 13.49*B*). The right sacrocardinal vein becomes the sacrocardinal segment of the inferior vena cava. When the renal segment of the inferior vena cava connects with the hepatic segment, which is derived from the right vitelline vein, the inferior vena cava, consisting of hepatic, renal, and sacrocardinal segments, is complete. Hence, some portions of these additional veins and their anastomosis regresses and disappears leading to the formation of final definitive inferior vena cava (Table 13.3; Fig. 13.49*B*).

With obliteration of the major portion of the posterior cardinal veins, the supracardinal veins assume a greater role in draining the body wall. The 4th to 11th right intercostal veins empty into the right supracardinal vein, which together with a portion of the posterior cardinal vein forms the **azygos vein** (Fig. 13.49). On the left, the 4th to 7th intercostal veins enter into the left supracardinal vein, and the left supracardinal

| Table 13.3 | Developmental Component of IVC |
|---|---|
| Right hepatocardiac channel [**Hepatic Segment**] | |
| Subcardinal vein and right hepatocardiac channel anastomosis | |
| Right subcardinal vein (between supracardinal and subcardinal vein anastomosis and anastomosis between subcardinal vein and right hepatocardiac channel) [**Renal Segment**] | |
| Right supracardinal vein and subcardinal vein anastomosis | |
| Right supracardinal vein (between the junction of the right supracardinal vein with the posterior cardinal vein and supracardinal vein–subcardinal vein anastomosis) | |
| Right posterior cardinal vein (between the junction of the right posterior cardinal vein with the supracardinal vein and anastomosis between posterior cardinal veins) [**Sacrocardinal Segment**] | |

Part 2

## Clinical Correlates

### Venous System Defects

The complicated development of the vena cava may account for the fact that deviations from the normal pattern are common. Also, the fact that the original pattern of venous return is established bilaterally and then shifts to the right probably accounts for the fact that vena cava abnormalities are often observed in individuals with laterality (sidedness) defects.

A **double inferior vena cava** occurs when the left sacrocardinal vein fails to lose its connection with the left subcardinal vein (Fig. 13.50*A*). The left common iliac vein may or may not be present, but the left gonadal vein remains as in normal conditions.

**Absence of the inferior vena cava** arises when the right subcardinal vein fails to make its connection with the liver and shunts its blood directly into the right supracardinal vein (Figs. 13.49 and 13.50*B*). Hence, the bloodstream from the caudal part of the body reaches the heart by way of the azygos vein and superior vena cava. The hepatic vein enters into the right atrium at the site of the inferior vena cava. Usually, this abnormality is associated with other heart malformations.

**Left superior vena cava** is caused by persistence of the left anterior cardinal vein and obliteration of the common cardinal and proximal part of the anterior cardinal veins on the right (Fig. 13.51*A*). In such a case, blood from the right is channeled toward the left by way of the brachiocephalic vein. The left superior vena cava drains into the right atrium by way of the left sinus horn, that is, the coronary sinus.

A **double superior vena cava** is characterized by the persistence of the left anterior cardinal vein and failure of the left brachiocephalic vein to form (Fig. 13.51*B*). The persistent left anterior cardinal vein, the **left superior vena cava**, drains into the right atrium by way of the coronary sinus.

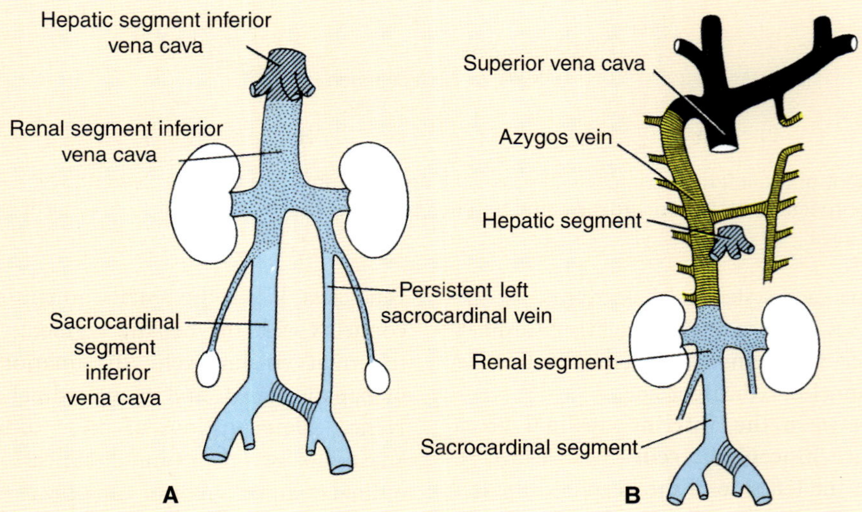


**FIGURE 13.50** **A.** Double inferior vena cava at the lumbar level arising from the persistence of the left sacrocardinal vein. **B.** Absent inferior vena cava. The lower half of the body is drained by the azygos vein, which enters the superior vena cava. The hepatic vein enters the heart at the site of the inferior vena cava.

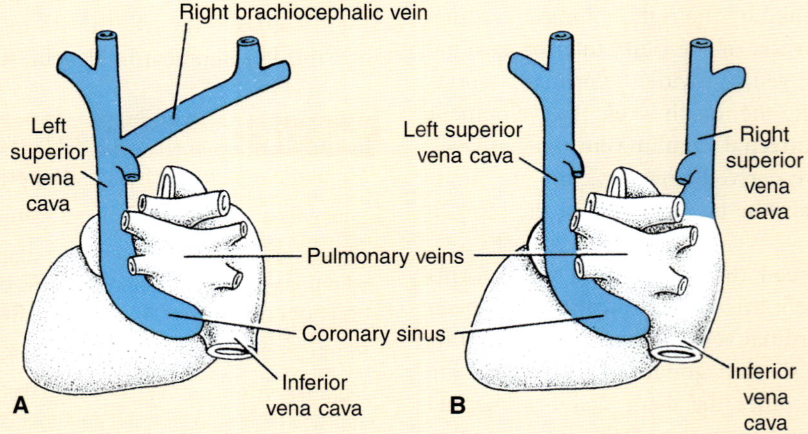


**FIGURE 13.51** **A.** Left superior vena cava draining into the right atrium by way of the coronary sinus (dorsal view). **B.** Double superior vena cava. The communicating (brachiocephalic) vein between the two anterior cardinals has failed to develop (dorsal view).

vein, then known as the **hemiazygos vein**, empties into the azygos vein (Fig. 13.49*B*).

## CIRCULATION BEFORE AND AFTER BIRTH

### Fetal Circulation

Before birth, blood from the placenta, about 80% saturated with oxygen, returns to the fetus by way of the umbilical vein. On approaching the liver, most of this blood flows through the ductus venosus directly into the inferior vena cava, short-circuiting the liver. A smaller amount enters the liver sinusoids and mixes with blood from the portal circulation (Fig. 13.52). A **sphincter mechanism** in the **ductus venosus**, close to the entrance of the umbilical vein, regulates flow of umbilical blood through the liver sinusoids. This sphincter closes when a uterine contraction renders the venous return too high, preventing a sudden overloading of the heart.

After a short course in the inferior vena cava, where placental blood mixes with deoxygenated blood returning from the lower limbs, it enters the right atrium. Here, it is guided toward the oval foramen by the valve of the inferior vena cava, and most of the blood passes directly into the left atrium. A small amount is prevented from doing so by the lower edge of the septum secundum, the **crista dividens**, and remains in the right atrium. Here, it mixes with desaturated blood returning from the head and arms by way of the superior vena cava.

From the left atrium, where it mixes with a small amount of desaturated blood returning from the lungs, blood enters the left ventricle and ascending aorta. Because the coronary and carotid arteries are the first branches of the ascending aorta, the heart musculature and the brain are supplied with well-oxygenated blood. Desaturated blood from the superior vena cava flows by way of the right ventricle into the pulmonary trunk. During fetal life, resistance in the pulmonary vessels is high, such that most of this blood passes directly through the **ductus arteriosus** into the descending aorta, where it mixes with blood from the proximal aorta. After coursing through the descending aorta, blood flows toward the placenta by way of the two umbilical arteries. The oxygen saturation in the umbilical arteries is approximately 58%.

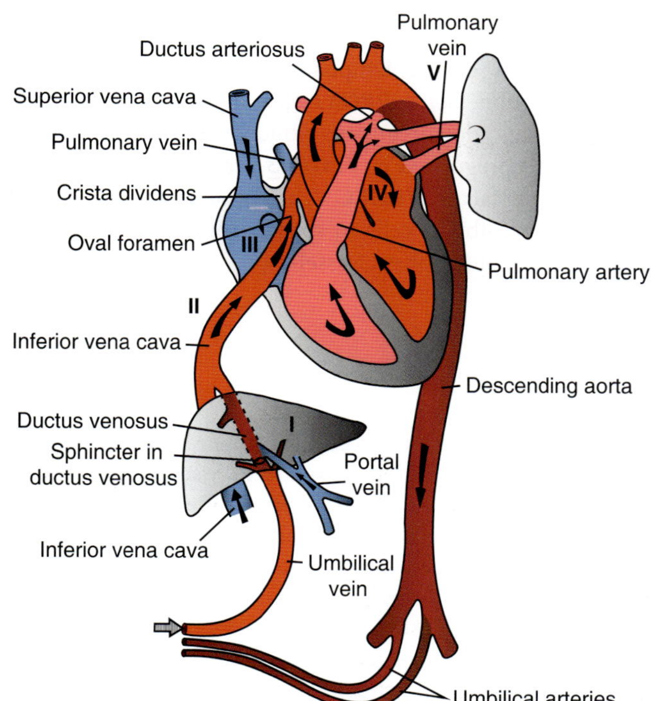


**FIGURE 13.52** Fetal circulation before birth. *Arrows*, direction of blood flow. Note where oxygenated blood mixes with deoxygenated blood in the liver (*I*), the inferior vena cava (*II*), the right atrium (*III*), the left atrium (*IV*), and at the entrance of the ductus arteriosus into the descending aorta (*V*).

During its course from the placenta to the organs of the fetus, blood in the umbilical vein gradually loses its high oxygen content as it mixes with desaturated blood. Theoretically, mixing may occur in the following places (Fig. 13.52, *I* to *V*):

I. Liver, by mixture with a small amount of blood returning from the portal system
II. Inferior vena cava, which carries deoxygenated blood returning from the lower extremities, pelvis, and kidneys
III. Right atrium, by mixture with blood from the head and upper limbs
IV. Left atrium, by mixture with blood returning from the lungs
V. The entrance of the ductus arteriosus into the descending aorta

### Circulatory Changes at Birth

Changes in the vascular system at birth are caused by cessation of placental blood flow and the beginning of respiration. Because the ductus arteriosus closes by muscular contraction of its wall, the amount of blood flowing through the lung vessels increases rapidly. This, in turn, raises pressure in the left atrium. Simultaneously, pressure in the right atrium decreases as a result of interruption of placental blood flow. The septum primum is then apposed to the septum secundum, and functionally, the oval foramen closes.

To summarize, the following changes occur in the vascular system after birth (Fig. 13.53):

**Closure of the umbilical arteries**, accomplished by contraction of the smooth musculature in their walls, is probably caused by thermal and mechanical stimuli and a change in oxygen tension. Functionally, the arteries close a few minutes after birth, although the actual obliteration of the lumen by fibrous proliferation may take 2 to 3 months. Distal parts of the umbilical arteries form the **medial umbilical ligaments**, and the proximal portions remain open as the **superior vesical arteries** (Fig. 13.53).

**Closure of the umbilical vein and ductus venosus** occurs shortly after that of the umbilical arteries. Hence, blood from the placenta may enter the newborn for some time after birth. After obliteration, the umbilical vein forms the **ligamentum teres hepatis** in the lower margin of the falciform ligament. The ductus venosus, which courses from the ligamentum teres to the inferior vena cava, is also obliterated and forms the **ligamentum venosum**.

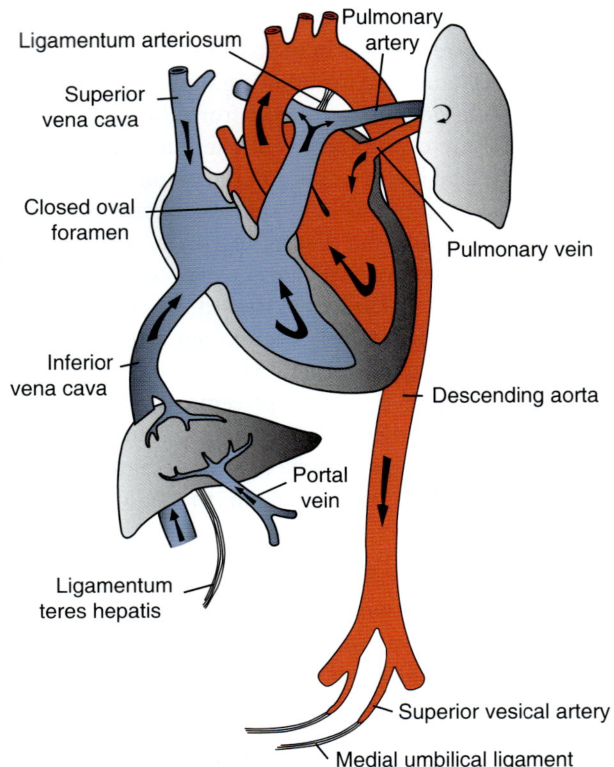


**FIGURE 13.53** Human circulation after birth. Note the changes occurring as a result of the beginning of respiration and interruption of placental blood flow. *Arrows*, direction of blood flow.

**Closure of the ductus arteriosus** by contraction of its muscular wall occurs almost immediately after birth; it is mediated by **bradykinin**, a substance released from the lungs during initial inflation. Complete anatomical obliteration by proliferation of the intima is thought to take 1 to 3 months. In the adult, the obliterated ductus arteriosus forms the **ligamentum arteriosum.**

**Closure of the oval foramen** is caused by an increased pressure in the left atrium, combined with a decrease in pressure on the right side. The first breath presses the septum primum against the septum secundum. During the first days of life, however, this closure is reversible. Crying by the baby creates a shunt from right to left, which accounts for cyanotic periods in the newborn. Constant apposition gradually leads to fusion of the two septa in about 1 year. In 20% of individuals, however, perfect anatomical closure may never be obtained (**probe patent foramen ovale**).

### Lymphatic System

The lymphatic system begins its development later than the cardiovascular system, not appearing until the fifth week of gestation. Lymphatic vessels arise as saclike outgrowths from the endothelium of veins. Six primary lymph sacs are formed: two **jugular**, at the junction of the subclavian and anterior cardinal veins; two **iliac**, at the junction of the iliac and posterior cardinal veins; one **retroperitoneal**, near the root of the mesentery; and one **cisterna chyli**, dorsal to the retroperitoneal sac. Numerous channels connect the sacs with each other and drain lymph from the limbs, body wall, head, and neck. Two main channels, the right and left thoracic ducts, join the jugular sacs with the cisterna chyli, and soon, an anastomosis forms between these ducts. The **thoracic duct** then develops from the distal portion of the right thoracic duct, the anastomosis, and the cranial portion of the left thoracic duct. The **right lymphatic duct** is derived from the cranial portion of the right thoracic duct. Both ducts maintain their original connections with the venous system and empty into the junction of the internal jugular and subclavian veins. Numerous anastomoses produce many variations in the final form of the thoracic duct.

Specification of the lymphatic lineage is regulated by the transcription factor ***PROX1*** that upregulates lymphatic vessel genes and downregulates blood vessel genes. A critical gene that is upregulated is ***VEGFR3*** that is the receptor for the paracrine factor **VEGFC**. This protein causes *PROX1* expressing endothelial cells to sprout from existing veins to initiate growth of lymphatic vessels.

## SUMMARY

- On approximately day 16, **heart progenitor cells** migrate through the primitive streak to a position cranial to the neural folds where they establish a horseshoe-shaped region in the visceral layer of lateral plate mesoderm called the **primary heart field (PHF)** (Fig. 13.1).
- As the heart progenitor cells migrate, these cells are specified by the laterality pathway (Fig. 13.3) to contribute to right and left sides of the heart and to form specific heart regions, including part of the atria and the left ventricle. (Fig. 13.1A).
- The remainder of the heart, including part of the atria, the right ventricle, conus cordis, and truncus arteriosus (the outflow tract), is derived from cells in the **secondary heart field (SHF)** (Fig. 13.2).
- The SHF arises from cells that migrate through the primitive streak and then reside in visceral mesoderm near the floor of the posterior part of the pharynx. These cells are also patterned by laterality signaling and regulate neural crest cell contributions to septation of the outflow tract, including the spiraling of the conotruncal septum (Figs. 13.2 and 13.30).
- Disruption of the laterality pathway results in many different types of heart defects, whereas disruption of the SHF results in defects of the outflow tract, including transposition of the great arteries, pulmonary stenosis, double outlet right ventricle (DORV), and others (see Table 13.1, p. 168).

- Induction of the cardiogenic region is initiated by anterior endoderm underlying progenitor heart cells and causes the cells to become myoblasts and vessels. **BMPs** secreted by this endoderm in combination with inhibition of ***WNT*** expression induce expression of ***NKX2.5***, the master gene for heart development.
- Some cells in the PHF become endothelial cells and form a horseshoe-shaped tube, whereas others form myoblasts surrounding the tube. By the 22nd day of development, lateral body wall folds bring the two sides of the horseshoe (Fig. 13.5) toward the midline where they fuse (except for their caudal [atrial] ends) to form a single, slightly bent heart tube (Fig. 13.7) consisting of an inner endocardial tube and a surrounding myocardial mantle (Figs. 13.5C and 13.15).
- During the fourth week, the heart undergoes **cardiac looping**. This process causes the heart to fold on itself and assume its normal position in the left part of the thorax with the atria posteriorly and the ventricles in a more anterior position. Failure of the heart to loop properly results in **dextrocardia** and the heart lies on the right side. Dextrocardia can also be induced at an earlier time when laterality is established.
- Septum formation in the heart in part arises from development of **endocardial cushion** tissue in the atrioventricular canal (**atrioventricular cushions**) and in the conotruncal region (**conotruncal swellings**). Because of the key location of cushion tissue, many cardiac malformations are related to abnormal cushion morphogenesis.
- Atrial development is dependent upon expansion of the original atrial region and incorporation of additional structures. On the right, the **sinus venosus** is incorporated and forms the **smooth-walled portion** of the right atrium (Figs. 13.11 and 13.13), which is separated from the trabeculated portion by the **crista terminalis** (Fig. 13.13).
- On the left, the **pulmonary vein**, which forms in the **dorsal mesocardium**, is positioned into the posterior wall of the left atrium when cells in the **dorsal mesenchymal protrusion (DMP)** proliferate and accompany the septum primum as this structure grows toward the floor of the atrium (Fig. 13.17).
- Later, the root of the pulmonary vein is incorporated into the left atrium by atrial expansion until the vein's four branches enter the atrium on its posterior wall. This portion constitutes the smooth-walled region of the left atrium (Fig. 13.18).
- Development of the pulmonary vein begins in the midline and then shifts to the left, a result of laterality signaling. **Total anomalous pulmonary venous return (TAPVR)** in which the vein is shifted to the right and enters the right atrium or even the superior vena cava or brachiocephalic vein, arises in cases of **heterotaxy** where left–right patterning is disrupted.
- **Septum Formation in the Atrium.** The **septum primum**, a sickle-shaped crest descending from the roof of the atrium, begins to divide the atrium in two but leaves a lumen, the **ostium primum**, for communication between the two sides (Fig. 13.16). Later, when the ostium primum is obliterated by fusion of the septum primum with the endocardial cushions, the **ostium secundum** is formed by cell death that creates an opening in the septum primum. Finally, a **septum secundum** forms, but an interatrial opening, the **oval foramen**, persists. Only **at birth**, when pressure in the left atrium increases, do the two septa press against each other and close the communication between the two. Abnormalities in the atrial septum may vary from total absence (Fig. 13.23) to a small opening known as **probe patency** of the oval foramen.
- **Septum Formation in the Atrioventricular Canal.** Four **endocardial cushions** surround the atrioventricular canal. Fusion of the opposing superior and inferior cushions divides the orifice into right and left atrioventricular canals (Fig. 13.16*B–D*). Cushion tissue then becomes fibrous and forms the mitral (bicuspid) valve on the left and the tricuspid valve on the right (Fig. 13.16*F*). Persistence of the common atrioventricular canal (Fig. 13.24) and abnormal formation of the valves are defects that occur due to abnormalities in this endocardial cushion tissue.
- **Septum Formation in the Ventricles.** The interventricular septum consists of a thick **muscular** part and a thin **membranous** portion (Figs. 13.16*F* and 13.29) formed by (1) the inferior endocardial atrioventricular cushion, (2) the right conus swelling, and (3) the left conus swelling (Fig. 13.27). In many cases, these three components fail to fuse, resulting in an open interventricular foramen. Although this abnormality may be isolated, it is commonly combined with other compensatory defects (Figs. 13.33 and 13.34).
- **Septum Formation in the Bulbus.** The bulbus is divided into the smooth-walled portion of the right ventricle and the conus and truncus arteriosus. The truncus region is divided by the spiral **aorticopulmonary septum** into the proximal segments of the aorta and pulmonary artery (Fig. 13.27). Conus cushions divide the outflow tract regions of the aortic and pulmonary channels from the left and right ventricles, respectively and also, together with tissue from the inferior endocardial cushion, close the interventricular foramen (Fig. 13.27).
- Many vascular abnormalities, such as **transposition of the great vessels** and **pulmonary valvular atresia**, result from abnormal division of the conotruncal region; their origin may involve **neural crest cells** that contribute to septum formation in the conotruncal region (Fig. 13.30).
- **The conduction system** for the heart is derived from myocardial cells and the heart begins to beat at approximately 21 days of gestation. Initially, **pacemaker** activity for the heart is located in the caudal part of the left side of the cardiac tube. Later, the sinus venosus assumes this function, and when this structure is incorporated into the right atrium, the **sinuatrial node (SAN)** is formed. The **atrioventricular node (AVN)** is formed from cells surrounding the atrioventricular canal. Later, impulses

*(Continued)*

from the AVN pass to the **atrioventricular bundle** and **left and right bundle branches** and finally to the **Purkinje fiber network** surrounding and activating the ventricles. All of the cells for the heart's conduction system are derived from primary cardiac myocytes that differentiate into nodes, bundle branches, and Purkinje fibers. Expression of the transcription factor *TBX3* inhibits differentiation of these primary myocytes into ventricular muscle cells and allows them instead to differentiate into the conducting system.

- The **aortic arches** lie in each of the five pharyngeal arches (Figs. 13.38 and 13.40). Four important derivatives of the original aortic arch system are (1) the carotid arteries (third arches); (2) the arch of the aorta (left fourth aortic arch); (3) the pulmonary artery (sixth aortic arch), which during fetal life is connected to the aorta through the ductus arteriosus; and (4) the right subclavian artery formed by the right fourth aortic arch, distal portion of the right dorsal aorta, and the seventh intersegmental artery (Fig. 13.40*B*). The most common vascular aortic arch abnormalities include (1) open ductus arteriosus and coarctation of the aorta (Fig. 13.42) and (2) persistent right aortic arch and abnormal right subclavian artery (Figs. 13.43 and 13.44), which may cause respiratory and swallowing complaints.
- The **vitelline arteries** initially supply the yolk sac but later form the **celiac and superior mesenteric arteries. The inferior mesenteric arteries are derived from the umbilical arteries. These three arteries** supply the **foregut**, **midgut**, and **hindgut** regions, respectively.
- The paired **umbilical arteries** arise from the common iliac arteries. After birth, the distal portions of these arteries are obliterated to form the **medial umbilical ligaments**, whereas the proximal portions persist as the **internal iliac** and **vesicular arteries**.
- **Venous System.** Three systems can be recognized: (1) the **vitelline system**, which develops into the **portal system**; (2) the cardinal system, which forms the **caval system**; and (3) the **umbilical system**, which disappears after birth. The complicated caval system is characterized by many abnormalities, such as double inferior and superior vena cava and left superior vena cava (Fig. 13.51), which are also associated with laterality defects.
- **Changes at Birth.** During prenatal life, the placental circulation provides the fetus with its oxygen, but after birth, the lungs take on gas exchange. In the circulatory system, the following changes take place at birth and in the first postnatal months: (1) The ductus arteriosus closes, (2) the oval foramen closes, (3) the umbilical vein and ductus venosus close and remain as the **ligamentum teres hepatis** and **ligamentum venosum**, and (4) the umbilical arteries form the **medial umbilical ligaments**.
- **Lymphatic System.** The lymphatic system develops later than the cardiovascular system, originating from the endothelium of veins as six sacs: two jugular, two iliac, one retroperitoneal, and one cisterna chyli. Numerous channels form to connect the sacs and provide drainage from other structures. Ultimately, the **thoracic duct** forms from anastomosis of the right and left thoracic ducts, the distal part of the right thoracic duct, and the cranial part of the left thoracic duct. The **right lymphatic duct** develops from the cranial part of the right thoracic duct.

**Adult Derivatives of the Parts of the Heart Tube**

| Heart Tube | Derivatives |
|---|---|
| Truncus arteriosus (distal part of bulbus cordis) | Roots and proximal portion of aorta and pulmonary artery |
| Conus cordis (middle part of bulbus cordis) | Outflow part of both ventricles |
| Proximal part of bulbus cordis | Trabeculated (rough) part of the right ventricle |
| Sinus venosus | • Right horn: Smooth part of right atrium |
| | • Left horn: Oblique vein of left atrium, coronary sinus |
| Right venous valve | • Crista terminalis<br>• Valve of IVC<br>• Valve of coronary sinus |
| Left venous valve | Merges with septum secundum along with septum spurium |

**Adult Derivatives of the Developmental Components of the Septum of the Heart**

| | Developmental Component | Adult Derivative |
|---|---|---|
| Interatrial septum | Septum primum | Fossa ovalis |
| | Septum secundum | Limbus fossa ovalis |
| Interventricular septum | Muscular part | Muscular part |
| | Membranous part | • Right conus cushion<br>• Left conus cushion<br>• Proliferation of inferior endocardial (atrioventricular) cushion |

**Developmental Components of the Major Blood Vessels of the Pharyngeal Arch Arteries**

| Arteries | Embryological Developmental Component |
|---|---|
| Ascending aorta and pulmonary trunk | Truncus arteriosus |
| Arch of aorta | Aortic sac, left horn of aortic sac and left fourth arch artery |

| | |
|---|---|
| Descending aorta | Left dorsal aorta and fused dorsal aorta |
| Brachiocephalic artery | Right horn of aortic sac |
| Right subclavian artery | • Right fourth arch artery<br>• Right dorsal aorta between right fourth arch artery and right seventh cervical intersegmental artery<br>• Right seventh cervical intersegmental artery |
| Left subclavian artery | Left seventh cervical intersegmental artery |
| Common carotid artery | Third arch artery (proximal part) |
| Internal carotid artery | • Third arch artery (distal part)<br>• Dorsal aorta cranial to third arch artery |
| External carotid artery | Proliferating bud from third arch artery |
| Pulmonary artery | Sixth arch artery |
| Ductus arteriosus | Left sixth arch artery portion between lung bud and dorsal aorta |

**Adult Derivatives of the Umbilical Vessels and the Ductus Vessels**

| Developmental Components | Adult Derivative |
|---|---|
| Umbilical arteries | • Distal parts: Medial umbilical ligaments<br>• Proximal parts: Superior vesical arteries |
| Left umbilical vein | Ligamentum teres hepatis |
| Right umbilical vein | Degenerates |
| Ductus venosus | Ligamentum venosum. |
| Ductus arteriosus | Ligamentum arteriosum |

## Self-Assessment

### Comprehensive Questions

1. Discuss fetal circulation and the changes taking place after birth.
2. Discuss the embryological basis of Fallot's tetralogy.
3. Discuss the embryological basis of patent ductus arteriosus (PDA).

### Problem Solving Questions

1. A prenatal ultrasound of a 35-year-old woman in her 12th week of gestation reveals an abnormal image of the fetal heart. Instead of a four-chambered view provided by the typical cross, a portion just below the crosspiece is missing. What structures constitute the cross, and what defect does this infant probably have?
2. A child is born with severe craniofacial defects and transposition of the great vessels. What cell population may play a role in both abnormalities, and what type of insult might have produced this effect?
3. What type of tissue is critical for dividing the heart into four chambers and the outflow tract into pulmonary and aortic channels?
4. A patient complains about having difficulty swallowing. What vascular abnormality or abnormalities might produce this complaint? What is its embryological origin?
5. A 20-year-old primigravida, 18 weeks of pregnant, presented for routine prenatal ultrasound scan. The scan revealed interventricular septal defect in the fetus. The left ventricular outflow tract (aorta) was also observed to be arising directly from the ventricular septal defect. This was confirmed by the color Doppler images demonstrating filling of aorta from both the left and the right ventricles. The right ventricular outflow tract was observed to be narrow with hypertrophy of the right ventricle. Both the atrias were normal. The tricuspid and mitral valves were normal. What is the diagnosis in this condition?

### Multiple Choice Questions

1. Primary heart field forms
   (a) Right and left atrium
   (b) Right ventricle
   (c) Pulmonary trunk
   (d) Left ventricle
2. Which of the following is not derived from secondary heart field (SHF)?
   (a) Conus cordis
   (b) Truncus arteriosus
   (c) Left ventricle
   (d) Right ventricle
3. Which of the following does not develop from bulbous cordis?
   (a) Atrium
   (b) Right ventricle
   (c) Ascending aorta
   (d) Pulmonary trunk
4. All of the following statements are correct about heart tube folding except
   (a) Bulboventricular tube shifts ventrally, caudally, and to right.
   (b) Primitive atrium shifts anteriorly and superiorly.
   (c) Sinus venosus moves superiorly and posteriorly.
   (d) Conotruncal part shifts from right side of pericardial cavity to medial position.
5. Tetralogy of Fallot includes all of the following cardiac defects except
   (a) Overriding aorta
   (b) Aortic stenosis

(Continued)

(c) Ventricular septal defect
(d) Pulmonary stenosis

6. Left horn of sinus venosus forms
   (a) Left atrium
   (b) Pulmonary trunk
   (c) Coronary artery
   (d) Coronary sinus
7. Right horn forms
   (a) Superior vena cava
   (b) Smooth part of right atrium
   (c) Rough part of right atrium
   (d) Coronary sinus
8. Which of the following is the event taking place after birth in fetal circulation?
   (a) Obliteration of left umbilical vein
   (b) Patency of ductus venosus
   (c) Opening of umbilical arteries
   (d) Patency of foramen ovale
9. Artery of the fourth arch on the left side forms
   (a) Arch of aorta
   (b) Internal carotid artery
   (c) Pulmonary trunk
   (d) Internal thoracic artery
10. Portal vein forms around the
    (a) Stomach
    (b) Duodenum
    (c) Transverse colon
    (d) Liver
11. Which of the following vessels obliterates?
    (a) Right umbilical vein
    (b) Left umbilical vein
    (c) Right umbilical arteries
    (d) Left umbilical arteries
12. Primitive right ventricle is formed from
    (a) Trabeculated proximal third of the bulbus cordis
    (b) Smooth part of the bulbus cordis
    (c) Conus cordis
    (d) Primitive ventricular chamber
13. Which of the following statements is false regarding transposition of great vessels?
    (a) The conotruncal septum fails to follow its normal spiral course and runs straight down.
    (b) Both aorta and pulmonary trunk originate from the left ventricle.
    (c) It is associated with a defect in the membranous part of the interventricular septum.
    (d) Neural crest cells contribute to this defect in the outflow tract.

**Answers**

1. (d) 2. (c) 3. (a) 4. (c) 5. (b) 6. (d) 7. (b) 8. (a) 9. (a) 10. (b) 11. (a) 12. (d) 13. (b)

Part 2

CHAPTER

# 14 Respiratory System

## Specific Learning Objectives

- Development of lung and pleura
  - Formation of lung bud
  - Stages of maturation of lung: Pseudoglandular, canalicular, terminal sac, and alveolar
- Congenital anomalies/defects of the respiratory system:
  - Tracheoesophageal fistula
  - Respiratory distress syndrome (RDS)

## Competencies Covered

AN25.2 Describe about the development of the pleura and lung.
AN25.4 Describe the embryological basis of tracheoesophageal fistula.

Part 2

## FORMATION OF THE LUNG BUDS

When the embryo is approximately 4 weeks old, the **respiratory diverticulum (lung bud)** appears as an outgrowth from the ventral wall of the foregut (Fig. 14.1*A*). The appearance and location of the lung bud are dependent upon an increase in **retinoic acid (RA)** produced by adjacent mesoderm. This increase in RA causes upregulation of the transcription factor ***TBX4*** expressed in the endoderm of the gut tube at the site of the respiratory diverticulum. ***TBX4*** induces formation of the **bud** and the continued growth and differentiation of the lungs. Hence, **epithelium** of the internal lining of the larynx, trachea, and bronchi, as well as that of the lungs, is entirely of **endodermal origin**. The **cartilaginous**, **muscular**, and **connective tissue** components of the trachea and lungs are derived from **visceral (splanchnic) mesoderm** surrounding the foregut.

Initially, the lung bud is in open communication with the foregut (Fig. 14.1*B*). When the diverticulum expands caudally, however, two longitudinal ridges, the **tracheoesophageal ridges**, separate it from the foregut (Fig. 14.2*A*). Subsequently, when these ridges fuse to form the **tracheoesophageal septum**, the foregut is divided into a dorsal portion, the **esophagus**, and a ventral portion, the **trachea** (Fig. 14.2*B*,*C*). The respiratory

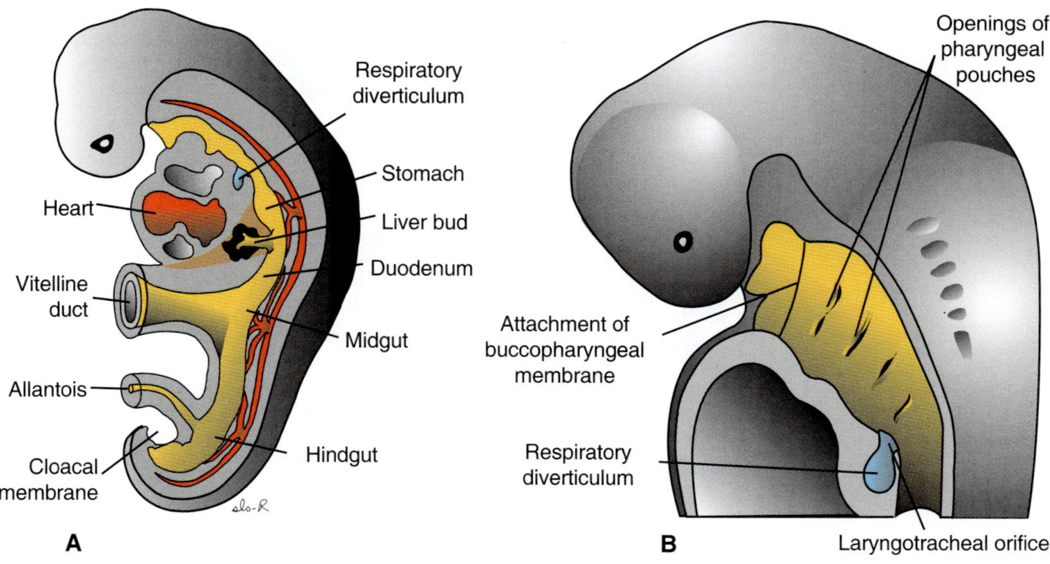


**FIGURE 14.1 A.** Embryo of approximately 25 days' gestation showing the relation of the respiratory diverticulum to the heart, stomach, and liver. **B.** Sagittal section through the cephalic end of a 5-week embryo showing the openings of the pharyngeal pouches and the laryngotracheal orifice.

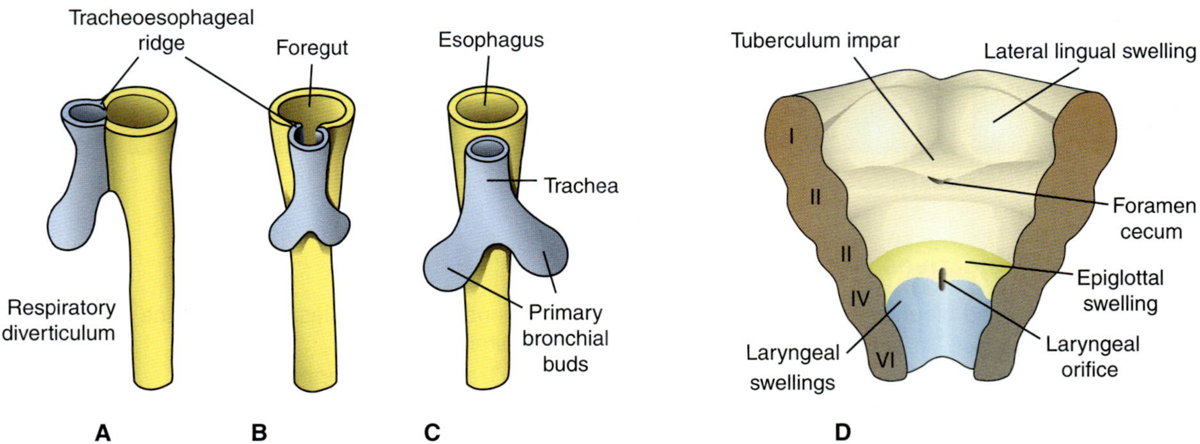


**FIGURE 14.2 A–C.** Successive stages in development of the respiratory diverticulum (lung bud) showing the tracheoesophageal ridges and formation of the septum, splitting the foregut into esophagus and trachea with bronchial buds. **D.** The ventral portion of the pharynx seen from above showing the laryngeal orifice and surrounding swelling.

## *Clinical Correlates*

Abnormalities in partitioning of the esophagus and trachea by the tracheoesophageal septum result in **esophageal atresia** with or without **tracheoesophageal fistulas (TEFs)**. These defects occur in approximately 1/3,000 births, and 90% result in the upper portion of the esophagus ending in a blind pouch and the lower segment forming a fistula with the trachea (Fig. 14.3*A*). Isolated esophageal atresia (Fig. 14.3*B*) and H-type TEF without esophageal atresia (Fig. 14.3*C*) each account for 4% of these defects. Other variations (Fig. 14.3*D,E*) each account for approximately 1% of these defects. These abnormalities are associated with other birth defects, including cardiac abnormalities, which occur in 33% of these cases. In this regard, TEFs are a component of the **VACTERL** association (**V**ertebral anomalies, **A**nal atresia, **C**ardiac defects, **T**racheoesophageal fistula, **E**sophageal atresia, **R**enal anomalies, and **L**imb defects), a collection of defects of unknown causation, but occurring more frequently than predicted by chance alone.

A complication of some TEFs is polyhydramnios because in some types of TEF, amniotic fluid, when swallowed, does not pass to the stomach and intestines. Also, gastric contents and/or amniotic fluid at birth may enter the trachea through a fistula, causing pneumonitis and pneumonia.

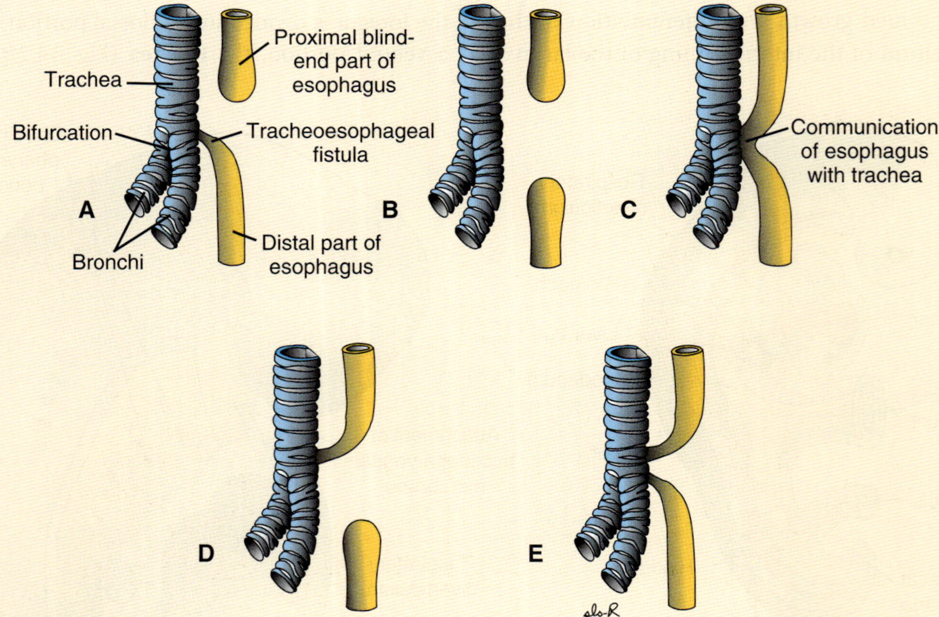


**FIGURE 14.3** Various types of esophageal atresia and/or TEFs. **A.** The most frequent abnormality (90% of cases) occurs with the upper esophagus ending in a blind pouch and the lower segment forming a fistula with the trachea. **B.** Isolated esophageal atresia (4% of cases). **C.** H-type TEF (4% of cases). **D,E.** Other variations (each 1% of cases).

primordium maintains its communication with the pharynx through the **laryngeal orifice** (Fig. 14.2*D*).

## LARYNX

The internal lining of the larynx originates from endoderm, but the cartilages and muscles originate from mesenchyme of the **fourth** and **sixth pharyngeal arches**. As a result of rapid proliferation of this mesenchyme, the laryngeal orifice changes in appearance from a sagittal slit to a T-shaped opening (Fig. 14.4*A*). Subsequently, when mesenchyme of the two arches transforms into the **thyroid**, **cricoid**, and **arytenoid cartilages**, the characteristic adult shape of the laryngeal orifice can be recognized (Fig. 14.4*B*).

At about the time that the cartilages are formed, the laryngeal epithelium also proliferates rapidly, resulting in a temporary occlusion of the lumen. Subsequently, vacuolization and recanalization produce a pair of lateral recesses, the **laryngeal ventricles**. These recesses are bounded by folds of tissue that differentiate into the **false** and **true vocal cords**.

Because musculature of the larynx is derived from mesenchyme of the fourth and sixth pharyngeal arches, all laryngeal muscles are innervated by branches of the 10th cranial nerve, the **vagus nerve**: The **superior laryngeal** nerve innervates derivatives of the fourth pharyngeal arch, and the **recurrent laryngeal nerve** innervates derivatives of the sixth pharyngeal arch. (For further details on the laryngeal cartilages, see Chapter 17, p. 238.)

## TRACHEA, BRONCHI, AND LUNGS

During its separation from the foregut, the **lung bud** forms the trachea and two lateral outpocketings, the **primary bronchial buds** (Fig. 14.2*B*,*C*). At the beginning of the fifth week, each of these buds enlarges to form right and left primary bronchi. The right then forms three secondary bronchi, and the left, two (Fig. 14.5*A*), thus foreshadowing the three lobes of the lung on the right side and two on the left (Fig. 14.5*B*,*C*).

With subsequent growth in caudal and lateral directions, the lungs expand into the body cavity (Fig. 14.6). **The spaces for the lungs, the pericardioperitoneal canals**, are narrow. They lie on each side of the foregut and are gradually filled by the expanding growth of the lungs. Ultimately, the pleuroperitoneal and pleuropericardial folds separate the pericardioperitoneal canals from the peritoneal and pericardial cavities, respectively, and the remaining spaces form the **primitive pleural cavities** (see Chapter 7). The mesoderm, which covers the outside of the lung, develops into the **visceral pleura**. The somatic mesoderm layer, covering the body wall from the inside, becomes the **parietal pleura** (Fig. 14.6*A*). The space between the parietal and visceral pleura is the **pleural cavity** (Fig. 14.7).

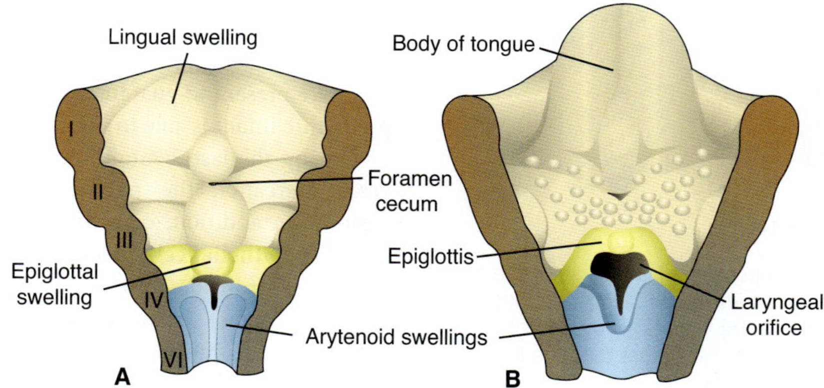


**FIGURE 14.4** Laryngeal orifice and surrounding swellings at successive stages of development. **A.** 6 weeks. **B.** 12 weeks.

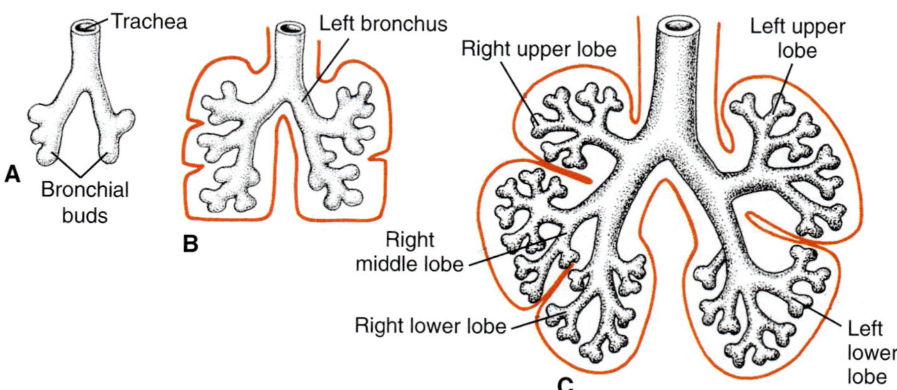


**FIGURE 14.5** Stages in development of the trachea and lungs. **A.** 5 weeks. **B.** 6 weeks. **C.** 8 weeks.

Part 2

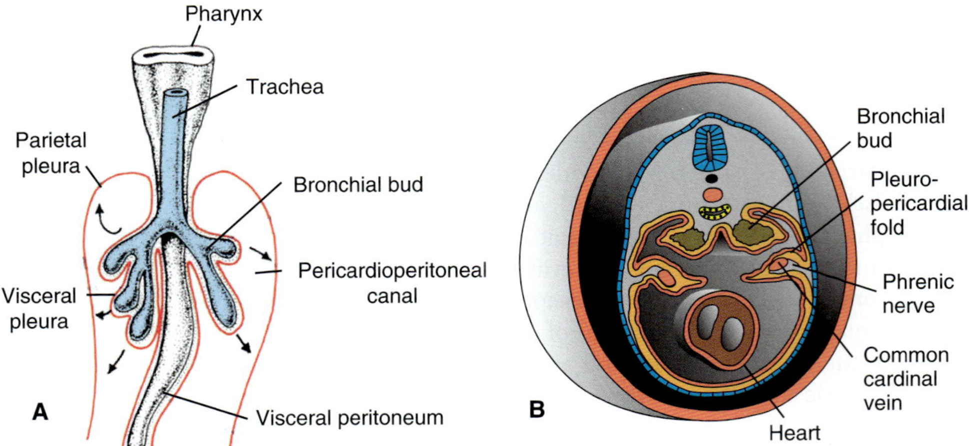


**FIGURE 14.6** Expansion of the bronchial buds into the pericardioperitoneal canals. At this stage, the canals are in communication with the peritoneal and pericardial cavities. **A.** Ventral view of the bronchial buds covered by visceral pleura. **B.** Transverse section through the bronchial buds showing the pleuropericardial folds that will divide the thoracic portion of the body cavity into the pleural and pericardial cavities.

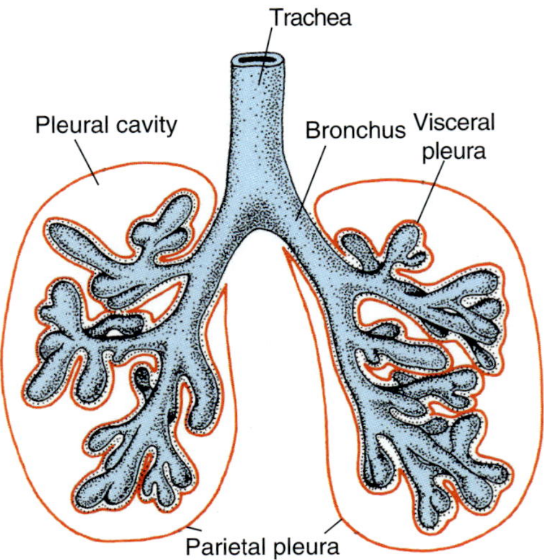


**FIGURE 14.7** Once the pericardioperitoneal canals separate from the pericardial and peritoneal cavities, respectively, the lungs expand in the pleural cavities. Note the visceral and parietal pleura and definitive pleural cavity. The visceral pleura extends between the lobes of the lungs.

During further development, secondary bronchi divide repeatedly in a dichotomous fashion, forming 10 **tertiary (segmental)** bronchi in the right lung and 8 in the left, creating the **bronchopulmonary segments** of the adult lung. By the end of the sixth month, approximately 17 generations of subdivisions have formed. Before the bronchial tree reaches its final shape, however, **an additional six divisions form during postnatal life**. Branching is regulated by epithelial–mesenchymal interactions between the endoderm of the lung buds and visceral mesoderm that surrounds them. Signals for branching, which emit from the mesoderm, involve members of the fibroblast growth factor family. While all of these new subdivisions are occurring and the bronchial tree is developing, the lungs assume a more caudal position, so that by the time of birth, the bifurcation of the trachea is opposite the fourth thoracic vertebra.

## MATURATION OF THE LUNGS

Up to the seventh prenatal month, the bronchioles divide continuously into more and smaller canals **(canalicular phase)** and the vascular supply increases steadily (Fig. 14.8*A*). **Terminal bronchioles** divide to form **respiratory bronchioles**, and each of these divides into three to six alveolar ducts (Fig. 14.8*B*). The ducts end in **terminal sacs (primitive alveoli)** that are surrounded by flat alveolar cells in close contact with neighboring capillaries (Fig. 14.8*B*). By the end of the seventh month, sufficient numbers of mature alveolar sacs and capillaries are present to guarantee adequate gas exchange, and the premature infant is able to survive (Fig. 14.9) (Table 14.1).

During the last 2 months of prenatal life and for several years thereafter, the number of terminal sacs increases steadily. In addition, cells lining the sacs, known as **type I alveolar epithelial cells**, become thinner, so that surrounding capillaries protrude into the alveolar sacs (Fig. 14.9). This intimate contact between epithelial and endothelial cells makes up the **blood–air barrier**. **Mature alveoli** are not present before birth. In addition to endothelial cells and flat alveolar epithelial cells, another cell type develops at the end of the sixth month. These cells, **type II alveolar epithelial cells**, produce **surfactant**, a phospholipid-rich fluid capable of lowering surface tension at the air–alveolar interface.

Before birth, the lungs are full of fluid that contains a high chloride concentration, little protein, some mucus from the bronchial glands, and surfactant from the alveolar epithelial cells (type II). The amount of surfactant in the fluid increases, particularly during the last 2 weeks before birth.

As concentrations of surfactant increase during the 34th week of gestation, some of this phospholipid enters the amniotic fluid and acts on macrophages in the amniotic cavity. Once "activated," evidence suggests that these macrophages migrate across the chorion into the uterus where they begin to produce immune system proteins, including **interleukin-1β (IL-1β)**. Upregulation of these proteins results in increased production of prostaglandins that cause uterine contractions.

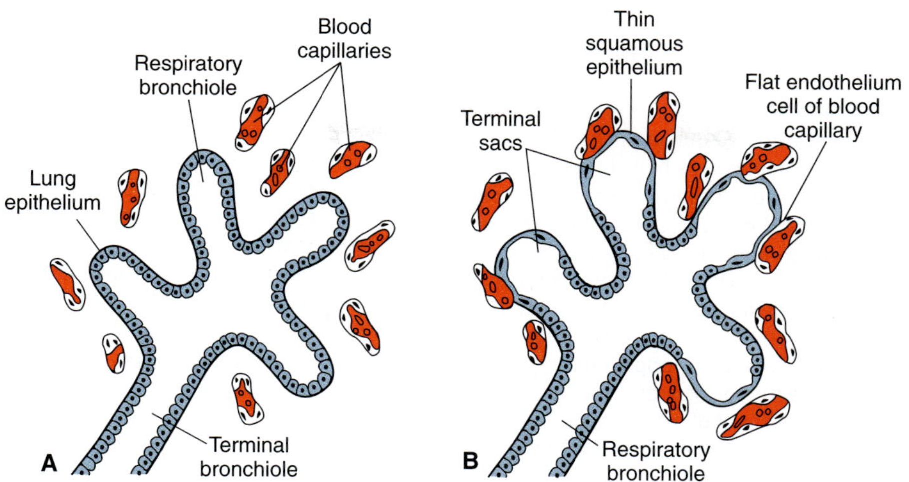


**FIGURE 14.8** Histological and functional development of the lung. **A.** The **canalicular** period lasts from the 16th to the 26th week. Note the cuboidal cells lining the respiratory bronchioli. **B.** The **terminal sac** period begins at the end of the sixth and beginning of the seventh prenatal month. Cuboidal cells become very thin and intimately associated with the endothelium of blood and lymph capillaries or form terminal sacs (primitive alveoli).

| Table 14.1 | Maturation of the Lungs | |
|---|---|---|
| Pseudoglandular period | 5–16 wk | Branching has continued to form terminal bronchioles. No respiratory bronchioles or alveoli are present. |
| Canalicular period | 16–26 wk | Each terminal bronchiole divides into two or more respiratory bronchioles, which in turn divide into three to six alveolar ducts. |
| Terminal sac period | 26 wk to birth | Terminal sacs (primitive alveoli) form, and capillaries establish close contact. |
| Alveolar period | 8 mo to childhood | Mature alveoli have well-developed epithelial endothelial (capillary) contacts. |



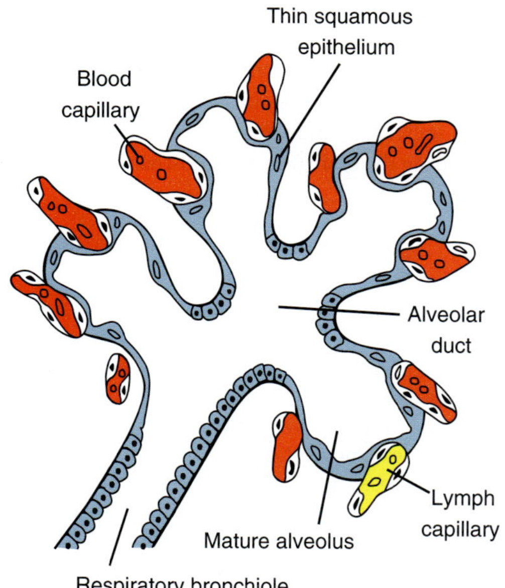


**FIGURE 14.9** Lung tissue in a newborn. Note the thin squamous epithelial cells (also known as **alveolar epithelial cells, type I**) and surrounding capillaries protruding into mature alveoli.

Thus, there may be signals from the fetus that participate in initiating labor and birth.

Fetal **breathing movements** begin before birth and cause aspiration of amniotic fluid. These movements are important for stimulating lung development and conditioning respiratory muscles. When respiration begins at birth, most of the lung fluid is rapidly resorbed by the blood and lymph capillaries, and a small amount is probably expelled via the trachea and bronchi during delivery. When the fluid is resorbed from alveolar sacs, surfactant remains deposited as a thin phospholipid coat on alveolar cell membranes. With air entering alveoli during the first breath, the surfactant coat prevents development of an air–water (blood) interface with high surface tension. Without the fatty surfactant layer, the alveoli would collapse during expiration (atelectasis).

Respiratory movements after birth bring air into the lungs, which expand and fill the pleural cavity. Although the alveoli increase somewhat in size, growth of the lungs after birth is due primarily to an increase in the number of respiratory bronchioles and alveoli. It is estimated that only one-sixth of the adult number of alveoli are present at birth. The remaining alveoli are formed during the first 10 years of postnatal life through the continuous formation of new primitive alveoli.

## Clinical Correlates

**Surfactant** is particularly important for survival of the **premature infant**. When surfactant is insufficient, the air–water (blood) surface membrane tension becomes high, bringing great risk that alveoli will collapse during expiration. As a result, **respiratory distress syndrome (RDS)** develops. This is a common cause of death in the premature infant. In these cases, the partially collapsed alveoli contain a fluid with a high protein content, many hyaline membranes, and lamellar bodies, probably derived from the surfactant layer. RDS, which was previously known as **hyaline membrane disease**, accounts for approximately 20% of deaths among newborns. Treatment of preterm babies with artificial surfactant as well as treatment of mothers with premature labor with glucocorticoids to stimulate surfactant production have reduced the mortality associated with RDS.

Although many abnormalities of the lung and bronchial tree have been described (e.g., blind-ending trachea with absence of lungs and agenesis of one lung), most of these gross abnormalities are rare. Abnormal divisions of the bronchial tree are more common; some result in supernumerary lobules. These variations of the bronchial tree have little functional significance, but they may cause unexpected difficulties during bronchoscopies.

More interesting are **ectopic lung lobes** arising from the trachea or esophagus. It is believed that these lobes are formed from additional respiratory buds of the foregut that develop independent of the main respiratory system.

Most important clinically are **congenital cysts of the lung**, which are formed by dilation of terminal or larger bronchi. These cysts may be small and multiple, giving the lung a honeycomb appearance on radiograph, or they may be restricted to one or more larger ones. Cystic structures of the lung usually drain poorly and frequently cause chronic infections.

## SUMMARY

- **The respiratory system** is an outgrowth of the ventral wall of the foregut, and the epithelium of the larynx, trachea, bronchi, and alveoli originates in the endoderm.
- The cartilaginous, muscular, and connective tissue components arise in the mesoderm.
- In the fourth week of development, the **tracheoesophageal septum** separates the trachea from the foregut, dividing the foregut into the **respiratory diverticulum (lung bud)** anteriorly and the esophagus posteriorly.
- Contact between the two is maintained through the **larynx**, which is formed by tissue of the **fourth and sixth pharyngeal arches**.
- The lung bud develops into two primary bronchi: The right forms three secondary bronchi and three lobes; the left forms two secondary bronchi and two lobes.
- Faulty partitioning of the foregut by the tracheoesophageal septum causes **esophageal atresias** and **tracheoesophageal fistulas (TEFs)** (Fig. 14.3).
- After a pseudoglandular (5 to 16 weeks) and canalicular (16 to 26 weeks) phase, cells of the cuboidal-lined respiratory bronchioles change into thin, flat cells, **type I alveolar epithelial cells**, intimately associated with blood and lymph capillaries.
- In the seventh month, gas exchange between the blood and the air in the **primitive alveoli** is possible.
- Before birth, the lungs are filled with fluid with little protein, some mucus, and **surfactant**, which is produced by type **II alveolar epithelial cells** and which forms a phospholipid coat on the alveolar membranes.
- At the beginning of respiration, the lung fluid is resorbed except for the surfactant coat, which prevents the collapse of the alveoli during expiration by reducing the surface tension at the air–blood capillary interface.
- Absent or insufficient surfactant in the premature baby causes **respiratory distress syndrome (RDS)** because of collapse of the primitive alveoli (**hyaline membrane** disease).
- Growth of the lungs after birth is primarily due to an increase in the **number** of respiratory bronchioles and alveoli and not due to an increase in the **size** of the alveoli. New alveoli are formed during the first 10 years of postnatal life.

## Self-Assessment

### Comprehensive Questions

1. Discuss the embryological basis of tracheoesophageal fistula.
2. Discuss the embryological basis of respiratory distress syndrome.
3. Briefly explain the histological maturation of the lungs.

### Problem Solving Questions

1. A prenatal ultrasound revealed polyhydramnios, and at birth, the baby had excessive fluids in its mouth. What type of birth defect might be present, and what is its embryological origin? Would you examine the child carefully for other birth defects? Why?
2. A 26-year-old primigravida female with 29 weeks of pregnancy presented in emergency with vaginal bleeding and early onset of labor pains. She was immediately administered a dose of dexamethasone (glucocorticoid) iv and was then rushed for an emergency cesarean section due to uncontrolled bleeding. A male infant was delivered with a weight of 1.1 kg. The infant was observed to have difficulty in breathing, occasional respiratory gasps, and grunting with deep chest wall retractions, blue discoloration of the skin, and a rapid heart rate of 110 bpm. What is the probable diagnosis of the infant?
3. A fetal ultrasound revealed agenesis of the right lung and diaphragmatic hernia with the liver in the thoracic

cage, scoliosis, and a mediastinal shift. The left lung was hypoplastic. What could be the case? Also, explain the embryological basis.

## Multiple Choice Questions

1. Respiratory diverticulum arises from
   (a) Dorsal wall of the foregut
   (b) Ventral wall of the midgut
   (c) Ventral wall of the foregut
   (d) Junction of the foregut and midgut
2. The correct sequence of maturation of the lungs is
   (a) Canalicular period, pseudoglandular period, alveolar period, terminal sac period
   (b) Pseudoglandular period, terminal sac period, canalicular period, alveolar period
   (c) Pseudoglandular period, canalicular period, terminal sac period, alveolar period
   (d) Alveolar period, terminal sac period, pseudoglandular period, canalicular period
3. Which is most common type of tracheoesophageal fistula (TEF)?
   (a) H-type TEF
   (b) Isolated esophageal atresia
   (c) The upper segment of the esophagus ending in a blind pouch and the lower segment forming a fistula with the trachea
   (d) The upper esophagus forming a fistula and the lower segment ending in a blind pouch
4. Surfactant is secreted by
   (a) Type II alveolar epithelial cells
   (b) Terminal sacs
   (c) Type I alveolar epithelial cells
   (d) Respiratory bronchioles
5. Pseudoglandular phase is present in which week of pregnancy?
   (a) 5–16
   (b) 17–20
   (c) 20–24
   (d) 25–30
6. At what age can gas exchange start in a preterm baby?
   (a) 5 months
   (b) 6 months
   (c) 7 months
   (d) 8 months
7. Transcription factor responsible for lung bud formation is
   (a) PAX
   (b) HOX
   (c) TBX4
   (d) FGF4
8. The respiratory primordium maintains its communication with the pharynx by the
   (a) Laryngeal orifice
   (b) Oropharynx
   (c) Nasopharynx
   (d) Cricopharynx
9. Surfactants are secreted by
   (a) Type I pneumocytes
   (b) Type II pneumocytes
   (c) Clara cells
   (d) Bronchiole-associated lymphatic tissue (BALT)

### Answers

1. (c) 2. (c) 3. (c) 4. (a) 5. (a) 6. (c) 7. (c) 8. (a) 9. (b)

Part 2

CHAPTER

# 15 Digestive System

## Specific Learning Objectives

- Gut tube and its divisions
- Molecular regulations of gut development
- Development of peritoneal folds
- Foregut development and associated clinical correlates
- Development of liver, gallbladder, and pancreas and molecular regulation
- Rotation of midgut and malrotation
- Hindgut and its derivatives

## Competency Covered

AN52.6 Describe the development and congenital anomalies of the foregut, midgut, and hindgut.



## DIVISIONS OF THE GUT TUBE

As a result of cephalocaudal and lateral folding of the embryo, a portion of the endoderm derived from gastrulation is incorporated into the embryo to form the **primitive gut**. The **yolk sac** and the **allantois** remain outside the embryo (Fig. 15.1*A–D*).

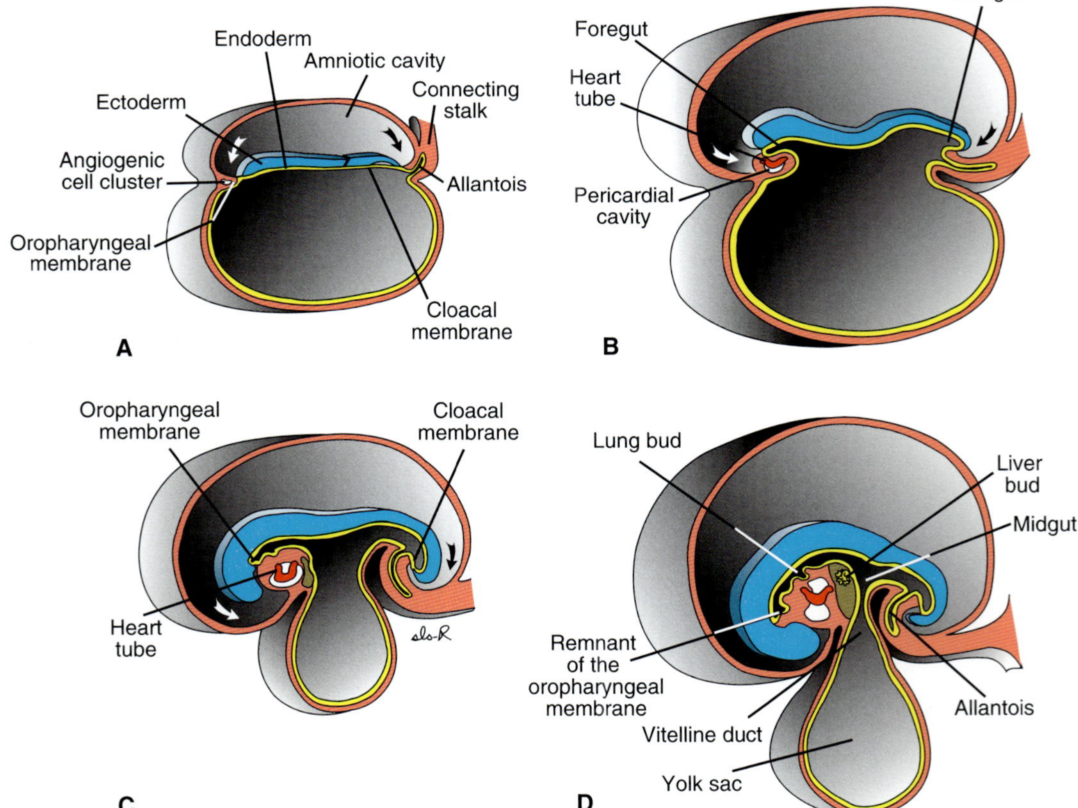


**FIGURE 15.1** Sagittal sections through embryos at various stages of development demonstrating the effect of cephalocaudal and lateral folding on the position of the endoderm-lined cavity. Note formation of the foregut, midgut, and hindgut. **A.** Presomite embryo. **B.** Embryo with seven somites. **C.** Embryo with 14 somites. **D.** At the end of the first month.

In the cephalic and caudal parts of the embryo, the primitive gut forms a blind-ending tube, the **foregut** and **hindgut**, respectively. The middle part, the **midgut**, remains temporally connected to the yolk sac by means of the **vitelline duct** or **yolk stalk** (Fig. 15.1*D*).

Development of the primitive gut and its derivatives is usually discussed in four sections:

1. The **pharyngeal gut**, or **pharynx**, extends from the oropharyngeal membrane to the respiratory diverticulum and is part of the foregut; this section is particularly important for development of the head and neck and is discussed in Chapter 17.
2. The remainder of the **foregut** lies caudal to the pharyngeal tube and extends caudally to the liver bud origin; this site corresponds to the second part of the duodenum where the bile duct and pancreatic duct open in adults.
3. The **midgut** begins caudal to the liver bud and extends to the junction of the right two-thirds and left third of the transverse colon in the adult.
4. The **hindgut** extends from the left third of the transverse colon to the cloacal membrane (Fig. 15.1).

**Endoderm** forms the epithelial lining of the digestive tract and gives rise to the specific cells (the **parenchyma**) of glands, such as hepatocytes and the exocrine and endocrine cells of the pancreas. The **stroma** (connective tissue) for the glands is derived from visceral mesoderm. Muscle, connective tissue, and peritoneal components of the wall of the gut also are derived from visceral mesoderm.

## MOLECULAR REGULATION OF GUT TUBE DEVELOPMENT

Regional specification of the gut tube into different components occurs during the time that the lateral body folds are bringing the two sides of the tube together (Figs. 15.2 and 15.3). Specification is initiated by a concentration gradient of retinoic acid (RA) from the pharynx, which is exposed to little or no RA, to the colon, that sees the highest concentration of RA. This RA gradient causes transcription factors to be expressed in different regions of the gut tube. Thus, ***SOX2*** "specifies" the esophagus and stomach; ***PDX1***, the duodenum; ***CDXC***, the small intestine; and ***CDXA***, the large intestine and rectum (Fig. 15.2*A*). This initial patterning is stabilized by reciprocal interactions between the endoderm and visceral



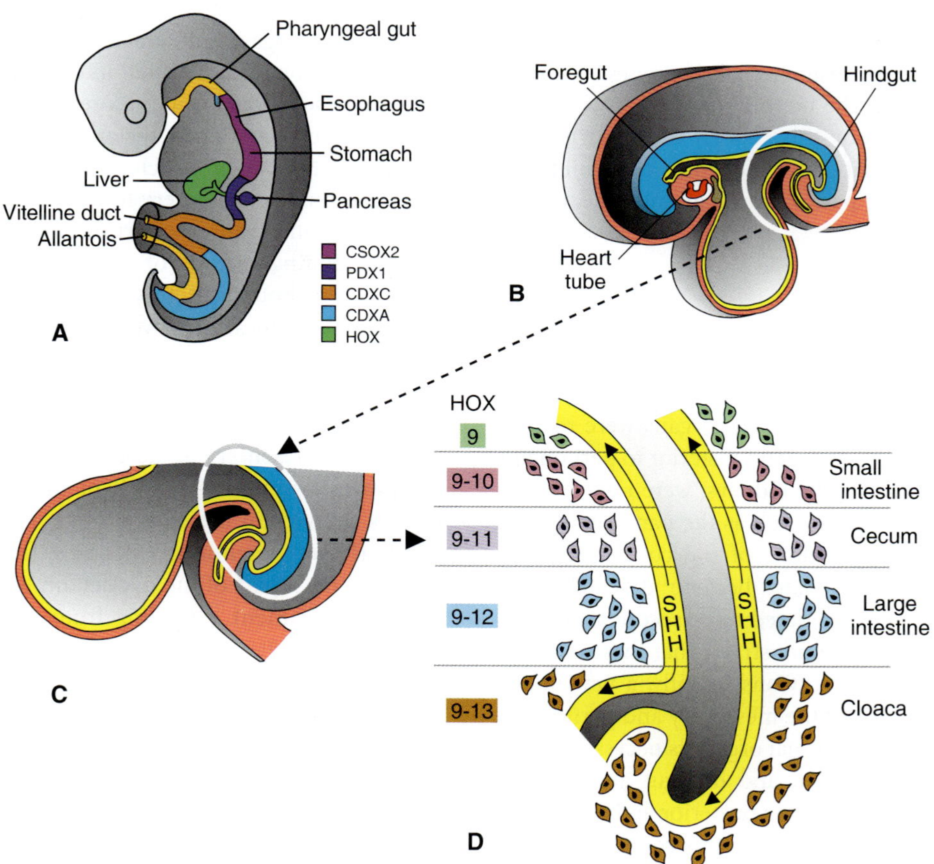


**FIGURE 15.2** Diagrams showing molecular regulation of gut development. **A.** Color-coded diagram that indicates genes responsible for initiating regional specification of the gut into esophagus, stomach, duodenum, etc. **B–D.** Drawings showing an example from the midgut and hindgut regions indicating how early gut specification is stabilized. Stabilization is effected by epithelial–mesenchymal interactions between gut endoderm and surrounding visceral (splanchnic) mesoderm. Endoderm cells initiate the stabilization process by secreting sonic hedgehog (SHH), which establishes a nested expression of *HOX* genes in the mesoderm. This interaction results in a genetic cascade that regulates specification of each gut region as is shown for the small and large intestine regions in these diagrams.

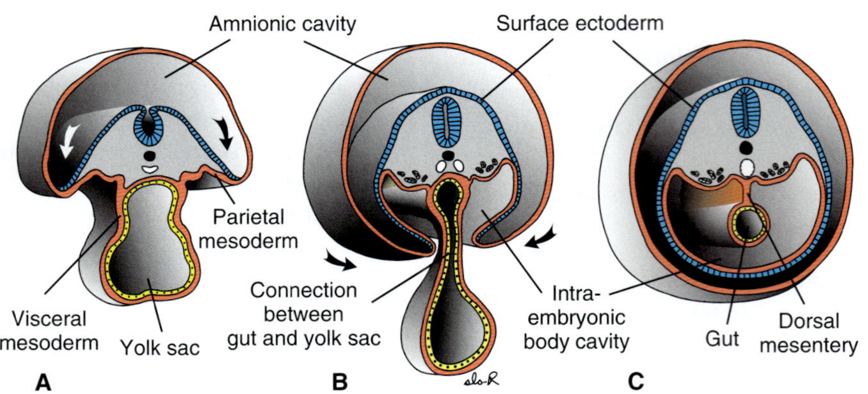


**FIGURE 15.3** Transverse sections through embryos at various stages of development. **A.** The intraembryonic cavity, bordered by visceral and parietal layers of lateral plate mesoderm, is in open communication with the extraembryonic cavity. **B.** The intraembryonic cavity is losing its wide connection with the extraembryonic cavity. **C.** At the end of the fourth week, visceral mesoderm layers are fused in the midline and form a double-layered membrane (dorsal mesentery) between right and left halves of the body cavity. Ventral mesentery exists only in the region of the septum transversum (not shown).

mesoderm adjacent to the gut tube (Fig. 15.2*B–D*). This **epithelial–mesenchymal interaction** is initiated by ***SONIC HEDGEHOG (SHH)*** expression throughout the gut tube. *SHH* expression upregulates factors in the mesoderm that then determine the type of structure that forms from the gut tube, such as the stomach, duodenum, small intestine, etc. For example, in the region of the caudal limit of the midgut and all of the hindgut, *SHH* expression establishes a nested expression of the ***HOX* genes** in the mesoderm (Fig. 15.2*D*). Once the mesoderm is specified by this code, it then instructs the endoderm to form the various components of the mid- and hindgut regions, including part of the small intestine, cecum, colon, and cloaca (Fig. 15.2).

Part 2

## MESENTERY

Formerly, a mesentery was defined as a double layer of peritoneum that encloses an organ and suspends it from the posterior abdominal wall. Such "suspended" organs were referred to as **intraperitoneal,** whereas organs posterior to peritoneum lining the body wall, such as the kidneys, were referred to as retroperitoneal. Finally, organs, such as the pancreas and the ascending and descending regions of the colon, that were originally intraperitoneal, but later became attached to the posterior body wall, were considered to be secondarily retroperitoneal. Recent evidence demonstrates that these concepts and definitions are not correct. Consequently, a new understanding of the embryology of the mesentery and peritoneum and their relationship to abdominal organs is necessary.

Initially, the foregut, midgut, and hindgut are in broad contact with the mesenchyme of the posterior abdominal wall (Fig. 15.3). By the fifth week, however, this connecting tissue bridge has narrowed, and the caudal part of the foregut, the midgut, and a major part of the hindgut are suspended from the abdominal wall by the **dorsal mesentery** (Figs. 15.3*C* and 15.4). This **mesentery** is a collection of connective tissues that maintains the gut tube and its derivatives in their normal anatomical positions. In the abdomen, **dorsal mesentery** extends from the lower portion of the esophagus to the rectum as a **continuous sheet** of tissue attached to the posterior body wall and providing a pathway for blood vessels, lymphatics, and nerves to the gut tube and its derivatives. Its various regions are named according to the parts of the gut tube to which they attach (Fig. 15.4). These regions include: the dorsal mesogastrium, greater omentum, mesoduodenum, mesentery proper to the small intestine, mesocolon, mesoappendix, mesosigmoid, and mesorectum. In some regions, this mesentery extends some distance from the posterior wall to a portion of the gut, such as the mesentery proper to the small intestine or mesentery to the transverse colon. In other cases when an organ or a part of one, such as the ascending and descending regions of the colon, become attached to the posterior body wall, the mesentery is short. When these attachments of mesentery to the posterior wall occur, a layer of fascia (**Toldt fascia**) forms between visceral peritoneum on the organ and parietal peritoneum covering the posterior body wall.

**Ventral mesentery** is derived from mesenchyme of the **septum transversum.** Growth of the liver into the septum divides the ventral mesentery into (1) the **ventral mesogastrium (lesser omentum)** extending from the stomach and proximal most part of the duodenum to the liver and (2) the **falciform ligament** extending from the liver to the ventral body wall (Fig. 15.4). Ventral mesentery is **continuous** with dorsal mesentery. The fact that the dorsal mesentery is a continuous structure and is also continuous with ventral mesentery is important clinically when surgeons are resecting tumors or organs in the abdominal cavity. Similarly, the fact that there is a fascial plane (Toldt fascia) between visceral and parietal peritoneum for organs that attach to the posterior body wall is important for surgery involving these organs and for understanding pathways for the spread of infections.

**Peritoneum** is a continuous serous membrane lining the inner surface of the abdominal cavity from which it is reflected onto the viscera. The layer in apposition to the viscera forms **visceral peritoneum**, whereas the layer attached to the

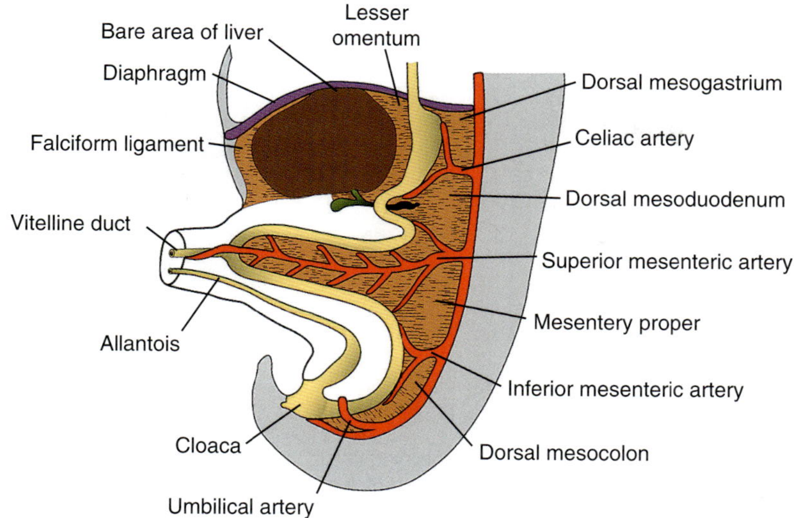


**FIGURE 15.4** Primitive dorsal and ventral mesenteries. The liver is connected to the ventral abdominal wall and to the stomach by the falciform ligament and lesser omentum, respectively. The superior mesenteric artery runs through the mesentery proper and continues toward the yolk sac as the vitelline artery.

abdominal wall forms **parietal peritoneum. Peritoneal reflections** (formerly called ligaments) occur where the peritoneum bridges the space between an organ and the inner surface of the posterior abdominal wall. For example, the coronary and triangular reflections on the surface of the liver or the lienorenal reflection between the spleen and left kidney. Knowledge of these reflections is important during surgery to divide planes of section to remove organs or to gain access to spaces and cavities associated with various organs.

## FOREGUT

### Esophagus

When the embryo is approximately 4 weeks old, the **respiratory diverticulum (lung bud)** appears at the ventral wall of the foregut at the border with the pharyngeal gut (Fig. 15.5). The **tracheoesophageal septum** gradually partitions this **diverticulum** from the dorsal part of the foregut (Fig. 15.6). In this manner, the foregut divides into a ventral portion, the **respiratory primordium** (see Chapter 14), and a dorsal portion, the **esophagus**.

At first, the esophagus is short (Fig. 15.5*A*), but with descent of the heart and lungs, it lengthens rapidly (Fig. 15.5*B*). The muscular coat, which is formed by surrounding visceral mesenchyme, is striated in its upper two-thirds and innervated by the vagus; the muscle coat is smooth in the lower third and is innervated by the splanchnic plexus.

### Stomach

The stomach begins its development from the foregut in the fourth week as a fusiform dilation in close approximation to the respiratory diverticulum in the primitive thoracic region.



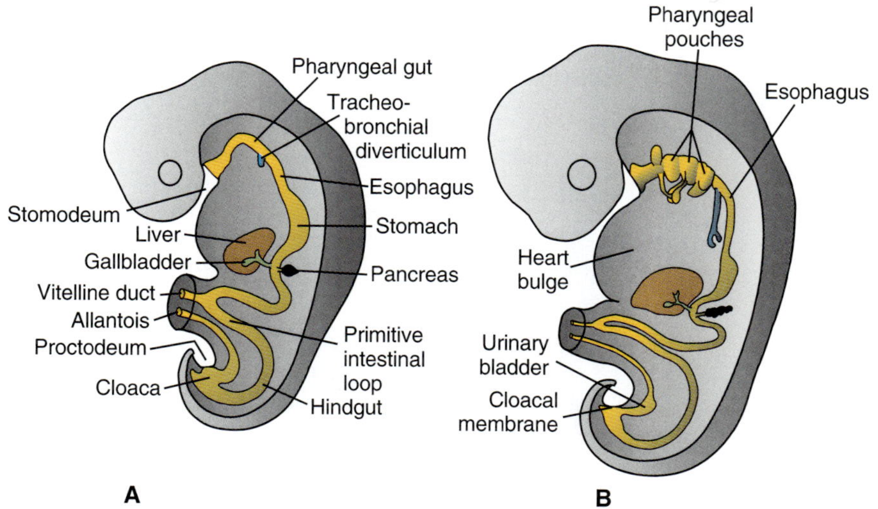


**FIGURE 15.5** Embryos during the fourth **(A)** and fifth **(B)** weeks of development showing formation of the gastrointestinal tract and the various derivatives originating from the endodermal germ layer.

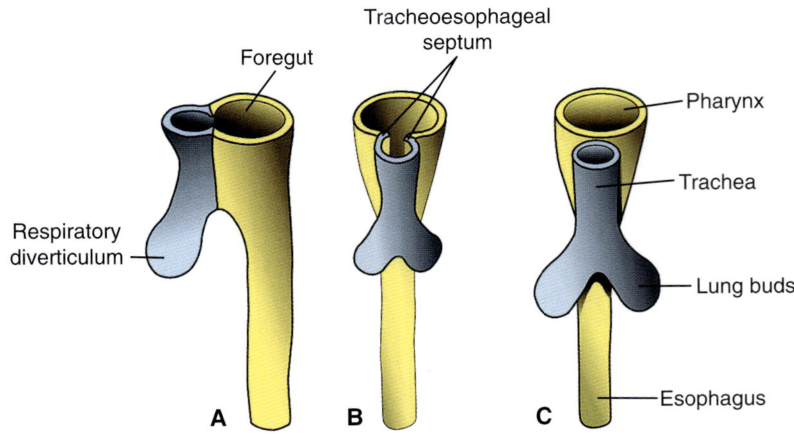


**FIGURE 15.6** Successive stages in development of the respiratory diverticulum and esophagus through partitioning of the foregut. **A.** At the end of the third week (lateral view). **B,C.** During the fourth week (ventral view).

## Clinical Correlates

### Esophageal Abnormalities

**Esophageal atresia** and/or **tracheoesophageal fistula** results either from spontaneous posterior deviation of the **tracheoesophageal septum** or from some mechanical factor pushing the dorsal wall of the foregut anteriorly. In its most common form, the proximal part of the esophagus ends as a blind sac, and the distal part is connected to the trachea by a narrow canal just above the bifurcation (Fig. 15.7*A*). Other types of defects in this region occur much less frequently (Fig. 15.7*B–E*) (see Chapter 14).

Atresia of the esophagus prevents normal passage of amniotic fluid into the intestinal tract, resulting in accumulation of excess fluid in the amniotic sac (**polyhydramnios**). In addition to atresias, the lumen of the esophagus may narrow, producing **esophageal stenosis**, usually in the lower third. Stenosis may be caused by incomplete recanalization, vascular abnormalities, or accidents that compromise blood flow. Occasionally, the esophagus fails to lengthen sufficiently, and the stomach is pulled up into the esophageal hiatus through the diaphragm. The result is a **congenital hiatal hernia**.

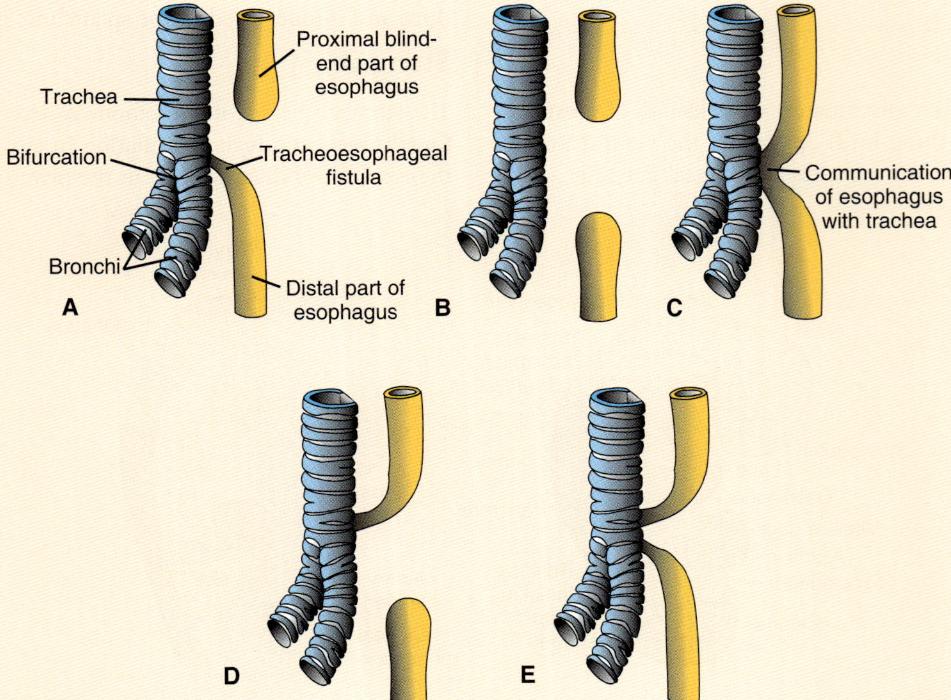


**FIGURE 15.7** Variations of esophageal atresia and/or tracheoesophageal fistula in order of their frequency of appearance: **(A)** 90%, **(B)** 4%, **(C)** 4%, **(D)** 1%, and **(E)** 1%.

Part 2

Growth to lengthen the esophageal region is essential for positioning the stomach in the abdominal cavity below the diaphragm. If this growth does not occur, a diaphragmatic hernia results with the stomach remaining in the thoracic cavity and compressing the lungs (see Chapter 7; p. 85) (Fig. 15.5*A*).

During the following weeks, after lengthening of the esophageal region of the foregut has occurred, the appearance and position of the stomach change greatly as a result of the different rates of growth in various regions of its wall and the changes in position of surrounding organs. Positional changes of the stomach are most easily explained by assuming that it rotates around a longitudinal and an anteroposterior axis (Fig. 15.8).

The stomach rotates 90° clockwise around its longitudinal axis, causing its left side to face anteriorly and its right side to face posteriorly (Fig. 15.8*A–C*). Hence, the left vagus nerve, initially innervating the left side of the stomach, now innervates the anterior wall; similarly, the right nerve innervates the posterior wall. During this rotation, the original posterior wall of the stomach grows faster than the anterior portion, forming the **greater** and **lesser curvatures** (Fig. 15.8*C*).

The cephalic and caudal ends of the stomach originally lie in the midline, but during further growth, the stomach rotates around an anteroposterior axis, such that the caudal or **pyloric part** moves to the right and upward, and the cephalic or **cardiac portion** moves to the left and slightly downward (Fig. 15.8*D,E*). The stomach thus assumes its final position, its axis running from above left to below right.

The stomach is attached to the dorsal body wall by the **dorsal mesogastrium** and to the ventral body wall by the **ventral mesogastrium**, which is part of the septum transversum. As the liver grows into this region, mesoderm forming the ventral mesogastrium becomes thinner and forms the two parts of the **ventral mesentery**: (1) the **lesser omentum**, connecting the stomach to the liver; and (2) the **falciform ligament**, connecting the liver to the ventral body wall (Figs. 15.4 and 15.9*A*). Due to the stomach's rotation and disproportionate growth, the position of the dorsal and ventral mesenteric connections is altered. Rotation about the longitudinal axis pulls the dorsal mesogastrium to the left, creating a space behind the stomach called the **omental bursa (lesser peritoneal sac)** (Figs. 15.9 and 15.10). This rotation also pulls the lesser omentum to the right. As this process continues in the fifth week of development, the spleen primordium appears as a mesodermal proliferation between the two leaves of the dorsal mesogastrium (Figs. 15.10 and 15.11). With continued rotation of the stomach, the dorsal mesogastrium lengthens, and the portion between the spleen and dorsal midline swings to the left and becomes attached to peritoneum of the posterior abdominal wall by a layer of fascia (Toldt fascia; see Figs. 15.10 and 15.11). The spleen becomes connected to the posterior body wall in the region of the left kidney by the **lienorenal reflection** of peritoneum and to the stomach by the **gastrolienal reflection** (Figs. 15.10 and 15.11). Lengthening and attachment of the dorsal mesogastrium to the posterior body wall also determines the final position of the pancreas. Initially, the organ grows into the dorsal mesoduodenum, but eventually, its tail extends into the dorsal mesogastrium (Fig. 15.10*A*). Because this portion of the dorsal mesogastrium becomes attached to the posterior



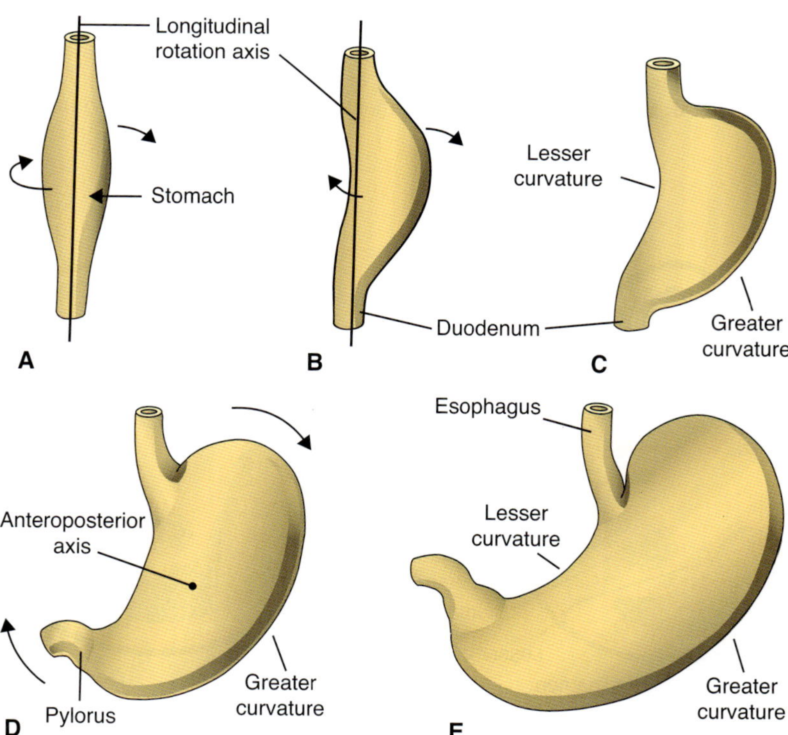


**FIGURE 15.8 A–C.** Rotation of the stomach along its longitudinal axis as seen anteriorly. **D,E.** Rotation of the stomach around the anteroposterior axis. Note the change in position of the pylorus and cardia.

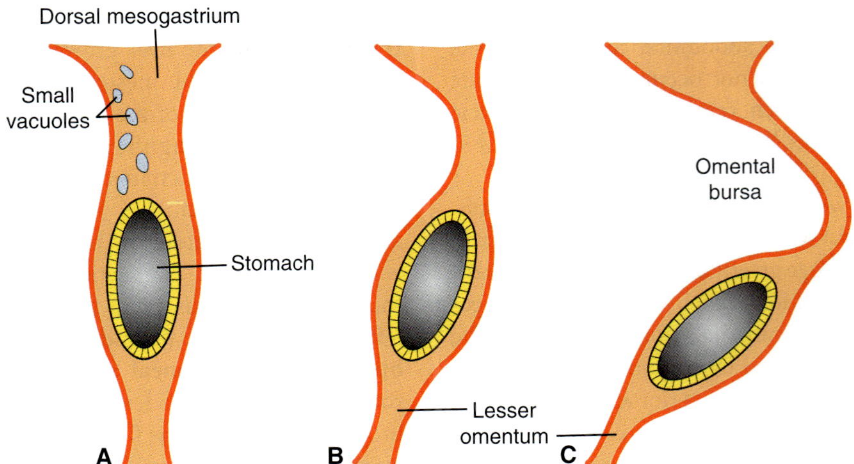


**FIGURE 15.9** **A.** Transverse section through a 4-week embryo showing intercellular clefts appearing in the dorsal mesogastrium. **B,C.** The clefts have fused, and the omental bursa is formed as an extension of the right side of the intraembryonic cavity behind the stomach.

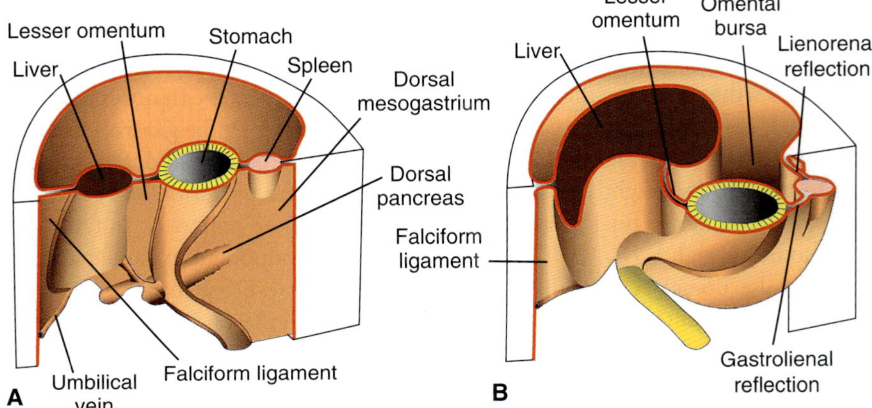


**FIGURE 15.10** **A.** The positions of the spleen, stomach, and pancreas at the end of the fifth week. Note the position of the spleen and pancreas in the dorsal mesogastrium. **B.** Position of spleen and stomach at the 11th week. Note formation of the omental bursa (lesser peritoneal sac).

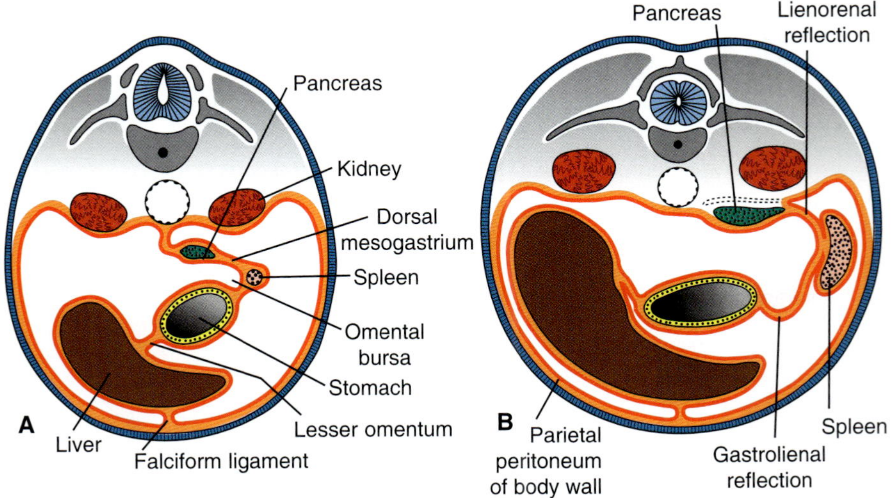


**FIGURE 15.11** Transverse sections through the region of the stomach, liver, and spleen, showing formation of the omental bursa (lesser peritoneal sac), rotation of the stomach, and position of the spleen and tail of the pancreas between the two leaves of the dorsal mesogastrium. With further development, the pancreas attaches to the posterior body wall.

body wall, the tail of the pancreas lies against this region (Fig. 15.11).

As a result of rotation of the stomach about its anteroposterior axis, the dorsal mesogastrium bulges down (Fig. 15.12). It continues to grow down and forms a double-layered sac extending over the transverse colon and small intestinal loops like an apron (Fig. 15.13*A*). This double layered apron is the **greater omentum**; later, its layers fuse to form a single sheet hanging from the greater curvature of the stomach (Fig. 15.13*B*). The posterior layer of the greater omentum also fuses with mesentery of the transverse colon (Fig. 15.13*B*).

**Ventral mesentery**, which includes the **lesser omentum** and **falciform ligament**, forms from the ventral mesogastrium, which itself is derived from mesoderm of the **septum transversum**. When liver cords grow into the septum, it thins to form (1) the peritoneum of the liver; (2) the **falciform ligament**, extending from the liver to the ventral body wall; and (3) the **lesser omentum**, extending from the stomach and proximal part of the duodenum to the liver (Figs. 15.14 and 15.15). The free margin of the falciform ligament contains the **umbilical vein** (Fig. 15.10*A*), which is obliterated after birth to form the **round ligament of the liver (ligamentum teres hepatis)**. The free margin of the lesser omentum connecting the duodenum and liver is thickened to form the **portal pedicle**. The pedicle contains the bile duct, portal vein, and hepatic artery (**portal triad**) and also forms the roof of the **epiploic foramen (of Winslow)**, which is the opening connecting the **omental bursa (lesser sac)** with the rest of the peritoneal cavity (**greater sac**) (Fig. 15.16).

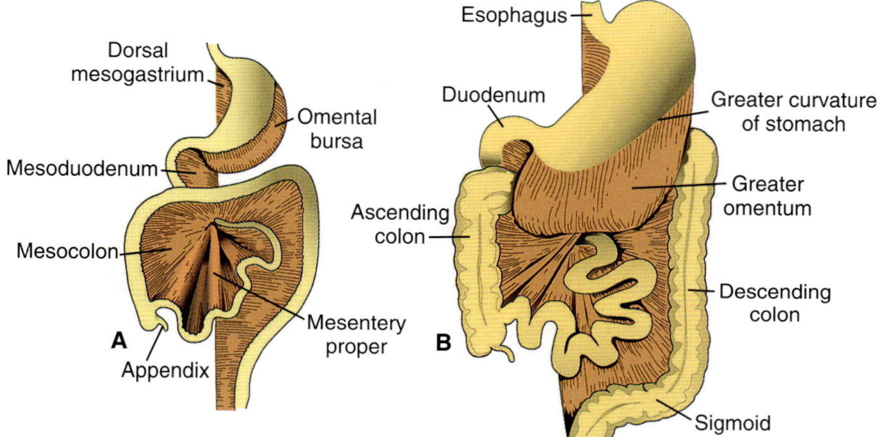


**FIGURE 15.12 A.** Derivatives of the dorsal mesentery at the end of the third month. The dorsal mesogastrium bulges out on the left side of the stomach, where it forms part of the border of the omental bursa. **B.** The greater omentum hangs down from the greater curvature of the stomach in front of the transverse colon.

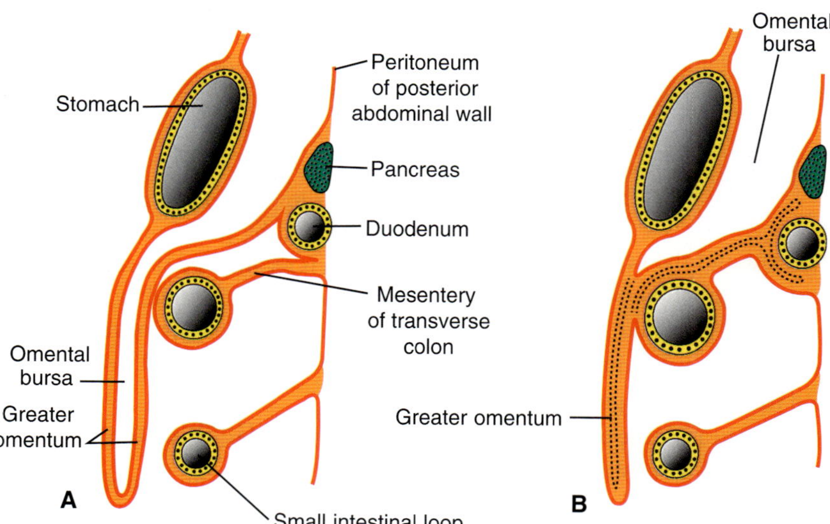


**FIGURE 15.13 A.** Sagittal section showing the relation of the greater omentum, stomach, transverse colon, and small intestinal loops at 4 months. The pancreas and duodenum have already become attached to the posterior abdominal wall. **B.** Similar section as in **(A)** in the newborn. The leaves of the greater omentum have fused with each other and with the transverse mesocolon. The transverse mesocolon covers the duodenum, which attaches to the posterior body wall.

Part 2

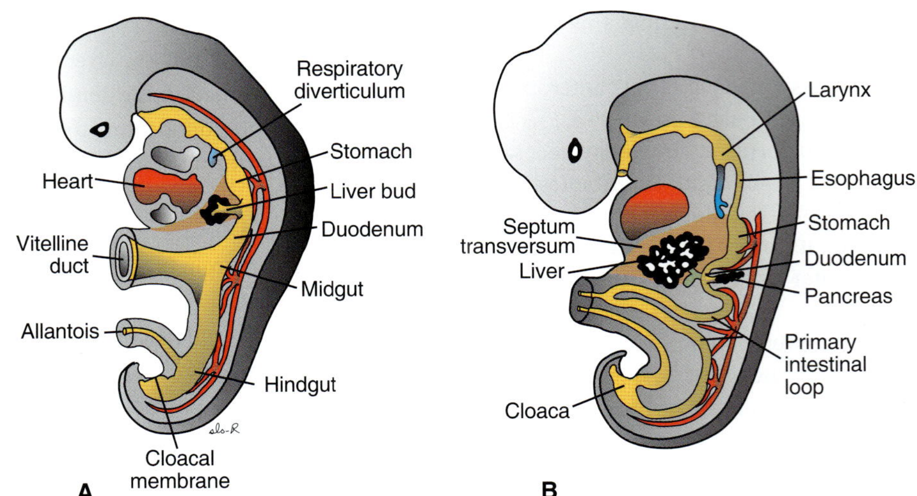


**FIGURE 15.14** **A.** A 3-mm embryo (approximately 25 days) showing the primitive gastrointestinal tract and formation of the liver bud. The bud is formed by endoderm lining the foregut. **B.** A 5-mm embryo (approximately 32 days). Epithelial liver cords penetrate the mesenchyme of the septum transversum.

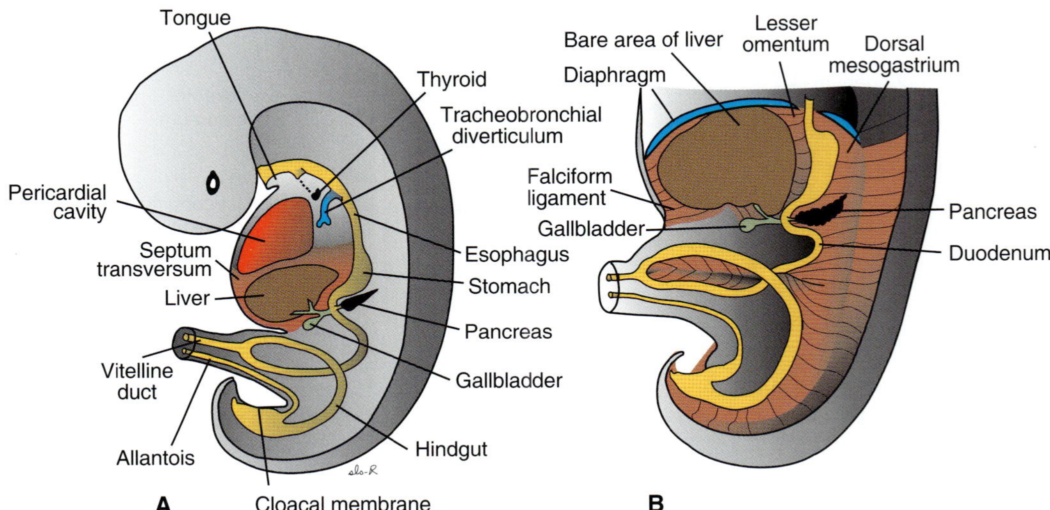


**FIGURE 15.15** **A.** A 9-mm embryo (approximately 36 days). The liver expands caudally into the abdominal cavity. **B.** A slightly older embryo. Note the falciform ligament extending between the liver and the anterior abdominal wall and the lesser omentum extending between the liver and the foregut (stomach and duodenum). The liver is entirely surrounded by peritoneum except in its contact area with the diaphragm. This is the bare area of the liver.

## Duodenum

The terminal part of the foregut and the cephalic part of the midgut form the duodenum. The junction of the two parts is directly distal to the origin of the liver bud (Figs. 15.14 and 15.15). As the stomach rotates, the duodenum takes on the form of a C-shaped loop and rotates to the right. This rotation, together with rapid growth of the head of the pancreas, swings the duodenum from its initial midline position to the right side of the abdominal cavity (Figs. 15.10*A* and 15.17). The pancreas and most of the duodenum become attached to the posterior body wall. A small portion of the distal region of the duodenum (**duodenal cap**) retains an extension of mesentery and remains unattached to the posterior body wall.

During the second month, the lumen of the duodenum is obliterated by proliferation of cells in its walls. However, the lumen is recanalized shortly thereafter (Fig. 15.18*A*,*B*). Because the **foregut** is supplied by the **celiac artery** and the midgut is supplied by the **superior mesenteric artery**, the duodenum is supplied by branches of both arteries (Fig. 15.14).

## Liver and Gallbladder

The liver primordium appears in the middle of the third week as an outgrowth of the endodermal epithelium at the distal end of the foregut (Figs. 15.14 and 15.15). This outgrowth, the **hepatic diverticulum** or **liver bud**, consists of rapidly proliferating cells that penetrate the **septum transversum**, that is, the mesodermal plate between the pericardial cavity and the stalk

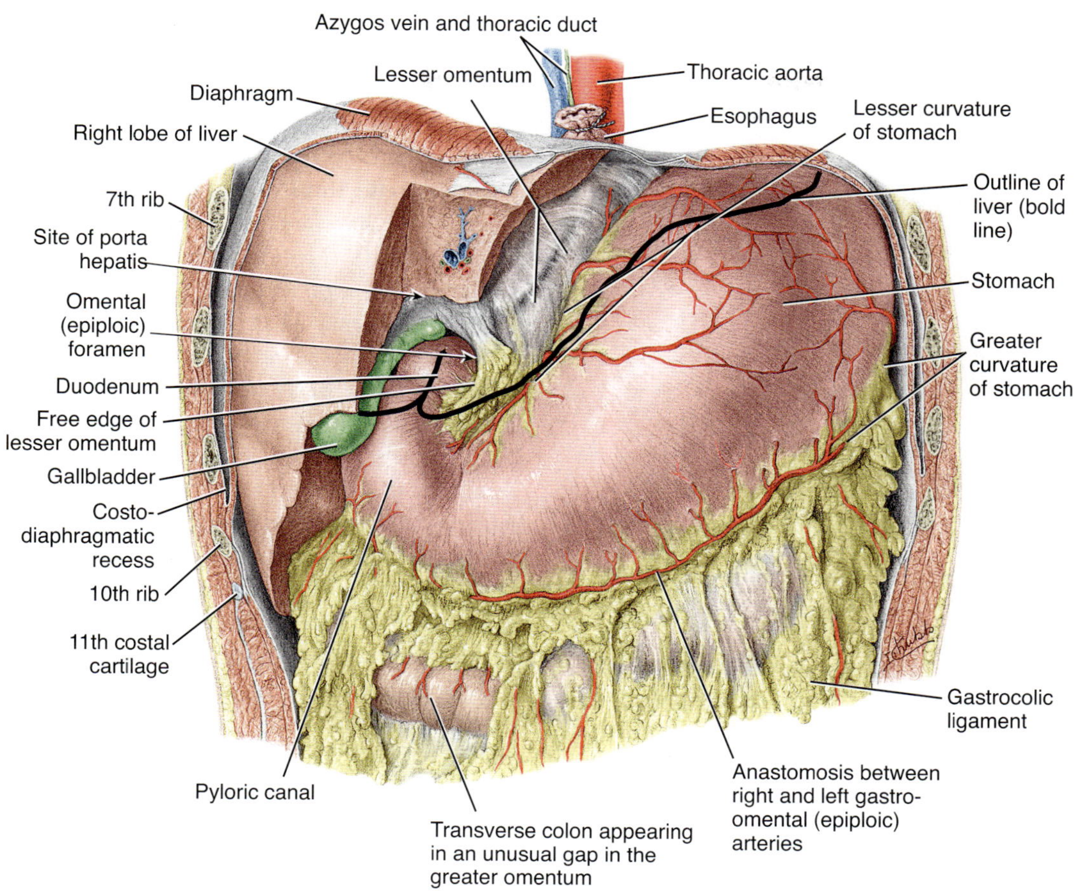


**FIGURE 15.16** Lesser omentum extending from the liver to the lesser curvature of the stomach and to the duodenum where it thickens to form the portal pedicle. The pedicle lies anterior to the omental foramen (epiploic foramen of Winslow) and it contains the hepatic artery, portal vein, and bile duct (portal triad).



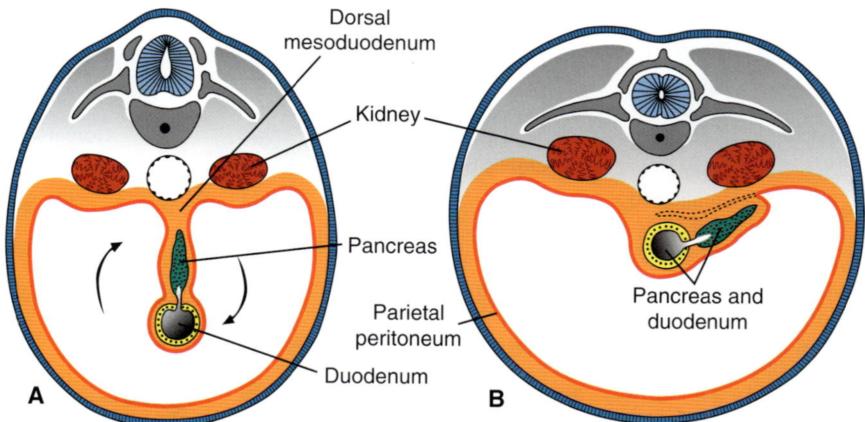


**FIGURE 15.17** Transverse sections through the region of the duodenum at various stages of development. At first, the duodenum and head of the pancreas are located in the median plane **(A)**, but later, they swing to the right and become attached to the posterior abdominal wall **(B)**.

of the yolk sac (Figs. 15.14 and 15.15). Whereas hepatic cells continue to penetrate the septum, the connection between the hepatic diverticulum and the foregut (duodenum) narrows, forming the **bile duct**. A small ventral outgrowth is formed by the bile duct, and this outgrowth gives rise to the **gallbladder** and the **cystic duct** (Fig. 15.15). During further development, epithelial liver cords intermingle with the vitelline and umbilical veins, which form hepatic sinusoids. Liver cords differentiate into the **parenchyma (liver cells)** and form the lining of the biliary ducts. **Hematopoietic cells**, **Kupffer cells**, and **connective tissue cells** are derived from mesoderm of the septum transversum.

When liver cells have invaded the entire septum transversum, so that the organ bulges caudally into the abdominal

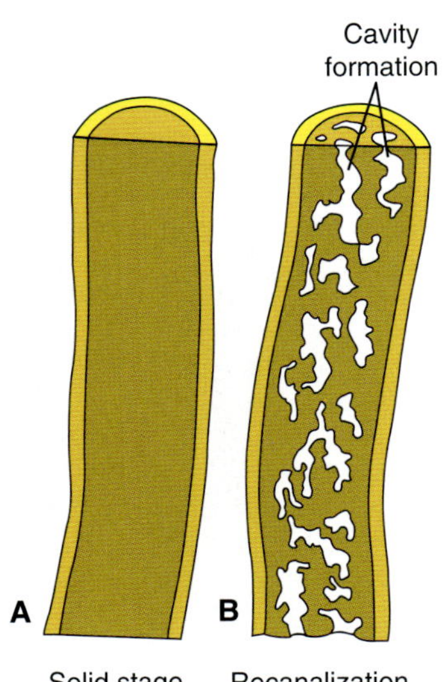


**FIGURE 15.18** Upper portion of the duodenum showing the solid stage **(A)** and cavity formation **(B)** produced by recanalization.

cavity, mesoderm of the septum transversum lying between the liver and the foregut and the liver and the ventral abdominal wall becomes membranous, forming the **lesser omentum** and **falciform ligament**, respectively. Together, they are known as the **ventral mesentery** and are continuous with the dorsal mesentery (Fig. 15.15).

Mesoderm on the surface of the liver differentiates into visceral peritoneum except on its cranial surface (Fig. 15.15*B*). In this region, the liver comes in contact with the central tendon of the diaphragm, such that this surface of the liver is never covered by peritoneum and forms the **bare area of the liver**. Reflections of peritoneum from the diaphragm to the liver form the **anterior** and **posterior coronary reflections** that in turn meet on the right and left sides of the bare area to form the **triangular reflections** (Fig. 15.15). In the 10th week of development, the weight of the liver is approximately 10% of the total body weight. Although this may be attributed partly to the large numbers of sinusoids, another important factor is its **hematopoietic function**. Large nests of proliferating cells, which produce red and white blood cells, lie between hepatic cells and walls of the vessels. This activity gradually subsides during the last 2 months of intrauterine life, and only small hematopoietic islands remain at birth. The weight of the liver is then only 5% of the total body weight.

Another important function of the liver begins at approximately the 12th week, when bile is formed by hepatic cells. Meanwhile, because the **gallbladder** and **cystic duct** have developed and the cystic duct has joined the hepatic duct to form the **bile duct** (Fig. 15.15), bile can enter the gastrointestinal tract. As a result, its contents take on a dark green color. Because of positional changes of the duodenum, the entrance of the bile duct gradually shifts from its initial anterior position to a posterior one, and consequently, the bile duct passes behind the duodenum (Figs. 15.19 and 15.20).

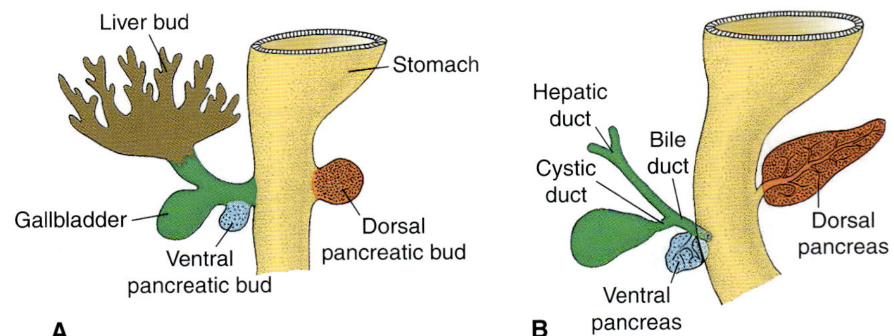


**FIGURE 15.19** Stages in development of the pancreas. **A.** 30 days (approximately 5 mm). **B.** 35 days (approximately 7 mm). Initially, the ventral pancreatic bud lies close to the liver bud, but later, it moves posteriorly around the duodenum toward the dorsal pancreatic bud.

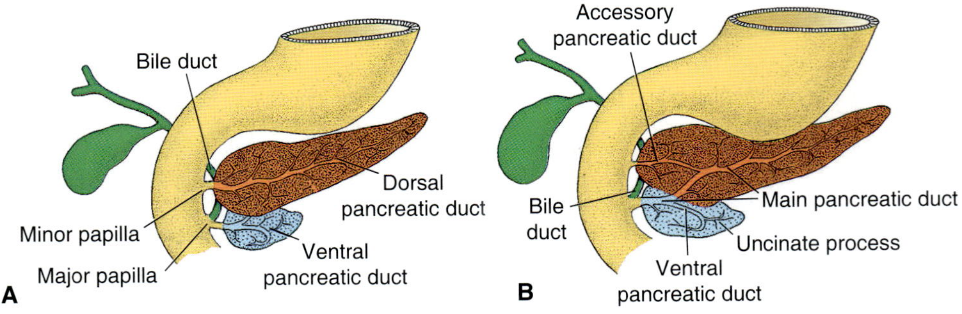


**FIGURE 15.20 A.** Pancreas during the sixth week of development. The ventral pancreatic bud is in close contact with the dorsal pancreatic bud. **B.** Fusion of the pancreatic ducts. The main pancreatic duct enters the duodenum in combination with the bile duct at the major papilla. The accessory pancreatic duct (when present) enters the duodenum at the minor papilla.

## Clinical Correlates

### Stomach Abnormalities

**Pyloric stenosis** occurs when the circular and, to a lesser degree, the longitudinal musculature of the stomach in the region of the pylorus hypertrophies. One of the most common abnormalities of the stomach in infants, pyloric stenosis was previously believed to develop only during fetal life, despite the fact that most cases present 3 to 5 days after birth. However, recent data indicate that a postnatal exposure (e.g., treatment with erythromycin in the newborn period) substantially increases the risk for pyloric stenosis, suggesting that in some cases, the defect may develop later. Pyloric stenosis is characterized by an extreme narrowing of the pyloric lumen, and the passage of food is obstructed, resulting in severe projectile vomiting. In a few cases, the pylorus is atretic. Other malformations of the stomach, such as duplications and a prepyloric septum, are rare.

## MOLECULAR REGULATION OF LIVER INDUCTION

All of the foregut endoderm has the potential to express liver-specific genes and to differentiate into liver tissue. However, this expression is blocked by factors produced by surrounding tissues, including ectoderm, noncardiac mesoderm, and particularly the notochord (Fig. 15.21). The

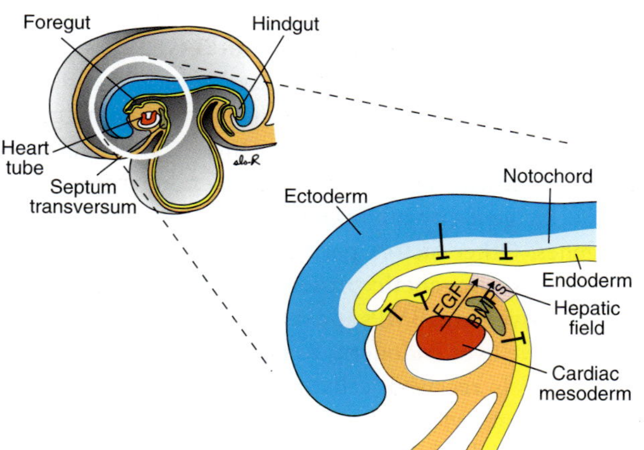


**FIGURE 15.21** Diagrams of the cardiac- and hepatic-forming regions illustrating induction of liver development. All of the gut endoderm has the potential to form liver tissue, but this capacity is repressed by inhibitors secreted by neighboring mesoderm, ectoderm, and the notochord. Stimulation of hepatic development is achieved by secretion of bone morphogenetic proteins (BMPs) by the septum transversum and fibroblast growth factor 2 (FGF2) by cardiac mesoderm. BMPs enhance the competence of prospective liver endoderm to respond to FGF2. Then, FGF2 inhibits activity of the inhibitors, thereby specifying the hepatic field and initiating liver development. This interaction demonstrates that not all inductive processes are a result of direct signaling by an inducing molecule but instead may occur by removal of a repressor signal.

Part 2

## Clinical Correlates

### Liver and Gallbladder Abnormalities

Variations in liver lobulation are common but not clinically significant. **Accessory hepatic ducts** and **duplication of the gallbladder** (Fig. 15.22) are also common and usually asymptomatic. However, they become clinically important under pathological conditions. In some cases, the ducts, which pass through a solid phase in their development, fail to recanalize (Fig. 15.22). This defect, **extrahepatic biliary atresia**, occurs in 1/15,000 live births. Among patients with extrahepatic biliary atresia, 15% to 20% have patent proximal ducts and a correctable defect, but the remainder usually die unless they receive a liver transplant. Another problem with duct formation lies within the liver itself, it is **intrahepatic biliary duct atresia** and **hypoplasia**. This rare abnormality (1/100,000 live births) may be caused by fetal infections. It may be lethal but usually runs an extended benign course.

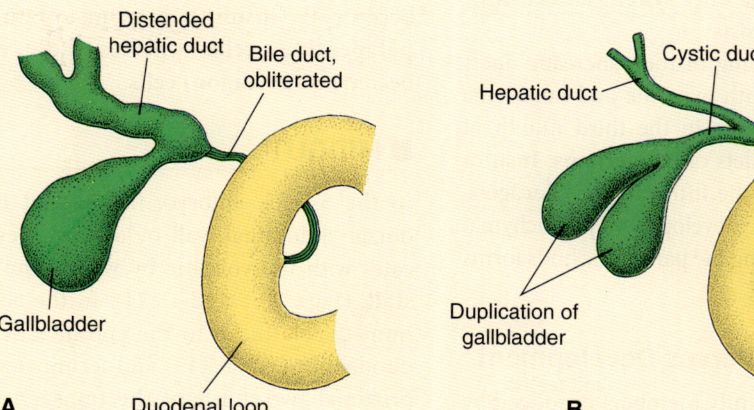


**FIGURE 15.22** **A.** Obliteration of the bile duct resulting in distention of the gallbladder and the hepatic ducts distal to the obliteration. **B.** Duplication of the gallbladder.

action of these inhibitors is blocked in the prospective hepatic region by **fibroblast growth factors (FGF2)** secreted by cardiac mesoderm and by blood vessel–forming endothelial cells adjacent to the gut tube at the site of liver bud outgrowth. Thus, the cardiac mesoderm together with neighboring vascular endothelial cells "instructs" gut endoderm to express liver-specific genes by inhibiting an inhibitory factor of these same genes. Other factors participating in this "instruction" are **bone morphogenetic proteins (BMPs)** secreted by the septum transversum. BMPs appear to enhance the competence of prospective liver endoderm to respond to FGF2. Once this "instruction" is received, cells in the liver field differentiate into both hepatocytes and biliary cell lineages, a process that is at least partially regulated by ***HEPATOCYTE NUCLEAR TRANSCRIPTION FACTORS (HNF3 and HNF4)***.

## PANCREAS

The pancreas is formed by two buds, dorsal and ventral, originating from the endodermal lining of the duodenum (Fig. 15.19). Whereas the **dorsal pancreatic bud** is in the dorsal mesentery, the **ventral pancreatic bud** is close to the bile duct (Fig. 15.19). When the duodenum rotates to the right and becomes C-shaped, the ventral pancreatic bud moves dorsally in a manner similar to the shifting of the entrance of the bile duct (Fig. 15.19). Finally, the ventral bud comes to lie immediately below and behind the dorsal bud (Fig. 15.20). Later, the parenchyma and the duct systems of the dorsal and ventral pancreatic buds fuse (Fig. 15.20*B*). The ventral bud forms the **uncinate process** and inferior part of the head of the pancreas. The remaining part of the gland is derived from the dorsal bud. The **main pancreatic duct** (of **Wirsung**) is formed by the distal part of the dorsal pancreatic duct and the entire ventral pancreatic duct (Fig. 15.20*B*). The proximal part of the dorsal pancreatic duct either is obliterated or persists as a small channel, the **accessory pancreatic duct** (of **Santorini**). The main pancreatic duct, together with the bile duct, enters the duodenum at the site of the **major papilla**; the entrance of the accessory duct (when present) is at the site of the **minor papilla**. In about 10% of cases, the duct system fails to fuse, and the original double system persists.

The cells in the endodermal lining of the pancreatic ducts proliferate and differentiate into both exocrine and endocrine cells. The endocrine cells differentiate in the third month of fetal life and form the pancreatic islets of **Langerhans**. **Insulin secretion** begins at approximately the fifth month. Glucagon- and somatostatin-secreting cells also develop from parenchymal cells. Visceral mesoderm surrounding the pancreatic buds forms the pancreatic connective tissue.

### Molecular Regulation of Pancreas Development

**FGF2** and **ACTIVIN** (a TGF-β family member) produced by the notochord and endothelium of the dorsal aorta repress at ***SHH*** expression in gut endoderm destined to form the dorsal pancreatic bud. The ventral bud is induced by visceral mesoderm. As a result, expression of the ***PANCREATIC AND DUODENAL HOMEOBOX 1 (PDX) gene*** is upregulated. Although all of the downstream effectors of pancreas development have not been determined, it appears that expression of the paired homeobox genes ***PAX4*** and ***PAX6*** specifies the endocrine cell lineage, such that cells expressing both genes become β (**insulin**), **δ** (somatostatin), and γ (**pancreatic polypeptide) cells**; whereas those expressing only *PAX6* become α **(glucagon) cells**.

### *Clinical Correlates*

#### Pancreatic Abnormalities

The ventral pancreatic bud consists of two components that normally fuse and rotate around the duodenum so that they come to lie below the dorsal pancreatic bud. Occasionally, however, the right portion of the ventral bud migrates along its normal route, but the left migrates in the opposite direction. In this manner, the duodenum is surrounded by pancreatic tissue, and an **annular pancreas** is formed (Fig. 15.23). The malformation sometimes constricts the duodenum and causes complete obstruction.

**Accessory pancreatic tissue** may be anywhere from the distal end of the esophagus to the tip of the primary intestinal loop. Most frequently, it lies in the mucosa of the stomach and in Meckel diverticulum, where it may show all of the histological characteristics of the pancreas itself.

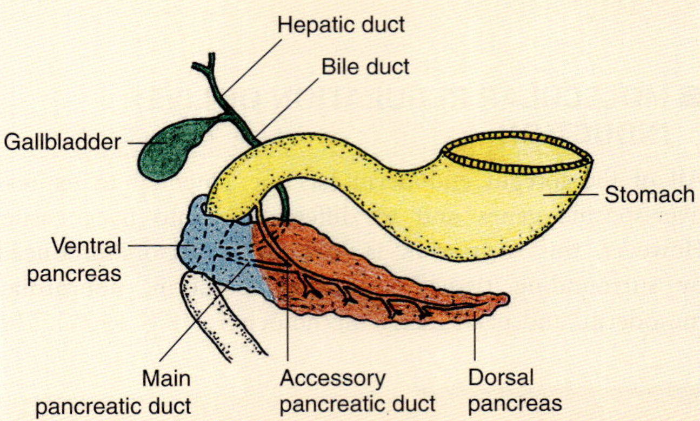


**FIGURE 15.23** Annular pancreas. The ventral pancreas splits and forms a ring around the duodenum, occasionally resulting in duodenal stenosis.

## MIDGUT

In the 5-week embryo, the midgut is suspended from the dorsal abdominal wall by a short mesentery and communicates with the yolk sac by way of the **vitelline duct** or **yolk stalk** (Figs. 15.1 and 15.24). In the adult, the midgut begins immediately distal to the entrance of the bile duct into the duodenum (Fig. 15.15) and terminates at the junction of the proximal two-thirds of the transverse colon with the distal third. Over its entire length, the midgut is supplied by the **superior mesenteric artery** (Fig. 15.24).

Development of the midgut is characterized by rapid elongation of the gut and its mesentery, resulting in formation

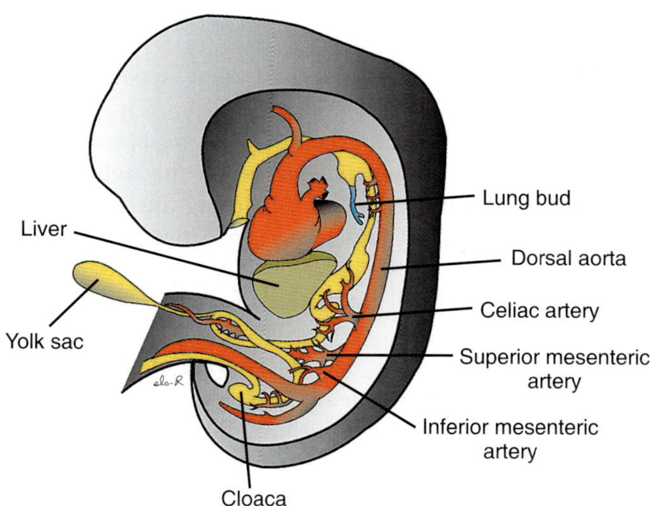


**FIGURE 15.24** Embryo during the sixth week of development, showing blood supply to the segments of the gut and formation and rotation of the primary intestinal loop. The superior mesenteric artery forms the axis of this rotation and supplies the midgut. The celiac and inferior mesenteric arteries supply the foregut and hindgut, respectively.

of the **primary intestinal loop** (Figs. 15.24 and 15.25). At its apex, the loop remains in open connection with the yolk sac by way of the narrow **vitelline duct** (Fig. 15.24).

**Derivatives of the cephalic limb:**

- Distal part of the duodenum
- Jejunum
- Part of the ileum

**Derivatives of the caudal limb:**

- Lower portion of the ileum
- Cecum
- Appendix
- Ascending colon
- Proximal two-third of the transverse colon

## Physiological Herniation

Development of the primary intestinal loop is characterized by rapid elongation, particularly of the cephalic limb. As a result of the rapid growth and expansion of the liver, the abdominal cavity temporarily becomes too small to contain all the intestinal loops, and they enter the extraembryonic cavity in the umbilical cord during the sixth week of development (**physiological umbilical herniation**) (Fig. 15.26).

## Rotation of the Midgut

Coincident with growth in length, the primary intestinal loop rotates around an axis formed by the **superior mesenteric artery** (Fig. 15.25). When viewed from the front, this rotation is counterclockwise, and it amounts to approximately 270° when it is complete (Figs. 15.25 and 15.27). Even during rotation, elongation of the small intestinal loop continues, and the jejunum and ileum form a number of coiled loops (Fig. 15.26). The large intestine likewise lengthens considerably but does not participate in the coiling phenomenon. Rotation occurs during herniation (about 90°) as well as during return of the intestinal loops into the abdominal cavity (remaining 180°) (Fig. 15.27).

## Retraction of Herniated Loops

During the 10th week, herniated intestinal loops begin to return to the abdominal cavity. Although the factors responsible for this return are not precisely known, the following are the factors that those that play important roles are as follows:

- Regression of the mesonephric kidney
- Reduced growth of the liver
- Expansion of the abdominal cavity

The cecal bud hinders reduction of the caudal loop. Therefore, the proximal portion of the jejunum, the first part to reenter the abdominal cavity, comes to lie on the left side (Fig. 15.27*A*). The later returning loops gradually settle more and more to the right.



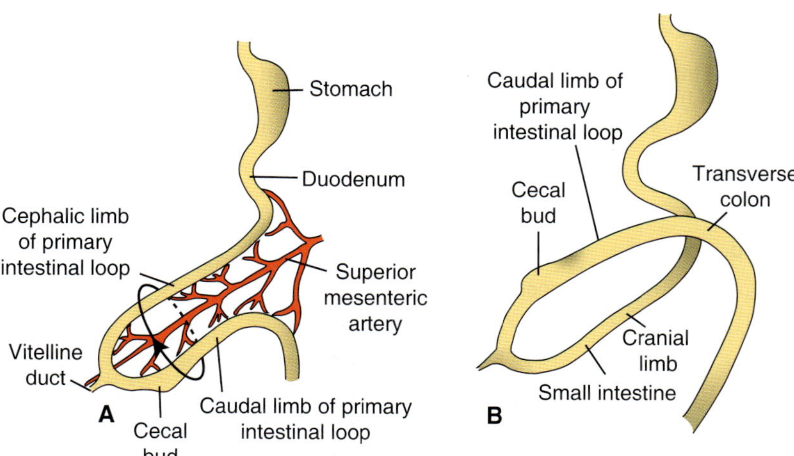


**FIGURE 15.25** **A.** Primary intestinal loop before rotation (lateral view). The superior mesenteric artery forms the axis of the loop. *Arrow*, counterclockwise rotation. **B.** Similar view as in **(A)** showing the primary intestinal loop after 90° counterclockwise rotation. The transverse colon passes in front of the duodenum.

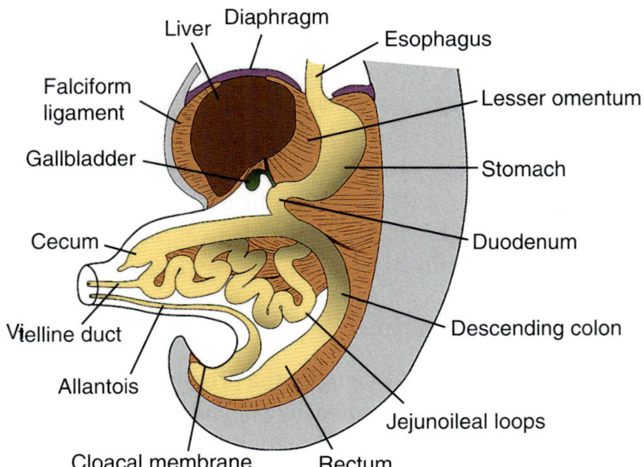


**FIGURE 15.26** Umbilical herniation of the intestinal loops in an embryo of approximately 8 weeks (crown-rump length, 35 mm). Coiling of the small intestinal loops and formation of the cecum occur during the herniation. The first 90° of rotation occurs during herniation; the remaining 180° occurs during the return of the gut to the abdominal cavity in the third month.

The **cecal bud**, which appears at about the sixth week as a small conical dilation of the caudal limb of the primary intestinal loop, is the last part of the gut to reenter the abdominal cavity.

## Fixation of the Midgut

Temporarily, the cecum lies in the right upper quadrant directly below the right lobe of the liver (Fig. 15.27*A*). From here, it descends into the right iliac fossa, placing the **ascending colon** and **hepatic flexure** on the right side of the abdominal cavity (Fig. 15.27*B*). During this process, the distal end of the cecal bud forms a narrow diverticulum, the **appendix** (Fig. 15.28). After birth, the cecal walls grow unequally, the lateral wall grows much more, and the appendix comes to lie medially.

Because the appendix develops during descent of the colon, its final position frequently is posterior to the cecum or colon. These positions of the appendix are called **retrocecal** or **retrocolic**, respectively (Fig. 15.29).

## Mesenteries of the Intestinal Loops

The mesentery of the primary intestinal loop, the **mesentery proper**, undergoes profound changes with rotation and coiling of the bowel. When the caudal limb of the loop moves to the right side of the abdominal cavity, the dorsal mesentery twists around the origin of the **superior mesenteric artery** (Fig. 15.24). Despite these changes in position, mesentery to the midgut and hindgut remains **continuous as a single**

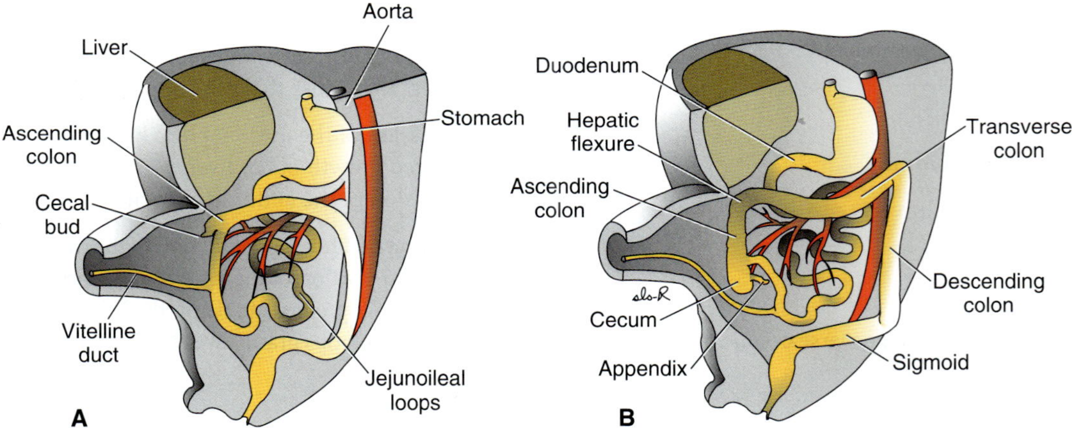


**FIGURE 15.27** **A.** Anterior view of the intestinal loops after 270° counterclockwise rotation. Note the coiling of the small intestinal loops and the position of the cecal bud in the right upper quadrant of the abdomen. **B.** Similar view as in **(A)** with the intestinal loops in their final position. Displacement of the cecum and appendix caudally places them in the right lower quadrant of the abdomen.

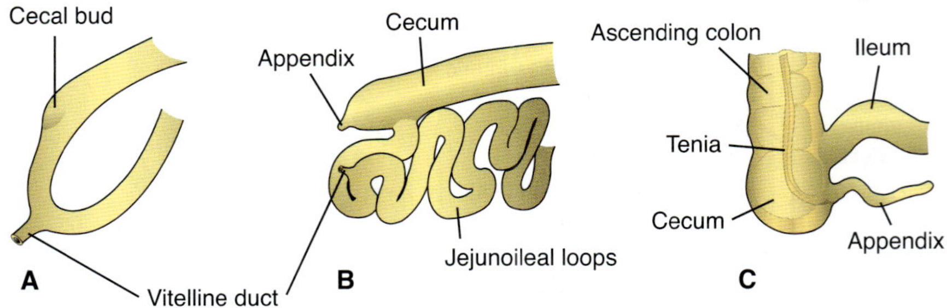


**FIGURE 15.28** Successive stages in development of the cecum and appendix. **A.** 7 weeks. **B.** 8 weeks. **C.** Newborn.

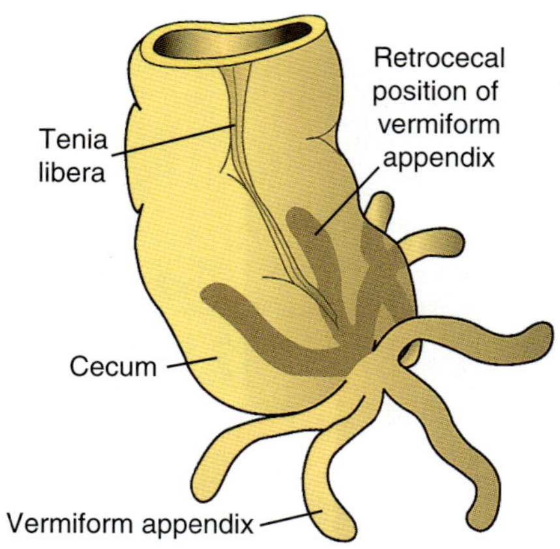


**FIGURE 15.29** Various positions of the appendix. In about 50% of cases, the appendix is retrocecal or retrocolic.

**entity** from the duodenojejunal flexure to the mesorectal level. In some regions, it is retained as a free mesentery. These regions include the mesentery proper to the jejunum and ileum, the transverse mesocolon, mesoappendix, mesosigmoid, and mesorectum (Fig. 15.30). In other regions, such as the ascending and descending segments of the colon, the mesentery becomes attached to the peritoneum on the posterior wall of the body cavity with a layer of fascia (**Toldt fascia**) intervening between the two peritoneal layers (Fig. 15.30). The fact that the entire mesentery is continuous is important for surgical procedures involving this tissue as is the fascial plane created by Toldt fascia.

## HINDGUT

The hindgut gives rise to the distal third of the transverse colon, the descending colon, the sigmoid, the rectum, and the upper part of the anal canal. The endoderm of the hindgut also forms the internal lining of the bladder and urethra (see Chapter 16).

A urorectal septum is formed by the condensation of mesoderm. It divides the cloaca into an anterior urogenital sinus and a posterior hindgut proper. The terminal portion

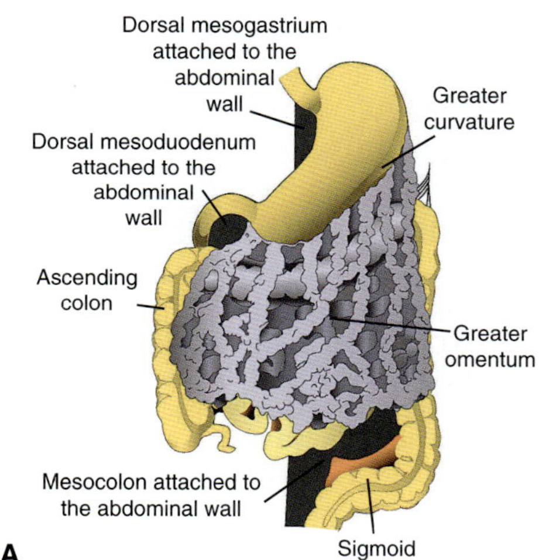


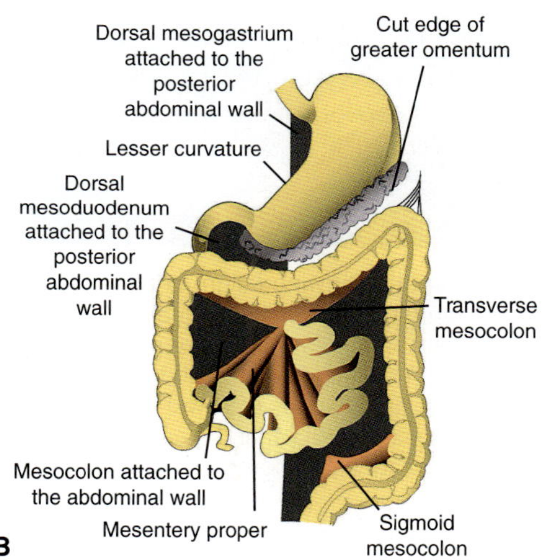


**FIGURE 15.30** Frontal view of the intestinal loops with **(A)** and after removal of **(B)** the greater omentum. *Gray areas*, parts of the dorsal mesentery that become attached to the posterior abdominal wall, including the ascending and descending segments of the colon. *Brown areas*, parts of the mesentery that remain free and do not become attached to the posterior wall of the body cavity, including the transverse mesocolon, mesentery proper, and sigmoid mesocolon (the free mesentery to the rectum is not illustrated). Despite having attached and unattached segments, it should be noted that the mesentery is continuous as one structure from the caudal end of the esophagus to the mesorectum.

### *Clinical Correlates*

#### Abnormalities of the Mesenteries

Normally, the ascending colon, except for its most caudal part (approximately 1 in.), attaches to the posterior abdominal wall. If the ascending portion of the colon fails to attach to the posterior abdominal wall, a mobile colon results, which may allow it to twist upon itself causing **volvulus** of the cecum and colon. Similarly, incomplete attachment of this region of the colon to the posterior body wall may give rise to **retrocolic pockets** behind the ascending colon. A **retrocolic hernia** is formed when entrapment of portions of the small intestine posterior to the ascending portion of the colon occurs.

#### Body Wall Defects

**Omphalocele** (Fig. 15.31*A,B*) involves herniation of abdominal viscera through an enlarged umbilical ring. The viscera, which may include liver, small and large intestines, stomach, spleen, or gallbladder, are covered by amnion. The origin of the defect is a failure of the bowel to return to the body cavity from its physiological herniation during the 6th to 10th weeks. It can be diagnosed in utero later in gestation by ultrasound (Fig. 15.31*D*). Omphalocele occurs in 2.5/10,000 births and is associated with a high rate of mortality (25%) and severe malformations, such as cardiac anomalies (50%) and neural tube defects (40%).

(*Continued*)

Part 2

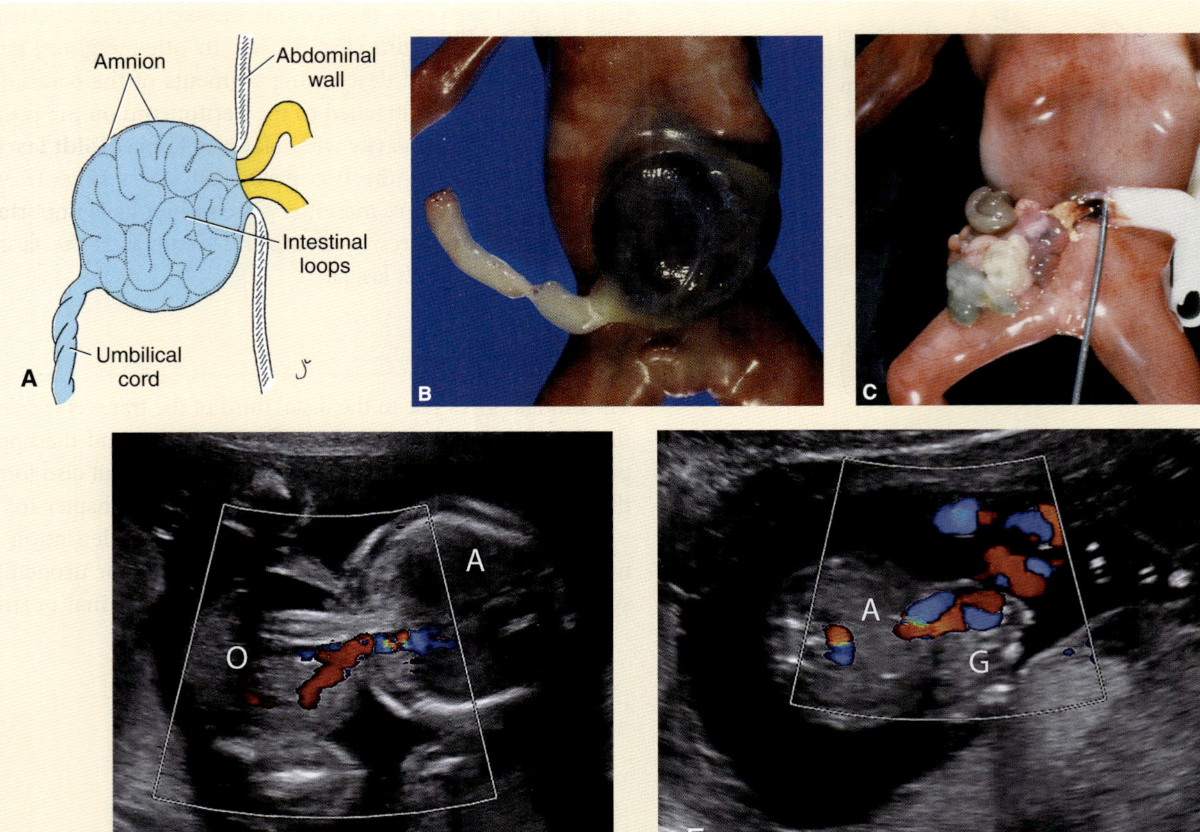


**FIGURE 15.31** **A.** Omphalocele showing failure of the intestinal loops to return to the body cavity after physiological herniation. The herniated loops are covered by amnion. **B.** Omphalocele in a newborn. **C.** Newborn with gastroschisis. Loops of bowel extend through a closure defect in the ventral body wall and are not covered by amnion (see Chapter 7). **D.** Ultrasound at 22 weeks showing a fetus with an omphalocele (*O*) protruding from the abdominal wall (*A*). The spherical nature of the defect is due to the fact that there is a covering of amnion that holds the loops of bowel in place. **E.** Ultrasound at 16 weeks of a fetus with gastroschisis (*G*). Loops of bowel protrude through the abdominal wall (*A*) and are not covered by amnion and so have a more ragged appearance. In both **(D)** and **(E)**, the *red* and *blue* colors indicate blood flow in the umbilical circulation.

Approximately 15% of live-born infants with omphalocele have chromosomal abnormalities.

**Gastroschisis** (Fig. 15.31*C*) refers to a protrusion of abdominal contents through the body wall directly into the amniotic cavity. It occurs lateral to the umbilicus usually on the right, and the defect is most likely due to abnormal closure of the body wall around the connecting stalk (see Chapter 7). Viscera are not covered by peritoneum or amnion, and the bowel may be damaged by exposure to amniotic fluid. Like omphalocele, it can be diagnosed later in pregnancy by ultrasound (Fig. 15.31*E*). Gastroschisis occurs in 1/10,000 births but is increasing in frequency, especially among young women (<20 years old). The reason for this increase and why the defect is more prevalent in babies born to younger women is not known. Unlike omphalocele, gastroschisis is not associated with chromosome abnormalities or other severe defects, so the survival rate is excellent. Volvulus (rotation of the bowel) resulting in a compromised blood supply may, however, kill large regions of the intestine and lead to fetal death.

## Vitelline Duct Abnormalities

In 2% to 4% of people, a small portion of the **vitelline duct** persists, forming an outpocketing of the ileum, **Meckel diverticulum** or **ileal diverticulum** (Fig. 15.32*A*). In the adult, this diverticulum, approximately 40 to 60 cm from the ileocecal valve on the antimesenteric border of the ileum, does not usually cause any symptoms. However, when it contains heterotopic pancreatic tissue or gastric mucosa, it may cause ulceration, bleeding, or even perforation. Sometimes, both ends of the vitelline duct transform into fibrous cords, and the middle portion forms a large cyst, an **enterocystoma**, or a **vitelline**

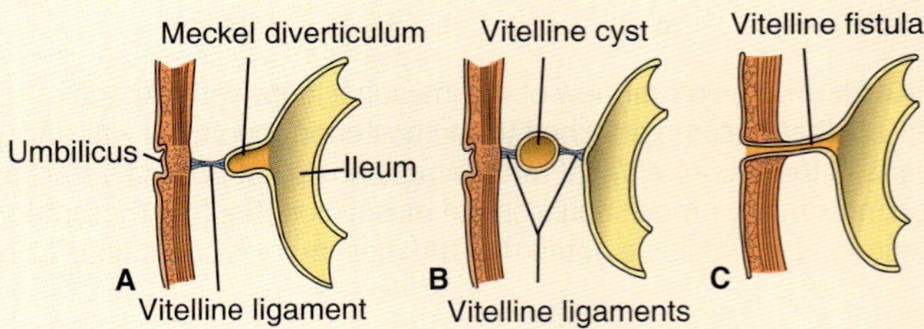


**FIGURE 15.32** Remnants of the vitelline duct. **A.** Meckel, or ileal, diverticulum combined with fibrous cord (vitelline ligament). **B.** Vitelline cyst attached to the umbilicus and wall of the ileum by vitelline ligaments. **C.** Vitelline fistula connecting the lumen of the ileum with the umbilicus.

**cyst** (Fig. 15.32*B*). Because the fibrous cords traverse the peritoneal cavity, intestinal loops may twist around the fibrous strands and become obstructed, causing strangulation or volvulus. In another variation, the vitelline duct remains patent over its entire length, forming a direct communication between the umbilicus and the intestinal tract. This abnormality is known as an **umbilical fistula**, or a **vitelline fistula** (Fig. 15.32*C*). A fecal discharge may then be found at the umbilicus.

## Gut Rotation Defects

Malrotation of the intestinal loop may result in twisting of the intestine (**volvulus**) and a compromise of the blood supply. Normally, the primary intestinal loop rotates 270° counterclockwise. Occasionally, however, rotation amounts to 90° only. When this occurs, the colon and cecum are the first portions of the gut to return from the umbilical cord, and they settle on the left side of the abdominal cavity (Fig. 15.33*A*). The later returning loops then move more and more to the right, resulting in a **left-sided colon**.

**Reversed rotation of the intestinal loop** occurs when the primary loop rotates 90° clockwise. In this abnormality, the transverse colon passes behind the duodenum (Fig. 15.33*B*) and lies behind the superior mesenteric artery.

**Duplications of intestinal loops and cysts** may occur anywhere along the length of the gut tube. They are most frequently found in the region of the ileum, where they may vary from a long segment to a small diverticulum. Symptoms usually occur early in life, and 33% are associated with other defects, such as intestinal atresias, imperforate anus, gastroschisis, and omphalocele. Their origin is unknown, although they may result from abnormal proliferations of gut parenchyma.

## Gut Atresias and Stenoses

**Atresias and stenoses** may occur anywhere along the intestine. Most occur in the duodenum, fewest occur in the colon, and equal numbers occur in the jejunum and ileum (1/1,500 births). Atresias in the upper duodenum are probably due to a lack of recanalization (Fig. 15.18). From the distal portion of the duodenum caudally, however, stenoses and atresias were thought to be caused by **vascular "accidents"** that resulted in compromised blood flow and tissue necrosis in a section of the gut resulting in the defects. It was suggested that these accidents could be caused by malrotation, volvulus, gastroschisis, omphalocele, and other factors. However, new evidence suggests that problems with gut differentiation can also cause these defects. Thus, misexpression of some *HOX* genes and of genes and receptors in the *FGF* family result in gut atresias. In 50% of cases, a region of the bowel is lost, and in 20%, a fibrous cord remains (Fig. 15.34*A*,*B*). In another 20%, there is narrowing, with a thin diaphragm separating the larger and smaller pieces of bowel (Fig. 15.34*C*). Stenoses and multiple atresias account for the remaining 10% of these defects, with a frequency of 5% each (Fig. 15.34*D*). **Apple peel atresia** accounts for 10% of atresias. The atresia is in the proximal jejunum, and the intestine is short, with the portion distal to the lesion coiled around a mesenteric remnant (Fig. 15.35). Effects of atresias on newborns depend on the amount of bowel that has been damaged and its location. Some babies with extensive gut involvement have low birth weight and other abnormalities.

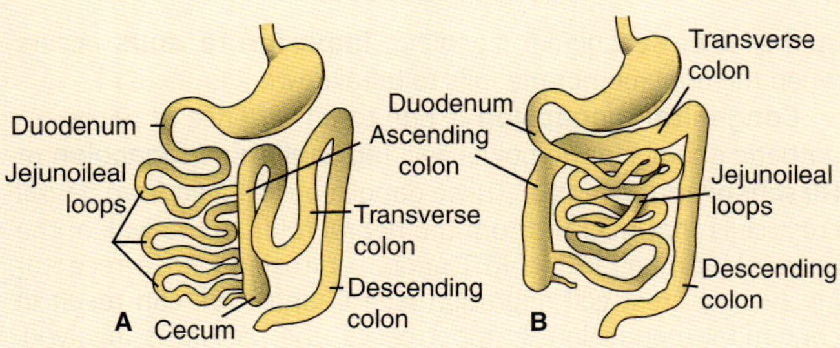


**FIGURE 15.33** **A.** Abnormal rotation of the primary intestinal loop. The colon is on the left side of the abdomen, and the small intestinal loops are on the right. The ileum enters the cecum from the right. **B.** The primary intestinal loop is rotated 90° clockwise (reversed rotation). The transverse colon passes behind the duodenum.

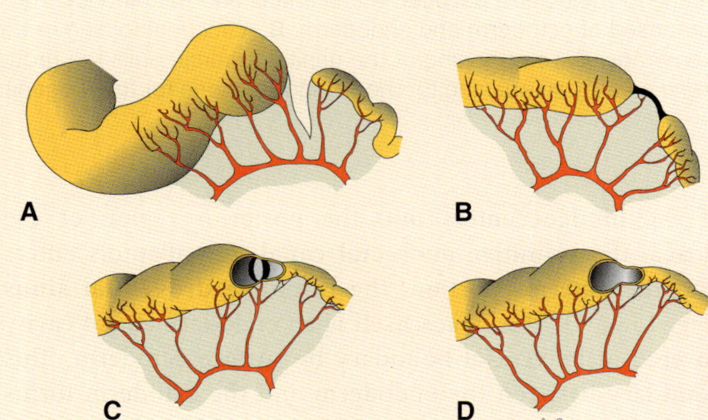


**FIGURE 15.34** The most commonly occurring bowel atresias and stenoses. **(A)** The most common, occurs in 50% of cases; **(B)** and **(C)** occur in 20% each of cases, and **(D)** occurs in 5% of cases. They may be caused by problems with expression of *HOX* and *FGFs* and certain FGF receptors during gut differentiation or by vascular accidents; those in the upper duodenum may be caused by a lack of recanalization. Atresias **(A–C)** occur in 95% of cases, and stenoses **(D)** in only 5%.

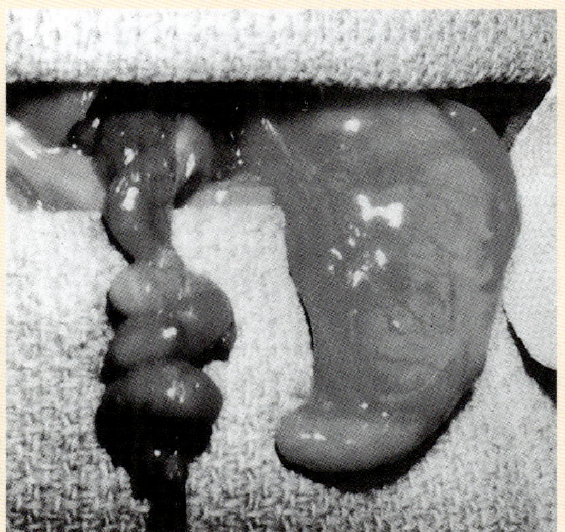

**FIGURE 15.35** Apple peel atresia, which occurs in the jejunum and accounts for 10% of bowel atresias. The affected portion of the bowel is coiled around a remnant of mesentery.

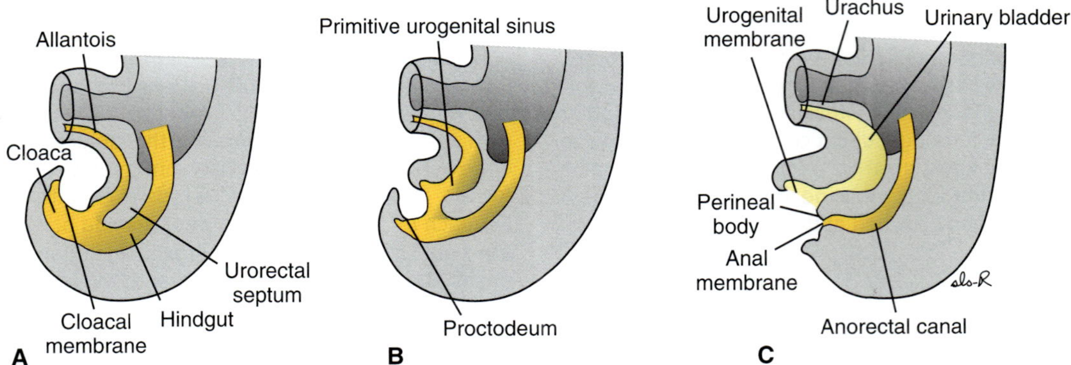


**FIGURE 15.36** Cloacal region in embryos at successive stages of development. **A.** The hindgut enters the posterior portion of the cloaca, the future anorectal canal; the allantois enters the anterior portion, the future urogenital sinus. The urorectal septum is formed by a wedge of mesoderm between the allantois and the hindgut. The cloacal membrane, which forms the ventral boundary of the cloaca, is composed of ectoderm and endoderm. **B.** As caudal folding of the embryo continues, the urorectal septum moves closer to the cloacal membrane. **C.** Lengthening of the genital tubercle pulls the urogenital portion of the cloaca anteriorly; breakdown of the cloacal membrane creates an opening for the hindgut and one for the urogenital sinus. The tip of the urorectal septum forms the perineal body.

of the hindgut enters into the posterior region of the cloaca, the primitive **anorectal canal**; the allantois enters into the anterior portion, the primitive **urogenital sinus** (Fig. 15.36*A*). The cloaca itself is an endoderm-lined cavity covered at its ventral boundary by surface ectoderm. This boundary between the endoderm and the ectoderm forms the **cloacal membrane** (Fig. 15.36). As the embryo grows and caudal folding continues, the tip of the urorectal septum comes to lie close to the cloacal membrane (Fig. 15.36*B,C*). At the end of the seventh week, the cloacal membrane ruptures, creating the anal opening for the hindgut and a ventral opening for the urogenital sinus. Between the two, the tip of the urorectal septum forms the perineal body (Fig. 15.36*C*). The upper part (two-thirds) of the anal canal is derived from endoderm of the hindgut; the lower part (one-third) is derived from ectoderm around the **proctodeum** (Fig. 15.36*B,C*). Ectoderm in the region of the proctodeum on the surface of part of the cloaca proliferates and invaginates to create the **anal pit** (Fig. 15.37*D*). Subsequently, degeneration of the **cloacal membrane** (now called the **anal membrane**) establishes continuity between the upper and lower parts of the anal canal. Because the caudal part of the anal canal originates from ectoderm, it is supplied by the **inferior rectal arteries**, branches of the **internal pudendal arteries**. However, the cranial part of the anal canal originates from endoderm and is therefore supplied by **the superior rectal artery**, a continuation of the **inferior mesenteric artery**, the artery of the hindgut. The junction between the endodermal and ectodermal regions of the anal canal is delineated by the **pectinate line**, just below the anal columns. At this line, the epithelium changes from columnar to stratified squamous epithelium.

## *Clinical Correlates*

### Hindgut Abnormalities

Rectourethral and **rectovaginal fistulas**, which occur in 1/5,000 live births, may be caused by abnormalities in formation of the cloaca and/or the urorectal septum. For example, if the cloaca is too small or if the urorectal septum does not extend far enough caudally, then opening of the hindgut shifts anteriorly leading to an opening of the hindgut into the urethra or vagina (Fig. 15.37*A,B*). **Rectoanal fistulas and atresias** vary in severity and may leave a narrow tube or fibrous remnant connected to the perineal surface (Fig. 15.37*C*). These defects are probably due to misexpression of genes during epithelial–mesenchymal signaling. **Imperforate anus** occurs when the anal membrane fails to breakdown (Fig. 15.37*D*).

**Congenital megacolon** is due to an absence of parasympathetic ganglia in the bowel wall (**aganglionic megacolon** or **Hirschsprung disease**). These ganglia are derived from neural crest cells that migrate from the neural folds to the wall of the bowel. Mutations in the *RET* gene, a tyrosine kinase receptor involved in crest cell migration (see Chapter 18), can result in congenital megacolon. In most cases, the rectum is involved, and in 80%, the defect extends to the midpoint of the sigmoid. In only 10% to 20% are the transverse and right-side colonic segments involved, and in 3%, the entire colon is affected.

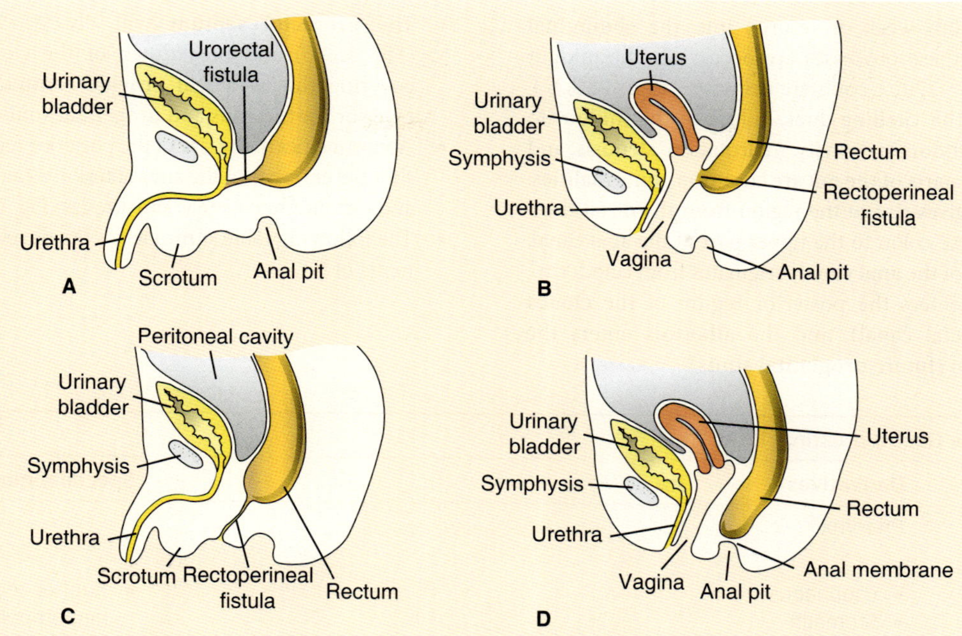


**FIGURE 15.37** Urorectal **(A)** and rectovaginal **(B)** fistulas that result from incomplete separation of the hindgut from the urogenital sinus by the urorectal septum. These defects may also arise if the cloaca is too small, which causes the opening of the hindgut to shift anteriorly. **C.** Rectoperineal (fistula). These defects probably result from misexpression of genes during epithelial–mesenchymal signaling in this region. **D.** Imperforate anus resulting from failure of the anal membrane to break down.

## SUMMARY

- The epithelium of the digestive system and the **parenchyma** of its derivatives originate in the endoderm; connective tissue, muscular components, and peritoneal components originate in the mesoderm.
- Different regions of the gut tube such as the esophagus, stomach, duodenum, etc., are specified by an RA gradient that causes transcription factors unique to each region to be expressed (Fig. 15.2A).
- Differentiation of the gut and its derivatives depends upon reciprocal interactions between the gut endoderm (epithelium) and its surrounding mesoderm (an epithelial–mesenchymal interaction).
- *HOX* genes in the mesoderm are induced by *SHH* secreted by gut endoderm and regulate the craniocaudal organization of the gut and its derivatives. The gut system extends from the oropharyngeal membrane to the cloacal membrane (Fig. 15.5) and is divided into the pharyngeal gut, foregut, midgut, and hindgut.
- The pharyngeal gut gives rise to the pharynx and related glands (see Chapter 17).
- The **foregut** gives rise to the esophagus, the trachea and lung buds, the stomach, and the duodenum proximal to the entrance of the bile duct. In addition, the liver, pancreas, and biliary apparatus develop as outgrowths of the endodermal epithelium of the upper part of the duodenum (Fig. 15.15).
- Because the upper part of the foregut is divided by a septum (the **tracheoesophageal septum**) into the esophagus posteriorly and the trachea and lung buds anteriorly, deviation of the septum may result in abnormal openings between the trachea and esophagus.
- Liver: The epithelial liver cords and biliary system growing out into the septum transversum (Fig. 15.15) differentiate into parenchyma. **Hematopoietic cells** (present in the liver in greater numbers before birth than afterward), the Kupffer cells, and connective tissue cells originate in the mesoderm.
- Pancreas: The **pancreas** develops from a **ventral bud** and a **dorsal bud** that later fuse to form the definitive pancreas (Figs. 15.19 and 15.20). Sometimes, the two parts surround the duodenum (annular pancreas), causing constriction of the gut (see Fig. 15.23).
- **The midgut** forms the **primary intestinal loop** (Fig. 15.24), gives rise to the duodenum distal to the entrance of the bile duct, and continues to the junction of the proximal two-thirds of the transverse colon with the distal third.
- At its apex, the primary loop remains temporarily in open connection with the yolk sac through the **vitelline duct**.
- During the sixth week, the loop grows so rapidly that it protrudes into the umbilical cord (**physiological herniation**) (Fig. 15.26).

(Continued)

Part 2

- During the 10th week, it returns into the abdominal cavity. While these processes are occurring, the midgut loop rotates 270° counterclockwise (Fig. 15.27). Remnants of the vitelline duct, failure of the midgut to return to the abdominal cavity, malrotation, stenosis, and duplication of parts of the gut are common abnormalities.
- **The hindgut** gives rise to the region from the distal third of the transverse colon to the upper part of the anal canal; the distal part of the **anal canal;** originates from ectoderm.
- The hindgut enters the posterior region of the **cloaca** (future anorectal canal), and the **allantois** enters the anterior region (future **urogenital sinus**).
- The **urorectal septum** will divide the two regions (Fig. 15.36) and breakdown of the cloacal membrane covering this area will provide communication to the exterior for the anus and urogenital sinus.
- Abnormalities in the size of the posterior region of the cloaca shift the entrance of the anus anteriorly, causing rectovaginal and rectourethral fistulas and atresias (Fig. 15.37).
- The following table summarizes the development components of GIT.

**Derivatives of the Gastrointestinal Tract**

| Gut | | Derivatives | Special remarks |
|---|---|---|---|
| **Pharyngeal gut** (Chapter 17) | | Pharynx | |
| **Foregut** | | • Esophagus<br>• Stomach<br>• Duodenum (proximal part)<br>• Liver<br>• Gallbladder<br>• Bile duct<br>• Pancreas<br>• Trachea and lung bud | • Kupffer cells, hematopoietic cells, and connective tissue cells of liver are derived from the mesoderm of septum transversum |
| **Midgut** | Cephalic limb | • Distal part of the duodenum<br>• Jejunum<br>• Part of the ileum | • Nil |
| | Caudal limb | • Lower portion of the ileum<br>• Cecum<br>• Appendix<br>• Ascending colon<br>• Proximal two-thirds of the transverse colon | |
| **Hindgut** | | • Distal one-third of the transverse colon<br>• Descending colon<br>• Sigmoid<br>• Rectum<br>• Upper part of anal canal<br>• Endoderm also forms the internal lining of the bladder and urethra | • Distal part of anal canal: From ectoderm |

## Self-Assessment

### Comprehensive Questions

1. Write down the embryological basis of malrotation defects of the midgut.
2. Write down the embryological basis of annular pancreas.
3. Name the derivatives of secondary yolk sac.

### Problem Solving Questions

1. Prenatal ultrasound showed polyhydramnios at 36 weeks, and at birth, the infant had excessive fluids in its mouth and difficulty breathing. What birth defect might cause these conditions?
2. Prenatal ultrasound at 20 weeks revealed a midline mass that appeared to contain intestines and was membrane bound. What diagnosis would you make, and what would be the prognosis for this infant?
3. At birth, a baby girl has meconium in her vagina and no anal opening. What type of birth defect does she have, and what was its embryological origin?

### Multiple Choice Questions

1. Which of the following is a derivative of midgut?
   (a) Esophagus
   (b) Stomach
   (c) Ascending colon
   (d) Descending colon

2. Which organ forms in the dorsal mesogastrium?
   (a) Liver
   (b) Spleen
   (c) Stomach
   (d) Gallbladder
3. In normal gut rotation, the part of the midgut to enter the abdomen first is
   (a) Ileum and jejunum
   (b) Ascending colon
   (c) Transverse colon
   (d) Cecum
4. The stomach rotates during development in which of the following ways?
   (a) 90° clockwise in the anteroposterior axis
   (b) 90° anticlockwise in the anteroposterior axis
   (c) 90° in a transverse plane
   (d) 180° in the anteroposterior axis
5. Umbilical fistula is associated with
   (a) Allantois duct
   (b) Vitelline duct
   (c) Ductus venosus
   (d) Neural tube
6. The part of the pancreas derived from the ventral pancreatic bud is
   (a) Upper part of the head
   (b) Lower part of the head
   (c) Body
   (d) Tail
7. The stomach acquires its adult shape as it rotates around its longitudinal axis. Which of the following events does not result from this rotation?
   (a) The ventral border of the stomach moves to the right.
   (b) The dorsal border moves to the left.
   (c) The pyloric part moves to the left.
   (d) The posterior wall of the stomach grows faster than the anterior wall.
8. Physiological umbilical hernia occur at
   (a) 6th month
   (b) 10th month
   (c) 10th week
   (d) 6th week
9. In subhepatic cecum
   (a) The cecum ascends up to the inferior border of the liver.
   (b) The cecum fails to descend to the right iliac fossa.
   (c) The cecum enters the abdomen first following the physiological hernia.
   (d) The cecum is stuck at the prearterial segment and fails to move.
10. Transcription factor for differentiation of the duodenum in the gut tube is
   (a) SHH
   (b) FGF
   (c) PTX1
   (d) PDX2
11. The fascial plane between the visceral peritoneum and the parietal peritoneum in the abdomen is
   (a) Toldt fascia
   (b) Iliolumbar fascia
   (c) Falciform ligament
   (d) Phrenicocolic ligament
12. All of the following statements are true for annular pancreas except
   (a) Pancreatic tissue envelops the second part of the duodenum.
   (b) It can cause obstructive jaundice.
   (c) Migration of the dorsal pancreatic bud is to the right side
   (d) The ventral pancreas has two parts; one part rotates to the left and the other part goes in the opposite direction.
13. In a left-sided colon
   (a) The cecum is the first to enter after physiological hernia.
   (b) The cecum is the last to enter.
   (c) Transverse colon lies posterior.
   (d) Ascending and descending colon are intraperitoneal.
14. Which of the following is a derivative of ventral mesogastrium?
   (a) Greater omentum
   (b) Transverse mesocolon
   (c) Mesentery
   (d) Lesser omentum
15. Anal canal is formed by
   (a) Cloaca
   (b) Hindgut
   (c) Surface ectoderm and endoderm
   (d) Upper two-thirds from the endoderm and lower one-third from the proctodeum
16. Angiogenesis starts in
   (a) Secondary yolk sac
   (b) Liver
   (c) Spleen
   (d) Amniotic cavity

**Answers**

1. (c) 2. (b) 3. (a) 4. (a) 5. (b) 6. (b) 7. (c) 8. (d) 9. (b) 10. (d) 11. (a) 12. (c) 13. (a) 14. (d) 15. (d) 16. (a)

Part 2

CHAPTER

# 16 Urogenital System

## Specific Learning Objectives

- The sequential development of three excretory systems: pronephros, mesonephros, metanephros
- Formation of the mesonephric duct
- Structures formed from the ureteric bud and metanephros
- Formation of permanent kidney, its positional changes, and time of onset of function
- Disorders associated with kidney development
- Division of cloaca
- Adult derivatives of the various parts of the urogenital sinus in males and females
- Formation of the paramesonephric duct
- Fate of mesonephric and paramesonephric ducts in male and female
- Formation of external genitalia
- Anatomical basis of hypospadias and epispadias

## Competencies Covered

AN52.7 Describe the development of the urinary system.
AN52.8 Describe the development of the male and female reproductive system.



Functionally, the urogenital system can be divided into two entirely different components: the **urinary system** and the **genital system**. Embryologically and anatomically, however, they are intimately interwoven. Both develop from a common mesodermal ridge (**intermediate mesoderm**) along the posterior wall of the abdominal cavity, and initially, the excretory ducts of both systems enter a common cavity, the cloaca (Fig. 16.1). The intermediate mesoderm lies between the paraxial mesoderm on the medial side and the lateral plate mesoderm on the lateral side (Fig. 16.1).

## URINARY SYSTEM

### Kidney Systems

Three slightly overlapping kidney systems are formed in a cranial-to-caudal sequence during intrauterine life in humans:

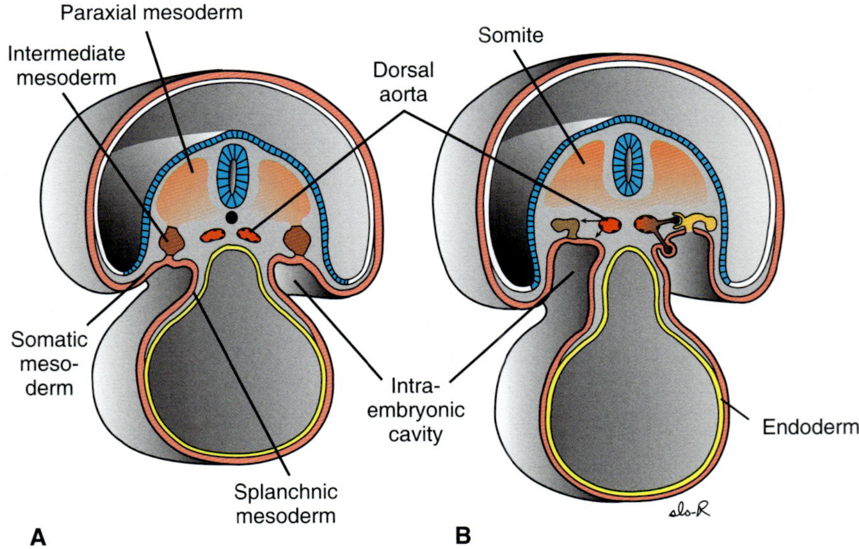


**FIGURE 16.1** Transverse sections through embryos at various stages of development showing formation of nephric tubules. **A.** 21 days. **B.** Transverse section through embryo at 21 days showing the position of the intermediate mesoderm. Note formation of external and internal glomeruli and the open connection between the intraembryonic cavity and the nephric tubule.

**Table 16.1 Sequential Development of the Three Nephric Systems in the Fetus**

| Excretory Organ | Time | Position | Function |
|---|---|---|---|
| Pronephros | Fourth week | Cervical region | Non-functioning |
| Mesonephros | Fourth week | Thoracic and upper lumbar regions | Functions |
| Metanephros | Fifth week | Lower lumbar and sacral regions | Permanent kidney |

the **pronephros**, **mesonephros**, and **metanephros**. The first of these systems is rudimentary and nonfunctional; the second may function for a short time during the early fetal period; the metanephros forms the permanent kidney (Table 16.1).

### Pronephros

At the beginning of the fourth week, the pronephros is represented by 7 to 10 solid cell groups in the cervical region (Figs. 16.1 and 16.2). These groups form vestigial excretory units that regress before more caudal ones are formed. By the end of the fourth week, all indications of the pronephric system have disappeared.

### Mesonephros

The mesonephros and mesonephric ducts are derived from intermediate mesoderm from upper thoracic to upper lumbar (L3) segments (Fig. 16.2). Early in the fourth week of development, during regression of the pronephric system, the first excretory tubules of the mesonephros appear. They lengthen rapidly, form an S-shaped loop, and acquire a tuft of capillaries that will form a **glomerulus** at their medial extremity (Fig. 16.3*A*). Around the glomerulus, the tubules form **Bowman capsule**, and together these structures constitute a **renal corpuscle.** Laterally, the tubule enters the longitudinal collecting duct known as the **mesonephric** or **Wolffian duct** (Figs. 16.2 and 16.3).

In the middle of the second month, the mesonephros forms a large ovoid organ on each side of the midline (Fig. 16.3). Because the developing gonad is on its medial side, the ridge formed by both organs is known as the **urogenital ridge** (Fig. 16.3). The mesonephric kidney is functional until 12 weeks when the metanephric kidney takes over the urine production. While caudal tubules are still differentiating, cranial tubules and glomeruli show degenerative changes, and by the end of the second month, the majority have disappeared. In the male, a few of the caudal tubules and the mesonephric duct persist and participate in formation of the genital system, but they disappear in the female.

### Metanephros: The Definitive Kidney

The third urinary organ, the **metanephros** or **permanent kidney**, appears in the fifth week. Its excretory units develop from **metanephric mesoderm** (Fig. 16.4) in the same manner as in the mesonephric system. The development of the duct system differs from that of the other kidney systems.

### Collecting System

Collecting ducts of the permanent kidney develop from the **ureteric bud**, an outgrowth of the mesonephric duct close



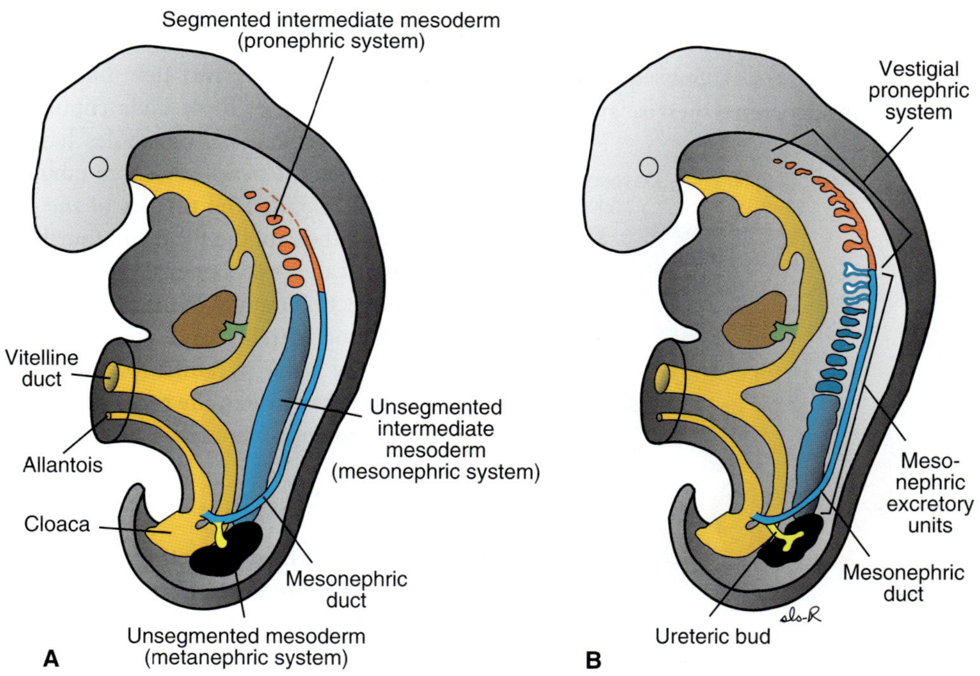


**FIGURE 16.2 A.** Relationship of the intermediate mesoderm of the pronephric, mesonephric, and metanephric systems. In cervical and upper thoracic regions, intermediate mesoderm is segmented; in lower thoracic, lumbar, and sacral regions, it forms a solid, unsegmented mass of tissue, the nephrogenic cord. Note the longitudinal collecting duct, formed initially by the pronephros but later by the mesonephros (mesonephric duct). **B.** Excretory tubules of the pronephric and mesonephric systems in a 5-week embryo.

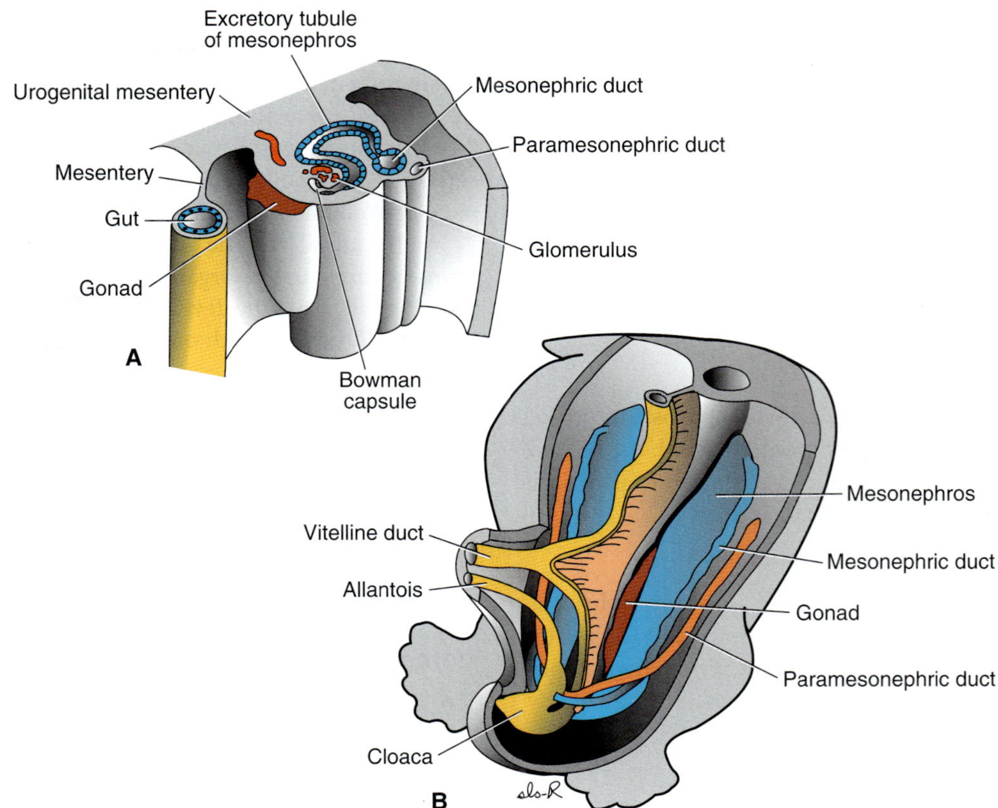


**FIGURE 16.3 A.** Transverse section through the urogenital ridge in the lower thoracic region of a 5-week embryo showing formation of an excretory tubule of the mesonephric system. Note the appearance of Bowman capsule and the gonadal ridge. The mesonephros and gonad are attached to the posterior abdominal wall by a broad urogenital mesentery. **B.** Relation of the gonad and the mesonephros. Note the size of the mesonephros. The mesonephric duct (Wolffian duct) runs along the lateral side of the mesonephros.



to its entrance to the cloaca (Fig. 16.4). The bud penetrates the metanephric tissue, which is molded over its distal end as a metanephric tissue cap (Fig. 16.4). Subsequently, the bud dilates, forming the primitive **renal pelvis**, and splits into cranial and caudal portions, the future **major calyces** (Fig. 16.5*A,B*).

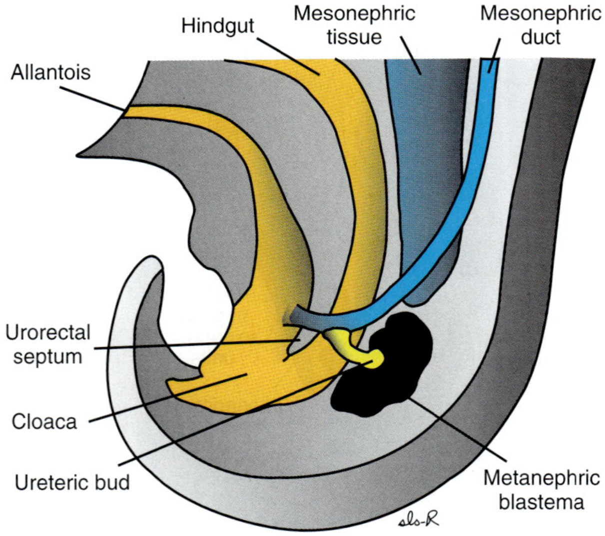

**FIGURE 16.4** Relation of the hindgut and cloaca at the end of the fifth week. The ureteric bud penetrates the metanephric mesoderm (blastema).

Each calyx forms two new buds while penetrating the metanephric tissue. These buds continue to subdivide until 12 or more generations of tubules have formed (Fig. 16.5). Meanwhile, at the periphery, more tubules form until the end of the fifth month. The tubules of the second order enlarge and absorb those of the third and fourth generations, forming the **minor calyces** of the renal pelvis. During further development, collecting tubules of the fifth and successive generations elongate considerably and converge on the minor calyx, forming the **renal pyramid** (Fig. 16.5*D*). **The ureteric bud gives rise to the ureter, the renal pelvis, the major and minor calyces, and approximately 1 to 3 million collecting tubules.**

## Excretory System

Each newly formed collecting tubule is covered at its distal end by a **metanephric tissue cap** (Fig. 16.6*A*). Under the inductive influence of the tubule, cells of the tissue cap form small vesicles, the **renal vesicles**, which in turn give rise to small S-shaped tubules (Fig. 16.6*B,C*). Capillaries grow into the pocket at one end of the S and differentiate into **glomeruli**. These tubules, together with their glomeruli, form **nephrons** or **excretory units**. The proximal end of each nephron forms

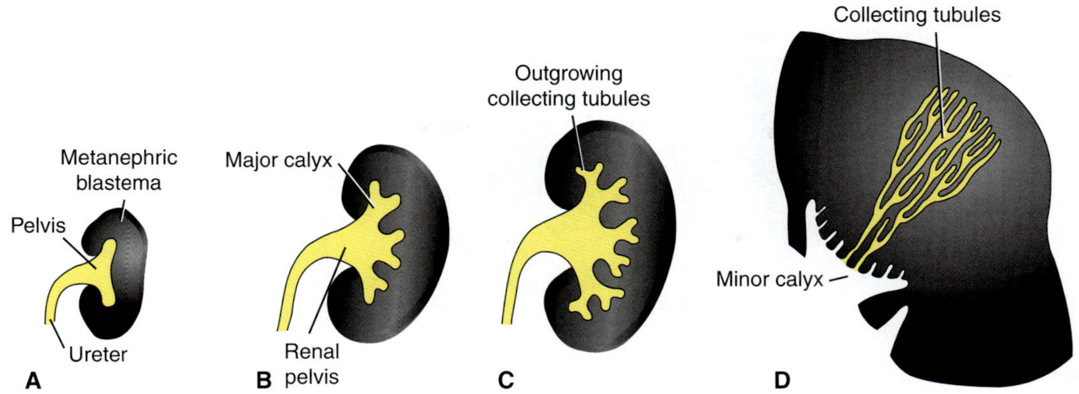


**FIGURE 16.5** Development of the renal pelvis, calyces, and collecting tubules of the metanephros. **A.** 6 weeks. **B.** At the end of the sixth week. **C.** 7 weeks. **D.** Newborn. Note the pyramid form of the collecting tubules entering the minor calyx.

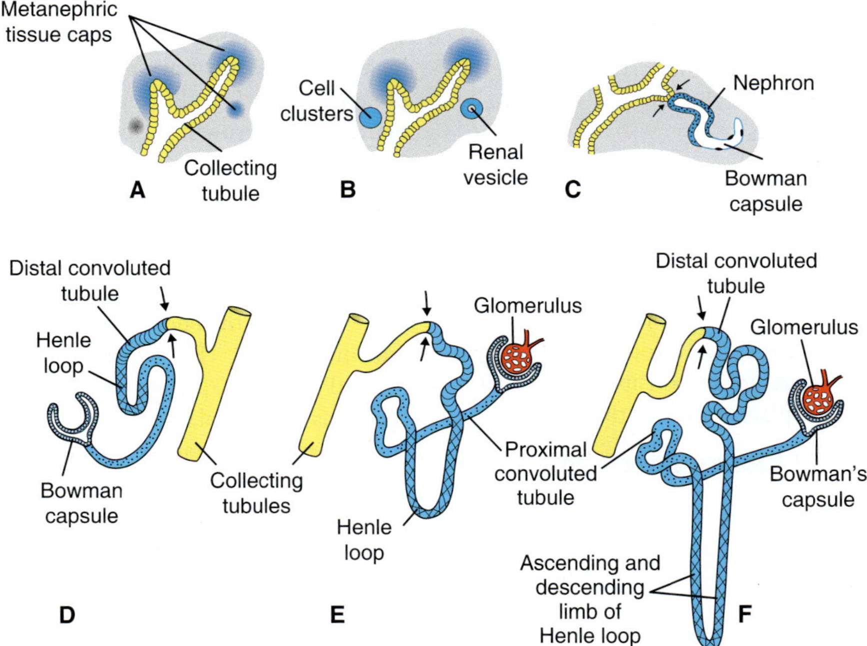


**FIGURE 16.6** **A–F.** Development of a metanephric excretory unit. *Arrows*, the place where the excretory unit (*blue*) establishes an open communication with the collecting system (*yellow*), allowing flow of urine from the glomerulus into the collecting ducts.

**Bowman capsule**, which is deeply indented by a glomerulus (Fig. 16.6*C,D*). The distal end forms an open connection with one of the collecting tubules, establishing a passageway from Bowman capsule to the collecting unit. Continuous lengthening of the excretory tubule results in formation of the **proximal convoluted tubule**, **loop of Henle**, and **distal convoluted tubule** (Fig. 16.6*E,F*). Hence, the permanent kidney develops from two sources: (1) **metanephric mesoderm**, and (2) the **ureteric bud**, which gives rise to the collecting system.

Nephrons are formed until birth, at which time there are approximately 1 million in each kidney. Urine production begins in the 12th week, following differentiation of the glomerular capillaries, which start to form by the 10th week. At birth, the kidneys have a lobulated appearance, but the lobulation disappears during infancy as a result of further growth of the nephrons, although there is no increase in their number.

The process of nephron formation (nephrogenesis) is complete by birth in humans. Studies have demonstrated that there are approximately 250,000 to more than 2 million nephrons in human beings. The wide variation of nephrons is probably influenced by factors like genetic, environmental, sex, racial, and ethnic background. There are a number of nephrons lost during aging. Suboptimal nephron endowment has been associated with an increased risk of cardiovascular and renal diseases in adults.

## Position of the Kidney

The kidney, initially in the pelvic region, later shifts to a more cranial position in the abdomen. This **ascent of the kidney** is caused by diminution of body curvature and by growth

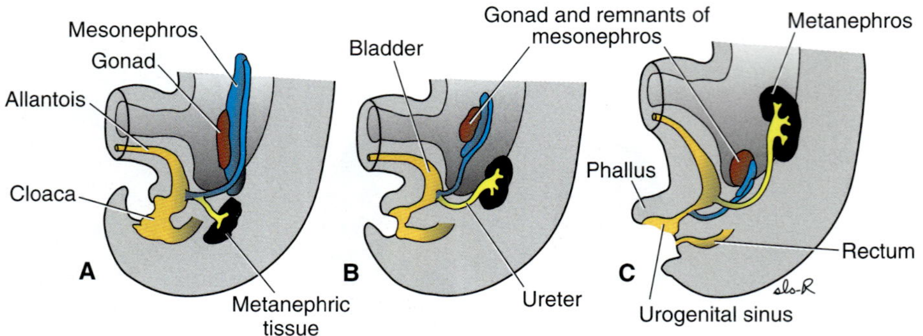


**FIGURE 16.7 A–C.** Ascent of the kidneys. Note the change in position between the mesonephric and metanephric systems. The mesonephric system degenerates almost entirely, and only a few remnants persist in close contact with the gonad. In both male and female embryos, the gonads descend from their original level to a much lower position.

of the body in the lumbar and sacral regions (Fig. 16.7). In the pelvis, the metanephros receives its arterial supply from a pelvic branch of the aorta. During its ascent to the abdominal level, it is vascularized by arteries that originate from the aorta at continuously higher levels. The lower vessels usually degenerate, but some may remain.

## Function of the Kidney

The definitive kidney formed from the metanephros becomes functional near the 12th week. Urine is passed into the amniotic cavity and mixes with the amniotic fluid. The fluid is swallowed by the fetus and recycles through the kidneys. During fetal life, the kidneys are not responsible for excretion of waste products because the placenta serves this function.

## Molecular Regulation of Kidney Development

As with most organs, differentiation of the kidney involves epithelial mesenchymal interactions. In this example, epithelium of the ureteric bud from the mesonephros interacts with mesenchyme of the metanephric blastema (Fig. 16.8). The mesenchyme expresses ***WT1***, a transcription factor that makes this tissue competent to respond to induction by the ureteric bud. *WT1* also regulates production of **glial-derived neurotrophic growth factor (GDNF)** and **hepatocyte growth factor (HGF**, or **scatter factor**) by the mesenchyme, and these proteins stimulate branching and growth of the ureteric buds (Fig. 16.8*A*). The **tyrosine kinase receptors RET**, for GDNF, and **MET**, for HGF, are synthesized by the epithelium of the ureteric buds, establishing signaling pathways between the two tissues. In turn, the buds induce the mesenchyme via fibroblast growth factor 2 (FGF2) and bone morphogenetic protein 7 (BMP7) (Fig. 16.8*A*). Both of these growth factors block apoptosis and stimulate proliferation in the metanephric mesenchyme while maintaining production of *WT1*. Conversion of the mesenchyme to an epithelium for nephron formation is also mediated by the ureteric buds through expression of ***WNT9B*** and ***WNT6***, which upregulate ***PAX2*** and ***WNT4*** in



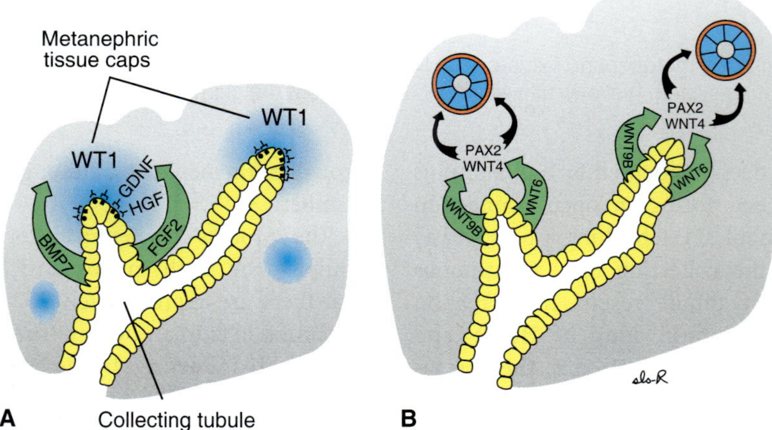


**FIGURE 16.8** Genes involved in differentiation of the kidney. **A.** *WT1*, expressed by the mesenchyme, enables this tissue to respond to induction by the ureteric bud. Glial-derived neurotrophic factor (GDNF) and hepatocyte growth factor (HGF), also produced by the mesenchyme, interact through their receptors, RET and MET, respectively, in the ureteric bud epithelium, to stimulate growth of the bud and maintain the interactions. The growth factors fibroblast growth factor 2 (FGF2) and bone morphogenetic protein 7 (*BMP7*) stimulate proliferation of the mesenchyme and maintain *WT1* expression. **B.** WNT9B and WNT6 secreted by branches of the ureteric bud epithelium cause upregulation of *PAX2* and *WNT4* in the surrounding mesenchyme. In turn, these genes cause the mesenchyme to epithelialize (*PAX2*) and to then form tubules (*WNT4*). Changes in the extracellular matrix also occur, such that laminin and type IV collagen form a basement membrane (*orange*) for the epithelial cells.

## Clinical Correlates

### Renal Tumors and Defects

**Wilms tumor** is a cancer of the kidneys that usually affects children by 5 years of age but may also occur in the fetus. Wilms tumor is due to mutations in the *WT1* gene on 11p13, and it may be associated with other abnormalities and syndromes. For example, **WAGR syndrome** is characterized by **W**ilms tumor, **a**niridia, **g**onadoblastomas (tumors of the gonads), and mental **r**etardation (intellectual disability). The constellation of defects is due to a microdeletion in chromosome 11 that includes both the *PAX6* (aniridia) and *WT1* genes that are only 700 kb apart. Similarly, **Denys-Drash syndrome** consists of renal failure, ambiguous genitalia, and Wilms tumor.

**Renal dysplasias** and **agenesis** are a spectrum of severe malformations that represent the primary diseases requiring dialysis and transplantation in the first years of life. **Multicystic dysplastic kidney** is one example of this group of abnormalities in which numerous ducts are surrounded by undifferentiated cells. Nephrons fail to develop, and the ureteric bud fails to branch, so that the collecting ducts never form. In some cases, these defects cause involution of the kidneys and **renal agenesis**. Renal agenesis may also arise if the interaction between the metanephric mesoderm and the ureteric bud fails to occur. Normally, during the interaction, **GDNF** produced by the metanephric mesoderm produces branching and growth of the ureteric bud. Thus, mutations in genes that regulate *GDNF* expression of signaling may result in renal agenesis. Examples include the gene *SALL1*, responsible for Townes-Brock syndrome; *PAX2* that causes renal coloboma syndrome; and *EYA1* that results in branchiootorenal syndrome. Bilateral renal agenesis, which occurs in 1/10,000 births, results in renal failure. The baby presents with **Potter sequence**, characterized by anuria, oligohydramnios (decreased volume of amniotic fluid), and hypoplastic lungs secondary to the oligohydramnios. In 85% of cases, other severe defects, including absence or abnormalities of the vagina and uterus, vas deferens, and seminal vesicles, accompany this condition. Common associated defects in other systems include cardiac anomalies, tracheal and duodenal atresias, cleft lip and palate, and brain abnormalities. Because of the oligohydramnios, the uterine cavity is compressed resulting in a characteristic appearance of the fetus, including a flattened face (Potter facies) and club feet.

In **congenital polycystic kidney disease** (Fig. 16.9), numerous cysts form. It may be inherited as an autosomal recessive or autosomal dominant disorder or may be caused by other factors. **Autosomal recessive polycystic kidney disease (ARPKD)**, which occurs in 1/5,000 births, is a progressive disorder in which cysts form from collecting ducts. The kidneys become very large, and renal failure occurs in infancy or childhood. In **autosomal dominant polycystic kidney disease (ADPKD)**, cysts form from all segments of the nephron and usually do not cause renal failure until adulthood. The autosomal dominant disease is more common (1/500 to 1/1,000 births) but less progressive than the autosomal recessive disease. Both types of disease are linked to mutations in genes that encode proteins localized in cilia and that are important for ciliary function. These abnormalities belong to a growing group of diseases called the **ciliopathies** that are due to mutations in cilia-related proteins. These disorders include **Bardet-Biedl syndrome**, characterized by renal cysts, obesity, intellectual disability, and limb defects, and **Meckel-Gruber syndrome**, characterized by renal cysts, hydrocephalus, microphthalmia, cleft palate, absence of the olfactory tract, and polydactyly. Because cilia are present on most cell types and in most tissues, many organ systems can be affected by abnormalities in ciliary structure and function.

Duplication of the ureter results from early splitting of the ureteric bud (Fig. 16.10). Splitting may be partial or complete, and metanephric tissue may be divided into two parts, each with its own renal pelvis and ureter. More frequently, however, the two parts have a number of lobes in common as a result of intermingling of collecting tubules. In rare cases, one ureter opens into the bladder, and the other is ectopic, entering the vagina, urethra, or vestibule (Fig. 16.10*C*). This abnormality results from development of two ureteric buds. One of the buds usually has a normal position, whereas the abnormal bud moves down together with the mesonephric duct. Thus, it has a low, abnormal entrance in the bladder, urethra, vagina, or epididymal region.

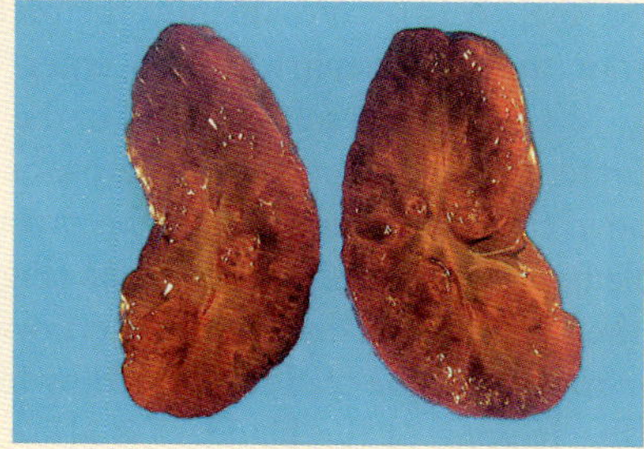

**FIGURE 16.9** Surface view of a fetal kidney with multiple cysts characteristic of polycystic kidney disease.

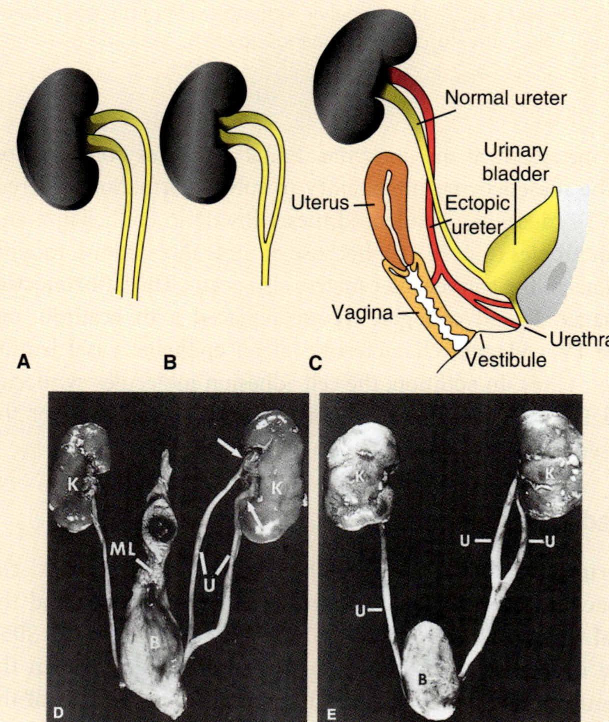


**FIGURE 16.10 A,B.** A complete and a partial double ureter (*U*). **C.** Possible sites of ectopic ureteral openings in the vagina, urethra, and vestibule. **D,E.** Photomicrographs of complete and partial duplications of the ureters. *Arrows*, duplicated hilum; *B*, bladder; *K*, kidneys; *ML*, median umbilical ligament.

Part 2

## Clinical Correlates

### Abnormal Location of the Kidneys

During their ascent, the kidneys pass through the arterial fork formed by the umbilical arteries, but occasionally, one of them fails to do so. Remaining in the pelvis close to the common iliac artery, it is known as a **pelvic kidney** (Fig. 16.11*A*). Sometimes, the kidneys are pushed so close together during their passage through the umbilical arterial fork, that the lower poles fuse, forming a **horseshoe kidney** (Fig. 16.11*B,C*). The horseshoe kidney is usually at the level of the lower lumbar vertebrae because its ascent is prevented by the root of the inferior mesenteric artery (Fig. 16.11*B*). The ureters arise from the anterior surface of the kidney and pass ventral to the isthmus in a caudal direction. Horseshoe kidney is found in 1/600 people.

**Accessory renal arteries** are common; they derive from the persistence of embryonic vessels that formed during ascent of the kidneys. These arteries usually arise from the aorta and enter the superior or inferior poles of the kidneys.

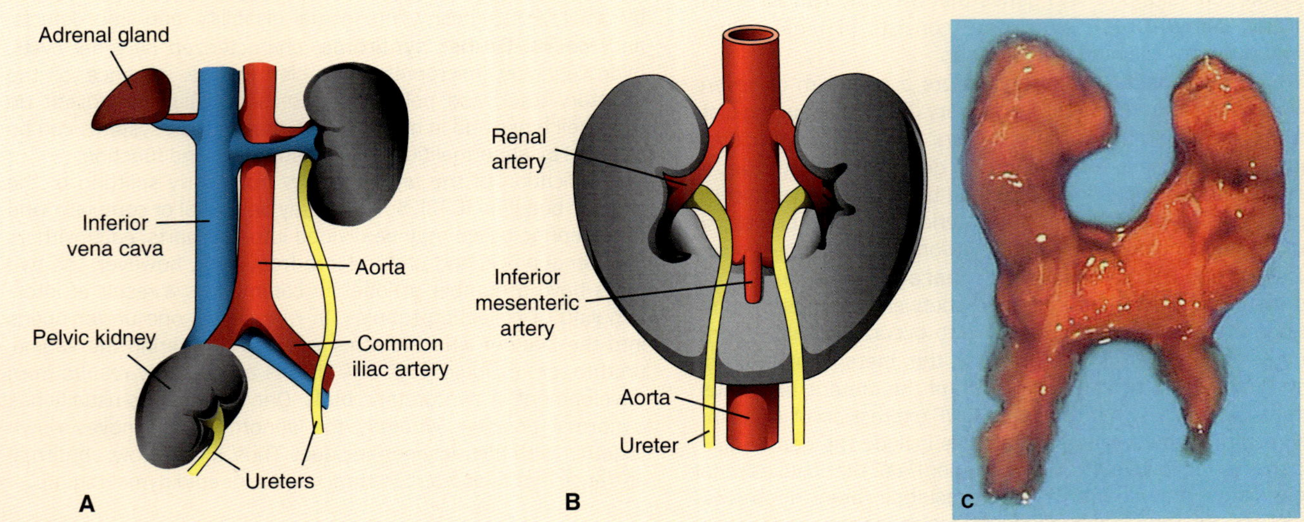


**FIGURE 16.11 A.** Unilateral pelvic kidney showing the position of the adrenal gland on the affected side. **B,C.** Drawing and photomicrograph, respectively, of horseshoe kidneys showing the position of the inferior mesenteric artery.

the metanephric mesenchyme. *PAX2* promotes condensation of the mesenchyme preparatory to tubule formation, whereas *WNT4* causes the condensed mesenchyme to epithelialize and form tubules (Fig. 16.8*B*). Because of these interactions, modifications in the extracellular matrix also occur. Thus, **fibronectin**, **collagen I**, and **collagen III** are replaced with **laminin** and **type IV collagen**, characteristic of an epithelial basal lamina (Fig. 16.8*B*). In addition, the cell adhesion molecules **syndecan** and **E-cadherin**, which are essential for condensation of the mesenchyme into an epithelium, are synthesized.

## Bladder and Urethra

During the fourth to seventh weeks of development, the **cloaca** divides into the **urogenital sinus** anteriorly and the **anal canal** posteriorly (Fig. 16.12) (see Chapter 15, p. 205). **The urorectal septum** is a layer of mesoderm between the primitive anal canal and the urogenital sinus. The tip of the septum will form the **perineal body**, **a site of insertion of several perineal muscles** (Fig. 16.12*C*). Three portions of the urogenital sinus can be distinguished; the upper and largest part is the **urinary bladder** (Fig. 16.13*A*). Initially, the bladder is continuous with the allantois, but when the lumen of the allantois is obliterated, a thick, fibrous cord, the **urachus** (Fig. 16.13*B*), remains and connects the apex of the bladder with the umbilicus (Fig. 16.13*B*). In the adult, it forms the **median umbilical ligament**. The next part is a rather narrow canal, the **pelvic part of the urogenital sinus**, which in the male gives rise to the **prostatic** and **membranous** parts of the **urethra**. The last part is the **phallic part** of the urogenital sinus. It is flattened from side to side, and as the genital tubercle grows, this part of the sinus will be pulled ventrally (Fig. 16.13*A*). (Development of the phallic part of the urogenital sinus differs greatly between the two sexes.)

During differentiation of the cloaca, the caudal portions of the mesonephric ducts are absorbed into the wall of the urinary bladder (Fig. 16.14). Consequently, the ureters, initially outgrowths from the mesonephric ducts, enter the bladder separately (Fig. 16.14*B*). As a result of ascent of the kidneys, the orifices of the ureters move farther cranially; those of the mesonephric ducts move close together to enter the prostatic urethra and in the male become the **ejaculatory ducts** (Fig. 16.14*C,D*). Because both the mesonephric ducts and ureters originate in the mesoderm, the mucosa of the bladder formed by incorporation of the ducts (the **trigone** of the bladder) is also mesodermal. With time, the mesodermal lining of the trigone is replaced by endodermal epithelium, so that finally, the inside of the bladder is completely lined with endodermal epithelium.

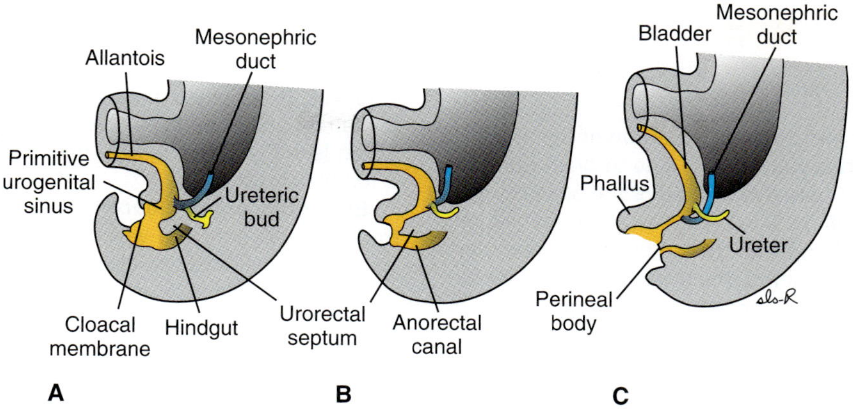


**FIGURE 16.12** Divisions of the cloaca into the urogenital sinus and anorectal canal. The mesonephric duct is gradually absorbed into the wall of the urogenital sinus, and the ureters enter separately. **A.** At the end of the fifth week. **B.** 7 weeks. **C.** 8 weeks.

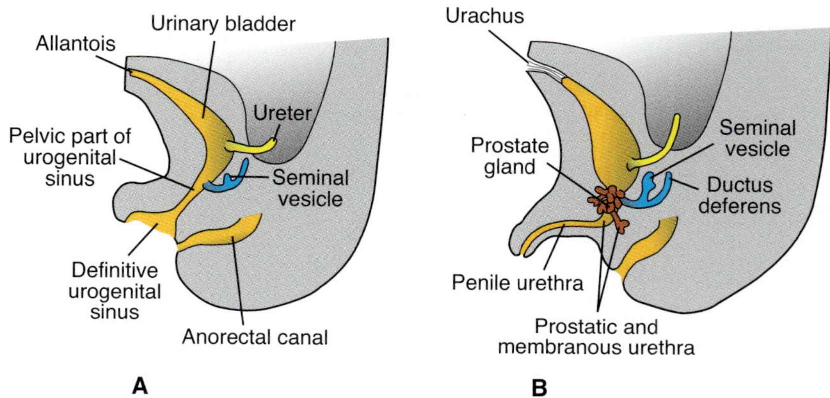


**FIGURE 16.13 A.** Development of the urogenital sinus into the urinary bladder and definitive urogenital sinus. **B.** In the male, the definitive urogenital sinus develops into the penile urethra. The prostate gland is formed by buds from the urethra, and seminal vesicles are formed by budding from the ductus deferens.



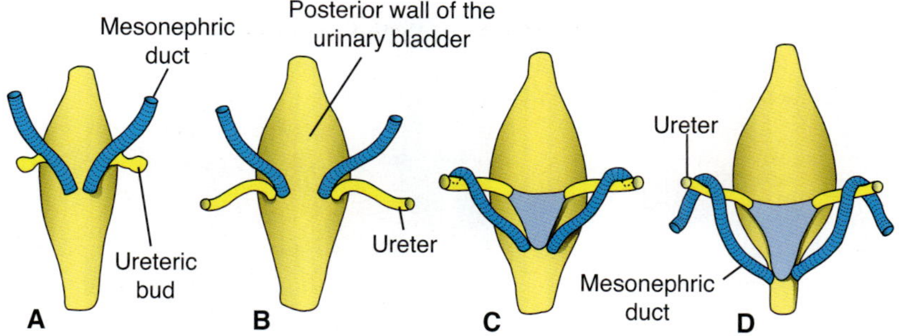


**FIGURE 16.14** Dorsal views of the bladder showing the relation of the ureters and mesonephric ducts during development. Initially, the ureters are formed by an outgrowth of the mesonephric duct **(A)**, but with time, they assume a separate entrance into the urinary bladder **(B–D)**. Note the trigone of the bladder formed by incorporation of the mesonephric ducts **(C,D)**.

The epithelium of the urethra in both sexes originates in the endoderm; the surrounding connective and smooth muscle tissue is derived from visceral mesoderm. At the end of the third month, epithelium of the prostatic urethra begins to proliferate and forms a number of outgrowths that penetrate the surrounding mesenchyme. In the male, these buds form the **prostate gland** (Fig. 16.13*B*). In the female, the cranial part of the urethra gives rise to the **urethral** and **paraurethral glands.**

## GENITAL SYSTEM

Sex differentiation is a complex process that involves many genes, including some that are autosomal. The key to sexual dimorphism is the Y chromosome, which contains the testis-determining gene called the ***SRY* (sex-determining region on Y) gene** on its short arm (Yp11). The protein product of this gene is a transcription factor initiating a cascade of downstream genes that determine the fate of rudimentary

## Clinical Correlates

### Bladder Defects

When the lumen of the intraembryonic portion of the allantois persists, a **urachal fistula** may cause urine to drain from the umbilicus (Fig. 16.15*A*). If only a local area of the allantois persists, secretory activity of its lining results in a cystic dilation, a **urachal cyst** (Fig. 16.15*B*). When the lumen in the upper part persists, it forms a **urachal sinus**. The sinus is usually not continuous with the lumen of the urinary bladder but the fistula is (Fig. 16.15*A,C*).

**Exstrophy of the bladder** (Fig. 16.16*A*) is a ventral body wall defect in which the bladder mucosa is exposed. Epispadias is a constant feature (Fig. 16.16*A*), and the open urinary tract extends along the dorsal aspect of the penis through the bladder to the umbilicus. Exstrophy of the bladder is probably due to failure of the lateral body wall folds to close in the midline in the pelvic region (see Chapter 7, p. 81). This anomaly is rare, occurring in 2/10,000 live births.

**Exstrophy of the cloaca** (Fig. 16.16*B*) is a more severe ventral body wall defect in which progression and closure of the lateral body wall folds are disrupted to a greater degree than is observed in bladder exstrophy (see Chapter 7, p. 81). In addition to the closure defect, normal development of the urorectal septum is altered, such that anal canal malformations and imperforate anus occur (see Chapter 15, p. 208). Furthermore, because the body folds do not fuse, the genital swellings are widely spaced resulting in defects in the external genitalia (Fig. 16.16*B*). Occurrence of the defect is rare (1/30,000).

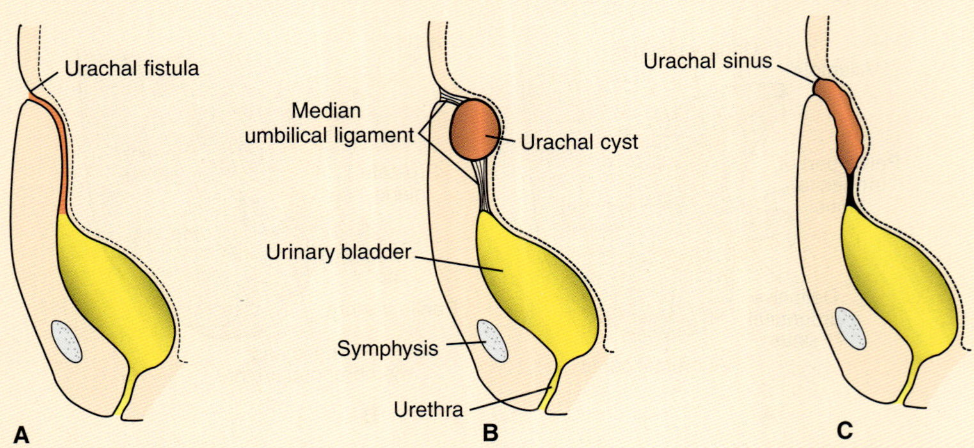


**FIGURE 16.15 A.** Urachal fistula. **B.** Urachal cyst. **C.** Urachal sinus. The sinus may or may not be in open communication with the urinary bladder.

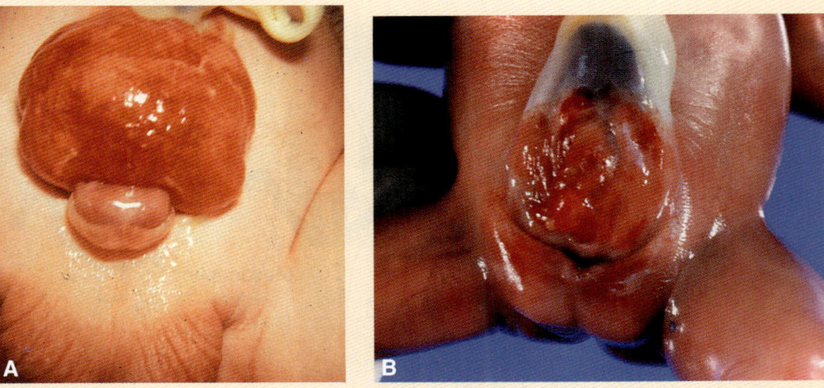


**FIGURE 16.16 A.** Exstrophy of the bladder. **B.** Cloacal exstrophy in a newborn.

sexual organs. The SRY protein is the **testis-determining factor**; under its influence, male development occurs; in its absence, female development is established.

## Gonads

Although the sex of the embryo is determined genetically at the time of fertilization, the gonads do not acquire male or female morphological characteristics until the seventh week of development.

Gonads appear initially as a pair of longitudinal ridges, the **genital** or **gonadal ridges** (Fig. 16.17). They are formed by proliferation of the epithelium and a condensation of underlying mesenchyme. **Germ cells** do not appear in the genital ridges until the sixth week of development.

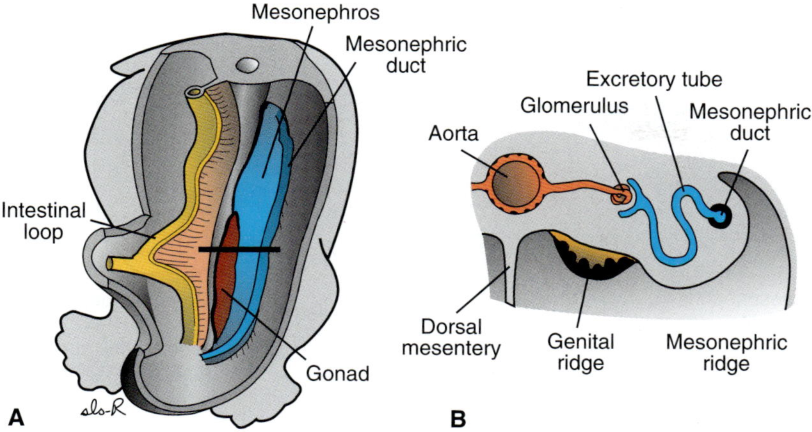


**FIGURE 16.17 A.** Relation of the genital ridge and the mesonephros showing location of the mesonephric duct. **B.** Transverse section through the mesonephros and genital ridge at the level indicated in **(A)**.

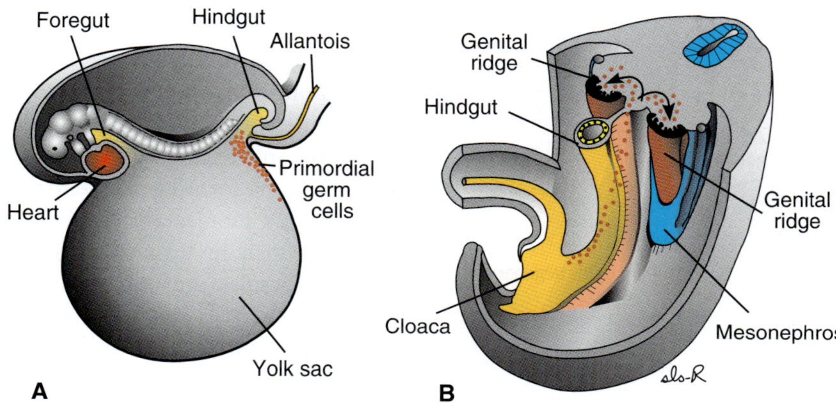


**FIGURE 16.18 A.** A 3-week embryo showing the primordial germ cells in the wall of the yolk sac close to the attachment of the allantois. **B.** Migrational path of the primordial germ cells along the wall of the hindgut and the dorsal mesentery into the genital ridge.

**Primordial germ cells** originate in the epiblast, migrate through the primitive streak, and by the third week, reside among endoderm cells in the wall of the yolk sac close to the allantois (Fig. 16.18*A*). During the fourth week, they migrate by ameboid movement along the dorsal mesentery of the hindgut (Fig. 16.18*A,B*), arriving at the primitive gonads at the beginning of the fifth week and invading the genital ridges in the sixth week. If they fail to reach the ridges, the gonads do not develop. Hence, the primordial germ cells have an inductive influence on development of the gonad into ovary or testis.

Shortly before and during arrival of primordial germ cells, the epithelium of the genital ridge proliferates, and epithelial cells penetrate the underlying mesenchyme. Here they form a number of irregularly shaped cords, the **primitive sex cords** (Fig. 16.19). In both male and female embryos, these cords are connected to surface epithelium, and it is impossible to differentiate between the male and female gonad. Hence, the gonad is known as the **indifferent gonad**.

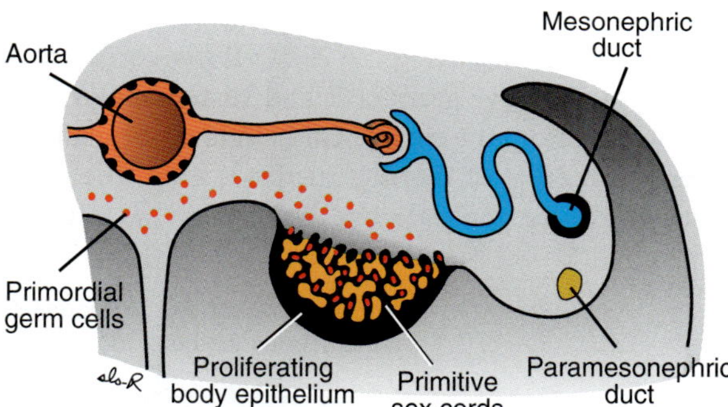


**FIGURE 16.19** Transverse section through the lumbar region of a 6-week embryo showing the indifferent gonad with the primitive sex cords. Some of the primordial germ cells are surrounded by cells of the primitive sex cords.

## *Testis*

If the embryo is genetically male, the primordial germ cells carry an XY sex chromosome complex. Under influence of the *SRY* gene on the Y chromosome, which encodes the testis-determining factor, the primitive sex cords continue to proliferate and penetrate deep into the medulla to form the **testis** or **medullary cords** (Figs. 16.20*A* and 16.21). Toward the hilum of the gland, the cords break up into a network of tiny cell strands that later give rise to tubules of the **rete testis** (Fig. 16.20*A,B*). During further development, a dense layer of fibrous connective tissue, the **tunica albuginea**, separates the testis cords from the surface epithelium (Fig. 16.20).

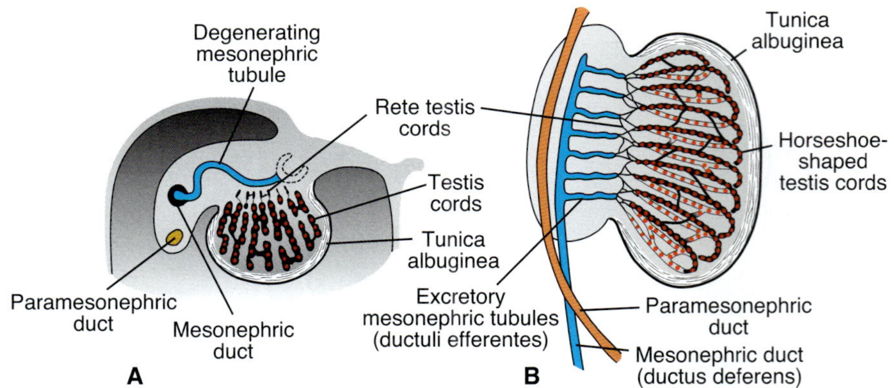


**FIGURE 16.20** **A.** Transverse section through the testis in the eighth week, showing the tunica albuginea, testis cords, rete testis, and primordial germ cells. The glomerulus and Bowman capsule of the mesonephric excretory tubule are degenerating. **B.** Testis and genital duct in the fourth month. The horseshoe-shaped testis cords are continuous with the rete testis cords. Note the ductuli efferentes (excretory mesonephric tubules), which enter the mesonephric duct.

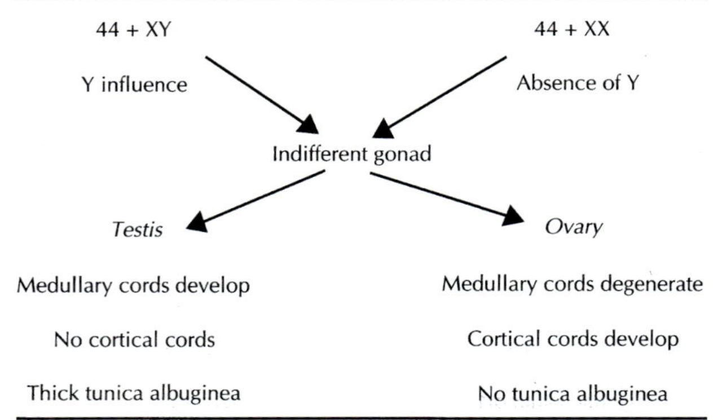


**FIGURE 16.21** Influence of primordial germ cells on indifferent gonad.

In the fourth month, the testis cords become horseshoe-shaped, and their extremities are continuous with those of the rete testis (Fig. 16.20*B*). Testis cords are now composed of primitive germ cells and **sustentacular cells of Sertoli** derived from the surface epithelium of the gland.

**Interstitial cells of Leydig**, derived from the original mesenchyme of the gonadal ridge, lie between the testis cords. They begin development shortly after onset of differentiation of these cords. By the eighth week of gestation, Leydig cells begin production of **testosterone** and the testis is able to influence sexual differentiation of the genital ducts and external genitalia.

Testis cords remain solid until puberty, when they acquire a lumen, thus forming the **seminiferous tubules**. Once the seminiferous tubules are canalized, they join the rete testis tubules, which in turn enter the **ductuli efferentes**. These efferent ductules are the remaining parts of the excretory tubules of the mesonephric system. They link the rete testis and the mesonephric or Wolffian duct, which becomes the **ductus deferens** (Fig. 16.20*B*).

### *Ovary*

In female embryos with an XX sex chromosome complement and no Y chromosome, primitive sex cords dissociate into irregular cell clusters (Figs. 16.21 and 16.22*A*). These clusters, containing groups of primitive germ cells, occupy the medullary part of the ovary. Later, they disappear and are replaced by a vascular stroma that forms the **ovarian medulla** (Fig. 16.22).

The surface epithelium of the female gonad, unlike that of the male, continues to proliferate. In the seventh week, it gives

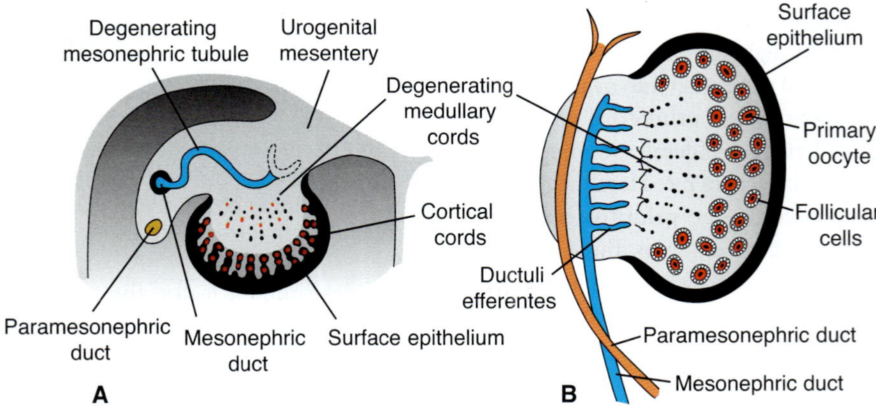


**FIGURE 16.22** **A.** Transverse section of the ovary at the seventh week, showing degeneration of the primitive (medullary) sex cords and formation of the cortical cords. **B.** Ovary and genital ducts in the fifth month. Note degeneration of the medullary cords. The excretory mesonephric tubules (efferent ductules) do not communicate with the rete. The cortical zone of the ovary contains groups of oogonia surrounded by follicular cells.

rise to a second generation of cords, **cortical cords**, which penetrate the underlying mesenchyme but remain close to the surface (Fig. 16.22*A*). In the third month, these cords split into isolated cell clusters. Cells in these clusters continue to proliferate and begin to surround each oogonium with a layer of epithelial cells called **follicular cells**. Together, the oogonia and follicular cells constitute a **primordial follicle** (Fig. 16.22*B*; see Chapter 2, p. 10).

It may thus be stated that the genetic sex of an embryo is determined at the time of fertilization, depending on whether the spermatocyte carries an X or a Y chromosome. In embryos with an XX sex chromosome configuration, medullary cords of the gonad regress, and a secondary generation of cortical cords develops (Figs. 16.21 and 16.22). In embryos with an XY sex chromosome complex, medullary cords develop into testis cords, and secondary cortical cords fail to develop (Figs. 16.20 and 16.21).

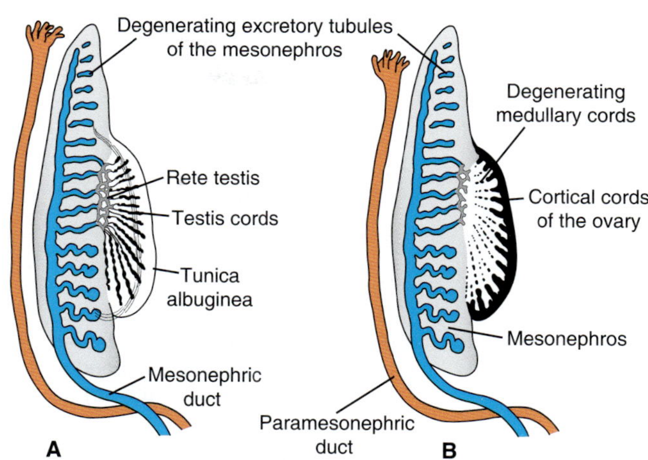


**FIGURE 16.23** Genital ducts in the sixth week in the male **(A)** and female **(B)**. The mesonephric and paramesonephric ducts are present in both. Note the excretory tubules of the mesonephros and their relation to the developing gonad in both sexes.

## Genital Ducts

### *Indifferent Stage*

Initially, both male and female embryos have two pairs of genital ducts: **mesonephric (Wolffian) ducts** and **paramesonephric (müllerian) ducts**. The paramesonephric duct arises as a longitudinal invagination of the epithelium on the anterolateral surface of the urogenital ridge (Fig. 16.23). Cranially, the duct opens into the abdominal cavity with a funnel-like structure. Caudally, it first runs lateral to the mesonephric duct, then crosses it ventrally to grow caudomedially (Fig. 16.23). In the midline, it comes in close contact with the paramesonephric duct from the opposite side. The caudal tip of the combined ducts projects into the posterior wall of the **urogenital sinus**, where it causes a small swelling, the **sinus tubercle** (Fig. 16.24*A*). The mesonephric ducts open into the urogenital sinus on either side of the sinus tubercle.

### *Genital Ducts in the Male*

Genital ducts in the male are stimulated to develop by testosterone and are derived from parts of the mesonephric kidney system (Fig. 16.25). Some of the original excretory tubules, the **epigenital tubules**, establish contact with cords of the rete testis and form the **efferent ductules** of the testis (Fig. 16.26). Excretory tubules along the caudal pole of the testis, the **paragenital tubules**, do not join the cords of the rete testis (Fig. 16.26). Their vestiges are collectively known as the **paradidymis**.

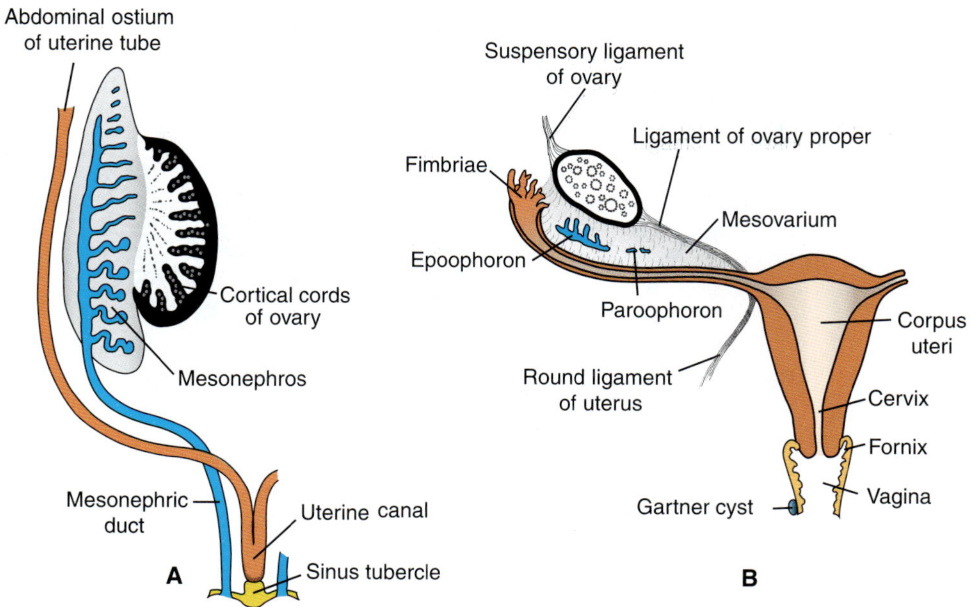


**FIGURE 16.24 A.** Genital ducts in the female at the end of the second month. Note the paramesonephric (müllerian) tubercle and formation of the uterine canal. **B.** Genital ducts after descent of the ovary. The only parts remaining from the mesonephric system are the epoophoron, paroophoron, and Gartner cyst. Note the suspensory ligament of the ovary, ligament of the ovary proper, and round ligament of the uterus.

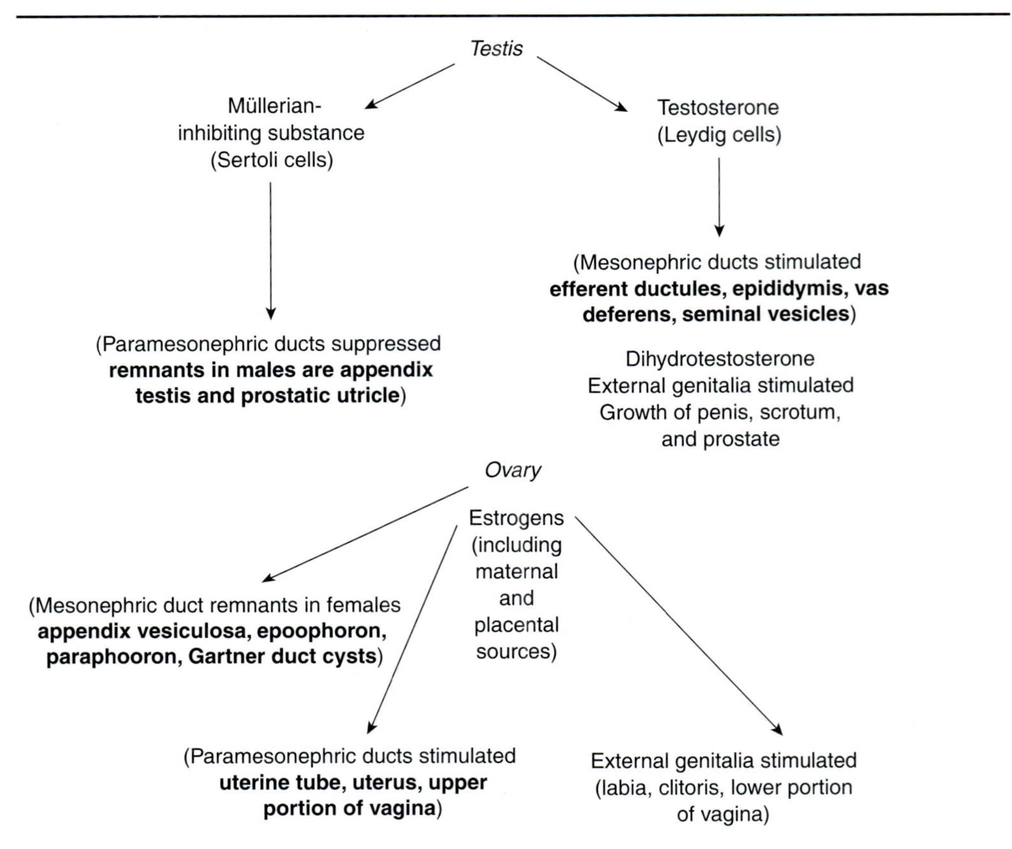


**FIGURE 16.25** Influence of the sex glands on further sex differentiation.

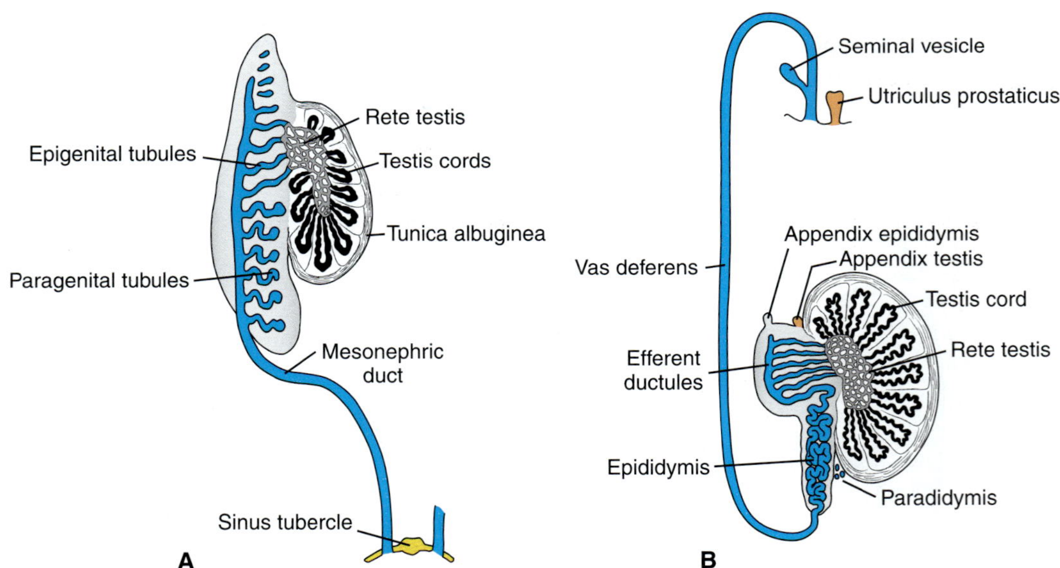


**FIGURE 16.26** **A.** Genital ducts in the male in the fourth month. Cranial and caudal (paragenital tubule) segments of the mesonephric system regress. **B.** Genital ducts after descent of the testis. Note the horseshoe-shaped testis cords, rete testis, and efferent ductules entering the ductus deferens. The paradidymis is formed by remnants of the paragenital mesonephric tubules. The paramesonephric duct has degenerated except for the appendix testis. The prostatic utricle is an outpocketing from the urethra.

Except for the most cranial portion, the **appendix epididymis**, the mesonephric ducts persist and form the main **genital ducts** (Fig. 16.26). Immediately below the entrance of the efferent ductules, the mesonephric ducts elongate and become highly convoluted, forming the (**ductus**) **epididymis**. From the tail of the epididymis to the outbudding of the **seminal vesicle**, the mesonephric ducts obtain a thick muscular coat and form the **ductus deferens**. The region of the ducts beyond the seminal vesicles is the **ejaculatory duct**. Under the influence of anti-müllerian hormone (**AMH**; also called **müllerian inhibiting substance** [**MIS**]) produced by **Sertoli cells**, paramesonephric ducts in the male degenerate except for a small portion at their cranial ends, the **appendix testis** (Figs. 16.25 and 16.26*B*).

### Genital Ducts in the Female

In the presence of **estrogen** and the absence of testosterone and AMH (MIS), **paramesonephric ducts** develop into the main genital ducts of the female (Fig. 16.25). Initially, three parts can be recognized in each duct: (1) a cranial vertical portion that opens into the abdominal cavity, (2) a horizontal part that crosses the mesonephric duct, and (3) a caudal vertical part that fuses with its partner from the opposite side (Fig. 16.24*A*). With descent of the ovary, the first two parts develop into the **uterine tube** (Fig. 16.24*B*), and the caudal parts fuse to form the **uterine canal**. When the second part of the paramesonephric ducts moves mediocaudally, the urogenital ridges gradually come to lie in a transverse plane (Fig. 16.27*A*,*B*). After the ducts fuse in the midline, a broad transverse pelvic fold is established (Fig. 16.27*C*). This fold, which extends from the lateral sides of the fused paramesonephric ducts toward the wall of the pelvis, is **the broad ligament of the uterus**. The uterine tube lies in its upper border, and the ovary lies on its posterior surface (Fig. 16.27*C*). The uterus and broad ligaments divide the pelvic cavity into the **uterorectal pouch** and the **uterovesical pouch**. The fused paramesonephric ducts give rise to the **corpus** and **cervix** of the uterus and the upper portion of the **vagina**. The uterus is surrounded by a layer of mesenchyme that forms both its muscular coat, the **myometrium**, and its peritoneal covering, the **perimetrium**. In the absence of testosterone, mesonephric ducts in the female degenerate.

### Vagina

Shortly after the solid tip of the paramesonephric ducts contacts the urogenital sinus (Figs. 16.28*A* and 16.29*A*), two solid evaginations grow out from the pelvic part of the sinus (Figs. 16.28*B* and 16.29*B*). These evaginations, the

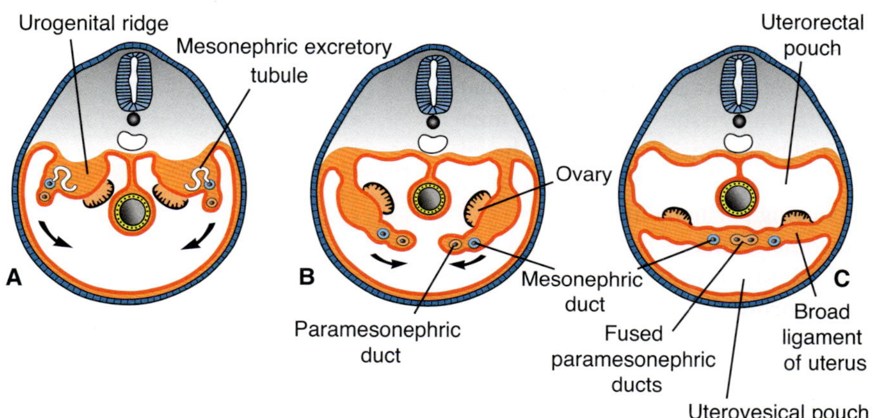


**FIGURE 16.27** Transverse sections through the urogenital ridge at progressively lower levels. **A,B.** The paramesonephric ducts approach each other in the midline and fuse. **C.** As a result of fusion, a transverse fold, the broad ligament of the uterus, forms in the pelvis. The gonads come to lie at the posterior aspect of the transverse fold.

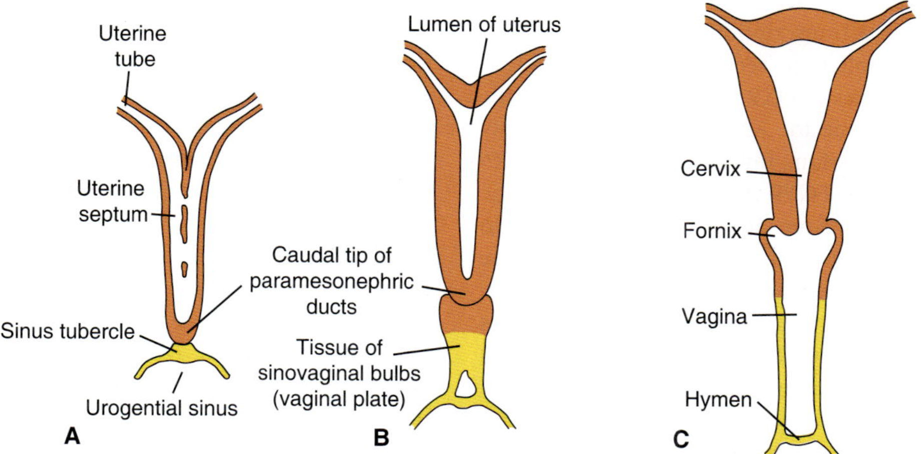


**FIGURE 16.28** Formation of the uterus and vagina. **A.** 9 weeks. Note the disappearance of the uterine septum. **B.** At the end of the third month. Note the tissue of the sinovaginal bulbs. **C.** Newborn. The fornices and the upper portion of the vagina are formed by vacuolization of the paramesonephric tissue, and the lower portion of the vagina is formed by vacuolization of the sinovaginal bulbs.

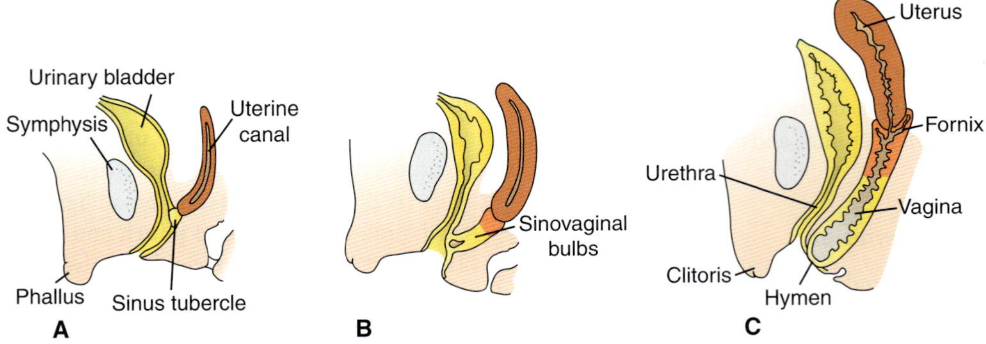


**FIGURE 16.29** Sagittal sections showing formation of the uterus and vagina at various stages of development. **A.** 9 weeks. **B.** End of third month. **C.** Newborn.

**sinovaginal bulbs**, proliferate and form a solid **vaginal plate**. Proliferation continues at the cranial end of the plate, increasing the distance between the uterus and the urogenital sinus. By the fifth month, the vaginal outgrowth is entirely canalized. The wing-like expansions of the vagina around the end of the uterus, the **vaginal fornices**, are of paramesonephric origin (Fig. 16.29*C*). Thus, the vagina has a dual origin, with the upper portion derived from the uterine canal and the lower portion derived from the urogenital sinus.

The lumen of the vagina remains separated from that of the urogenital sinus by a thin tissue plate, the **hymen** (Figs. 16.28*C* and 16.29*C*), which consists of the epithelial lining of the sinus and a thin layer of vaginal cells. It usually develops a small opening during perinatal life.

The female may retain some remnants of the cranial and caudal excretory tubules in the mesovarium where they form the **epoophoron** and **paroophoron**, respectively (Fig. 16.24*B*). The mesonephric duct disappears except for a small cranial portion found in the epoophoron and occasionally a small caudal portion that may be found in the wall of the uterus or vagina. Later in life, it may form **Gartner cyst** (Fig. 16.24*B*).

## Molecular Regulation of Genital Duct Development

***SRY*** is a transcription factor and the master gene for testes development. It appears to act in conjunction with the **autosomal gene *SOX9***, a transcriptional regulator, that can also induce testes differentiation (see Fig. 16.30 for a potential pathway for these genes). SOX9 is known to bind to the promoter region of the gene for AMH (MIS) and probably regulates this gene's expression. Initially, *SRY* and/or *SOX9* induce the testes to secrete **FGF9** that acts as a chemotactic factor that causes tubules from the mesonephric duct to penetrate the gonadal ridge. Without penetration by these tubules, differentiation of the testes does not continue. Next, *SRY* either directly or indirectly (through *SOX9*) upregulates production of **STEROIDOGENESIS FACTOR 1 (SF1)** that stimulates differentiation of Sertoli and Leydig cells. SF1 working with *SOX9* elevates the concentration of **AMH** leading to **regression** of the **paramesonephric (müllerian) ducts**. In Leydig cells, SF1 upregulates the genes for enzymes that synthesize **testosterone**. Testosterone enters cells of target tissues where it may remain intact or be converted

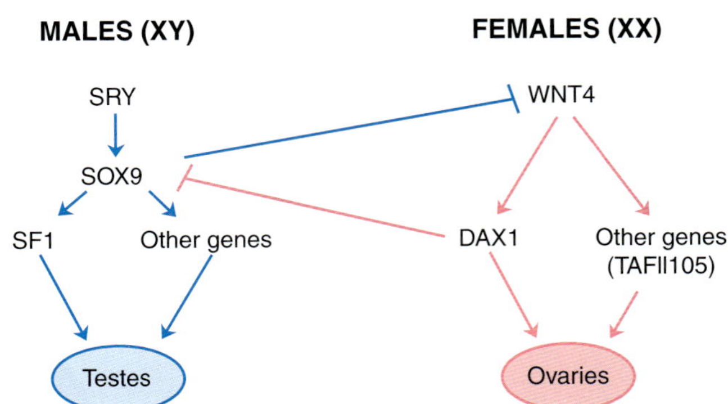


**FIGURE 16.30** Schematic showing genes responsible for differentiation of the testes and ovaries. In both males and females, *SOX9* and *WNT4* are expressed in the gonadal ridges. In males, the expression of *SRY* upregulates *SOX9*, which in turn activates expression of *SF1* and other genes responsible for testes differentiation while inhibiting expression of *WNT4*. In females, the uninhibited expression of *WNT4* upregulates *DAX1* that in turn inhibits *SOX9* expression. Then, under the continued influence of *WNT4*, other downstream target genes (perhaps *TAFII105*) induce ovarian differentiation.

to **dihydrotestosterone** by a **5-α reductase enzyme**. Testosterone and dihydrotestosterone bind to a specific high-affinity intracellular receptor, and this **hormone receptor complex** is transported to the nucleus where it binds to DNA to regulate transcription of tissue-specific genes and their protein products. **Testosterone receptor complexes mediate differentiation of the mesonephric ducts** to form the vas deferens, seminal vesicles, efferent ductules, and epididymis. **Dihydrotestosterone receptor complexes modulate differentiation of the male external genitalia** (Fig. 16.25).

***WNT4*** is the ovary-determining gene. This gene upregulates ***DAX1***, a member of the **nuclear hormone receptor family**, that inhibits the function of *SOX9*. In addition, *WNT4* regulates expression of other genes responsible for ovarian differentiation, but these target genes have not been identified. One target may be the *TAFII105* gene, whose protein product is a subunit for the TATA-binding protein for RNA polymerase in ovarian follicular cells. Female mice that do not synthesize this subunit do not form ovaries.

**Estrogens** are also involved in sexual differentiation, and under their influence, the **paramesonephric (müllerian) ducts** are stimulated to form the uterine tubes, uterus, cervix,

## Clinical Correlates

### Uterine and Vaginal Defects

**Duplications of the uterus** result from lack of fusion of the paramesonephric ducts in a local area or throughout their normal line of fusion. In its extreme form, the uterus is entirely double (**uterus didelphys**) (Fig. 16.31*A*); in the least severe form, it is only slightly indented in the middle (**uterus arcuatus**) (Fig. 16.31*B*). One of the relatively common anomalies is the **uterus bicornis**, in which the uterus has two horns entering a common vagina (Fig. 16.31*C*). This condition is normal in many mammals below the primates.

In patients with complete or partial atresia of one of the paramesonephric ducts, the rudimentary part lies as an appendage to the well-developed side. Because its lumen usually does not communicate with the vagina, complications are common (uterus bicornis unicollis with one rudimentary horn) (Fig. 16.31*D*). If the atresia involves both sides, an atresia of the cervix may result (Fig. 16.31*E*). If the sinovaginal bulbs fail to fuse or do not develop at all, a double vagina or atresia of the vagina, respectively, results (Fig. 16.31*A,F*). In the latter case, a small vaginal pouch originating from the paramesonephric ducts usually surrounds the opening of the cervix.

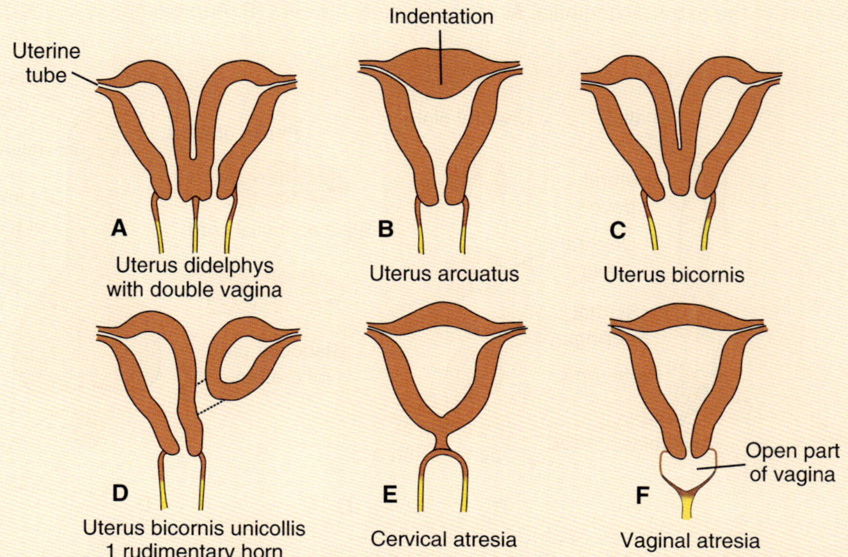


**FIGURE 16.31** Main abnormalities of the uterus and vagina caused by persistence of the uterine septum or obliteration of the lumen of the uterine canal.

and upper vagina. In addition, estrogens act on the external genitalia at the indifferent stage to form the labia majora, labia minora, clitoris, and lower vagina (Fig. 16.25).

## External Genitalia

### Indifferent Stage

In the third week of development, mesenchyme cells originating in the region of the primitive streak migrate around the cloacal membrane to form a pair of slightly elevated **cloacal folds** (Fig. 16.32*A*). Cranial to the cloacal membrane, the folds unite to form the **genital tubercle**. Caudally, the folds are subdivided into **urethral folds** anteriorly and **anal folds** posteriorly (Fig. 16.32*B*).

In the meantime, another pair of elevations, the **genital swellings**, becomes visible on each side of the urethral folds. These swellings later form the **scrotal swellings** in the male (Fig. 16.33A) and the **labia majora** in the female. At the end of the sixth week, however, it is impossible to distinguish between the two sexes.

### External Genitalia in the Male

Development of the external genitalia in the male is under the influence of androgens secreted by the fetal testes and is characterized by rapid elongation of the genital tubercle, which is now called the **phallus** (Fig. 16.33*A*). During this elongation, the phallus pulls the urethral folds forward so that they form the lateral walls of the **urethral groove**. This groove extends along the ventral aspect of the elongated phallus but does not reach the most distal part, the glans. The epithelial lining of the groove, which originates in the endoderm, forms the **urethral plate** (Fig. 16.33*B*).

At the end of the third month, the two urethral folds close over the urethral plate, forming the **penile urethra** (Fig. 16.33*B*). This canal does not extend to the tip of the phallus. This most distal portion of the urethra is formed during the fourth month, when ectodermal cells from the tip of the glans penetrate inward and form a short epithelial cord. This cord later obtains a lumen, thus forming the **external urethral meatus** (Fig. 16.33*C*).

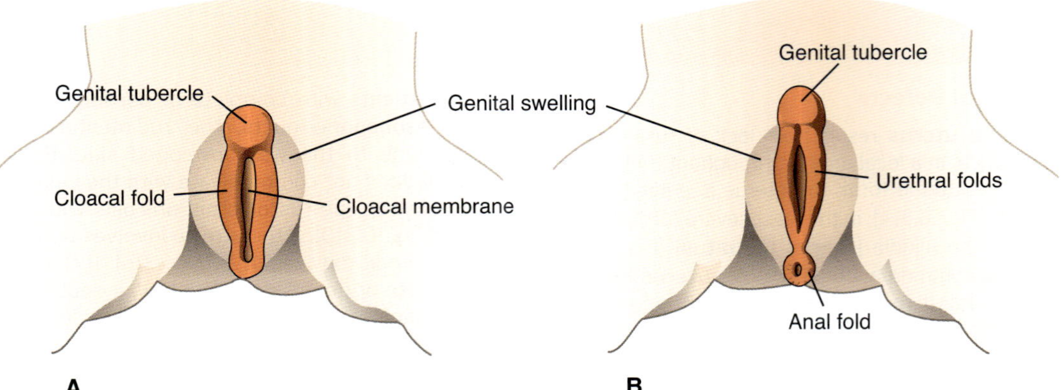


**FIGURE 16.32** Indifferent stages of the external genitalia. **A.** Approximately 4 weeks. **B.** Approximately 6 weeks.

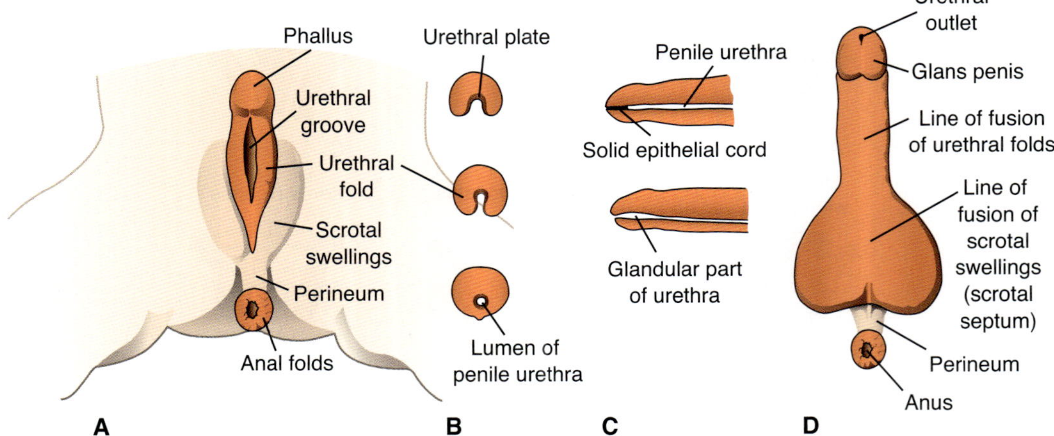


**FIGURE 16.33** **A.** Development of external genitalia in the male at 10 weeks. Note the deep urethral groove flanked by the urethral folds. **B.** Transverse sections through the phallus during formation of the penile urethra. The urogenital groove is bridged by the urethral folds. **C.** Development of the glandular portion of the penile urethra. **D.** Newborn.



The genital swellings, known in the male as the **scrotal swellings**, arise in the inguinal region. With further development, they move caudally, and each swelling then makes up half of the scrotum. The two are separated by the **scrotal septum** (Fig. 16.33*D*).

## *External Genitalia in the Female*

Estrogens stimulate development of the external genitalia of the female. The genital tubercle elongates only slightly and forms the **clitoris** (Fig. 16.35*A*); urethral folds do not fuse,

## *Clinical Correlates*

### Defects in the Male Genitalia

In **hypospadias**, fusion of the urethral folds is incomplete, and abnormal openings of the urethra occur along the ventral aspect of the penis, usually near the glans, along the shaft, or near the base of the penis (Fig. 16.34). In rare cases, the urethral meatus extends along the scrotal raphe. When fusion of the urethral folds fails entirely, a wide sagittal slit is found along the entire length of the penis and the scrotum. The two scrotal swellings then closely resemble the labia majora. The incidence of hypospadias is 3 to 5/1,000 births, and this rate represents a doubling over the past 15 to 20 years. Reasons for the increase are not known, but one hypothesis suggests it could be a result of a rise in environmental estrogens (endocrine disrupters; see Chapter 9).

**Epispadias** is a rare abnormality (1/30,000 births) in which the urethral meatus is found on the dorsum of the penis (Fig. 16.34*D*). Although epispadias may occur as an isolated defect, it is most often associated with exstrophy of the bladder and abnormal closure of the ventral body wall (Fig. 16.16).

**Micropenis** occurs when there is insufficient androgen stimulation for growth of the external genitalia. Micropenis is usually caused by primary hypogonadism or hypothalamic or pituitary dysfunction. By definition, the penis is 2.5 standard deviations below the mean in length as measured along the dorsal surface from the pubis to the tip with the penis stretched to resistance. **Bifid penis** or **double penis** may occur if the genital tubercle splits.

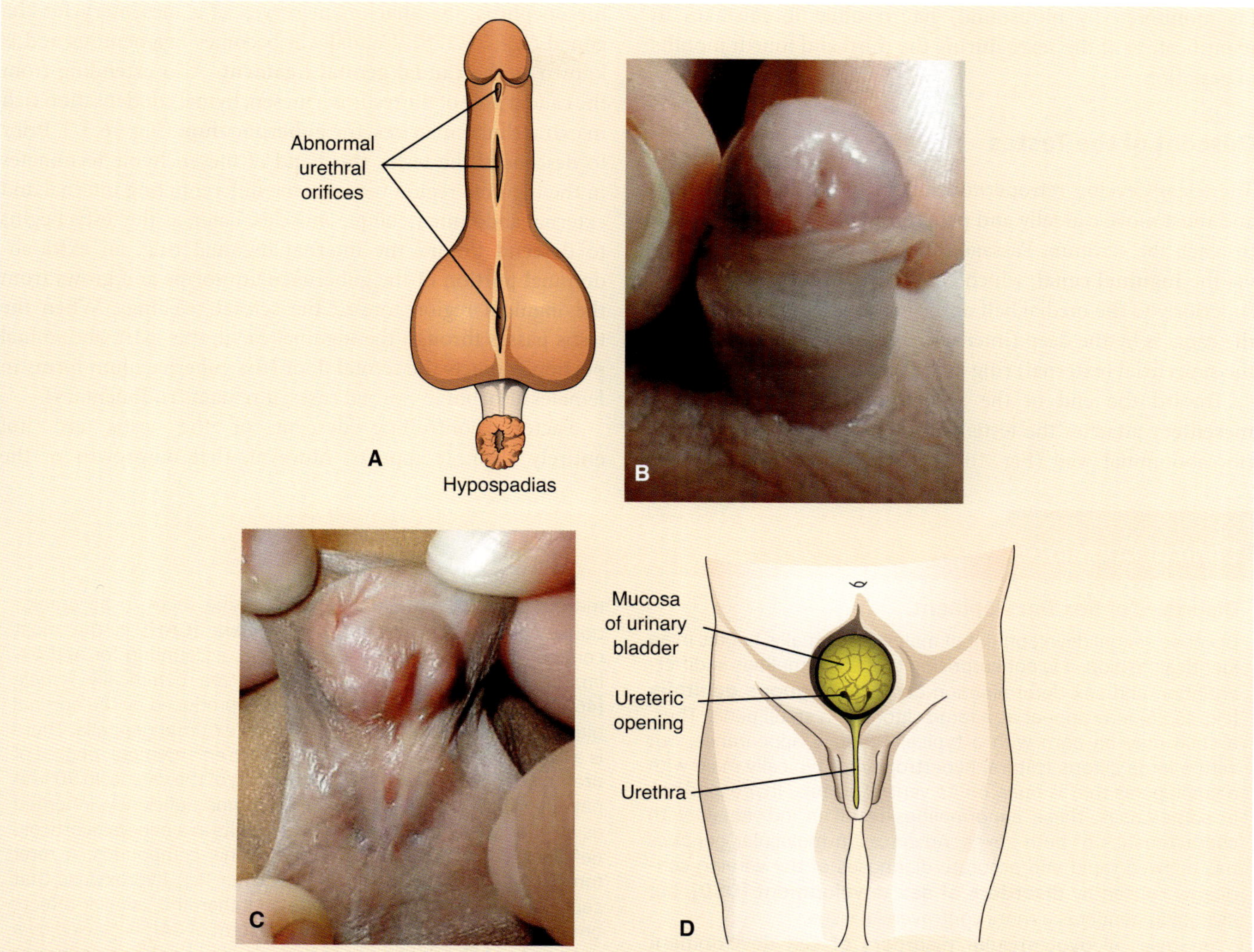

Abnormal urethral orifices
A
Hypospadias
B
Mucosa of urinary bladder
Ureteric opening
Urethra
C
D

**FIGURE 16.34** **A.** Hypospadias showing the various locations of abnormal urethral orifices. **B.** Patient with glandular hypospadias. The urethra is open on the ventral surface of the glans penis. **C.** Patient with hypospadias involving the glans and shaft of the penis. **D.** Epispadias combined with exstrophy of the bladder. Bladder mucosa is exposed.



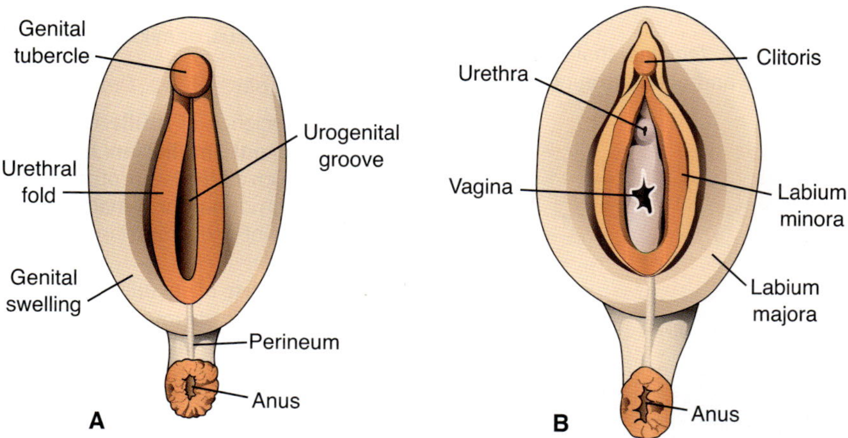


**FIGURE 16.35** Development of the external genitalia in the female at 5 months **(A)** and in the newborn **(B)**.

as in the male, but develop into the **labia minora**. Genital swellings enlarge and form the **labia majora**. The urogenital groove is open and forms the **vestibule** (Fig. 16.35*B*). Although the genital tubercle does not elongate extensively in the female, it is larger than in the male during the early stages of development. In fact, using tubercle length as a criterion (as monitored by ultrasound) has resulted in mistakes in identification of the sexes during the third and fourth months of gestation.

## Descent of the Testes

The testes develop retroperitoneally in the abdominal region and must move caudally and pass through the abdominal wall to reach the scrotum. Passage through the abdominal wall is via the **inguinal canal**, which is about 4 cm long and lies just superiorly to the medial half of the inguinal ligament. Entry to the canal is by the deep (internal) inguinal ring, and exit is by the superficial (external) ring near the pubic tubercle.

Toward the end of the second month, the **urogenital mesentery** attaches the testis and mesonephros to the posterior abdominal wall (Fig. 16.3*A*). With degeneration of the mesonephros, the attachment serves as a mesentery for the gonad (Fig. 16.27*B*). Caudally, it becomes ligamentous and is known as the **caudal genital ligament**. Also extending from the caudal pole of the testis is a mesenchymal condensation rich in extracellular matrices, the **gubernaculum** (Fig. 16.37). Prior to descent of the testis, this band of mesenchyme terminates in the inguinal region between the differentiating internal and external abdominal oblique muscles. Later, as the testis begins to descend toward the internal inguinal ring, an extra-abdominal portion of the gubernaculum forms and grows from the inguinal region toward the scrotal swellings. When the testis passes through the inguinal canal, this extra-abdominal portion contacts the scrotal floor (the gubernaculum forms in females also, but in normal cases, it remains rudimentary).

Factors controlling descent of the testis are not entirely clear. It appears, however, that outgrowth of the

### Clinical Correlates

#### Disorders of Sex Development

Because sexual development of males and females begins in an identical fashion, it is not surprising that abnormalities in differentiation and sex determination occur. **Ambiguous genitalia** (Fig. 16.36) may appear as a large clitoris or a small penis. Thus, a child may be born with a typically female appearance, but with a large clitoris (clitoral hypertrophy) or typically male with a small penis that is open on its ventral surface (hypospadias). In some cases, these abnormalities result in individuals with characteristics of both sexes. Advances in molecular genetics has allowed rapid and accurate diagnoses of the varying conditions caused by **disorders of sex development (DSD)**, but assigning gender is a more controversial issue.

In cases of **ovotesticular disorders of sex development** (formerly called true hermaphrodism), both ovarian and testicular tissues are present. Thus, gonadal tissue may be any combination of ovary, testis, or ovotestis, which is present in two-thirds of cases. Genitalia are always ambiguous, but there is a tendency toward masculinization. In 70% of cases, the karyotype is 46,XX.

#### *46,XX Disorders of Sex Development*

**Individuals with 46,XX DSD** are females that have been exposed to excessive amounts of androgenic compounds that masculinize the external genitalia causing them to be ambiguous. **Congenital adrenal hyperplasia (CAH)** is the most common cause of ambiguous genitalia, accounting for approximately 60% of all DSDs. Individuals are genetically female (46,XX), but excessive androstenedione produced by the adrenal glands results in masculinization of the external genitalia. There is a spectrum of defects, involving phallic enlargement, degree of urethral fold fusion, and size and opening of the vagina. In 90% of patients, there is a 21-hydroxylase enzyme deficiency, inherited as an autosomal recessive trait that results in a mineralocorticoid deficiency and an increase in androgenic compounds. A rarer form of CAH is caused by a deficiency of 11-$\beta$-hydroxylase that causes similar biochemical effects and, therefore, similar effects on the external genitalia. Yet, another form of CAH is caused by a deficiency of 17-$\alpha$-hydroxylase that results in a decrease in prenatal and pubertal sex steroids. Females have normal internal and external anatomy, but at puberty, neither the adrenal glands nor the ovaries produce sex steroids. Consequently, there is no breast development or growth of pubic hair. A similar deficiency in males causes a moderate to severe reduction in testosterone production. As a result external genitalia may appear as normal female, ambiguous, or mildly underdeveloped.

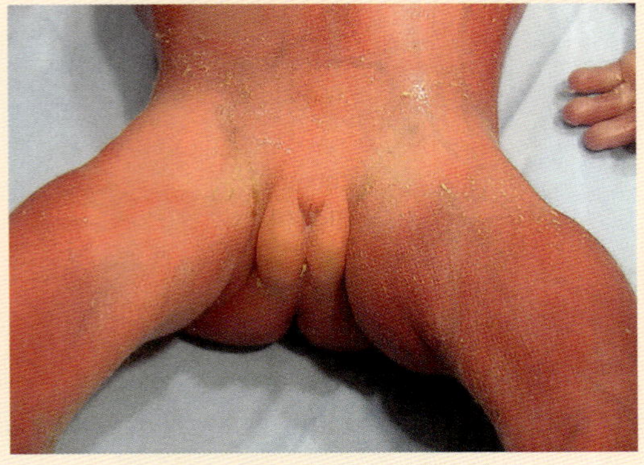

**FIGURE 16.36** Male (46,XY) infant with ambiguous genitalia. Note partial fusion of the scrotal swellings and a small penis with hypospadias.

#### *46,XY Disorders of Sex Development*

Isolated deficiency of **müllerian inhibiting substance (MIS; also called anti-müllerian hormone [AMH])** is a rare disorder in which there is no production of MIS. As a result, the genitalia are normal for a male, but there are varying degrees of remnants of the müllerian system, including a uterus and uterine tubes.

Another cause of sexual ambiguity in males is the **androgen insensitivity syndrome (AIS)**. In these individuals there is a lack of androgen receptors or failure of tissues to respond to receptor–dihydrotestosterone complexes. Consequently, androgens produced by the testes are ineffective in inducing differentiation of male genitalia. Because these patients have testes and MIS is present, the paramesonephric system is suppressed, and uterine tubes and uterus are absent. In patients with **complete androgen insensitivity syndrome (CAIS)**, a vagina is present but usually short or poorly developed. The testes are frequently found in the inguinal or labial regions, but spermatogenesis does not occur. Furthermore, there is an

Part 2

increased risk of testicular tumors, and 33% of these individuals develop malignancies prior to age 50 years. Other patients have **mild androgen insensitivity syndrome (MAIS)** or **partial androgen insensitivity syndrome (PAIS)** forms of the disorder. With the mild form, there is virilization to varying degrees, but with the partial form, ambiguous genitalia may be present, including clitoromegaly or a small penis with hypospadias. Testes are usually undescended in these cases.

**5-α-Reductase deficiency (5-ARD)** is another condition that causes ambiguous genitalia in males and is due to an inability to convert testosterone to dihydrotestosterone because of a lack of the reductase enzyme. Without dihydrotestosterone, external genitalia do not develop normally and may appear male but be underdeveloped with hypospadias, or they may appear to be female with clitoromegaly.

Other conditions may be associated with abnormal sexual differentiation. For example, **Klinefelter syndrome**, with a karyotype of 47,XXY (or other variants, e.g., XXXY), is the most common sex chromosome disorder, occurring with a frequency of 1 per 1,000 males. Patients may have decreased fertility, small testes, and decreased testosterone levels. Gynecomastia (enlarged breasts) is present in approximately 33% of affected individuals. Nondisjunction of the XX homologues is the most common causative factor.

In **gonadal dysgenesis**, oocytes are absent, and the ovaries appear as streak gonads. Individuals are phenotypically female but may have a variety of chromosomal complements, including XY. **XY female gonadal dysgenesis (Swyer syndrome)** results from point mutations or deletions of the *SRY* gene. Individuals appear to be normal females but do not menstruate and do not develop secondary sexual characteristics at puberty. Patients with **Turner syndrome** also have gonadal dysgenesis. They have a 45,X karyotype and short stature, high-arched palate, webbed neck, shield-like chest, cardiac and renal anomalies, and inverted nipples (see Chapter 2, p. 19).

extra-abdominal portion of the gubernaculum produces intra-abdominal migration, that an increase in intra-abdominal pressure due to organ growth produces passage through the inguinal canal, and that regression of the extra-abdominal portion of the gubernaculum completes movement of the testis into the scrotum. Normally, the testes reach the inguinal region by approximately 12 weeks' gestation, migrate through the inguinal canal by 28 weeks, and reach the scrotum by 33 weeks (Fig. 16.37). The process is influenced by hormones, including androgens and MIS. During descent, blood supply to the testis from the aorta is retained, and testicular vessels extend from their original lumbar position to the testis in the scrotum.

Independently from descent of the testis, the peritoneum of the abdominal cavity forms an evagination on each side of the midline into the ventral abdominal wall. This evagination, the **processus vaginalis**, follows the course of the gubernaculum testis into the scrotal swellings (Fig. 16.37*B*). Hence, the processus vaginalis, accompanied by the muscular and fascial layers of the body wall, evaginates into the scrotal swelling, forming the **inguinal canal** (Fig. 16.38).

The testis descends through the inguinal ring and over the rim of the pubic bone and is present in the scrotum at birth. The testis is then covered by a reflected fold of the processus vaginalis (Fig. 16.37*D*). The peritoneal layer covering the testis is the **visceral layer of the tunica vaginalis**; the remainder of the peritoneal sac forms the **parietal layer of the tunica**



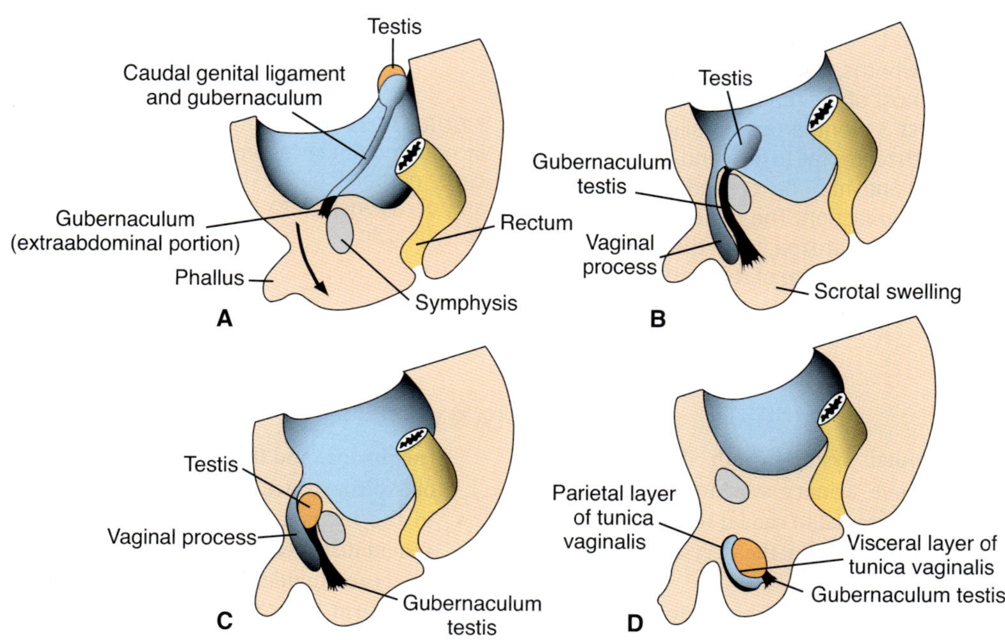


**FIGURE 16.37** Descent of the testis. **A.** During the second month. **B.** In the middle of the third month. Peritoneum lining the body cavity evaginates into the scrotal swelling, where it forms the vaginal process (tunica vaginalis). **C.** In the seventh month. **D.** Shortly after birth.

**vaginalis** (Fig. 16.37*D*). The narrow canal connecting the lumen of the vaginal process with the peritoneal cavity is obliterated at birth or shortly thereafter.

In addition to being covered by peritoneal layers derived from the processus vaginalis, the testis becomes ensheathed in layers derived from the anterior abdominal wall through which it passes. Thus, the **transversalis fascia** forms the **internal spermatic fascia**, the **internal abdominal oblique muscle** gives rise to the **cremasteric fascia and muscle**, and the **external abdominal oblique muscle** forms the **external spermatic fascia** (Fig. 16.38). The transversus abdominis muscle does not contribute a layer because it arches over this region and does not cover the path of migration.

## Descent of the Ovaries

Descent of the gonads is considerably less in the female than in the male, and the ovaries finally settle just below the rim of the true pelvis. The cranial genital ligament forms the **suspensory ligament** of the ovary, whereas the caudal genital ligament forms the **ligament of the ovary proper** and the **round ligament of the uterus** (Fig. 16.24). The latter extends into the labia majora.

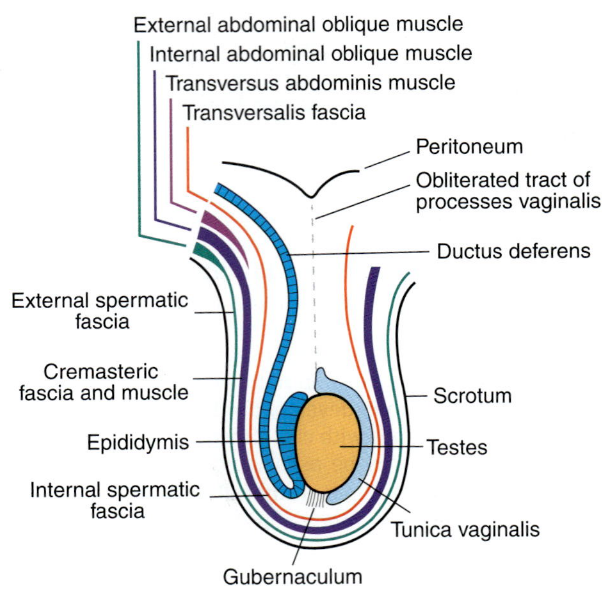


**FIGURE 16.38** Drawing showing the coverings of the testes that are derived from constituents of the abdominal wall. These coverings are formed as the testes migrate through the wall in route from their retroperitoneal location in the abdominal cavity to the scrotum.



## *Clinical Correlates*

### Hernias and Cryptorchidism

The connection between the abdominal cavity and the processus vaginalis through the inguinal canal and into the scrotal sac normally closes in the first year after birth (Fig. 16.37*D*). If this passageway remains open, intestinal loops may descend into the scrotum, causing a **congenital indirect inguinal hernia** (Fig. 16.39*A*). Sometimes, obliteration of this passageway is irregular, leaving small cysts along its course. Later, these cysts may secrete fluid, forming a **hydrocele of the testis and/or spermatic cord** (Fig. 16.39*B*).

In 97% of male newborns, testes are present in the scrotum before birth. In most of the remainder, descent will be completed during the first 3 months postnatally. However, in <1% of infants, one or both testes fail to descend. The condition is called **cryptorchidism** and may be caused by decreased androgen (testosterone) production. The undescended testes fail to produce mature spermatozoa, and the condition is associated with a 3% to 5% incidence of renal anomalies.

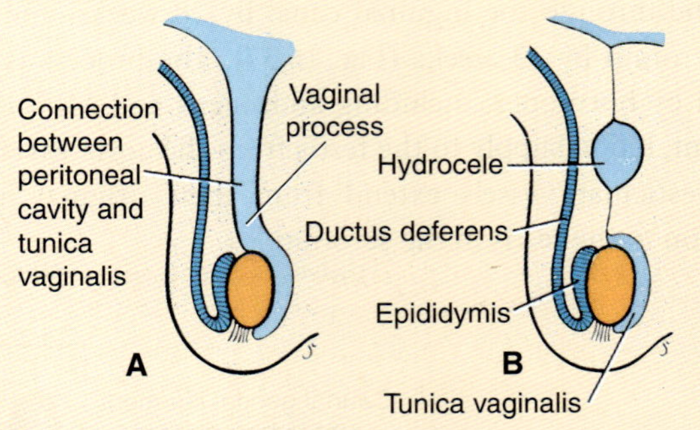


**FIGURE 16.39 A.** Inguinal hernia. The vaginal process remains in open communication with the peritoneal cavity. In such a case, portions of the intestinal loops often descend toward and occasionally into the scrotum, causing an inguinal hernia. **B.** Hydrocele.

## SUMMARY

- The urinary and genital systems both develop from mesodermal tissue. Three urinary systems develop in a temporal sequence from cranial to caudal segments:
- The **pronephros**, which forms in the cervical region, is vestigial.
- The **mesonephros**, which forms in the thoracic and lumbar regions, is large and is characterized by **excretory units (nephrons)** and its own collecting duct, the **mesonephric** or **Wolffian** duct.
- In the human, it may function briefly, but most of the system disappears.
- Ducts and tubules from the mesonephros form the conduit for sperm from the testes to the urethra. In the female, these ducts regress.

- The **metanephros**, or permanent kidney, develops from two sources. It forms its own excretory tubules or nephrons like the mesonephros, but its collecting system originates from the **ureteric bud**, an outgrowth of the mesonephric duct.
- This ureteric bud gives rise to the **ureter**, **renal pelvis**, **calyces**, and the entire **collecting system** (Fig. 16.5). Connection between the collecting and excretory tubule systems is essential for normal development (Fig. 16.6).
- ***WT1***, expressed by the mesenchyme, makes this tissue competent to respond to induction by the ureteric bud. Interactions between the bud and mesenchyme occur through production of GDNF and HGF by the mesenchyme with their tyrosine kinase receptors RET and MET, respectively, produced by the ureteric epithelium. PAX2 and WNT4, produced by metanephric mesenchyme, cause epithelialization and excretory tubule differentiation (Fig. 16.8).
- Early division of the ureteric bud may lead to bifid or supernumerary kidneys with **ectopic ureters** (Fig. 16.10). Because the kidneys develop in the pelvic region and then "ascend" to their location in the lumbar area, abnormal positions of the kidney, such as **pelvic** and **horseshoe kidney**, occur (Fig. 16.11).
- The **bladder** forms during the fourth to seventh weeks as the **cloaca**, the common repository for the primitive kidneys and gut system, is subdivided into the **urogenital sinus** anteriorly and the **anal canal** posteriorly by the **urorectal septum** (Fig. 16.12).
- The anterior portion of this sinus then differentiates into the bladder. The remaining portion of the sinus differentiates into the **prostatic** and **membranous** parts of the **urethra** in the male and the urethra in the female (Fig. 16.13).
- The **genital system** consists of (1) gonads or primitive sex glands, (2) genital ducts, and (3) external genitalia. All three components go through an **indifferent stage** in which they may develop into either a male or a female.
- The ***SRY* gene** on the Y chromosome produces **testes-determining factor** and regulates male sexual development. Genes downstream from *SRY* include ***SOX9*** and ***SF1*** that stimulate differentiation of **Sertoli** and **Leydig cells** in the testes.
- Expression of the *SRY* gene causes (1) development of the **medullary (testis) cords**, (2) formation of the **tunica albuginea**, and (3) **failure of the cortical (ovarian) cords to develop**.
- Ovarian development occurs in the absence of the *SRY* gene and in the presence of ***WNT4***, the master gene for this differentiation process. *WNT4* upregulates ***DAX1*** that inhibits the expression of *SOX9*.
- *WNT4*, together with other downstream genes, causes **formation of ovaries** with (1) **typical cortical cords**, (2) **disappearance of the medullary (testis) cords**, and (3) **failure of the tunica albuginea to develop** (Fig. 16.21).
- Development of both testes and ovaries is dependent upon induction by **primordial germ cells** that migrate from the yolk sac to the genital ridges during the **fourth to sixth weeks**. If these cells fail to reach the indifferent gonad, the gonad remains indifferent or is absent.
- The indifferent duct system and external genitalia develop under the influence of hormones. During the **indifferent stage**, there are two duct systems: the **mesonephric duct** and **paramesonephric duct**.
- **Testosterone**, produced by **Leydig cells** in the testes, stimulates development of the mesonephric ducts to form the efferent ducts, epididymis, **vas deferens**, and **ejaculatory duct**. **Müllerian inhibiting substance (MIS;** also called, **anti-müllerian hormone** [**AMH**]), produced by **Sertoli cells** in the testes, causes regression of the paramesonephric ducts.
- **Dihydrotestosterone** stimulates development of the external genitalia, including the penis and scrotum (Fig. 16.25). **Estrogens** (together with the absence of testosterone) regulate development of the paramesonephric ducts, which form the **uterine tube**, **uterus**, **cervix**, and **upper portion of the vagina**.
- Because there is no testosterone production to stimulate development of the mesonephric ducts, these structures regress. Estrogens also stimulate differentiation of the external genitalia, including the **clitoris**, **labia**, and **lower portion of the vagina** (Fig. 16.25). Errors in production of or sensitivity to hormones of the testes lead to a predominance of female characteristics under influence of the maternal and placental estrogens.
- External genitalia also begin in an indifferent stage.
  - Initially, a **genital tubercle**, two **genital swellings**, and two **cloacal folds** form on the exterior of the floor of the pelvis. When the urorectal septum reaches the interior of this floor to separate the anal canal from the primitive urogenital sinus (soon to form the bladder), the cloacal folds are now called the **urethral folds** (Fig. 16.32). In the male, the genital tubercle grows and is called the **phallus**. As it grows, it pulls the urethral folds together and these fuse forming the shaft of the penis. Meanwhile, the genital swellings become larger to form the **scrotal swellings**, and these also come together and fuse in the midline.
  - In females, the genital tubercle forms the **clitoris**, the urethral folds, the **labia minora**, and the genital swellings the **labia majora**. Note that in the female, there is a lack of fusion of the primordial structures.
  - Also note the **analogous structures** in the two sexes: penis/clitoris and scrotum/labia majora.

**Derivatives of Urogenital Sinus**

| Male | Female |
|---|---|
| Urinary bladder | Urinary bladder |
| Urethra | Urethra |
| Prostate and bulbourethral glands | Paraurethral and vestibular glands |

(*Continued*)

**Derivatives of Mesonephric Duct**

| Male | Female |
|---|---|
| Ureter, pelvis, major and minor calyces, and collecting ducts | Ureter, pelvis, major and minor calyces, and collecting ducts |
| Seminal vesicle | Duct of epoophoron |
| Ejaculatory ducts | |
| Ductus deferens | |
| Epididymis | |
| Appendix of epididymis | Appendix of ovary |
| Mesonephric tubules form vasa efferentia | Paroophoron |

**Derivatives of Paramesonephric Duct**

| Female | Male |
|---|---|
| Uterus | Appendix of testis |
| Uterine tubes | Prostatic utricle |
| Upper part of vagina | |

## Self-Assessment

### Comprehensive Questions

1. Write a note on polycystic kidney.
2. Write down the mechanism of descent of testis with the timeline.
3. Discuss the molecular regulation of the development of the female reproductive system.

### Problem Solving Questions

1. During development of the urinary system, three systems form. What are they, and what parts of each, if any, remain in the newborn?
2. At birth, an apparently male baby has no testicles in the scrotum. Later, it is determined that both are in the abdominal cavity. What is the term given to this condition? Explain the embryological origin of this defect.
3. It is said that male and female external genitalia have homologies. What are they, and what are their embryological origins?
4. After several years of trying to become pregnant, a young woman seeks consultation. Examination reveals a bicornuate uterus. How could such an abnormality occur?

### Multiple Choice Questions

1. Which of the following components of urinary system degenerates completely?
   (a) Pronephros
   (b) Mesonephros
   (c) Metanephros
   (d) Cloaca
2. Indifferent stage of sex determination extends till which week?
   (a) Third week
   (b) Fourth week
   (c) Fifth week
   (d) Sixth week
3. Which is the major sex-determining gene?
   (a) *SRY*
   (b) *SOX9*
   (c) *BMP*
   (d) *FGF*
4. Which syndrome results from malfunctioning or point mutation of *SRY* gene?
   (a) Turner syndrome
   (b) Down syndrome
   (c) Swyer syndrome
   (d) Klinefelter syndrome
5. Remnants of mesonephric ducts in males are all of the following except
   (a) Efferent ductules
   (b) Paroophoron
   (c) Epididymis
   (d) Vas deferens
6. Trigone of the urinary bladder is derived from
   (a) Endoderm
   (b) Metanephric blastema
   (c) Outpouching of mesonephric duct
   (d) Cloaca
7. In a horseshoe kidney, ascent of the kidney to the lumbar region is arrested due to which of the following arteries?
   (a) Superior mesenteric
   (b) Inferior mesenteric
   (c) Superior rectal
   (d) Renal artery
8. Upper one-third of the urogenital sinus forms
   (a) Urinary bladder
   (b) Membranous urethra
   (c) Ureter
   (d) Prostate
9. Ejaculatory ducts are formed by
   (a) Opening of mesonephric duct
   (b) Outpouchings of seminal vesicles
   (c) Ureteric bud
   (d) Paramesonephric duct

**Answers**

1. (a) 2. (d) 3. (a) 4. (c) 5. (b) 6. (c) 7. (a) 8. (a) 9. (a)

CHAPTER

# 17 Head and Neck



**Specific Learning Objectives**

- Formation of pharyngeal arches, clefts, and pouches
- Skeletal and muscular derivatives of each arch; nerve of each arch
- Derivatives of pharyngeal pouches and clefts
- Birth defects involving the pharyngeal region
- Development of tongue, thyroid, and face with their clinical correlates
- Development of teeth

**Competencies Covered**

AN39.1 Describe the embryological basis of nerve supply, blood supply, lymphatic drainage, and actions of extrinsic and intrinsic muscles of the tongue.

AN43.4 Describe the development and developmental basis of congenital anomalies of the face, palate, tongue, branchial apparatus, pituitary gland, thyroid gland, and eye.

Mesenchyme for formation of the head region is derived from **paraxial** and **lateral plate mesoderm**, **neural crest**, and thickened regions of ectoderm known as **ectodermal placodes**.

Paraxial mesoderm (**somites** and **somitomeres**) forms a large portion of the membranous and cartilaginous components of the neurocranium (skull) (Fig. 17.1; see also Chapter 10 and Fig. 10.4), all voluntary muscles of the craniofacial region (see Table 17.1, p. 236), the dermis and connective tissues in the dorsal region of the head, and the meninges caudal to the prosencephalon.

- Lateral plate mesoderm forms the laryngeal cartilages (arytenoid and cricoid) and connective tissue in this region.
- Neural crest cells originate in the neuroectoderm of forebrain, midbrain, and hindbrain regions and migrate ventrally into the pharyngeal arches and rostrally around the forebrain and optic cup into the facial region (Fig. 17.2).

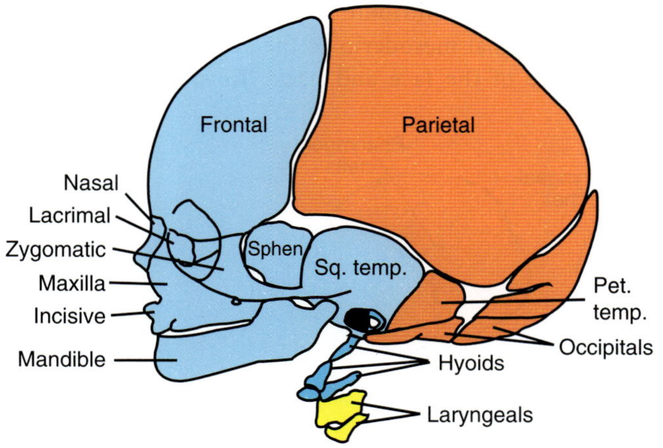

FIGURE 17.1 Skeletal structures of the head and face. Mesenchyme for these structures is derived from neural crest (*blue*), lateral plate mesoderm (*yellow*), and paraxial mesoderm (somites and somitomeres) (*red*).

In these locations, they form the entire viscerocranium (face) and parts of the membranous and cartilaginous regions of the neurocranium (skull) (Fig. 17.1; see also Chapter 10 and Fig. 10.4). They also form all other tissues in these regions, including cartilage, bone, dentin, tendon, dermis, pia and arachnoid, sensory neurons, and glandular connective tissue.

Cells from **ectodermal placodes (epipharyngeal placodes)**, together with neural crest, form neurons of the 5th, 7th, 9th, and 10th cranial sensory ganglia (Fig. 17.2).

## PHARYNGEAL ARCHES

The most distinctive feature in development of the head and neck is the presence of **pharyngeal arches** (the old term for these structures is **branchial arches** because they somewhat

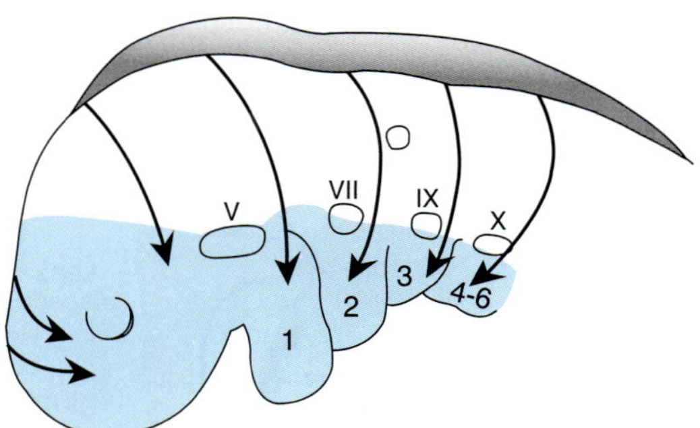


FIGURE 17.2 Migration pathways of neural crest cells from forebrain, midbrain, and hindbrain regions into their final locations (*blue areas*) in the pharyngeal arches and face. Regions of ectodermal thickenings (epipharyngeal placodes), which will assist crest cells in formation of the fifth (*V*), seventh (*VII*), ninth (*IX*), and tenth (*X*) cranial sensory ganglia, are also illustrated.

**Table 17.1 Derivatives of the Pharyngeal Arches and Their Innervation**

| Pharyngeal Arch | Nerve | Muscles | Skeleton |
|---|---|---|---|
| 1. Mandibular (maxillary and mandibular processes) | V. Trigeminal: maxillary and mandibular divisions | Mastication (temporal; masseter, medial, lateral pterygoids); mylohyoid, anterior belly of digastric, tensor palatine, tensor tympani | Premaxilla, maxilla, zygomatic bone, part of temporal bone, Meckel cartilage, mandible malleus, incus, anterior ligament of malleus, sphenomandibular ligament |
| 2. Hyoid | VII. Facial | Facial expression (buccinator, auricularis, frontalis, platysma, orbicularis oris, orbicularis oculi) posterior belly of digastric, stylohyoid, stapedius | Stapes, styloid process, stylohyoid ligament, lesser horn and upper portion of body of hyoid bone |
| 3. | IX. Glossopharyngeal | Stylopharyngeus | Greater horn and lower portion of body of hyoid bone |
| 4–6. | X. Vagus<br>■ Superior laryngeal branch (nerve to fourth arch)<br>■ Recurrent laryngeal branch (nerve to sixth arch) | Cricothyroid, levator veli palatini, constrictors of pharynx<br>Intrinsic muscles of larynx | Laryngeal cartilages (thyroid, cricoid, arytenoid, corniculate, cuneiform) |

resemble the gills [branchia] of a fish). These arches appear in the fourth and fifth weeks of development and contribute to the characteristic external appearance of the embryo (Table 17.1 and Fig. 17.3). Initially, they consist of bars of mesenchymal tissue separated by deep clefts known as **pharyngeal clefts** (Fig. 17.3C; see also Fig. 17.6). Simultaneously, with development of the arches and clefts, a number of outpocketings, the **pharyngeal pouches**, appear along the lateral walls of the pharynx, the most cranial part of the foregut (Fig. 17.4; see also Fig. 17.6). The pouches penetrate the surrounding mesenchyme but do not establish an open communication with the external clefts (Fig. 17.3C). Hence, although development of pharyngeal arches, clefts, and pouches resembles formation of gills in fishes and amphibians, in the human embryo, real gills are never formed. Therefore, the term **pharyngeal** (arches, clefts, and pouches) has been adopted for the human embryo.

## ■ DEVELOPMENT OF FACE

Pharyngeal arches not only contribute to formation of the neck but also play an important role in formation of the face. At the end of the fourth week, the center of the face is formed by the stomodeum, surrounded by the first pair of pharyngeal arches (Fig. 17.5). When the embryo is 42 days old, five mesenchymal prominences can be recognized: the **paired mandibular prominences** (first pharyngeal arch), caudal to the stomodeum; the **paired maxillary prominences** (dorsal portion of the first pharyngeal arch), lateral to the stomodeum; and the **frontonasal prominence**, a slightly rounded elevation cranial to the stomodeum. Development of the face is later complemented by formation of the **nasal prominences** (Fig. 17.5). In all cases, differentiation of structures derived from arches, pouches, clefts, and prominences is dependent on epithelial–mesenchymal interactions.

## ■ COMPONENTS OF PHARYNGEAL ARCHES

Each pharyngeal arch consists of a core of mesenchymal tissue covered on the outside by surface ectoderm and on the inside by epithelium of endodermal origin (Fig. 17.6). In addition to mesenchyme derived from paraxial and lateral plate mesoderm, the core of each arch receives substantial numbers of **neural crest cells**, which migrate into the arches to contribute to **skeletal components** of the face. The original mesoderm of the arches gives rise to the musculature of the face and neck. Thus, each pharyngeal

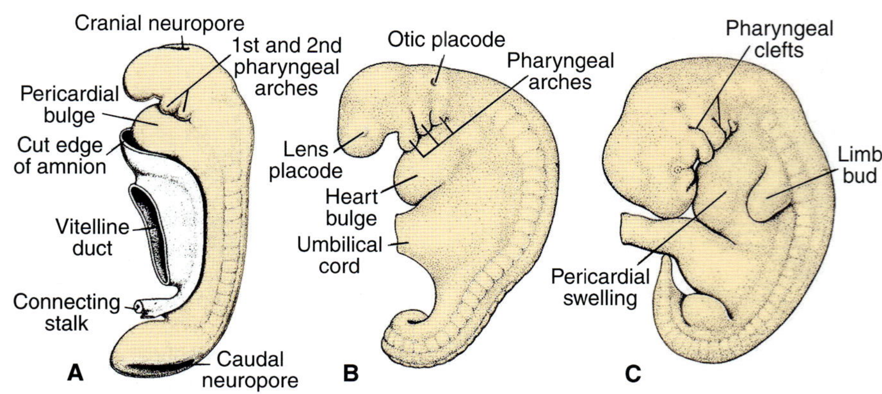


**FIGURE 17.3** Development of the pharyngeal arches. **A.** 25 days. **B.** 28 days. **C.** 5 weeks.

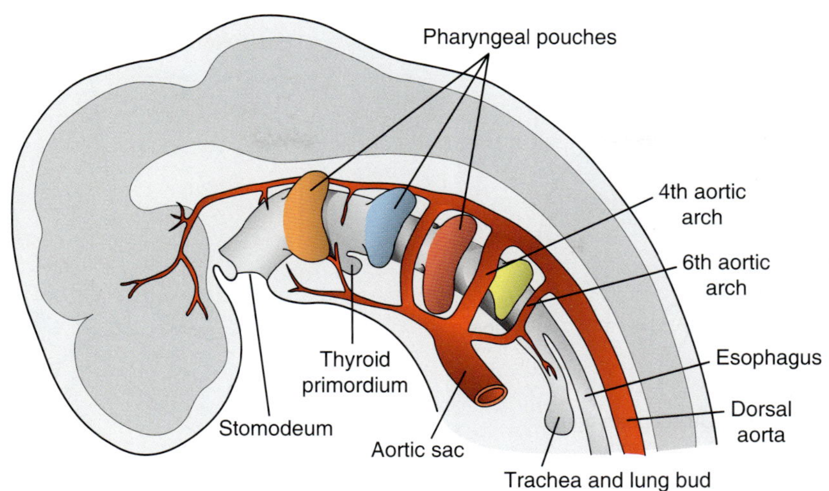


**FIGURE 17.4** Pharyngeal pouches as outpocketings of the foregut and the primordium of the thyroid gland and aortic arches.

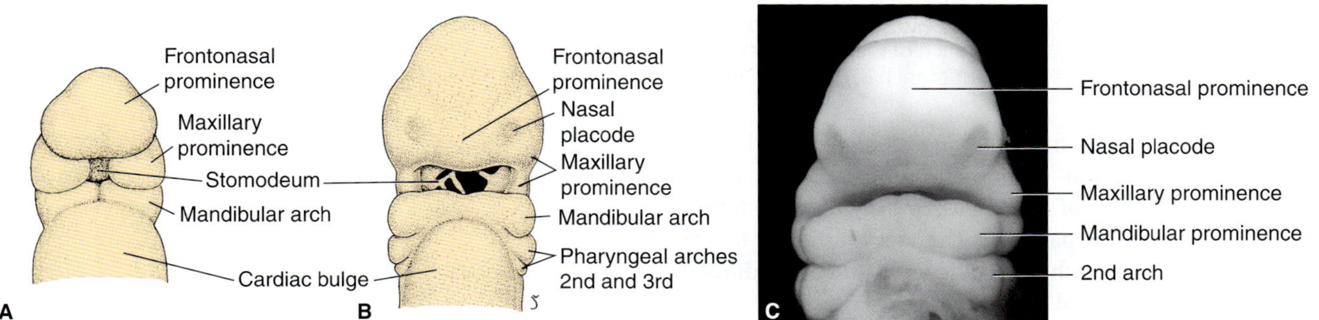


**FIGURE 17.5 A.** Frontal view of an embryo of approximately 24 days. The stomodeum, temporarily closed by the oropharyngeal membrane, is surrounded by five mesenchymal prominences. **B.** Frontal view of an embryo at approximately 30 days showing rupture of the oropharyngeal membrane and formation of the nasal placodes on the frontonasal prominence. **C.** Photograph of a human embryo at a stage (28 days) similar to that shown in **(B)**.

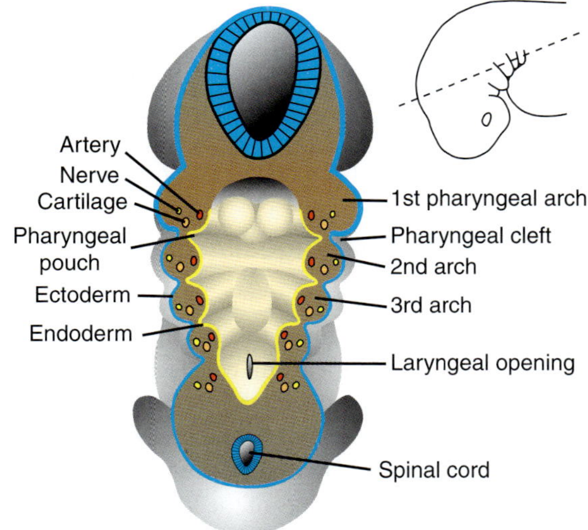


**FIGURE 17.6** Drawing shows the pharyngeal arches cut in cross section. Each arch consists of a mesenchymal core derived from mesoderm and neural crest cells and each is lined internally by endoderm and externally by ectoderm. Each arch also contains an artery (one of the aortic arches) and a cranial nerve and each will contribute specific skeletal and muscular components to the head and neck. Between the arches are pouches on the inner surface and clefts externally.

arch is characterized by its own **muscular components**. The muscular components of each arch have their own cranial nerve, and wherever the muscle cells migrate, they carry their **nerve component** with them (Figs. 17.6 and 17.7). In addition, each arch has its own **arterial component** (Figs. 17.4 and 17.6). (Derivatives of the pharyngeal arches and their nerve supply are summarized in Table 17.1.)

## First Pharyngeal Arch

The **first pharyngeal arch** consists of a dorsal portion, the **maxillary process**, which extends forward beneath the region of the eye, and a ventral portion, the mandibular process, which contains **Meckel cartilage** (Figs. 17.5 and 17.8*A*). During further development, Meckel cartilage disappears except for two small portions at its dorsal end that persist and form the **incus** and **malleus** (Figs. 17.8*B* and 17.9). Mesenchyme of the maxillary process gives rise to the **premaxilla**, **maxilla**, **zygomatic bone**, and part of the **temporal bone** through membranous ossification (Fig. 17.8*B*). The **mandible** is also formed by membranous ossification of mesenchymal tissue surrounding Meckel cartilage. In addition, the first arch contributes to formation of the bones of the middle ear, part of the external ear, and the external auditory meatus (see Chapter 19, p. 288).

Part 2

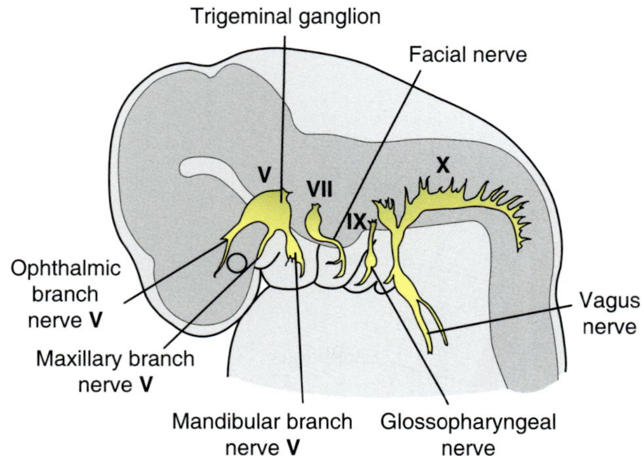


**FIGURE 17.7** Each pharyngeal arch is supplied by its own cranial nerve. The trigeminal nerve supplying the first pharyngeal arch has three branches: the ophthalmic, maxillary, and mandibular. The nerve of the second arch is the facial nerve; that of the third is the glossopharyngeal nerve. The musculature of the fourth arch is supplied by the superior laryngeal branch of the vagus nerve, and that of the sixth arch, by the recurrent branch of the vagus nerve.

Musculature of the first pharyngeal arch includes the **muscles of mastication** (temporalis, masseter, and pterygoids), **anterior belly of the digastric**, **mylohyoid**, **tensor tympani**, and **tensor palatini**. The **nerve** supply to the muscles of the first arch is provided by the **mandibular branch of the trigeminal nerve** (Fig. 17.7). Because mesenchyme from the first arch also contributes to the dermis of the face, sensory supply to the skin of the face is provided by **ophthalmic**, **maxillary**, and **mandibular branches of the trigeminal nerve**.

Muscles of the arches do not always attach to the bony or cartilaginous components of their own arch but sometimes migrate into surrounding regions. Nevertheless, the origin of these muscles can always be traced because their nerve supply is derived from the arch of origin.

## Second Pharyngeal Arch

The cartilage of the **second** or **hyoid arch (Reichert cartilage)** (Fig. 17.8*B*) gives rise to the **stapes**, **styloid process of the temporal bone**, **stylohyoid ligament**, and ventrally, the **lesser horn** and **upper part of the body of the hyoid bone** (Fig. 17.9). Mesenchyme of the arch also forms most of the external ear (see Chapter 19, p. 288). Muscles of the hyoid arch are the **stapedius**, **stylohyoid**, **posterior belly of the digastric**, **auricular**, **and muscles of facial expression**. The **facial nerve**, the nerve of the second arch, supplies all of these muscles.

## Third Pharyngeal Arch

The **cartilage** of the third pharyngeal arch produces the **lower part of the body** and **greater horn of the hyoid bone** (Fig. 17.9). The **musculature** is limited to the **stylopharyngeus muscles**. These muscles are innervated by the **glossopharyngeal nerve**, the nerve of the third arch (Fig. 17.7).

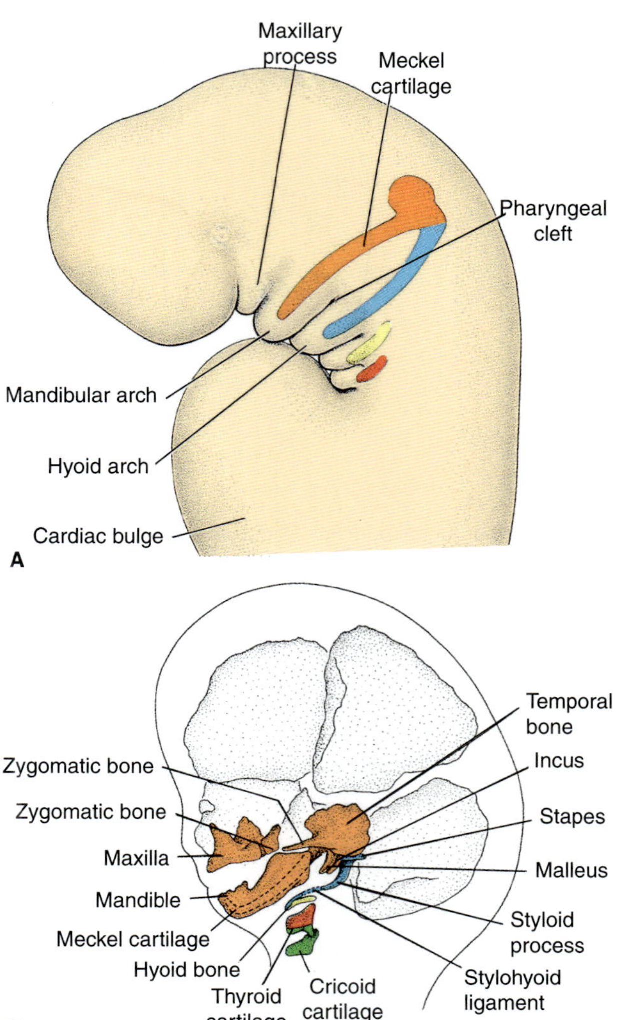


**FIGURE 17.8** **A.** Lateral view of the head and neck region demonstrating the cartilages of the pharyngeal arches participating in formation of the bones of the face and neck. **B.** Various components of the pharyngeal arches later in development. Some of the components ossify; others disappear or become ligamentous. The maxillary process and Meckel cartilage are replaced by the maxilla and mandible, respectively, which develop by membranous ossification.

## Fourth and Sixth Pharyngeal Arches

**Cartilaginous components** of the fourth and sixth pharyngeal arches fuse to form the **thyroid**, cricoid, arytenoid, corniculate, and cuneiform cartilages of the **larynx** (Fig. 17.9). **Muscles** of the fourth arch (**cricothyroid**, **levator veli palatini**, and **constrictors of the pharynx**) are innervated by the **superior laryngeal branch of the vagus**, the nerve of the fourth arch. Intrinsic muscles of the larynx are supplied by the **recurrent laryngeal branch of the vagus**, the nerve of the sixth arch.

# ■ PHARYNGEAL POUCHES

The human embryo has four pairs of pharyngeal pouches; the fifth is rudimentary (Figs. 17.6 and 17.10). Because the **epithelial endodermal lining** of the pouches gives rise

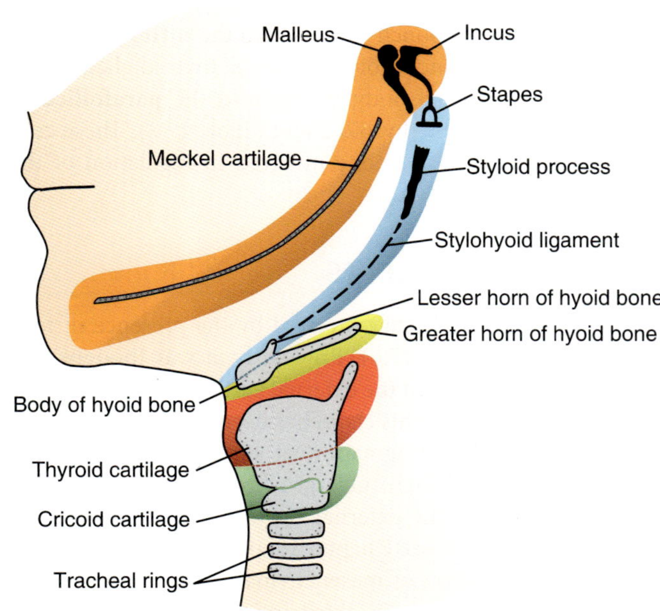


**FIGURE 17.9** Definitive structures formed by the cartilaginous components of the various pharyngeal arches.

to a number of important organs, the fate of each pouch is discussed separately. Derivatives of the pharyngeal pouches are summarized in Table 17.2.

## First Pharyngeal Pouch

The first pharyngeal pouch forms a stalklike diverticulum, the **tubotympanic recess**, which comes in contact with the epithelial lining of the first pharyngeal cleft (Fig. 17.10). The distal portion of the diverticulum widens into a saclike structure, the **primitive tympanic** or **middle ear cavity**, and the proximal part remains narrow, forming the **auditory (eustachian) tube**. The lining of the tympanic cavity later aids in formation of the **tympanic membrane** or **eardrum** (see Chapter 19, p. 288).

**Table 17.2 Derivatives of the Pharyngeal Pouches**

| Pharyngeal Pouch | Derivatives |
|---|---|
| 1 | Tympanic (middle ear) cavity<br>Auditory (eustachian) tube |
| 2 | Palatine tonsils<br>Tonsillar fossa |
| 3 | Inferior parathyroid gland<br>Thymus |
| 4 | Superior parathyroid gland<br>ultimobranchial body (parafollicular [C] cells of the thyroid gland) |

## Second Pharyngeal Pouch

The epithelial lining of the second pharyngeal pouch proliferates and forms buds that penetrate into the surrounding mesenchyme. The buds are secondarily invaded by mesodermal tissue, forming the primordium of the **palatine tonsils** (Fig. 17.10). During the third and fifth months, the tonsil is infiltrated by lymphatic tissue. Part of the pouch remains and is found in the adult as the **tonsillar fossa**.

## Third Pharyngeal Pouch

The third and fourth pouches are characterized at their distal extremity by a dorsal and a ventral wing (Fig. 17.10). In the fifth week, epithelium of the dorsal region of the third pouch differentiates into the **inferior parathyroid gland**, whereas the ventral region forms the **thymus** (Fig. 17.10). Both gland primordia lose their connection with the pharyngeal wall, and the thymus then migrates in a caudal and a medial direction, pulling the **inferior parathyroid** with it (Fig. 17.11). Although the main portion of the thymus moves rapidly to its final position in the anterior part of the thorax where it fuses with its counterpart from the opposite side, its tail portion sometimes persists either embedded in the thyroid gland or as isolated thymic nests.

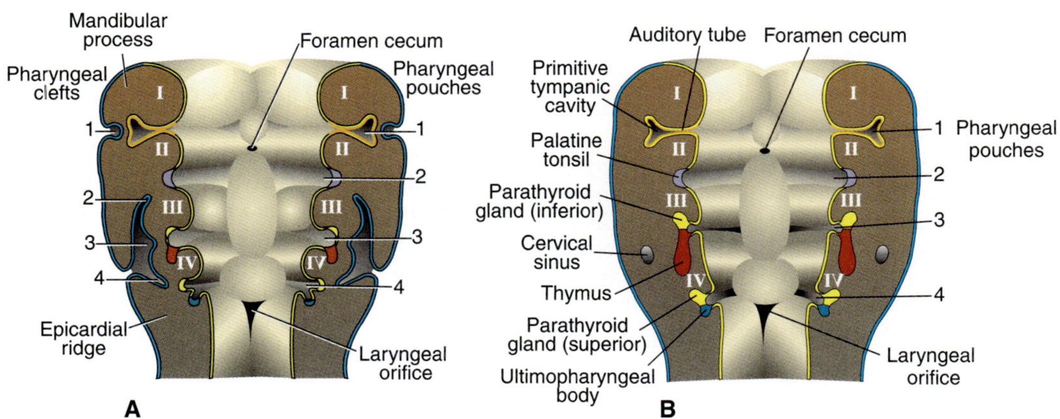


**FIGURE 17.10 A.** Development of the pharyngeal clefts and pouches. The second arch grows extensively to occlude all of the pharyngeal clefts. The first cleft is occluded when the second arch forms most of the external ear. Overgrowth of the second arch caudally covers the third and fourth arches, burying the second, third, and fourth pharyngeal clefts. **B.** Remnants of the second, third, and fourth pharyngeal clefts form the cervical sinus, which is normally obliterated. Note the structures formed by the various pharyngeal pouches.

Part 2

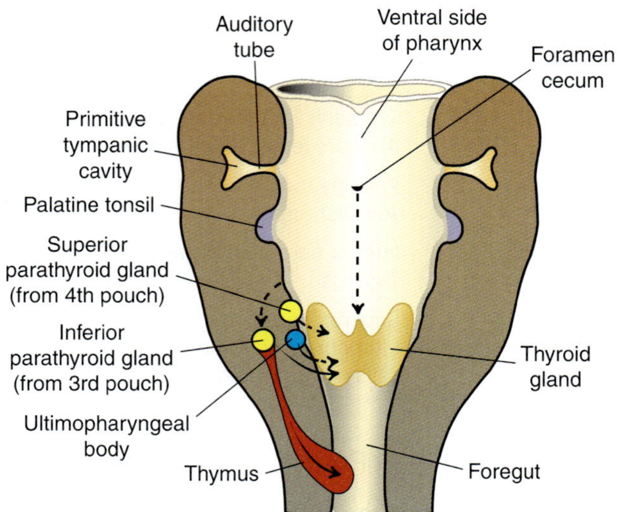


**FIGURE 17.11** Migration of the thymus, parathyroid glands, and ultimobranchial body. The thyroid gland originates in the midline at the level of the foramen cecum and descends to the level of the first tracheal rings.

Growth and development of the thymus continue until puberty. In the young child, the thymus occupies considerable space in the thorax and lies behind the sternum and anterior to the pericardium and great vessels. In older persons, it is difficult to recognize because it is atrophied and replaced by fatty tissue.

The parathyroid tissue of the third pouch finally comes to rest on the dorsal surface of the thyroid gland and forms the **inferior parathyroid gland** (Fig. 17.11).

### Fourth Pharyngeal Pouch

Epithelium of the dorsal region of the fourth pharyngeal pouch forms the **superior parathyroid gland**. When the parathyroid gland loses contact with the wall of the pharynx, it attaches itself to the dorsal surface of the caudally migrating thyroid as the **superior parathyroid gland** (Fig. 17.11). The ventral region of the fourth pouch gives rise to the **ultimobranchial body**, which is later incorporated into the thyroid gland. Cells of the ultimobranchial body give rise to the **parafollicular cells**, or **C cells**, of the thyroid gland (Table 17.2). These cells secrete **calcitonin**, a hormone involved in regulation of the calcium level in the blood.

## PHARYNGEAL CLEFTS

The 5-week embryo is characterized by the presence of four pharyngeal clefts (Fig. 17.6). Previously, it was thought that the first cleft contributed the external auditory meatus (EAM) of the external ear, but this claim has been disproved. Instead, the EAM forms by invagination of surface ectoderm from the first pharyngeal arch. Overgrowth of the second arch, as it forms most of the external ear, causes the first cleft to disappear (Fig. 17.10; see Chapter 19, p. 289).

Active proliferation of mesenchymal tissue in the second arch causes it to overlap the third and fourth arches. Finally, it merges with the **epicardial ridge** in the lower part of the neck (Fig. 17.10), and the second, third, and fourth clefts lose contact with the outside (Fig. 17.10*B*). The clefts form a cavity lined with ectodermal epithelium, the **cervical sinus**, but with further development, this sinus disappears.

## MOLECULAR REGULATION OF FACIAL DEVELOPMENT

Neural crest cells arise from neuroepithelial cells adjacent to the surface ectoderm all along the edges of the neural folds. Bone morphogenetic protein (BMP) signaling is important in establishing this edge region and then regulates *WNT1* expression to cause prospective crest cells to undergo an epithelial-to-mesenchymal transition and begin their migration into the surrounding mesenchyme (see Chapter 6, p. 60). In the hindbrain, crest cells originate in a specific

## *Clinical Correlates*

### Birth Defects Involving the Pharyngeal Region

#### *Ectopic Thymic and Parathyroid Tissue*

Because glandular tissue derived from the pouches undergoes migration, it is not unusual for accessory glands or remnants of tissue to persist along the pathway. This is true particularly for thymic tissue, which may remain in the neck, and for the parathyroid glands. The inferior parathyroids are more variable in position than the superior ones and are sometimes found at the bifurcation of the common carotid artery.

#### *Branchial Fistulas*

**Branchial fistulas** occur when the second pharyngeal arch fails to grow caudally over the third and fourth arches, leaving remnants of the second, third, and fourth clefts in contact with the surface by a narrow canal (Fig. 17.12*A*). Such a fistula, found on the lateral aspect of the neck directly **anterior** to the **sternocleidomastoid muscle**, usually provides drainage for a **lateral cervical cyst** (Fig. 17.12*B*). These cysts, remnants of the cervical sinus, are most often just below the angle of the jaw (Fig. 17.13), although they may be found anywhere along the anterior border of the sternocleidomastoid muscle. Frequently, a lateral cervical cyst is not visible at birth but becomes evident as it enlarges during childhood.

**Internal branchial fistulas** are rare; they occur when the cervical sinus is connected to the lumen of the pharynx by a small canal, which usually opens in the tonsillar region (Fig. 17.12*C*). Such a fistula results from a rupture of the membrane between the second pharyngeal cleft and pouch at some time during development.

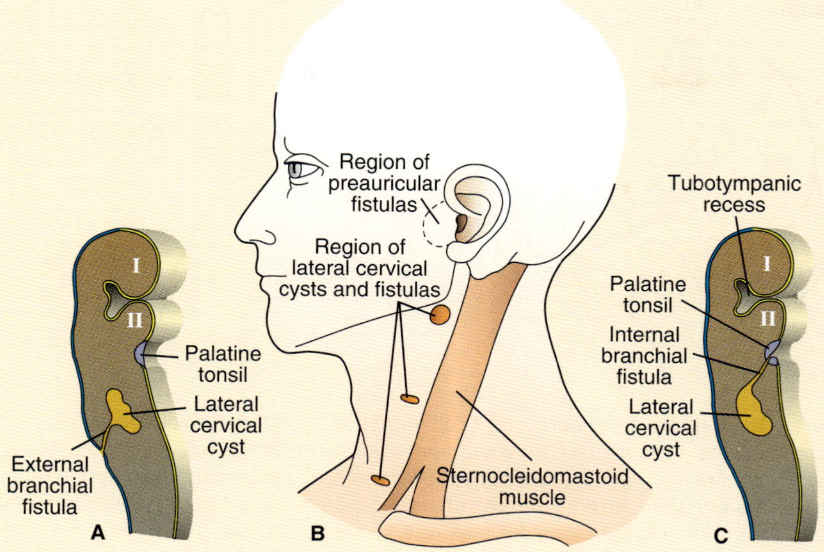


**FIGURE 17.12 A.** Lateral cervical cyst opening at the side of the neck by way of a fistula. **B.** Lateral cervical cysts and fistulas anterior to the sternocleidomastoid muscle. Note also the region of preauricular fistulas. **C.** A lateral cervical cyst opening into the pharynx at the level of the palatine tonsil.

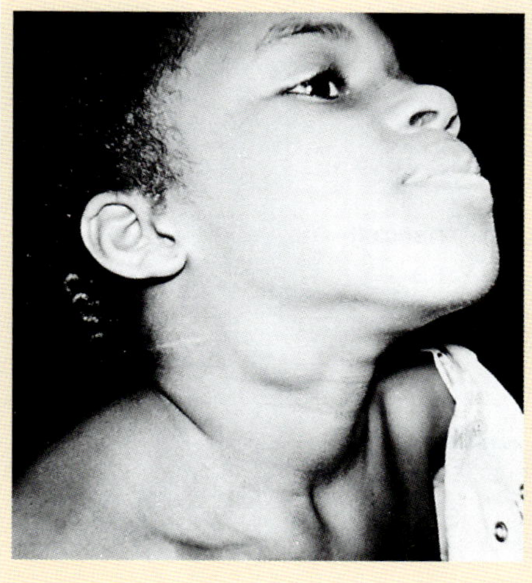

**FIGURE 17.13** Patient with a lateral cervical cyst. These cysts are always on the lateral side of the neck in front of the sternocleidomastoid muscle. They commonly lie under the angle of the mandible and do not enlarge until later in life.



pattern from segments called **rhombomeres** (Fig. 17.14). There are eight of these segments in the hindbrain (R1–R8), and neural crest cells from specific segments migrate to populate specific pharyngeal arches. These crest cells migrate in three streams: Those from R1 and R2 migrate to the first arch along with crest cells from the caudal midbrain region, crest from R4 migrate to the second arch, and cells from R6 and R7 migrate to arches 4 to 6 (Fig. 17.14). Segregation of the three streams is assisted by the fact that very few crest cells form from R3 and R5 segments and those that do enter adjoining streams of cells to migrate. Three distinct streams are important because they provide axonal guidance cues for axons from ganglia forming in the head and neck region, including the trigeminal, geniculate, vestibuloacoustic, petrosal, and nodose ganglia. These ganglia are formed from a combination of crest cells and cells from placodes in this region (see Chapter 18). Axons from the trigeminal ganglion enter the hindbrain at R2, those from the geniculate and vestibuloacoustic at R4, and those from the petrosal and nodose at R6 and R7, thus accounting for three streams of crest cells. No axons project to R3 or R5.

Neural crest cells that populate the pharyngeal arches form the skeletal components characteristic of each arch. Previously, it was thought that neural crest cells regulated patterning of these skeletal elements, but now, it is clear that this process is controlled by pharyngeal pouch endoderm. Formation of the pharyngeal pouches occurs prior to neural crest migration and takes place even in the absence of crest cells. Pouches are formed by migration of endoderm cells laterally, and this migration is stimulated by fibroblast growth factors (FGFs). As pouches form, they express a very characteristic pattern of genes (Fig. 17.15). *BMP7* is expressed

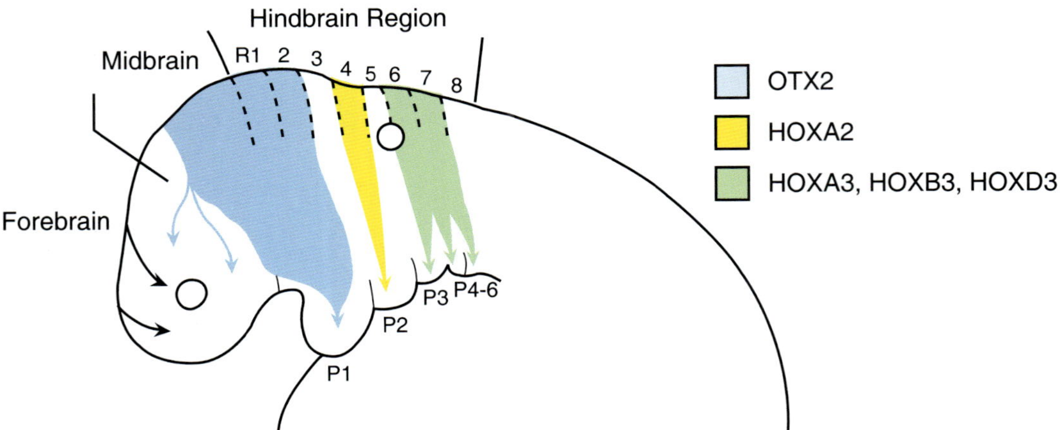


**FIGURE 17.14** Drawing showing the pathways of neural crest cell migration from the cranial neural folds into the face and pharyngeal arches. From the hindbrain region, crest cells migrate from segments called rhombomeres. Rhombomeres express a specific pattern of *HOX* genes (the midbrain and rhombomeres 1 and 2 express the homeodomain-containing transcription factor OTX2; see also Fig. 18.31), and neural crest cells carry these expression patterns into the pharyngeal arches. Also, notice that there are three streams of crest cells and that rhombomeres 3 and 5 do not contribute many (if any) cells to these streams. The three streams are important because they provide guidance cues for cranial nerves growing back from their ganglia to establish connections in the hindbrain (see also Fig. 18.40).



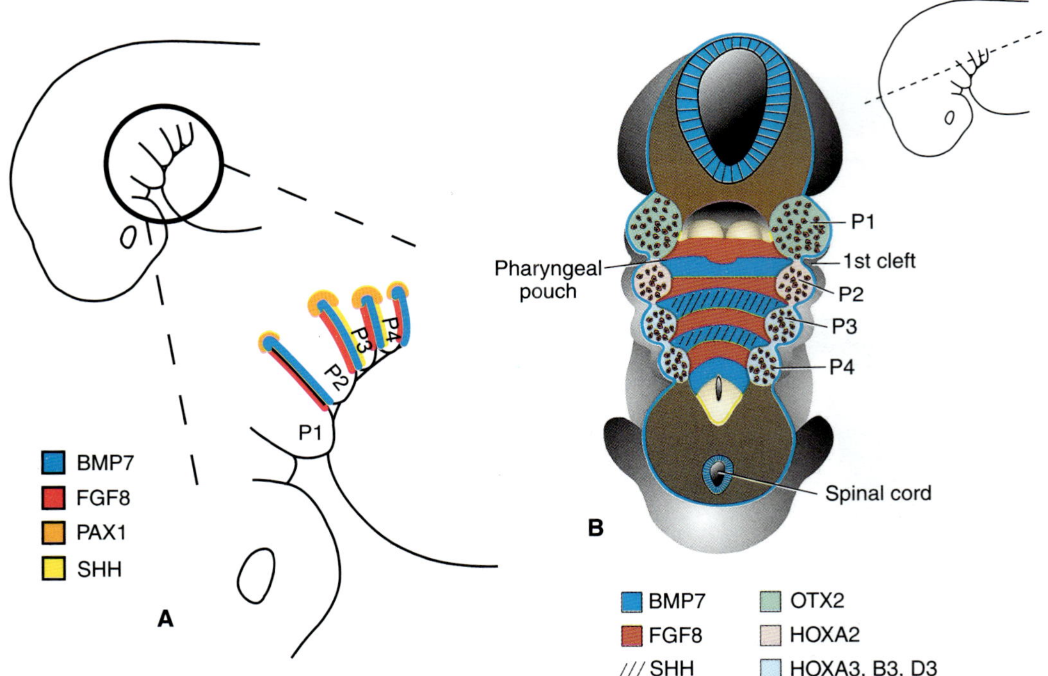


**FIGURE 17.15 A,B.** Drawings showing the gene expression patterns in pharyngeal arch endoderm and mesenchyme. Endoderm is responsible for patterning the skeletal derivatives of the arches, but the response of the mesenchyme to these signals is dictated by the genes that the mesenchyme expresses. Gene expression in the endoderm of the pouches shows a specific pattern: Fibroblast growth factor 8 (*FGF8*) is expressed in the anterior region of each pouch with bone morphogenetic protein 7 (*BMP7*) expressed in the posterior region; sonic hedgehog (*SHH*) is expressed in the posterior region of pouches 2 and 3, whereas *PAX1* is expressed in the dorsalmost area of each pouch **(A,B)**. Mesenchymal expression patterns are established by neural crest cells that migrate into the arches and carry the genetic code from their rhombomeres of origin (or also from the midbrain in the case of the first arch) to the arches **(B)** (see also Figs. 17.14 and 18.31).

in the posterior endoderm of each pouch, *FGF8* lies in the anterior endoderm, and *PAX1* expression is restricted to the dorsalmost endoderm of each pouch. In addition, *SONIC HEDGEHOG* (*SHH*) is expressed in the posterior endoderm of the second and third pouches. These expression patterns then regulate differentiation and patterning of pharyngeal arch mesenchyme into specific skeletal structures. This process, however, is also dependent on the mesenchyme and represents another example of an epithelial–mesenchymal interaction. In this case, the response of the mesenchyme to endodermal signals is dependent on transcription factors expressed in that mesenchyme. These transcription factors include *HOX* genes and others carried by neural crest cells into the arches. Crest cells acquire their specific gene expression patterns from the rhombomeres of their origin (Fig. 17.14). The pattern of rhombomeres itself is established by a nested code of *HOX* gene expression in the hindbrain (see Chapter 18) that crest cells carry with them when they migrate. The first arch is *HOX*-negative but does express *OTX2*, a homeodomain-containing transcription factor that is expressed in the midbrain; the second arch expresses *HOXA2*; and arches 3 to 6 express members of the third paralogous group of *HOX* genes, *HOXA3*, *HOXB3*, and *HOXD3* (Fig. 17.15*B*). The different expression patterns of these transcription factors allow each arch to respond differently to signals emanating from pouch endoderm, such that the first arch forms the maxilla and mandible, the second arch, the hyoid bone, etc.

The remainder of the skeleton of the face, the mid and upper facial regions, also is derived from neural crest cells that migrate into the frontonasal prominence (Fig. 17.14). In this region, signals emanating from the surface ectoderm and the underlying areas of the neuroepithelium dictate the fate of the mesenchyme. Again, it appears that *SHH* and *FGF8* play major roles in patterning this area, but the specific genetic interactions are not known.

## *Clinical Correlates*

### *Neural Crest Cells and Craniofacial Defects*

**Neural crest cells** (Fig. 17.2) are essential for formation of much of the craniofacial region. Consequently, disruption of crest cell development results in craniofacial malformations. Because neural crest cells also contribute to the **conotruncal endocardial cushions**, which septate the outflow tract of the heart into pulmonary and aortic channels, many infants with craniofacial defects also have cardiac abnormalities, including persistent truncus arteriosus, tetralogy of Fallot, and transposition of the great vessels. Unfortunately, crest cells appear to be a particularly vulnerable cell population and are easily killed by compounds such as alcohol and retinoic acid. Examples of craniofacial defects involving crest cells include the following.

**Treacher Collins syndrome (mandibulofacial dysostosis)** is a rare autosomal dominant disorder occurring in 1/50,000 live births with 60% of cases arising as new mutations. The syndrome is characterized by hypoplasia of the maxilla, mandible, and zygomatic arches, which may be absent. Cleft palate is common as are external ear defects accompanied by atresia of the auditory canals and abnormalities of the middle ear ossicles, such that bilateral conductive hearing loss is often present. The eyes are usually involved with down-slanting palpebral fissures and lower eyelid colobomas. Mutations in the *TCOF1* gene (5q32) are responsible for most cases. The product of this gene is a nucleolar protein called **treacle** that appears to be necessary for preventing apoptosis and maintaining proliferation in neural crest cells but not for regulating their migration, which occurs normally. Although most cases of the syndrome are due to genetic mutations, phenocopies can be produced in laboratory animals following exposure to teratogenic doses of retinoic acid, suggesting that some cases in humans may be caused by teratogens.

**Robin sequence** may occur independently or in association with other syndromes and malformations. Like Treacher Collins syndrome, Robin sequence alters first-arch structures, with development of the mandible most severely affected. Infants usually have a triad of micrognathia, cleft palate, and glossoptosis (posteriorly placed tongue) (Fig. 17.16*A*). Robin sequence may be due to genetic or environmental factors. It may also occur as a deformation, as for example, when the chin is compressed against the chest in cases of oligohydramnios. The primary defect includes poor growth of the mandible and, as a result, a posteriorly placed tongue that fails to drop from between the palatal shelves, preventing their fusion. Robin sequence occurs in approximately 1/8,500 births.

**22q11.2 Deletion syndrome** is the most common deletion syndrome in humans and has several presentations, including DiGeorge syndrome (Fig. 17.16*B*), DiGeorge anomaly, velocardiofacial syndrome (Fig. 17.16*C*), Shprintzen syndrome, conotruncal anomaly face syndrome, and congenital thymic aplasia and hypoplasia. The defects are the result of a deletion on the long arm

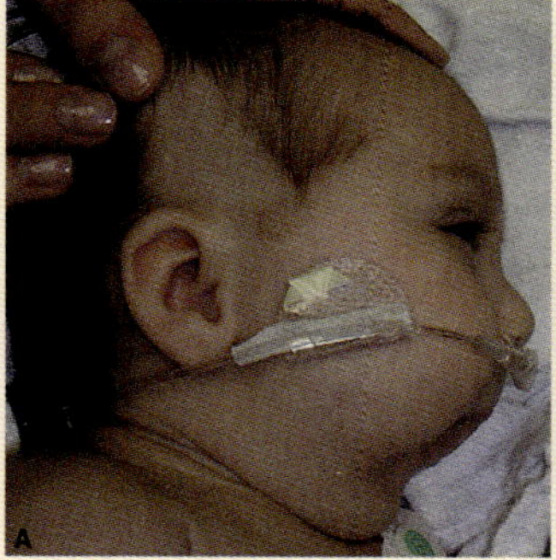

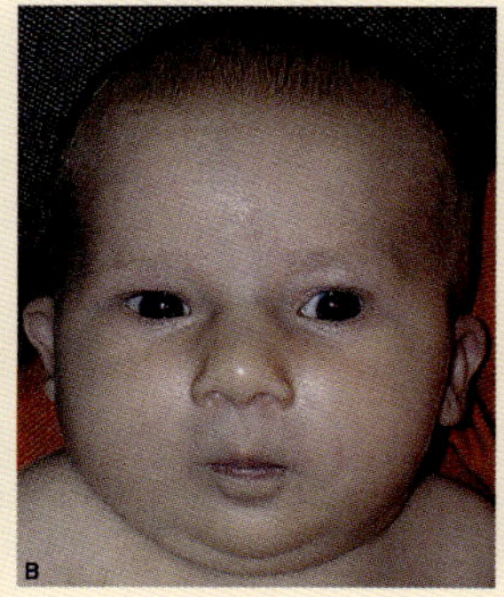

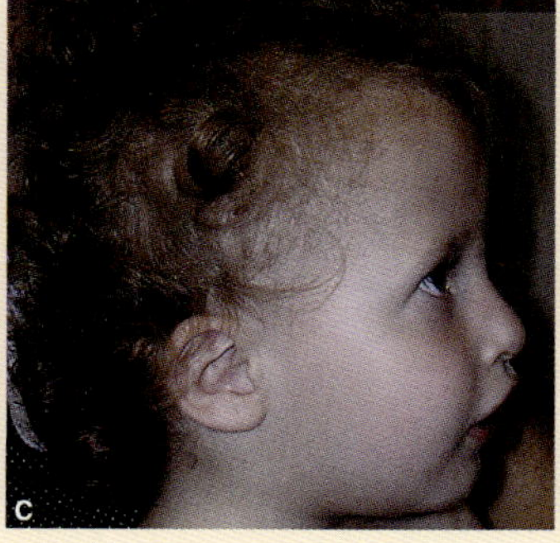

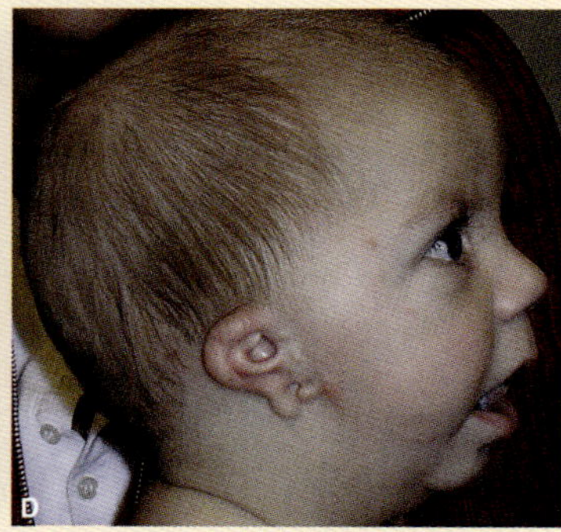


**FIGURE 17.16** Patients with craniofacial defects thought to arise from insults to neural crest cells. **A.** Robin sequence. Note the very small mandible (micrognathia) that keeps the tongue from "dropping" out of the way of the palatal shelves resulting in cleft palate. **B,C.** Examples of 22q11.2 deletion syndrome: DiGeorge syndrome. **B.** Note the small mouth, nearly smooth philtrum, micrognathia, prominent nasal bridge, and posteriorly rotated ears; velocardiofacial syndrome. **C.** This patient shows mild facial dysmorphology, including mild malar hypoplasia, micrognathia, prominent upper lip, and large ears. **D.** Hemifacial microsomia (oculoauriculovertebral spectrum, or Goldenhar syndrome). Note the abnormal ear with skin tags and the small chin.

(*Continued*)

of chromosome 22 and occur in approximately 1 per 4,000 births. Recent evidence shows that mutations in one of the genes in the deletion interval, *TBX1* (T-box DNA binding transcription factor 1), result in the same syndrome without a deletion. Furthermore, variability in regulation of the *TBX1* gene may explain the wide range of observed phenotypes. The syndrome is characterized by a variety of malformations and degrees of severity, but infants most often present with congenital heart and aortic arch defects, mild facial dysmorphology, learning disabilities, and frequent infections due to thymic hypoplasia or aplasia that disrupts the immune system's T cell–mediated response. Many of the infants also have seizures due to hypocalcemia caused by abnormal development of the parathyroid glands. Later in life, these individuals are more likely to have mental illnesses, including schizophrenia and depression. In part, origin of the defects is due to disruption of neural crest cells that contribute to many of the affected structures. Even the thymus and parathyroid defects are related to neural crest cells because these cells contribute the mesenchyme into which endoderm from the pharyngeal pouches migrates. Endoderm cells from the pouches make the thymus and parathyroid cells (see Fig. 17.10) and neural crest derived mesenchyme makes the connective tissue. Without this mesenchyme, the normal epithelial (endodermal)–mesenchymal interaction essential for differentiation of the glands does not occur.

**Hemifacial microsomia (oculoauriculovertebral spectrum or Goldenhar syndrome)** includes a number of craniofacial abnormalities that usually involve the maxillary, temporal, and zygomatic bones, which are small and flat. Ear (anotia, microtia), eye (tumors and dermoids in the eyeball), and vertebral (fused and hemivertebrae, spina bifida) defects are commonly observed in these patients (Fig. 17.16*D*). Asymmetry is present in 65% of the cases, which occur in 1/5,600 births. Other malformations, which occur in 50% of cases, include cardiac abnormalities, such as tetralogy of Fallot and ventricular septal defects. Causes of hemifacial microsomia are unknown.

## ■ TONGUE

The tongue appears in embryos of approximately 4 weeks in the form of two **lateral lingual swellings** and one **medial swelling**, the **tuberculum impar** (Fig. 17.17*A*). These three swellings originate from the first pharyngeal arch. A second median swelling, the **copula**, or **hypobranchial eminence**, is formed by mesoderm of the second, third, and part of the fourth arch. Finally, a third median swelling, formed by the posterior part of the fourth arch, marks development of the epiglottis. Immediately behind this swelling is the **laryngeal orifice**, which is flanked by the **arytenoid swellings** (Fig. 17.17).

As the lateral lingual swellings increase in size, they overgrow the tuberculum impar and merge, forming the anterior two-thirds, or body, of the tongue (Fig. 17.17; Table 17.3). Because the mucosa covering the body of the tongue originates from the first pharyngeal arch, **sensory innervation** to this area is by the **mandibular branch of the trigeminal nerve**. The

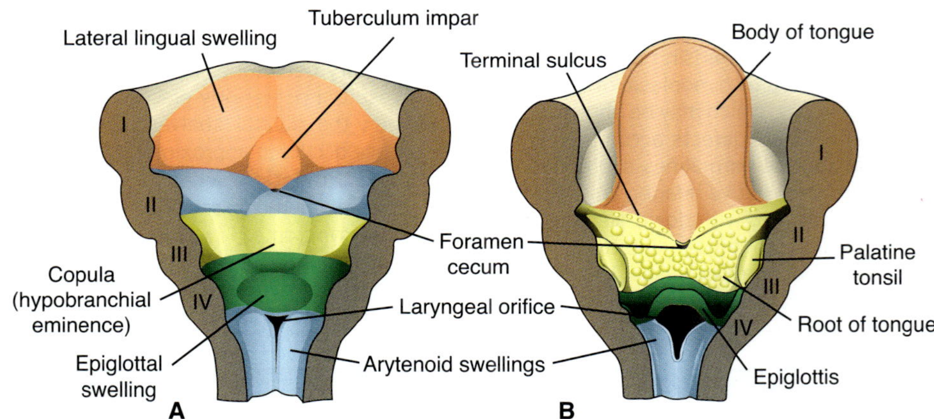


**FIGURE 17.17** Ventral portion of the pharyngeal arches seen from above showing development of the tongue. *I* to *IV*, the cut pharyngeal arches. **A.** 5 weeks (~6 mm). **B.** 5 months. Note the foramen cecum, site of origin of the thyroid primordium.

**Table 17.3 Structures Contributing to Formation of Tongue**

| S. No. | Pharyngeal Arches | Swellings of Arches | Adult Derivatives |
|---|---|---|---|
| 1 | First | Lateral swelling and tuberculum impar | Anterior two-thirds of the tongue and sensory innervation (by mandibular branch of trigeminal nerve) |
| 2 | Second | Hypobranchial eminence | Posterior one-third of the tongue and sensory innervation (by glossopharyngeal nerve) |
| 3 | Third | Hypobranchial eminence | Posterior one-third of the tongue and sensory innervation (by glossopharyngeal nerve) |
| 4 | Fourth | Hypobranchial eminence and third median swelling | Posterior-most part of the tongue (by vagus nerve) |

body of the tongue is separated from the posterior third by a V-shaped groove, the **terminal sulcus** (Fig. 17.17*B*).

The posterior part, or root, of the tongue originates from the second, third, and parts of the fourth pharyngeal arch. The fact that **sensory innervation** to this part of the tongue is supplied by the **glossopharyngeal nerve** indicates that tissue of the third arch overgrows that of the second.

The epiglottis and the extreme posterior part of the tongue are innervated by the **superior laryngeal nerve**, reflecting their development from the fourth arch. Some of the tongue muscles probably differentiate in situ, but most are derived from myoblasts originating in **occipital somites**. Thus, tongue musculature is innervated by the **hypoglossal nerve**.

The general sensory innervation of the tongue is easy to understand. The body is supplied by the trigeminal nerve, the nerve of the first arch; that of the root is supplied by the glossopharyngeal and vagus nerves, the nerves of the third and fourth arches, respectively. **Special sensory innervation (taste)** to the anterior two-thirds of the tongue is provided by the **chorda tympani branch of the facial nerve**, whereas the posterior third is supplied by the glossopharyngeal nerve.

### Clinical Correlates

#### Tongue-Tie

In **ankyloglossia (tongue-tie)**, the tongue is not freed from the floor of the mouth. Normally, extensive cell degeneration occurs, and the frenulum is the only tissue that anchors the tongue to the floor of the mouth. In the most common form of ankyloglossia, the frenulum extends to the tip of the tongue.

## THYROID GLAND

The thyroid gland appears as an epithelial proliferation in the floor of the pharynx between the tuberculum impar and the copula at a point later indicated by the **foramen cecum** (Figs. 17.17 and 17.18*A*). Subsequently, the thyroid descends in front of the pharyngeal gut as a bilobed diverticulum (Fig. 17.18). During this migration, the thyroid remains connected to the tongue by a narrow canal, the **thyroglossal duct**. This duct later disappears.

With further development, the thyroid gland descends in front of the hyoid bone and the laryngeal cartilages. It reaches its final position in front of the trachea in the seventh week (Fig. 17.18*B*). By then, it has acquired a small median isthmus and two lateral lobes. The thyroid begins to function at approximately the end of the third month, at which time the first follicles containing colloid become visible. **Follicular cells** produce the colloid that serves as a source of **thyroxine** and **triiodothyronine. Parafollicular cells**, or **C cells**, derived from the **ultimobranchial body** (Fig. 17.10) serve as a source of calcitonin.

## FACE

At the end of the fourth week, **facial prominences** consisting primarily of neural crest–derived mesenchyme and formed



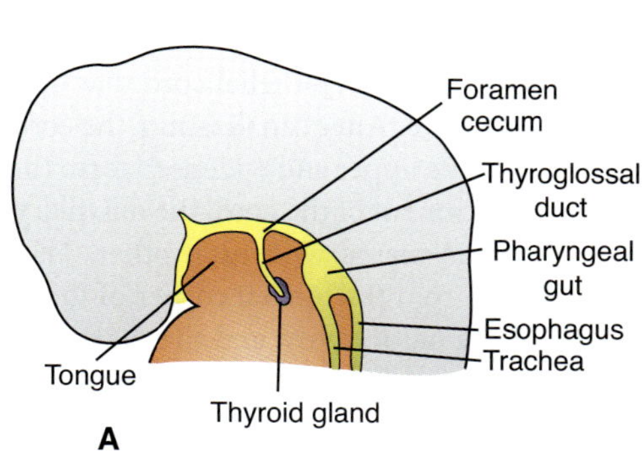


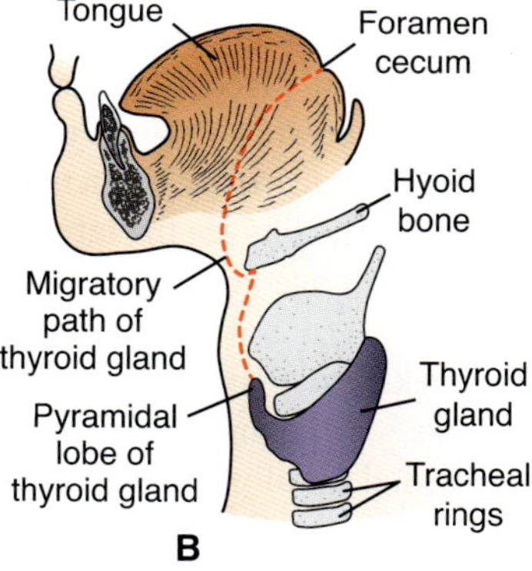


**FIGURE 17.18 A.** The thyroid primordium arises as an epithelial diverticulum in the midline of the pharynx immediately caudal to the tuberculum impar. **B.** Position of the thyroid gland in the adult. *Broken line*, the path of migration.

### Clinical Correlates

#### Thyroglossal Duct and Thyroid Abnormalities

A **thyroglossal cyst** may lie at any point along the migratory pathway of the thyroid gland but is always near or in the **midline** of the neck. As indicated by its name, it is a cystic remnant of the thyroglossal duct. Although approximately 50% of these cysts are close to or just inferior to the body of the hyoid bone (Figs. 17.19 and 17.20), they may also be found at the base of the tongue or close to the thyroid cartilage. Sometimes, a thyroglossal cyst is connected to the outside by a fistulous canal, a **thyroglossal fistula**. Such a fistula usually arises secondarily after rupture of a cyst but may be present at birth.

**Aberrant thyroid tissue** may be found anywhere along the path of descent of the thyroid gland. It is commonly found in the base of the tongue, just behind the foramen cecum, and is subject to the same diseases as the thyroid gland itself.

(Continued)

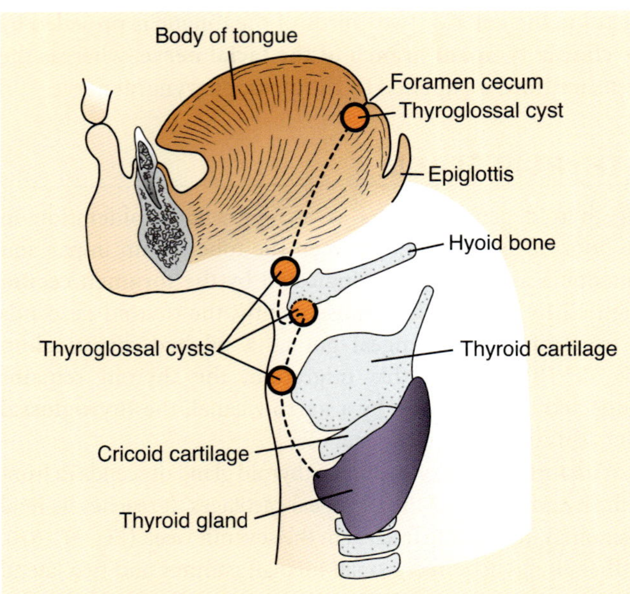


**FIGURE 17.19** Thyroglossal cysts. These cysts, most frequently found in the hyoid region, are always close to the midline.

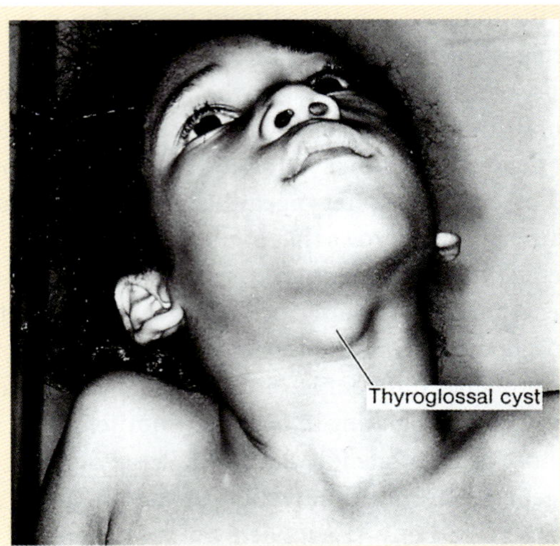


**FIGURE 17.20** Thyroglossal cyst. These cysts, which are remnants of the thyroglossal duct, may be anywhere along the migration pathway of the thyroid gland. They are commonly found behind the arch of the hyoid bone. An important diagnostic characteristic is their midline location.



mainly by the first pair of pharyngeal arches appear. **Maxillary prominences** can be distinguished lateral to the stomodeum, and **mandibular prominences** can be distinguished caudal to this structure (Fig. 17.21). The **frontonasal prominence**, formed by proliferation of mesenchyme ventral to the brain vesicles, constitutes the upper border of the stomodeum. On both sides of the frontonasal prominence, local thickenings of the surface ectoderm, the **nasal (olfactory) placodes**, originate under inductive influence of the ventral portion of the forebrain (Fig. 17.21).

During the fifth week, the nasal placodes invaginate to form **nasal pits**. In so doing, they create a ridge of tissue that surrounds each pit and forms the **nasal prominences**. The prominences on the outer edge of the pits are the **lateral nasal prominences**; those on the inner edge are the **medial nasal prominences** (Fig. 17.22).

During the following 2 weeks, the maxillary prominences continue to increase in size. Simultaneously, they grow medially, compressing the medial nasal prominences toward the midline. Subsequently, the cleft between the medial nasal prominence and the maxillary prominence is lost, and the two fuse (Fig. 17.23). Hence, the upper lip is formed by the two medial nasal prominences and the two maxillary prominences. The lateral nasal prominences do not participate in formation of the upper lip. The lower lip and jaw form from the mandibular prominences that merge across the midline.

Initially, the maxillary and lateral nasal prominences are separated by a deep furrow, the **nasolacrimal groove** (Figs. 17.22 and 17.23). Ectoderm in the floor of this groove forms a solid epithelial cord that detaches from the overlying ectoderm. After canalization, the cord forms the **nasolacrimal duct**; its upper end widens to form the **lacrimal sac**. Following detachment of the cord, the maxillary and lateral nasal prominences merge with each other. The nasolacrimal duct then runs from the medial corner of the eye to the inferior meatus of the nasal cavity, and the maxillary prominences enlarge to form the **cheeks** and **maxillae**.

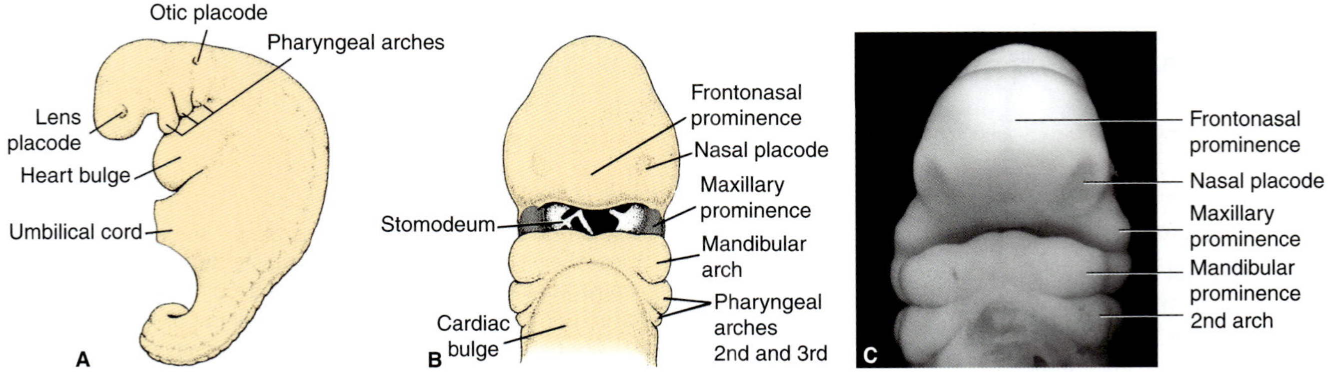


**FIGURE 17.21 A.** Lateral view of an embryo at the end of the fourth week, showing position of the pharyngeal arches. **B.** Frontal view of a 4.5-week embryo showing the mandibular and maxillary prominences. The nasal placodes are visible on either side of the frontonasal prominence. **C.** Photograph of a human embryo at a stage (4.5 weeks) similar to that of **(B)**.

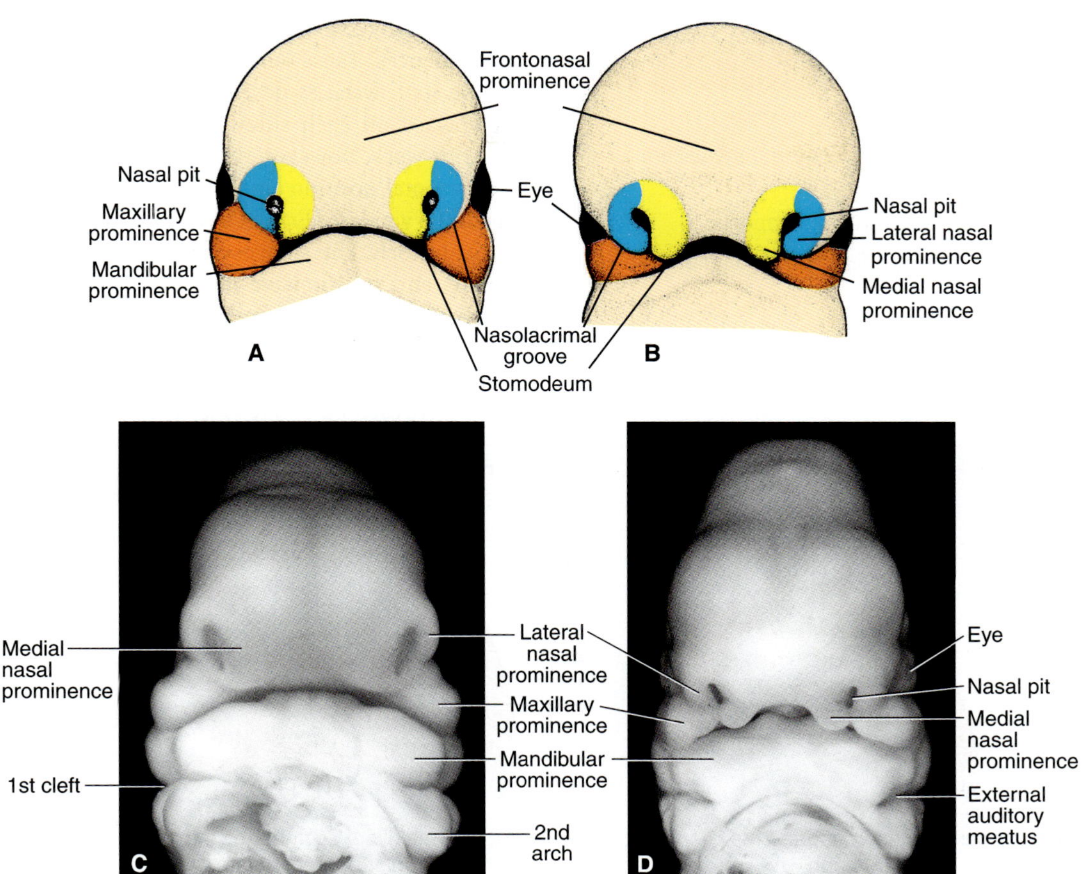


**FIGURE 17.22** Frontal aspect of the face. **A.** 5-week embryo. **B.** 6-week embryo. The nasal prominences are gradually separated from the maxillary prominence by deep furrows. **C,D.** Photographs of human embryos at stages similar to those depicted in **(A)** and **(B)**, respectively.

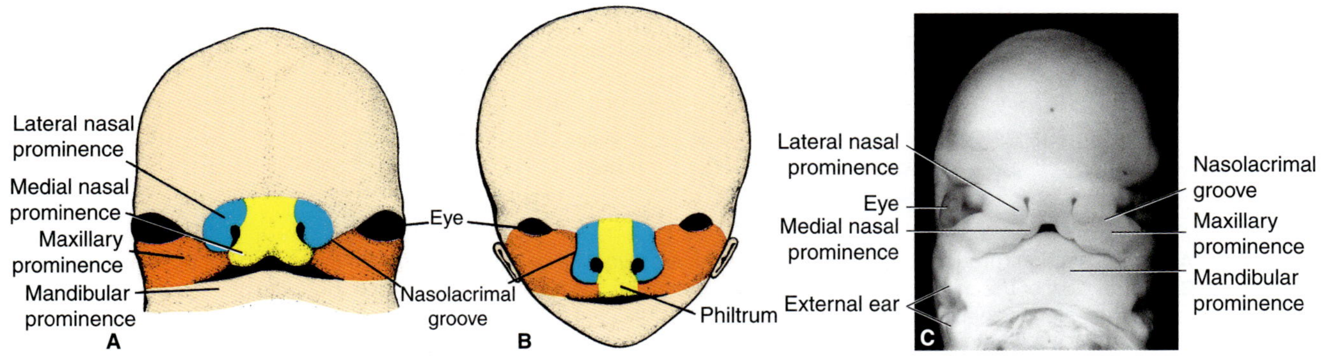


**FIGURE 17.23** Frontal aspect of the face. **A.** 7-week embryo. Maxillary prominences have fused with the medial nasal prominences. **B.** 10-week embryo. **C.** Photograph of a human embryo at a stage similar to that in **(A)**.

The **nose** is formed from five facial prominences (Fig. 17.23): the frontonasal prominence gives rise to the bridge, the merged medial nasal prominences provide the crest and tip, and the lateral nasal prominences form the sides (alae) (Table 17.4).

## ■ INTERMAXILLARY SEGMENT

As a result of medial growth of the maxillary prominences, the two medial nasal prominences merge not only at the surface but also at a deeper level. The structure formed by the two merged prominences is the **intermaxillary segment**. It is composed of (1) a **labial component**, which forms the philtrum of the upper lip; (2) an **upper jaw component**, which carries the four incisor teeth; and (3) a **palatal component**, which forms the triangular primary palate (Fig. 17.24). The intermaxillary segment is continuous with the rostral portion of the **nasal septum**, which is formed by the frontal prominence.

## ■ SECONDARY PALATE

Although the primary palate is derived from the intermaxillary segment (Fig. 17.24), the main part of the definitive palate

**Table 17.4 Structures Contributing to Formation of the Face**

| Prominence | Structures Formed |
|---|---|
| Frontonasal[a] | Forehead, bridge of nose, and medial and lateral nasal prominences |
| Maxillary | Cheeks, lateral portion of upper lip |
| Medial nasal | Philtrum of upper lip, crest, and tip of nose |
| Lateral nasal | Alae of nose |
| Mandibular | Lower lip |

[a]The frontonasal prominence is a single unpaired structure; the other prominences are paired.

is formed by two shelflike outgrowths from the maxillary prominences. These outgrowths, the **palatine shelves**, appear in the sixth week of development and are directed obliquely downward on each side of the tongue (Fig. 17.25). In the seventh week, however, the palatine shelves ascend to attain a horizontal position above the tongue and fuse, forming the **secondary palate** (Figs. 17.26 and 17.27).

Anteriorly, the shelves fuse with the triangular primary palate, and the **incisive foramen** is the midline landmark between the primary and secondary palates (Fig. 17.27*B*). At the same time as the palatine shelves fuse, the nasal septum grows down and joins with the cephalic aspect of the newly formed palate (Fig. 17.27).

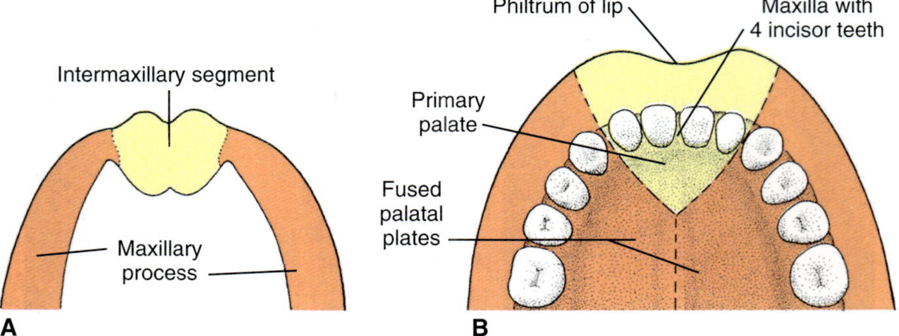


**FIGURE 17.24 A.** Intermaxillary segment and maxillary processes. **B.** The intermaxillary segment giving rise to the philtrum of the upper lip, the median part of the maxillary bone with its four incisor teeth, and the triangular primary palate.

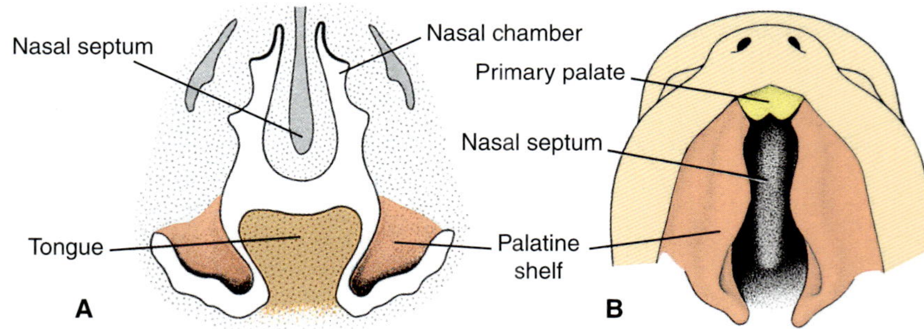


**FIGURE 17.25 A.** Frontal section through the head of a 6.5-week embryo. The palatine shelves are in the vertical position on each side of the tongue. **B.** Ventral view of the palatine shelves after removal of the lower jaw and the tongue. Note the clefts between the primary triangular palate and the palatine shelves, which are still vertical.

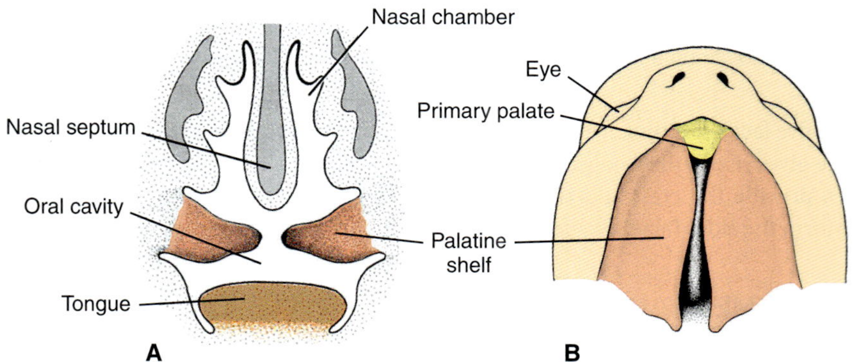


**FIGURE 17.26 A.** Frontal section through the head of a 7.5-week embryo. The tongue has moved downward, and the palatine shelves have reached a horizontal position. **B.** Ventral view of the palatine shelves after removal of the lower jaw and tongue. The shelves are horizontal. Note the nasal septum.

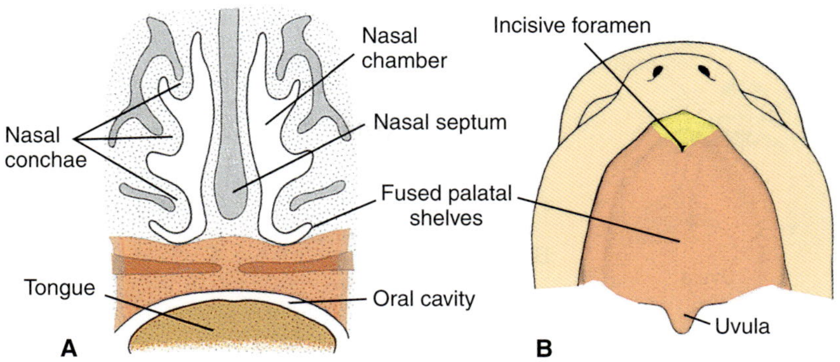


**FIGURE 17.27 A.** Frontal section through the head of a 10-week embryo. The two palatine shelves have fused with each other and with the nasal septum. **B.** Ventral view of the palate. The incisive foramen forms the midline between the primary and secondary palate.

## ■ NASAL CAVITIES

During the sixth week, the nasal pits deepen considerably, partly because of growth of the surrounding nasal prominences and partly because of their penetration into the underlying mesenchyme (Fig. 17.28*A*). At first, the **oronasal membrane** separates the pits from the primitive oral cavity by way of the newly formed foramina, the **primitive choanae** (Fig. 17.28*C*).

These choanae lie on each side of the midline and immediately behind the primary palate. Later, with formation of the secondary palate and further development of the primitive nasal chambers (Fig. 17.28*D*), the **definitive choanae** lie at the junction of the nasal cavity and the pharynx. **Paranasal air sinuses** develop as diverticula of the lateral nasal wall and extend into the maxilla, ethmoid, frontal, and sphenoid bones. They reach their maximum size during puberty and contribute to the definitive shape of the face.

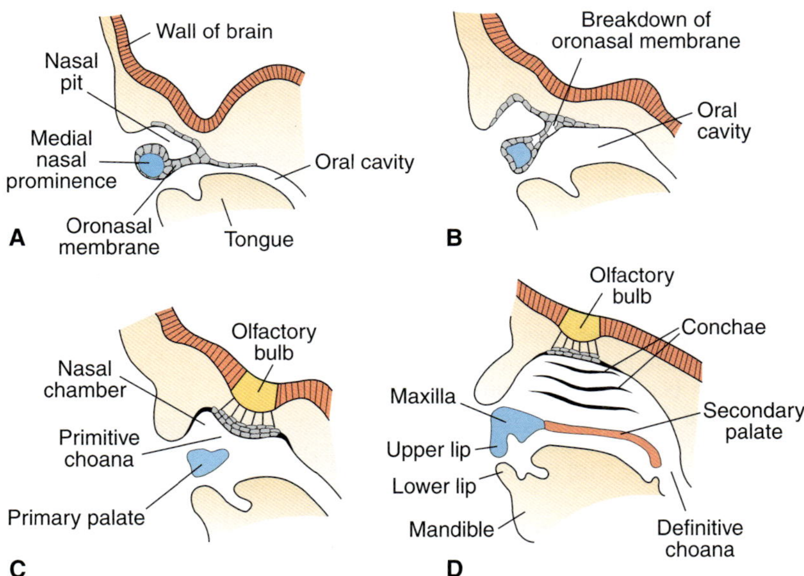


**FIGURE 17.28 A.** Sagittal section through the nasal pit and lower rim of the medial nasal prominence of a 6-week embryo. The primitive nasal cavity is separated from the oral cavity by the oronasal membrane. **B.** Similar section as in **(A)** showing the oronasal membrane breaking down. **C.** A 7-week embryo with a primitive nasal cavity in open connection with the oral cavity. **D.** Sagittal section through the face of a 9-week embryo showing separation of the definitive nasal and oral cavities by the primary and secondary palate. Definitive choanae are at the junction of the oral cavity and the pharynx.

### *Clinical Correlates*

#### Facial Clefts

Cleft lip and cleft palate are common defects that result in abnormal facial appearance and difficulties with speech. The **incisive foramen** is considered the dividing landmark between **anterior** and **posterior** cleft deformities. Those anterior to the incisive foramen include **lateral cleft lip**, **cleft upper**

*(Continued)*

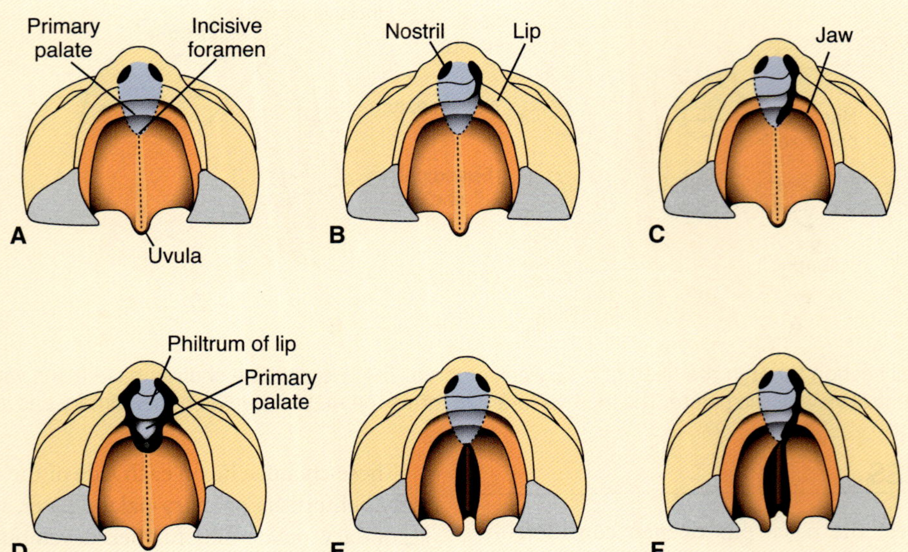


**FIGURE 17.29** Ventral view of the palate, gum, lip, and nose. **A.** Normal. **B.** Unilateral cleft lip extending into the nose. **C.** Unilateral cleft involving the lip and jaw and extending to the incisive foramen. **D.** Bilateral cleft involving the lip and jaw. **E.** Isolated cleft palate. **F.** Cleft palate combined with unilateral anterior cleft lip.



**jaw**, and **cleft** between the **primary and secondary palates** (Figs. 17.29*B–D* and 17.29*A*). Such defects are due to a partial or complete lack of fusion of the maxillary prominence with the medial nasal prominence on one or both sides. Those that lie posterior to the incisive foramen include **cleft (secondary) palate** and **cleft uvula** (Figs. 17.29*E* and 17.30*B*). Cleft palate results from a lack of fusion of the palatine shelves, which may be due to smallness of the shelves, failure of the shelves to elevate, inhibition of the fusion process itself, or failure of the tongue to drop from between the shelves because of micrognathia. The third category is formed by a combination of clefts lying anterior as well as posterior to the incisive foramen (Fig. 17.29*F*). Anterior clefts vary in severity from a barely visible defect in the vermilion of the lip to extension into the nose. In severe cases, the cleft extends to a deeper level, forming a cleft of the upper jaw, and the maxilla is split between the lateral incisor and the canine tooth (Fig. 17.30*A*). Frequently, such a cleft extends to the incisive foramen (Fig. 17.29*C,F*). Likewise, posterior clefts vary in severity from clefting of the entire secondary palate (Figs. 17.29*E* and 17.30*B*) to clefting of the uvula only.

**Van der Woude syndrome** is the most common syndrome associated with cleft lip with or without cleft palate. The syndrome is inherited as an autosomal dominant and is due to mutations in *INTERFERON REGULATORY FACTOR 6* (*IRF6*; 1p32-41) that is expressed in the medial (fusing) edge of the palatal shelves. Interestingly, 88% of affected infants will have pits in their lower lip, and in 64% of these individuals, this will be the only abnormality.

**Oblique facial clefts** are produced by failure of the maxillary prominence to merge with its corresponding lateral nasal prominence along the line of the nasolacrimal groove (Fig. 17.23*A,C*). When this occurs, the nasolacrimal duct is usually exposed to the surface (Fig. 17.30*C*).

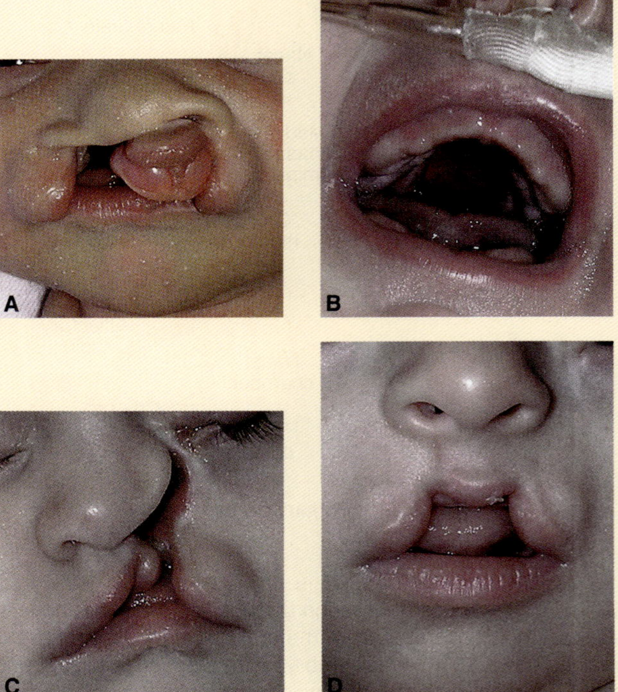


**FIGURE 17.30** **A.** Bilateral cleft lip (compare to Fig. 17.29*D*). **B.** Cleft palate (compare to Fig. 17.29*E*). **C.** Oblique facial cleft (see nasolacrimal groove, Fig. 17.23*A,C*). **D.** Midline cleft lip.

**Median (midline) cleft lip**, a rare abnormality, is caused by incomplete merging of the two medial nasal prominences in the midline (Figs. 17.30*D* and 17.31*A,B*). Infants with midline clefts are often **cognitively impaired** and may have brain abnormalities that include varying degrees of loss of midline structures. Loss of midline tissue may be so extensive that the lateral ventricles fuse (**holoprosencephaly**) (Fig. 17.31*C*). These defects are induced very early in development, at the beginning

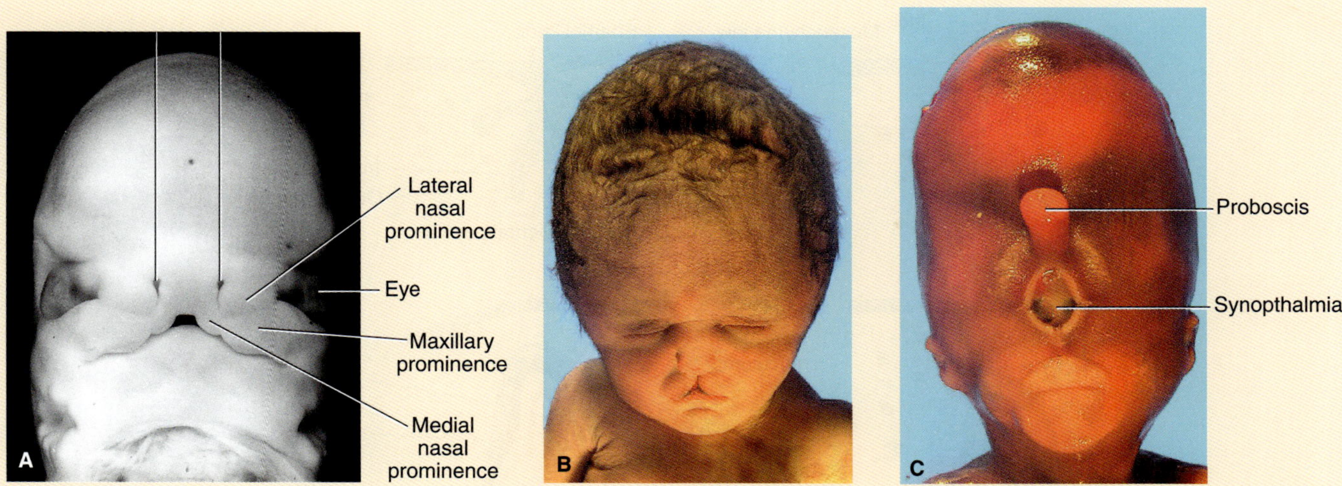


**FIGURE 17.31** Photographs demonstrating normal and abnormal development involving the midline of the face and brain. **A.** Normal face of an embryo at the beginning of the seventh week. Note the distance between the nasal openings (*vertical lines*) and between the medial nasal prominences. **B.** Face of a newborn with a midline cleft lip. In this case, there is insufficient tissue in the midline to fill in the space between the medial nasal prominences. **C.** Face of a newborn with holoprosencephaly characterized by such an extensive deficiency of midline tissue that the eyes have fused (synophthalmia), and a proboscis with a single nasal opening has formed from fusion of the lateral nasal processes. An upper lip is formed by fusion of the maxillary prominences. The head is narrow, and the brain would have a single ventricle (holoprosencephaly) due to such a loss of midline tissue that the two lateral ventricles fused. The condition may be caused by mutations in *SHH* (the gene that establishes the midline), by altered cholesterol biosynthesis, and by maternal exposure to teratogens, such as alcohol, in the third week of development (see also Chapter 18).

of neurulation (days 19 to 21) when the midline of the forebrain is being established (see Chapter 18).

Most cases of cleft lip with or without cleft palate are multifactorial. These conditions are usually classified as (1) cleft lip with or without cleft palate and (2) cleft palate are thought to be etiologically and pathogenetically distinct. Cleft lip with or without cleft palate (approximately 1/700 births) occurs more frequently in males (65%) than in females, and its incidence varies among populations. Asians and Native Americans have some of the highest rates (3.5/1,000), whereas African Americans have the lowest (1/1,000).

The frequency of isolated **cleft palate** is lower than that of cleft lip (1/1,500 births), occurs more often in females (55%) than in males. In females, the palatal shelves fuse approximately 1 week later than in males, which may be related to why isolated cleft palate occurs more frequently in females than in males.

Causes of cleft lip with or without cleft palate are not well defined. Some cases are syndromic and associated with certain syndromes and genes. Others are nonsyndromic but associated with some of the same genes that cause syndromes, such as *IRF6* (van der Woude syndrome) and *MSX1*. Still, other cases are caused by exposure to teratogenic compounds, such as anticonvulsant medications, particularly valproic acid. Cigarette smoking during pregnancy also increases the risk for having a baby with orofacial clefts.

Part 2

## TEETH

The shape of the face is determined not only by expansion of the paranasal sinuses but also by growth of the mandible and maxilla to accommodate the teeth. Teeth themselves arise from an epithelial–mesenchymal interaction between overlying oral epithelium and underlying mesenchyme derived from neural crest cells. By the sixth week of development, the basal layer of the epithelial lining of the oral cavity forms a C-shaped structure, the **dental lamina**, along the length of the upper and lower jaws. This lamina subsequently gives rise to a number of **dental buds** (Fig. 17.32*A*), 10 in each jaw, which form the primordia of the ectodermal components of the teeth. Soon, the deep surface of the buds invaginates, resulting in the **cap stage of tooth development** (Fig. 17.32*B*). Such a cap consists of an outer layer, the **outer dental epithelium**; an inner layer, the **inner dental epithelium**; and a central core of loosely woven tissue, the **stellate reticulum**. The **mesenchyme**, which originates in the **neural crest** in the indentation, forms the **dental papilla** (Fig. 17.32*B*).

As the dental cap grows and the indentation deepens, the tooth takes on the appearance of a bell (**bell stage**) (Fig. 17.32*C*). Mesenchyme cells of the papilla adjacent to the inner dental layer differentiate into **odontoblasts**, which later produce **dentin**. With thickening of the dentin layer, odontoblasts retreat into the dental papilla, leaving a thin cytoplasmic process (**dental process**) behind in the dentin (Fig. 17.32*D*). The odontoblast layer persists throughout the life of the tooth and continuously provides predentin. The remaining cells of the dental papilla form the **pulp** of the tooth (Fig. 17.32*D*).

In the meantime, epithelial cells of the inner dental epithelium differentiate into **ameloblasts (enamel formers)**. These cells produce long enamel prisms that are deposited over the dentin (Fig. 17.32*D*). Furthermore, a cluster of these cells

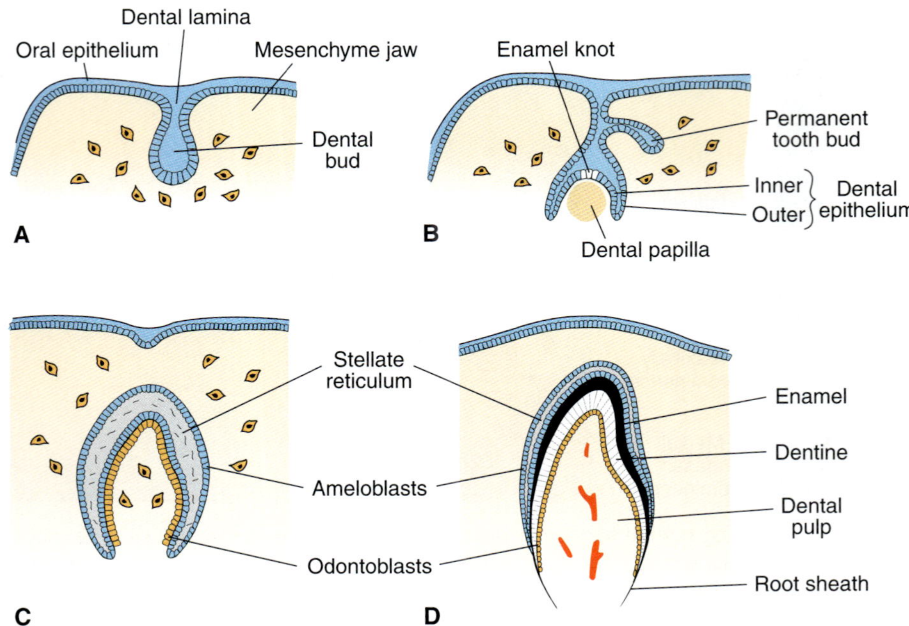


**FIGURE 17.32** Formation of the tooth at successive stages of development. **A.** Bud stage (8 weeks). **B.** Cap stage (10 weeks). **C.** Bell stage (3 months). **D.** 6 months.



in the inner dental epithelium forms the **enamel knot** that regulates early tooth development (Fig. 17.32*B*).

Enamel is first laid down at the apex of the tooth and from here spreads toward the neck. When the enamel thickens, the ameloblasts retreat into the stellate reticulum. Here they regress, temporarily leaving a thin membrane (**dental cuticle**) on the surface of the enamel. After eruption of the tooth, this membrane gradually sloughs off.

Formation of the root of the tooth begins when the dental epithelial layers penetrate into the underlying mesenchyme and form the **epithelial root sheath** (Fig. 17.32*D*). Cells of the dental papilla lay down a layer of dentin continuous with that of the crown (Fig. 17.33). As more and more dentin is deposited, the pulp chamber narrows and finally forms a canal containing blood vessels and nerves of the tooth.

Mesenchymal cells on the outside of the tooth and in contact with dentin of the root differentiate into **cementoblasts** (Fig. 17.33*A*). These cells produce a thin layer of specialized bone, the **cementum**. Outside of the cement layer, mesenchyme gives rise to the **periodontal ligament** (Fig. 17.33), which holds the tooth firmly in position and functions as a shock absorber.

With further lengthening of the root, the crown is gradually pushed through the overlying tissue layers into the oral cavity (Fig. 17.33*B*). The eruption of **deciduous** or **milk teeth** occurs 6 to 24 months after birth.

**Buds** for the **permanent teeth**, which lie on the lingual aspect of the milk teeth, are formed during the third month of development. These buds remain dormant until approximately the sixth year of postnatal life (Fig. 17.34). Then they begin to grow, pushing against the underside of the milk teeth

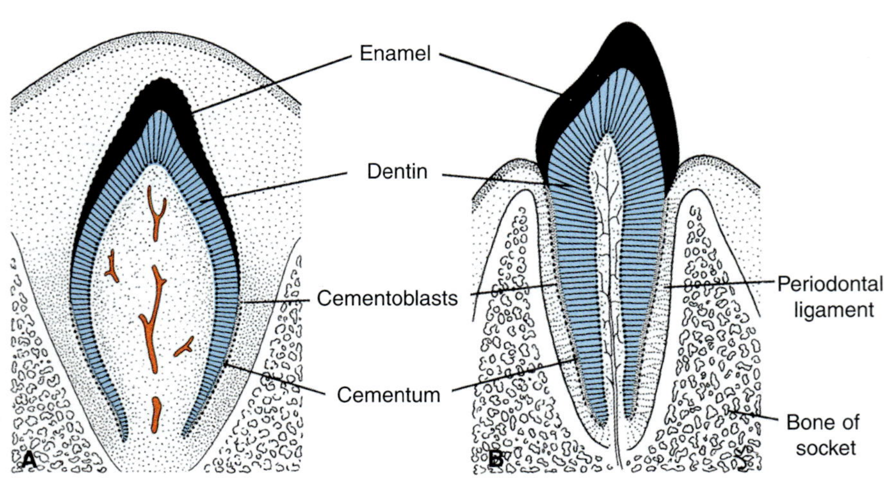


**FIGURE 17.33** The tooth just before birth **(A)** and after eruption **(B)**.

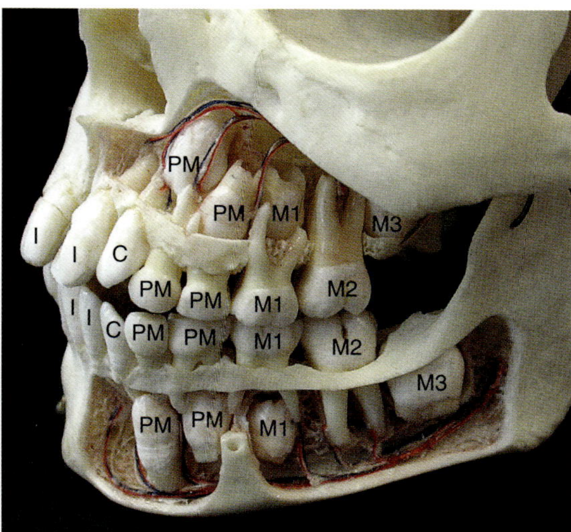


**FIGURE 17.34** Replacement of deciduous teeth with permanent teeth in a child. *I*, incisor; *C*, canine; *PM*, premolar; *M1*, *M2*, *M3*; first, second, and third molars.

and aiding in the shedding of them. As a permanent tooth grows, the root of the overlying deciduous tooth is resorbed by osteoclasts.

## MOLECULAR REGULATION OF TOOTH DEVELOPMENT

Teeth are present only in vertebrates and parallel the evolutionary appearance of the neural crest. Tooth development represents a classic example of an epithelial–mesenchymal interaction, in this case, between the overlying epithelium and underlying neural crest–derived mesenchyme. Regulation of tooth patterning from incisors to molars is generated by a combinatorial expression of ***HOX*** genes expressed in the mesenchyme. With respect to each tooth's individual development, the epithelium governs differentiation to the bud stage, at which time this regulatory function is transferred to the mesenchyme. Signals for development involve growth factors including **WNTs**, **BMPs**, and **FGFs**; the secreted factor **SHH**; and transcription factors, such as **MSX1 and MSX2**, that interact in a complex pathway to produce cell differentiation and patterning for each tooth. Teeth also appear to have a signaling center that represents the "organizer" for tooth development much like the activity of the node during gastrulation (see Chapter 5). This organizer region is called the **enamel knot**, and it appears in a circumscribed region of the dental epithelium at the tips of the tooth buds. It then enlarges at the cap stage into a tightly packed group of cells but undergoes apoptosis (cell death) and disappears by the end of this stage (Fig. 17.32*B*). While it is present, it expresses *FGF4*, *SHH*, and *BMP2* and *4*. FGF4 may regulate outgrowth of cusps much as it participates in limb outgrowth produced by the apical ectodermal ridge, whereas BMP4 may regulate the timing of apoptosis in knot cells.

### Clinical Correlates

#### Tooth Abnormalities

**Natal teeth** have erupted by the time of birth. Usually, they involve the mandibular incisors, which may be abnormally formed and have little enamel.

Teeth may be abnormal in number, shape, and size. They may be discolored by foreign substances, such as **tetracyclines**, or be deficient in enamel, a condition often caused by **vitamin D deficiency (rickets)**. Many factors affect tooth development, including genetic and environmental influences.

Part 2

## SUMMARY

- **Pharyngeal (branchial) arches**, consisting of bars of mesenchymal tissue separated by pharyngeal pouches and clefts, give the head and neck their typical appearance in the fourth week (Fig. 17.3).
- Each arch contains its own artery (Fig. 17.4), cranial nerve (Fig. 17.7), muscle element, and cartilage bar or skeletal element (Figs. 17.8 and 17.9; Table 17.1, p. 236).
- Endoderm of the **pharyngeal pouches** gives rise to a number of endocrine glands and part of the middle ear. In subsequent order, the pouches give rise to (1) the **middle ear cavity** and **auditory tube** (pouch 1), (2) the stroma of the **palatine tonsil** (pouch 2), (3) the **inferior parathyroid glands** and **thymus** (pouch 3), and (4) the **superior parathyroid glands** and **ultimobranchial body** (pouches 4 and 5) (Fig. 17.10).
- **Pharyngeal clefts** are transient structures that all disappear. The first cleft is occluded by overgrowth of the second pharyngeal arch when this arch forms most of the external ear. The second, third, and fourth clefts are occluded by growth of the second arch caudally that overlaps the third and fourth arches and merges with the epicardial ridge in the lower part of the neck. In some cases, remnants of the clefts remain as cervical cysts and/or fistulas.
- Patterning of the skeletal elements of the pharyngeal arches is regulated by gene expression in pharyngeal pouch endoderm.
- The process involves epithelial–mesenchymal signaling with endoderm of the pouches sending signals to the responding tissue, the mesenchyme.
- Mesenchymal gene expression is initially determined by homeodomain-containing transcription factors (*OTX2* and *HOX* genes) carried by pharyngeal arches by migrating neural crest cells. Crest cells originate from the caudal midbrain and from segments in the hindbrain called **rhombomeres**. These genes respond to endodermal signals and dictate the type of skeletal elements that form.
- The **thyroid gland** originates from an epithelial proliferation in the floor of the tongue and descends to its level in front of the tracheal rings in the course of development.

(Continued)

- The paired **maxillary** and **mandibular prominences** and the **frontonasal prominence** are the first prominences of the facial region.
- Later, medial and lateral nasal prominences form around the nasal placodes on the frontonasal prominence. All of these structures are important because they determine, through fusion and specialized growth, the size and integrity of the mandible, upper lip, palate, and nose (Table 17.4, p. 248).
- Formation of the upper lip occurs by fusion of the two maxillary prominences with the two medial nasal prominences (Figs. 17.22 and 17.23). The intermaxillary segment is formed by merging of the two medial nasal prominences in the midline.
- The intermaxillary segment is composed of (1) the **philtrum**; (2) the **upper jaw component**, which carries the four incisor teeth; and (3) the **palatal component**, which forms the triangular primary palate.
- The nose is derived from (1) the **frontonasal prominence**, which forms the **bridge**; (2) the **medial nasal prominences**, which provide the **crest and tip**; and (3) the **lateral nasal prominences**, which form the **alae** (Fig. 17.23).
- Fusion of the **palatal shelves**, which form from the **maxillary prominences**, creates the **hard (secondary)** and **soft palate**. A series of cleft deformities may result from partial or incomplete fusion of these mesenchymal tissues, which may be caused by hereditary factors and drugs (diphenylhydantoin).
- The adult form of the face is influenced by development of **paranasal sinuses**, **nasal conchae**, and **teeth**.
- Teeth develop from epithelial–mesenchymal interactions between oral epithelium and neural crest–derived mesenchyme. **Enamel** is made by **ameloblasts** (Figs. 17.32 and 17.33). It lies on a thick layer of **dentin** produced by **odontoblasts**, a neural crest derivative. **Cementum** is formed by **cementoblasts**, another mesenchymal derivative found in the root of the tooth.
- The first teeth (**deciduous teeth** or **milk teeth**) appear 6 to 24 months after birth, and the definitive or **permanent teeth**, which supplant the milk teeth, are formed during the third month of development (Fig. 17.34).

## Self-Assessment

### Comprehensive Questions

1. Correlate the development of the tongue with its nerve supply.
2. Discuss the development of the palate.

### Problem Solving Questions

1. Why are neural crest cells considered such an important cell population for craniofacial development?
2. You are called as a consultant for a child with a very small mandible and ears that are represented by small protuberances bilaterally. The baby has had numerous episodes of pneumonia and is small for its age. What might your diagnosis be, and what might have caused these abnormalities?
3. A child is born with a median cleft lip. Should you be concerned about any other abnormalities?
4. A child presents with a midline swelling beneath the arch of the hyoid bone. What might this swelling be, and what is its basis embryologically?
5. A newborn baby is having a thick discharge from the medial side of his right eye, with an oblique cleft on his face from medial canthus of eye to nose. What is the embryological basis of the condition?

### Multiple Choice Questions

1. A 4-year-old girl is reported to have a considerable conduction deficit in one ear during a routine hearing exam. A CT scan of the tympanic cavity reveals a complete agenesis of the stapes. Abnormal development of which of the following structures could lead to these findings?
   (a) First branchial arch
   (b) Second branchial arch
   (c) Third branchial arch
   (d) Frontonasal process
2. The glossopharyngeal nerves innervate the pharyngeal mucosa. Which of the following is the origin of the glossopharyngeal nerve?
   (a) First pharyngeal arch
   (b) Second pharyngeal arch
   (c) Third pharyngeal arch
   (d) Fourth pharyngeal arch
3. Select the correct statement with respect to muscular derivatives of the second pharyngeal arch.
   (a) All the muscles of mastication
   (b) Muscles of facial expression
   (c) Stylopharyngeus muscle
   (d) Constrictors of pharynx
4. Sensory supply of the anterior two-thirds of the tongue is derived from which of the following pharyngeal arches?
   (a) First arch
   (b) Second arch
   (c) Third arch
   (d) Fourth arch
5. Which of the following is incorrect with respect to derivatives of the first pharyngeal arch?
   (a) Sphenomandibular ligament
   (b) Zygomatic bone
   (c) Stapedius
   (d) Tensor tympani
6. Middle ear cavity is a derivative of which pharyngeal pouch?
   (a) First
   (b) Second
   (c) Third
   (d) Fourth

### Answers

1. (b) 2. (c) 3. (b) 4. (b) 5. (c) 6. (a)

Part 2

CHAPTER

# 18 Central Nervous System

## Specific Learning Objectives

- Neurulation
- Differentiation of neural tube into primary and secondary brain vesicles
- Development of the spinal cord
  - Histological differentiation of neuroepithelium: Neurons, glial cells
  - Formation of spinal nerves and dorsal root ganglia
  - Myelination of spinal nerves
  - Positional changes in cord
  - Clinical aspects: Neural tube defects
- Development of brain
  - Differentiation of brain vesicles
  - Differentiation of alar and basal lamina of rhombencephalon and mesencephalon
  - Prosencephalon: Formation of diencephalon and telencephalon
- Formation of meninges and CSF
- Development of the autonomic nervous system: Sympathetic, parasympathetic, and suprarenal glands

## Competencies Covered

AN64.2 Describe the development of neural tube, spinal cord, medulla oblongata, pons, midbrain, cerebral hemisphere, and cerebellum.

AN64.3 Describe the various types of open neural tube defects with their embryological bases.

Part 2

The central nervous system (CNS) appears at the beginning of the third week as a slipper-shaped plate of thickened ectoderm, **the neural plate** (actually a large **placode**; see definition and poem, p. iv) in the middorsal region in front of the **primitive node**. Its lateral edges soon elevate to form the **neural folds** (Fig. 18.1).

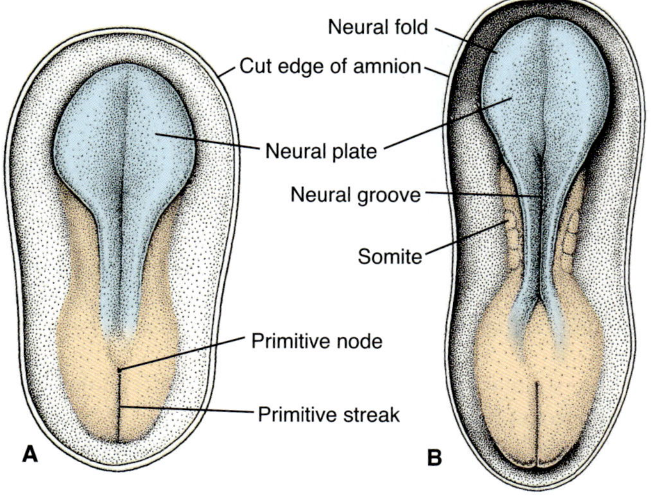


**FIGURE 18.1 A.** Dorsal view of a late presomite embryo at approximately 18 days. The amnion has been removed, and the neural plate is clearly visible. **B.** Dorsal view at approximately 20 days. Note the somites and the neural groove and neural folds.

With further development, the neural folds continue to elevate, approach each other in the midline, and finally fuse, forming the **neural tube** (Figs. 18.2 and 18.3). Fusion begins in the cervical region and proceeds in cephalic and caudal directions (Fig. 18.3*A*). Once fusion is initiated, the open ends of the neural tube form the **cranial** and **caudal neuropores** that communicate with the overlying amniotic cavity (Fig. 18.3*B*). Closure of the cranial neuropore proceeds cranially from the initial closure site in the cervical region (Fig. 18.3*A*) and from a site in the forebrain that forms later. This latter site proceeds cranially, to close the rostral-most region of the neural tube, and caudally to meet advancing closure from the cervical site (Fig. 18.3*B*). Final closure of the cranial neuropore occurs at the 18- to 20-somite stage (25th day); closure of the caudal neuropore occurs approximately 3 days later.

The cephalic end of the neural tube shows three dilations, the **primary brain vesicles**: (1) the **prosencephalon**, or **forebrain**; (2) the **mesencephalon**, or **midbrain**; and (3) the **rhombencephalon**, or **hindbrain** (Fig. 18.4). Simultaneously, it forms two flexures: (1) the **cervical flexure** at the junction of the hindbrain and the spinal cord and (2) the **cephalic flexure** in the midbrain region (Fig. 18.4).

By 5 weeks of development, the primary brain vesicles have differentiated into five **secondary vesicles**:

- The prosencephalon forms the **telencephalon** and **diencephalon**.

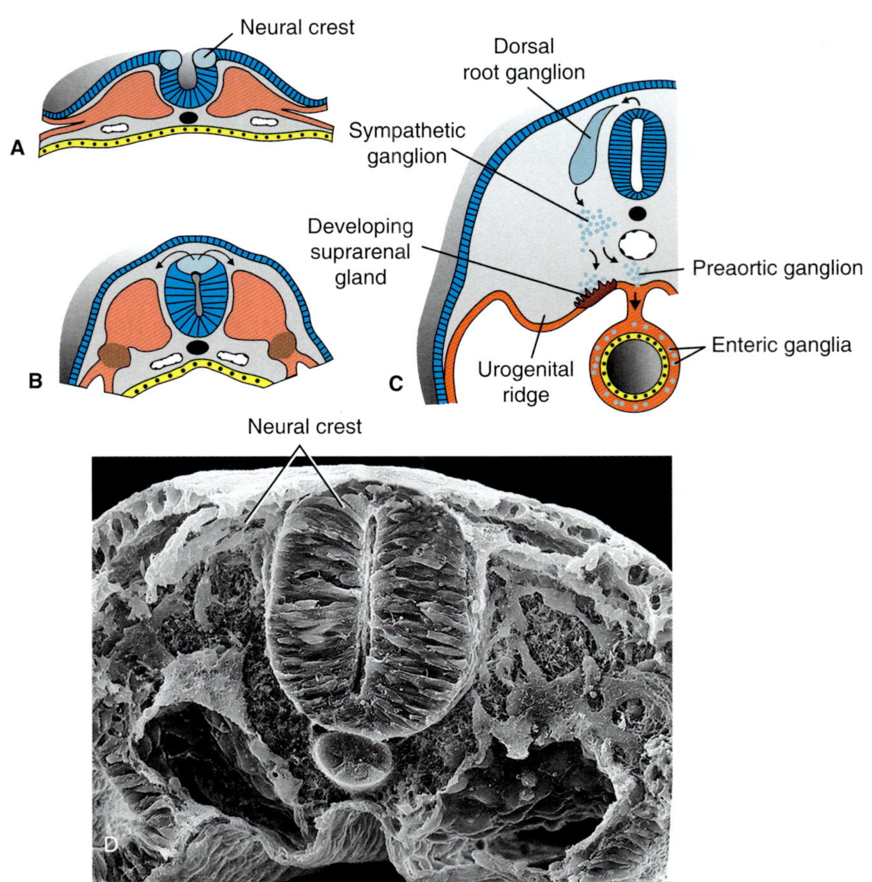


**FIGURE 18.2 A–C.** Transverse sections through successively older embryos showing formation of the neural groove, neural tube, and neural crest. Cells of the neural crest migrate from the edges of the neural folds and develop into spinal and cranial sensory ganglia. **D.** Scanning electron micrograph of a chick embryo showing the neural tube and neural crest cells migrating from the dorsal region of the tube (compare with **[B]** and **[C]**).

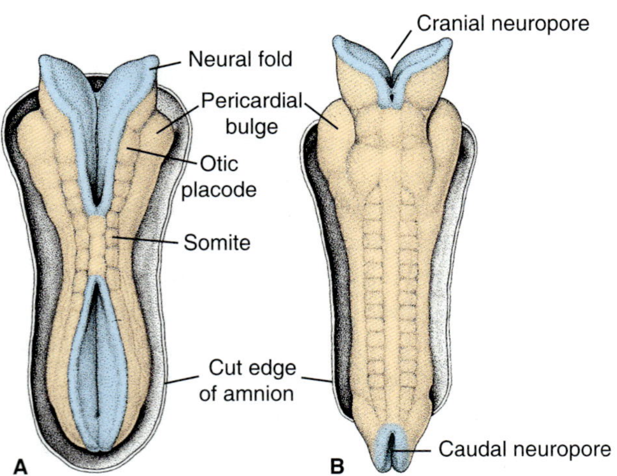


**FIGURE 18.3 A.** Dorsal view of a human embryo at approximately day 22. Seven distinct somites are visible on each side of the neural tube. **B.** Dorsal view of a human embryo at approximately day 23. The nervous system is in connection with the amniotic cavity through the cranial and caudal neuropores.

- The **mesencephalon** remains as such and forms the midbrain.

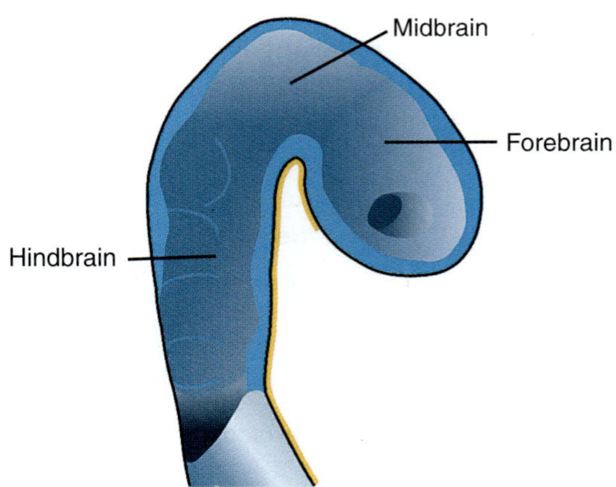


**FIGURE 18.4** Drawing of a sagittal section through the brain at approximately 28 days of human development. Three brain vesicles represent the forebrain, midbrain, and hindbrain.

- The rhombencephalon forms the **metencephalon** and **myelencephalon** (Fig. 18.5).
- A deep furrow, the **rhombencephalic isthmus** separates the mesencephalon from the metencephalon.
- The **pontine flexure** marks the boundary between the metencephalon and myelencephalon (Fig. 18.5).
- Each of the secondary vesicles will contribute a different part of the brain.

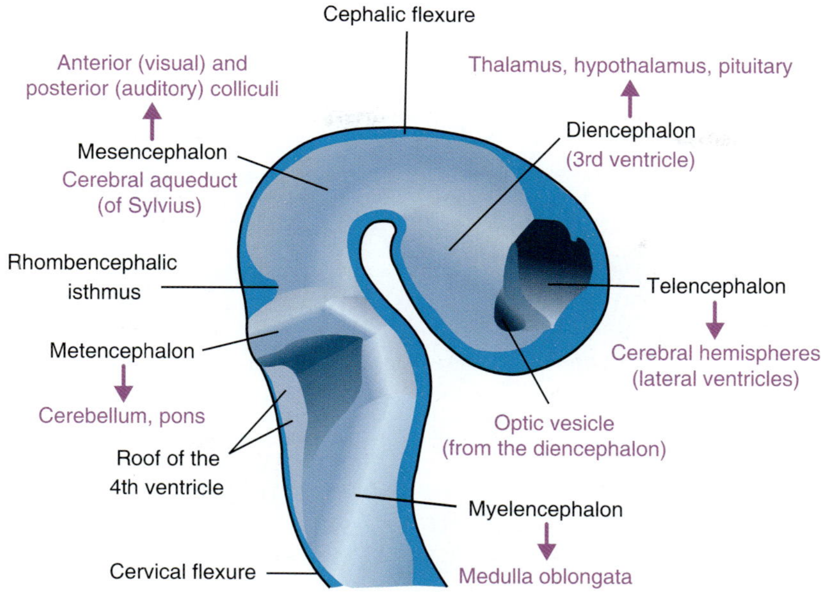


**FIGURE 18.5** Drawing of a sagittal section through the brain at approximately 32 days of human development. The three original brain vesicles have segregated into the telencephalon, diencephalon, mesencephalon, metencephalon, and myelencephalon. The major derivatives of each of these divisions are also indicated.

- The main derivatives of these vesicles are indicated in Figure 18.5 and include telencephalon (**cerebral hemispheres**), diencephalon (**optic vesicle**, **thalamus**, **hypothalamus**, **pituitary**), mesencephalon (**anterior [visual]** and **posterior [auditory] colliculi**), metencephalon (**cerebellum**, **pons**), and myelencephalon (**medulla oblongata**).

The lumen of the spinal cord, the **central canal**, is continuous with that of the brain vesicles. The cavity of the rhombencephalon is the **fourth ventricle**, that of the diencephalon is the **third ventricle**, and those of the cerebral hemispheres are the **lateral ventricles** (Fig. 18.5). The lumen of the mesencephalon connects the third and fourth ventricles. This lumen becomes very narrow and is then known as the **aqueduct of Sylvius**. Each lateral ventricle communicates with the third ventricle through the **interventricular foramina of Monro** (Fig. 18.5).

## ■ SPINAL CORD

### Neuroepithelial, Mantle, and Marginal Layers

The wall of a recently closed neural tube consists of **neuroepithelial cells**. These cells extend over the entire thickness of the wall and form a thick pseudostratified epithelium (Fig. 18.6). Junctional complexes at the lumen connect them. During the



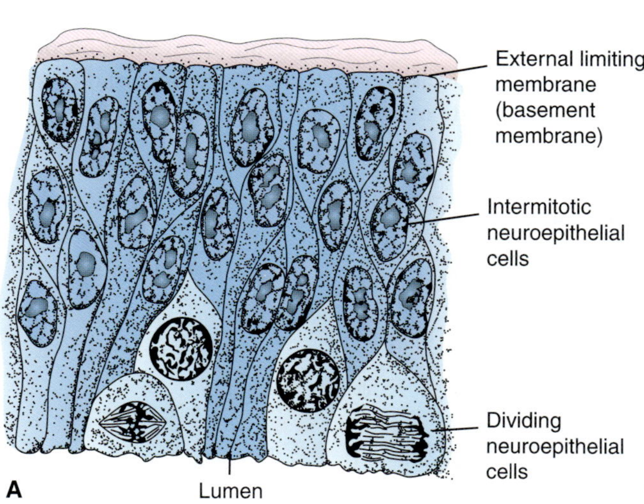


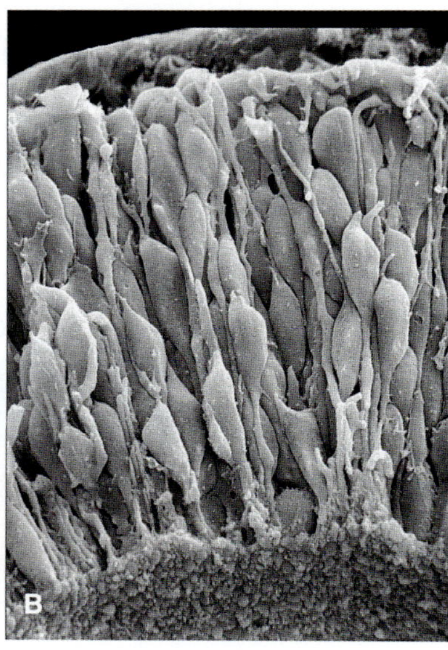


**FIGURE 18.6** **A.** Section of the wall of the recently closed neural tube showing neuroepithelial cells, which form a pseudostratified epithelium extending over the full width of the wall. Note the dividing cells at the lumen of the tube. **B.** Scanning electron micrograph of a section of the neural tube of a chick embryo similar to that in **(A)**.

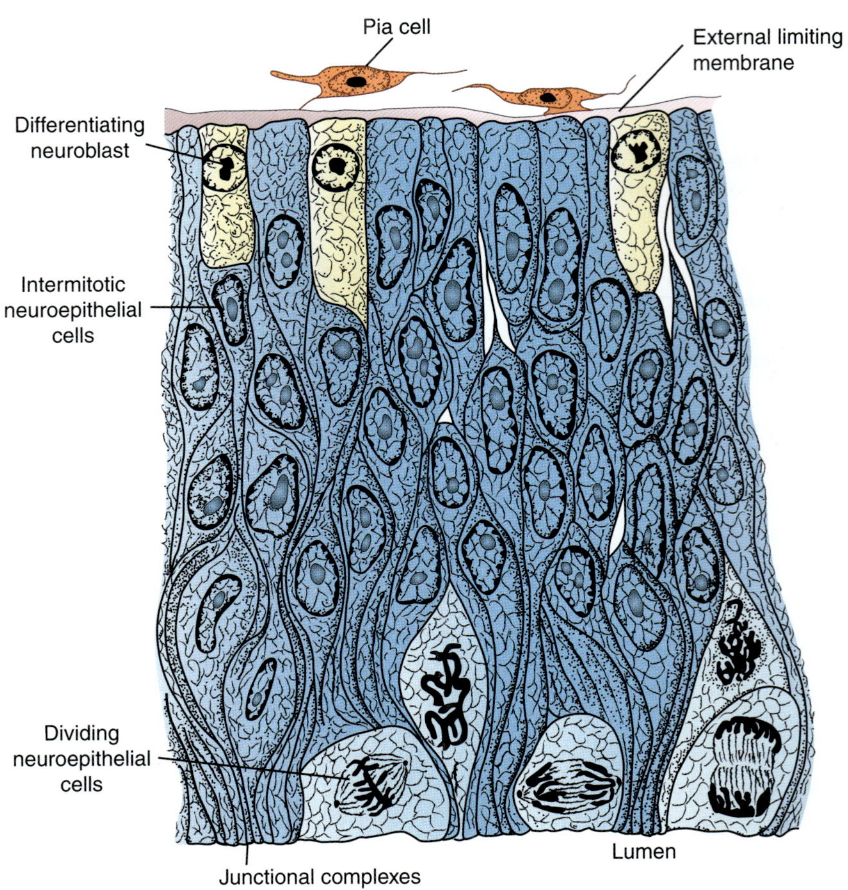


**FIGURE 18.7** Section of the neural tube at a slightly more advanced stage than in Figure 18.6. The major portion of the wall consists of neuroepithelial cells. On the periphery, immediately adjacent to the external limiting membrane, neuroblasts form (yellow cells). These cells, which are produced by the neuroepithelial cells in ever-increasing numbers, will migrate out of the dividing population of cells to form the mantle layer.



neural groove stage and immediately after closure of the tube, they divide rapidly, producing more and more neuroepithelial cells. Collectively, they constitute the **neuroepithelial layer** or **neuroepithelium**.

Once the neural tube closes, neuroepithelial cells begin to give rise to another cell type characterized by a large round nucleus with pale nucleoplasm and a dark-staining nucleolus. These are the primitive nerve cells, or **neuroblasts** (Fig. 18.7). They form the **mantle layer**, a zone around the neuroepithelial layer (Fig. 18.8). The mantle layer later forms the **gray matter of the spinal cord**.

The outermost layer of the spinal cord, the **marginal layer**, contains nerve fibers emerging from neuroblasts in the mantle layer. As a result of myelination of nerve fibers, this layer takes on a white appearance and therefore is called the **white matter of the spinal cord** (Fig. 18.8).

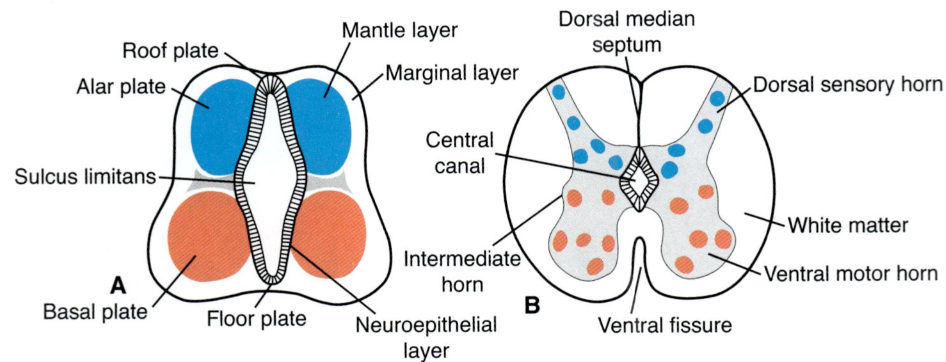


**FIGURE 18.8 A,B.** Two successive stages in the development of the spinal cord. Note formation of ventral motor and dorsal sensory horns and the **intermediate column**.

## Basal, Alar, Roof, and Floor Plates

As a result of continuous addition of neuroblasts to the mantle layer, each side of the neural tube shows a ventral and a dorsal thickening. The ventral thickenings, the **basal plates**, which contain ventral motor horn cells, form the motor areas of the spinal cord; the dorsal thickenings, the **alar plates**, form the **sensory areas** (Fig. 18.8*A*). A longitudinal groove, the **sulcus limitans**, marks the boundary between the two. The dorsal and ventral midline portions of the neural tube, known as the **roof** and **floor plates**, respectively, do not contain neuroblasts; they serve primarily as pathways for nerve fibers crossing from one side to the other.

In addition to the ventral motor horn and the dorsal sensory horn, a group of neurons accumulates between the two areas and forms a small **intermediate horn** (Fig. 18.8*B*). This horn, containing neurons of the sympathetic portion of the autonomic nervous system (ANS), is present only at thoracic (T1–T12) and upper lumbar levels (L2 or L3) of the spinal cord.

## Histological Differentiation

### *Nerve Cells*

**Neuroblasts**, or primitive nerve cells, arise exclusively by division of the neuroepithelial cells. Initially, they have a central process extending to the lumen (**transient dendrite**), but when they migrate into the mantle layer, this process disappears, and neuroblasts are temporarily round and **apolar** (Fig. 18.9*A*). With further differentiation, two new cytoplasmic processes appear on opposite sides of the cell body, forming a **bipolar neuroblast** (Fig. 18.9*B*). The process at one end of the cell elongates rapidly to form the **primitive axon**, and the process at the other end shows a number of cytoplasmic arborizations, the **primitive dendrites** (Fig. 18.9*C*). The cell is then known as a **multipolar neuroblast** and with further development becomes the adult nerve cell or **neuron**. Once neuroblasts form, they lose their ability to divide. Axons of neurons in the basal plate break through the marginal zone and become visible on the ventral aspect of the cord. Known collectively as the **ventral motor root of the spinal nerve**, they conduct motor impulses from the spinal cord to the muscles (Fig. 18.10).

Axons of neurons in the dorsal sensory horn (alar plate) behave differently from those in the ventral horn. They penetrate into the marginal layer of the cord, where they ascend to either higher or lower levels to form **association neurons**.

### *Glial Cells*

The majority of primitive supporting cells, the **glia blasts**, are formed by neuroepithelial cells after production of neuroblasts ceases. Glia blasts migrate from the neuroepithelial layer to the mantle and marginal layers. In the mantle layer, they differentiate into **protoplasmic astrocytes** and **fibrillar astrocytes** (Fig. 18.11). These cells are situated between blood vessels and neurons where they provide support and serve metabolic functions.

Another type of supporting cell possibly derived from glia blasts is the **oligodendroglial cell**. This cell, which is found primarily in the marginal layer, forms myelin sheaths around the ascending and descending axons in the marginal layer.

In the second half of development, a third type of supporting cell, the **microglial cell**, appears in the CNS. This highly phagocytic cell type is derived from vascular mesenchyme when blood vessels grow into the nervous system (Fig. 18.11). When neuroepithelial cells cease to produce neuroblasts and glia blasts, they differentiate into ependymal cells lining the central canal of the spinal cord.

### *Neural Crest Cells*

During elevation of the neural plate, a group of cells appears along each edge (the crest) of the neural folds (Fig. 18.2). These **neural crest cells** are ectodermal in origin and extend throughout the length of the neural tube. Crest cells migrate laterally and give rise to **sensory ganglia (dorsal root ganglia)** of the spinal nerves and other cell types (Fig. 18.2).

During further development, neuroblasts of the sensory ganglia form two processes (Fig. 18.10*A*). The centrally growing processes penetrate the dorsal portion of the neural tube. In the spinal cord, they either end in the dorsal horn or ascend through the marginal layer to one of the higher brain centers. These processes are known collectively as the **dorsal sensory root of the spinal nerve** (Fig. 18.10*B*). The peripherally growing processes join fibers of the ventral motor roots and thus participate in formation of the trunk of the spinal nerve. Eventually,

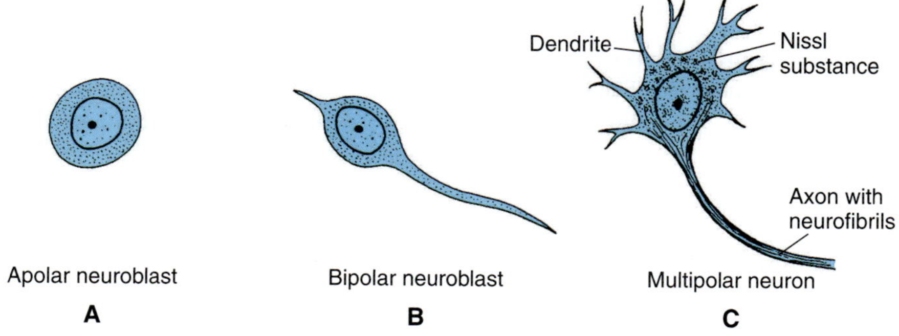


**FIGURE 18.9** Various stages of development of a neuroblast. A neuron is a structural and functional unit consisting of the cell body and all its processes.

Part 2

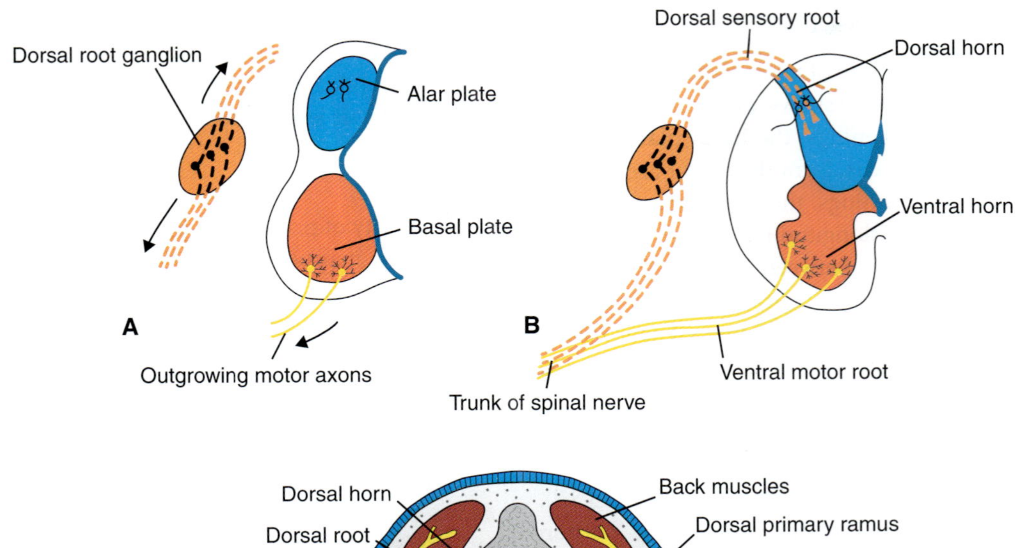


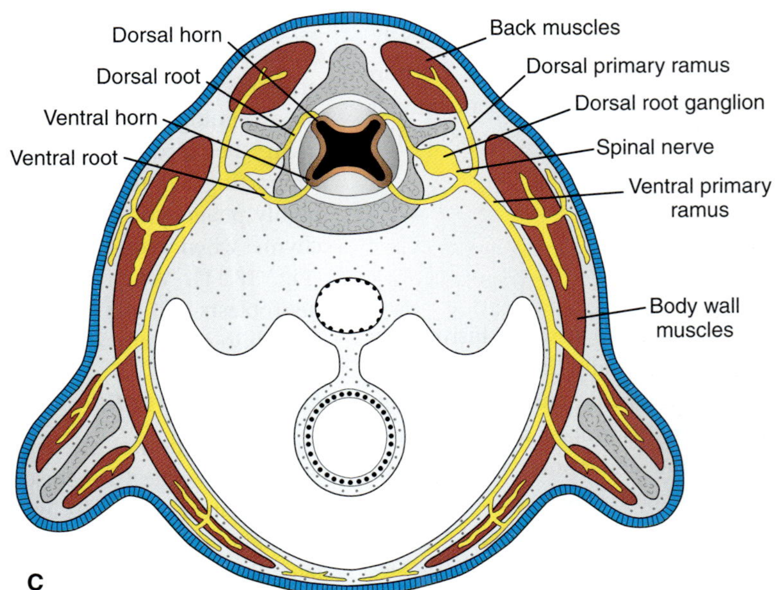


**FIGURE 18.10** **A.** Motor axons grow out from neurons in the basal plate, whereas neurons in dorsal root ganglia, positioned outside of the spinal cord, extend processes toward the dorsal horn of the spinal cord and to the periphery. **B.** Nerve fibers of the ventral motor roots and dorsal sensory roots join to form a spinal nerve. **C.** Cross section through an embryo showing dorsal and ventral roots coming together to form a spinal nerve. Almost immediately, spinal nerves divide into dorsal and ventral primary rami. Dorsal primary rami innervate back (epaxial) muscles and provide sensory innervation to the vertebral column and skin of the back. Ventral primary rami innervate muscles of the body wall and limbs (hypaxial muscles) and also carry sensory fibers to the skin and other structures. Thus, dorsal roots carry sensory fibers, ventral roots carry motor fibers, and spinal nerves and dorsal and ventral primary rami carry both motor and sensory fibers.

these processes terminate in the sensory receptor organs. Hence, neuroblasts of the sensory ganglia derived from neural crest cells give rise to the **dorsal root neurons**.

In addition to forming sensory ganglia, cells of the neural crest differentiate into autonomic neuroblasts, Schwann cells, pigment cells, odontoblasts, meninges, and mesenchyme of the pharyngeal arches.

### Spinal Nerves

Motor nerve fibers begin to appear in the fourth week, **arising from nerve cell bodies in the basal plates (ventral horns) of the spinal cord**. These fibers collect into bundles known as **ventral nerve roots** (Fig. 18.10). **Dorsal nerve roots** carrying **sensory** fibers originate from nerve cell bodies positioned **outside of the spinal cord** in **dorsal root ganglia (spinal ganglia) derived from neural crest cells**. Processes from these ganglia form bundles that grow into the dorsal horns of the spinal cord. Distal processes join the ventral nerve roots to form a **spinal nerve** (Fig. 18.10). Thus, dorsal root fibers carry sensory innervation, whereas ventral root fibers carry motor innervation and, therefore, spinal nerves contain both sensory and motor fibers. Almost immediately, spinal nerves divide into **dorsal** and **ventral primary rami, which contain both motor and sensory fibers**. Dorsal primary rami innervate dorsal axial musculature, vertebral joints, and the skin of the back. Ventral primary rami innervate the limbs and ventral body wall and form the major **nerve plexuses (brachial plexus and lumbosacral plexus)**.

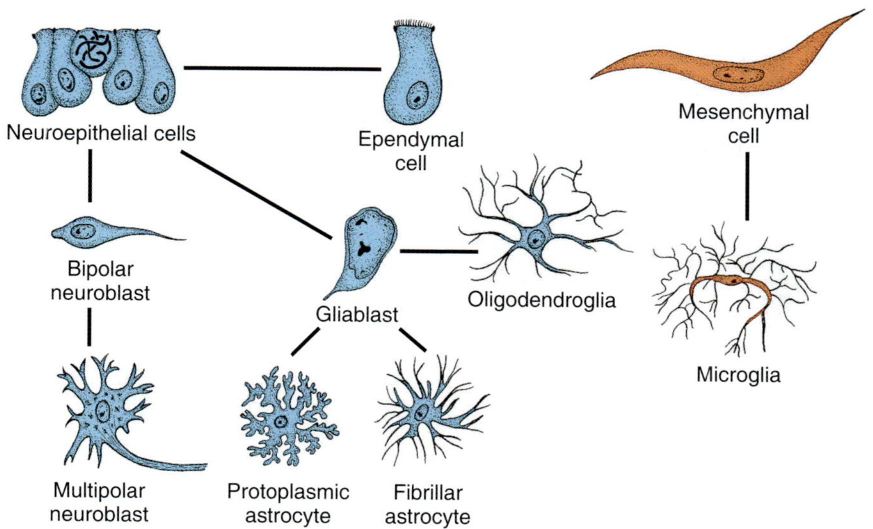


**FIGURE 18.11** Origin of the nerve cell and the various types of glial cells. Neuroblasts, fibrillar and protoplasmic astrocytes, and ependymal cells originate from neuroepithelial cells. Microglia develop from mesenchyme cells of blood vessels as the CNS becomes vascularized.

### *Myelination*

**Schwann cells** myelinate the peripheral nerves with each cell myelinating only a single axon. These cells originate from neural crest, migrate peripherally, and wrap themselves around axons, forming the **neurilemma sheath** (Fig. 18.12). Beginning at the fourth month of fetal life, many nerve fibers take on a whitish appearance as a result of deposition of **myelin**, which is formed by repeated coiling of the Schwann cell membrane around the axon (Fig. 18.12*C*).

The myelin sheath surrounding nerve fibers in the spinal cord has a completely different origin, the **oligodendroglial cells** (Fig. 18.12*B,C*). Unlike Schwann cells, a single oligodendrocyte can myelinate up to 50 axons. Although myelination of nerve fibers in the spinal cord begins in approximately the fourth month of intrauterine life, some of the motor fibers descending from higher brain centers to the spinal cord do not become myelinated until the first year of postnatal life. Tracts in the nervous system become myelinated at about the time they start to function.

## Positional Changes of the Cord

In the third month of development, the spinal cord extends the entire length of the embryo, and spinal nerves pass through the intervertebral foramina at their level of origin (Fig. 18.13*A*). With increasing age, however, the vertebral column and dura lengthen more rapidly than the neural tube, and the terminal end of the spinal cord gradually shifts to a higher level. At birth, this end is at the level of the third lumbar vertebra (Fig. 18.13*C*). As a result of this disproportionate growth, **dorsal and ventral roots of spinal nerves** run obliquely from their segment of origin in the spinal cord to the corresponding level of the vertebral column where the appropriate roots unite to form spinal nerves. The dura remains attached to the vertebral column at the coccygeal level.

In the adult, the spinal cord terminates at the level of L2–L3, whereas the dural sac and subarachnoid space extend to S2. At the end of the cord, a threadlike extension of pia mater passes caudally, goes through the dura, which provides a covering layer at S2 and extends to the first coccygeal vertebra. This structure is called the **filum terminale**, and it marks the tract of regression of the spinal cord as well as providing support for the cord (the part covered by dura and extending from S2 to the coccyx is also called the **coccygeal ligament**). Dorsal and ventral roots of spinal nerves below the terminal end of the cord at L2–L3 collectively constitute the **cauda equina (horse's tail)**. When cerebrospinal fluid is tapped during a **lumbar puncture**, the needle is inserted at the lower lumbar level (L4–L5), avoiding the lower end of the cord.

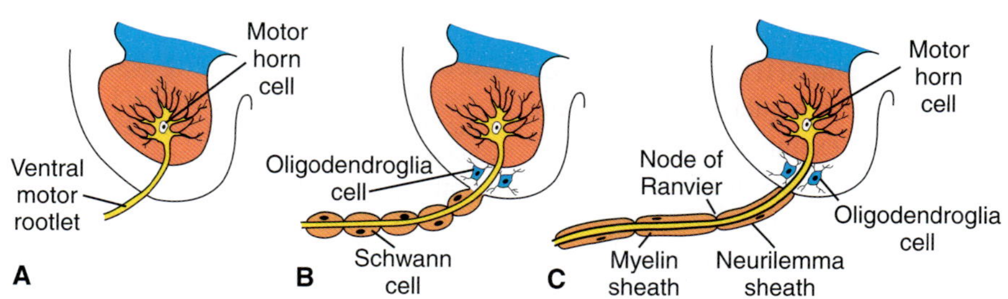


**FIGURE 18.12** **A.** Motor horn cell with naked rootlet. **B.** In the spinal cord, oligodendroglia cells surround the ventral rootlet; outside the spinal cord, Schwann cells begin to surround the rootlet. **C.** In the spinal cord, the myelin sheath is formed by oligodendroglia cells; outside the spinal cord, the sheath is formed by Schwann cells.

Part 2

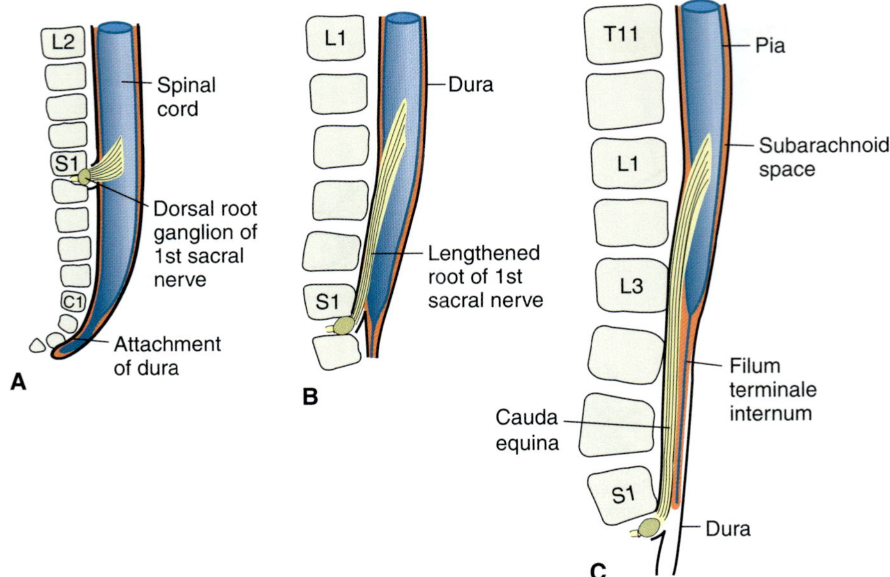


**FIGURE 18.13** Terminal end of the spinal cord in relation to that of the vertebral column at various stages of development. **A.** Approximately the third month. **B.** End of the fifth month. **C.** Newborn.



## Molecular Regulation of Nerve Differentiation in the Spinal Cord

Dorsal (sensory) and ventral (motor) regions of the developing spinal cord are dependent upon concentration gradients between members of the transforming growth factor β (TGF-β) family of growth factors secreted in the dorsal neural tube and sonic hedgehog (SHH) secreted by the notochord and floor plate (Fig. 18.14*A*). Initially, bone morphogenetic proteins (BMP) 4 and 7 are secreted by ectoderm overlying the neural tube, and the presence of these proteins establishes a second signaling center in the roof plate. Then, BMP4 in the roof plate induces a cascade of TGF-β proteins, including BMP5, BMP7, activin, and dorsalin in the roof plate and surrounding area. This cascade is organized in time and space such that a concentration gradient of these factors is established. As a result, cells near the roof plate are exposed to the highest concentrations with more ventrally positioned cells seeing less and less of these factors.

Similar events occur in the ventral region of the neural tube, only the signaling molecule is SHH. This factor is first expressed in the notochord followed by the establishment of a second signaling center in the floor plate (Fig. 18.14*A*). As a result, there is a diminishing concentration of SHH from the ventral to the dorsal region of the neural tube.

Thus, two overlapping concentrations are established between TGF-β family members and SHH. These gradients then activate transcription factors that regulate differentiation of sensory and motor neurons. For example, high concentrations of TGF-β factors and very low concentrations of SHH in the dorsal neural tube activate *PAX3* and *7* that control sensory neuron differentiation (Fig. 18.14*B*). Likewise, high concentrations of SHH and very low concentrations of TGF-β molecules in the ventral-most region result in activation of *NKX2.2* and *NKX6.1* and ventral neuron formation. Immediately dorsal to this region, where slightly lower

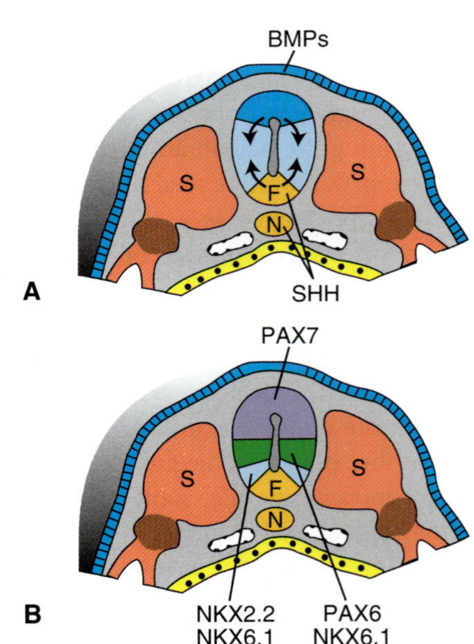


**FIGURE 18.14 A,B.** Drawings illustrating the molecular regulation of neuron differentiation in the spinal cord. **A.** Initially, bone morphogenetic protein 4 and 7 (BMP4 and 7) secreted in the ectoderm overlying the neural tube establish a signaling center in the roof plate. Then, BMP4 in the roof plate upregulates a cascade of TGF-β proteins, including BMP5 and 7, activin, and dorsalin in this region. Similarly, sonic hedgehog (SHH) secreted by the notochord establishes additional SHH signaling in the floor plate. In this manner, an overlapping gradient involving the dorsal and ventral factors is established in the neural tube. **B.** The gradient established by TGF-β proteins and SHH activates transcription factors that regulate neuronal differentiation. For example, high concentrations of TGF-β in the dorsal neural tube activate *PAX3* and *7* that control sensory neuron differentiation. High concentrations of SHH and very low concentrations of TGF-β near the floor plate activate *NKX2.2* and *NKX6.1* and ventral neuron formation. Slightly higher concentrations of TGF-β and slightly lower concentrations of SHH activate *NKX6.1* and *PAX6* and differentiation of ventral motor neurons and so on. *S*, somite; *N*, notochord; *F*, floorplate.

## Clinical Correlates

### Neural Tube Defects

Most defects of the spinal cord result from abnormal closure of the neural folds in the third and fourth weeks of development. The resulting abnormalities, **neural tube defects (NTDs)**, may involve the meninges, vertebrae, muscles, and skin. The birth prevalence of NTDs, including spina bifida and anencephaly, varies among different populations and may be as high as 1/200 births in some areas, such as northern China. The birth prevalence of NTDs in the United States has decreased by approximately 25% to 1/1,500 births because fortification of flour with folic acid was instituted in 1998. However, the prevalence of NTDs in India is very high, approximately 4.5 per 1,000 live births.

If the closure fails in the cranial region, it can result in the following defects:

- Anencephaly
- Hydranencephaly
- Encephalocele
- Iniencephaly

If the closure fails in the lower regions, it can result in:

- Congenital dermal sinus
- Spina bifida occulta
- Spina bifida cystica (with meningocele and meningomyelocele)
- Rachischisis

#### *Anencephaly*

Anencephaly results from failure of closure of the rostral neuropore in the fourth week of development. It is associated with defective development of the calvaria. Most of the brain extrudes from the cranium (EXENCEPHALY). Thus, the supratentorial nervous tissue undergoes degeneration. The disorder is incompatible with life. It is a common serious anomaly seen in still births.

#### *Spina Bifida*

**Spina bifida** is a general term for NTDs affecting the spinal region. It consists of a splitting of the vertebral arches and may or may not involve underlying neural tissue. **Spina bifida occulta** is a defect in the vertebral arches that is covered by skin and normally does not involve underlying neural tissue (Fig. 18.15*A*). Most often, the defect occurs in the sacral region (S1–S2) and is sometimes marked by a patch of hair overlying the affected region. The defect, which is due to a lack of fusion of the vertebral arches, affects about 10% of otherwise normal people. The malformation is not usually detected at birth and does not cause disability. Often, the defect is first noticed as an incidental finding diagnosed when an x-ray of the back is performed.

Spina bifida cystica includes meningocele and myelomeningocele. These are severe NTDs in which neural tissue and/or meninges protrude through a defect in the vertebral arches and skin to form a cyst-like sac (Fig. 18.15). Most lie in the lumbosacral region and result in neurological deficits, but they are usually not associated with intellectual disability. In some cases, only fluid-filled meninges protrude through the defect (**meningocele**) (Fig. 18.15*B*); in others, neural tissue is included in the sac (**myelomeningocele**) (Fig. 18.15*C*). Occasionally, the neural folds do not elevate but remain as a flattened mass of neural tissue (spina bifida with myeloschisis or **rachischisis**) (Figs. 18.15*D,E* and 18.16). **Hydrocephaly** requiring intervention develops in 80% to 90% of children born with severe NTDs and is often related to the presence

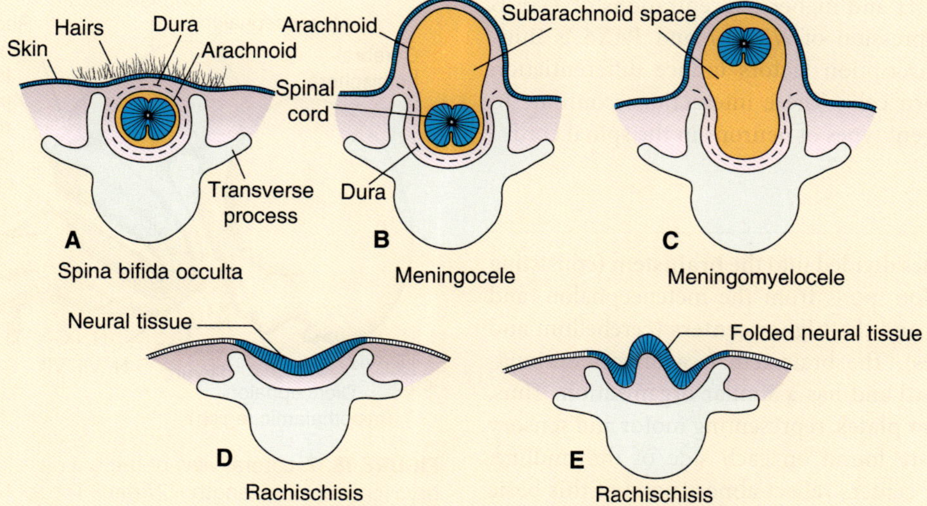


**FIGURE 18.15 A–E.** Drawings illustrating a variety of NTDs involving the spinal cord. The term *spina bifida* applies to all of the defects because the bony arch of one or more vertebrae has failed to fuse dorsal to the spinal cord. In some cases, the bony defect is covered by skin (spina bifida occulta **(A)**), but the spinal cord is intact. Often, this defect is noticeable because of a patch of dark hair that grows over the area. In cases of meningoceles **(B)**, only a fluid-filled sac of meninges protrudes from the defect, whereas myelomeningoceles include neural tissue in the sac **(C)**. *Rachischisis* refers to NTDs in which the neural tube fails to close, resulting in spina bifida and exposure of neural tissue that often becomes necrotic **(D,E)**. Rachischisis may occur in the spinal cord or brain regions of the neural tube and represents the most severe type of abnormality. Most spinal cord defects occur in the lumbosacral area, and 50% to 70% of all NTDs can be prevented by maternal use of folic acid (400 μg daily) prior to and during pregnancy.

(*Continued*)

Part 2

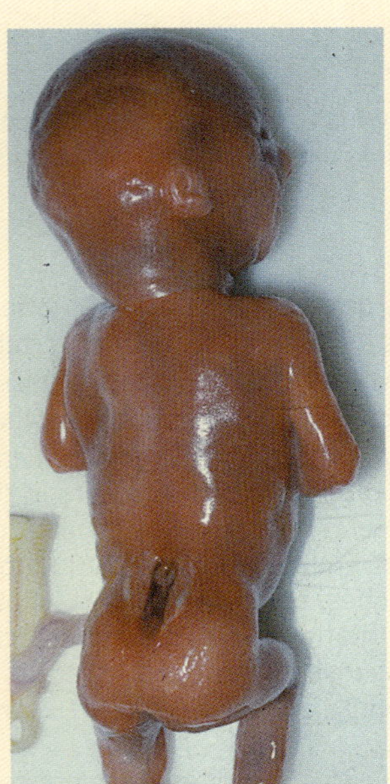

**FIGURE 18.16** Patient with a severe spina bifida involving several vertebrae in the lumbosacral region.

of an **Arnold-Chiari malformation** (herniation of part of the cerebellum into the foramen magnum), which obstructs the flow of cerebrospinal fluid and causes the hydrocephalus. Herniation of the cerebellum occurs because the spinal cord is tethered to the vertebral column due to its abnormal development. As the vertebral column lengthens, tethering of the cord pulls the cerebellum into the foramen magnum, cutting off the flow of cerebrospinal fluid. Hydrocephalus can be treated by inserting a ventriculoperitoneal shunt, which allows drainage of the cerebrospinal fluid from one of the cerebral ventricles to the peritoneal cavity.

### Antenatal Diagnosis of NTDs

Anencephaly can be easily diagnosed by ultrasound and MRI and also by raised α-fetoprotein levels in maternal serum.

Spina bifida can be diagnosed prenatally by ultrasound and by determination of α-fetoprotein levels in maternal serum and amniotic fluid. The vertebra can be visualized by 12 weeks of gestation, and defects in closure of the vertebral arches can be detected. Experimental treatment for the defect is to perform surgery in utero as early as 22 weeks of gestation. The fetus is exposed by an incision into the uterus, the defect is repaired, and the infant is placed back in the uterus.

### Predisposing Factors for NTDs

Hyperthermia, valproic acid, and hypervitaminosis A produce NTDs, as do a large number of other teratogens. The origin of most NTDs is multifactorial, and the likelihood of having a child with such a defect increases significantly once one affected offspring is **born**. Prevention of many NTDs is possible if women take **folic acid (400 μg/day)** starting at least 1 month prior to conception and then throughout their pregnancy. Such a protocol reduces the occurrence of NTDs by as much as 50% to 70%. Folic acid may also reduce the incidence of **autism spectrum disorder (ASD)**. Because approximately 50% of all pregnancies are unplanned, it is recommended that all women of childbearing age take a multivitamin containing 400 μg of folic acid daily. Furthermore, women who have had a child with an NTD or who have a family history of NTDs should take 400 μg of folic acid daily and then 4,000 μg (4 mg) per day starting at least 1 month before conception through the first 3 months of pregnancy.

concentrations of SHH and higher concentrations of TGF-β molecules occur, expression of *NKX6.1* and *PAX6* is initiated, and these transcription factors induce differentiation of ventral motor horn cells. These interactions continue to produce all the different types of neurons in the spinal cord.

## ■ BRAIN

The brain is sometimes divided into the **brainstem** (consisting of the myelencephalon, pons from the metencephalon, and the mesencephalon) and the **higher centers** (cerebellum and cerebral hemispheres). The brainstem is a direct continuation of the spinal cord and has a similar organization. Thus, distinct **basal** and **alar plates**, representing motor and sensory areas, respectively, are found on each side of the midline. However, the higher centers reflect almost none of this basic pattern and, instead, show accentuation of the alar plates and regression of the basal plates.

### Rhombencephalon: Hindbrain

The rhombencephalon consists of the **myelencephalon**, the most caudal of the brain vesicles, and the **metencephalon**, which extends from the pontine flexure to the rhombencephalic isthmus (Figs. 18.5 and 18.17).

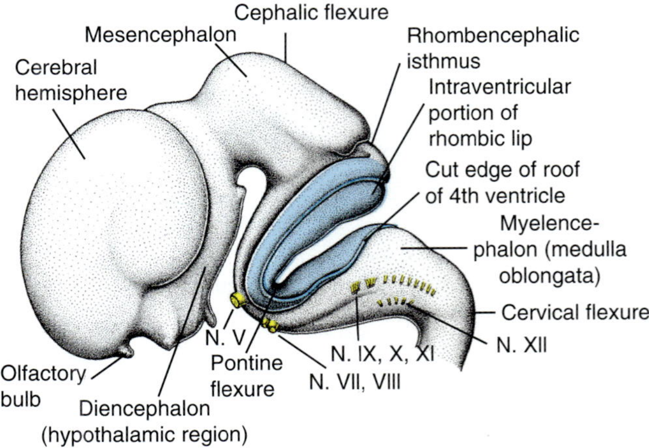


**FIGURE 18.17** Lateral view of the brain vesicles in an 8-week embryo (crown-rump length ~27 mm). The roof plate of the rhombencephalon has been removed to show the intraventricular portion of the rhombic lip. Note the origin of the cranial nerves.

### Myelencephalon

The myelencephalon gives rise to the **medulla oblongata**, a transitional zone between the brain and spinal cord. It differs from the spinal cord in that its lateral walls are everted (Fig. 18.18). As a result, the roof is stretched out. Alar and

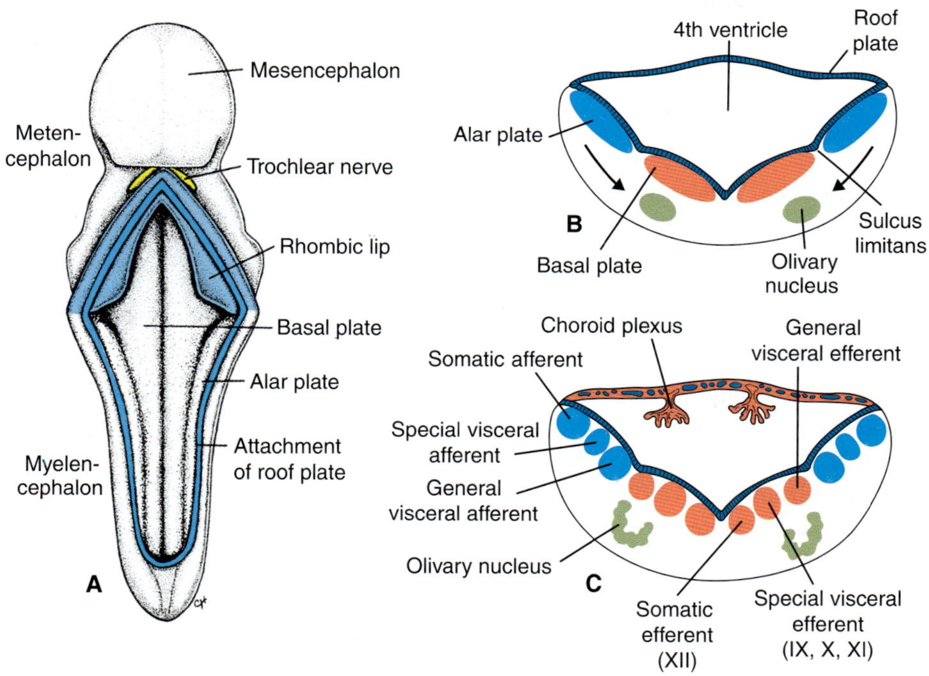


**FIGURE 18.18** **A.** Dorsal view of the floor of the fourth ventricle in a 6-week embryo after removal of the roof plate. Note the alar and basal plates in the myelencephalon. The rhombic lip is visible in the metencephalon. **B,C.** Position and differentiation of the basal and alar plates of the myelencephalon at different stages of development. Note formation of the nuclear groups in the basal and alar plates. *Arrows*, path followed by cells of the alar plate to the olivary nuclear complex. The choroid plexus produces cerebrospinal fluid.



basal plates separated by the sulcus limitans can be clearly distinguished. The basal plate, similar to that of the spinal cord, contains motor nuclei.

The alar lamina contains three groups of sensory relay nuclei (Fig. 18.18C; Table 18.1). Some cells from each alar lamina undergo ventral migration and come to lie ventrolateral to the basal lamina. These cells give rise to the **olivary nuclei**. The somatic afferent column in myelencephalon also gives rise to **nucleus gracilis** and **nucleus cuneatus**. The cavity of metencephalon forms the central canal of medulla and lower part of the fourth ventricle.

The roof plate of the myelencephalon consists of a single layer of ependymal cells covered by vascular mesenchyme, the **pia mater** (Fig. 18.18C). The two combined are known as the **tela choroidea**. Because of active proliferation of the vascular mesenchyme, a number of saclike invaginations project into

**Table 18.1** **Nuclei Derived from Basal and Alar Lamina in Myelencephalon**

| | | | |
|---|---|---|---|
| **Alar Lamina** | | | |
| Medial | General visceral afferent | Nucleus of IX and X nerves | Conveys visceral sensations from GIT and heart |
| ↓ | Special visceral afferent | Nucleus of tractus solitarius (accessory [XI], vagus [X], and glossopharyngeal [IX] nerves) | Conveys taste sensations from tongue, palate, epiglottis, and oropharynx |
| | General somatic afferent | Glossopharyngeal (IX) and vagus (X) nerves | Receives sensations of pain, temperature, and touch from pharynx via the glossopharyngeal nerve and from external ear via the vagus nerve |
| Lateral | Special somatic afferent | Vestibular and cochlear nuclei of the vestibulocochlear (VIII) nerve | Conveys sensations of hearing and balance from ears |
| **Basal Lamina** | | | |
| Medial | Somatic efferent | Nucleus of the hypoglossal nerve | Supplies musculature of tongue |
| ↓ | Special visceral efferent | Nuclei of accessory (XI), vagus (X), and glossopharyngeal (IX) nerves | Supply striated muscles of the pharyngeal arches |
| Lateral | General visceral efferent | Dorsal motor nucleus of the vagus nerve (X) | Motor neurons that supply involuntary musculature of the respiratory tract, intestinal tract, and heart (X nerve) |

the underlying ventricular cavity (Fig. 18.18*C*). These tuft-like invaginations form the choroid plexus, which produces cerebrospinal fluid.

### *Metencephalon*

The metencephalon, similar to the myelencephalon, is characterized by basal and alar plates (Fig. 18.19). From these regions, two new components form: (1) the **cerebellum**, derived from the alar plates and serving as a coordination center for posture and movement (Fig. 18.20), and (2) the **pons**, derived from the basal plates and serving as the pathway for nerve fibers between the spinal cord and the cerebral and cerebellar cortices. The cavity of metencephalon forms the upper part of the fourth ventricle.

Each basal plate of the metencephalon (Fig. 18.19) contains three groups of motor neurons. The alar plates of the mesencephalon contain three groups of sensory nuclei (Table 18.2).

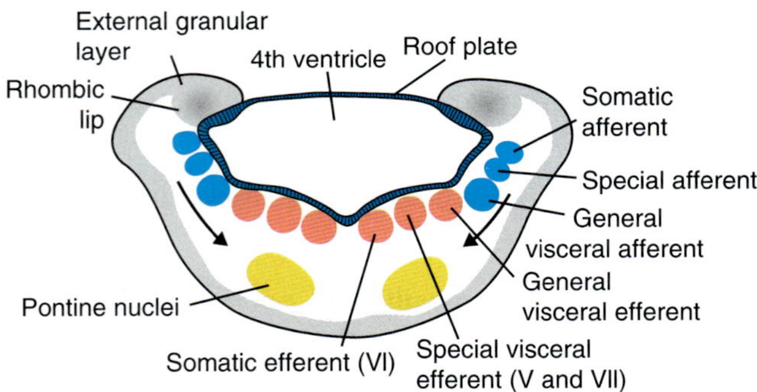


**FIGURE 18.19** Transverse section through the caudal part of the metencephalon. Note the differentiation of the various motor and sensory nuclear areas in the basal and alar plates, respectively, and the position of the rhombic lips, which project partly into the lumen of the fourth ventricle and partly above the attachment of the roof plate. *Arrows*, direction of migration of the pontine nuclei.

The marginal layer of the basal plates of the metencephalon expands as it makes a bridge for nerve fibers connecting the cerebral cortex and cerebellar cortex with the spinal cord. Hence, this portion of the metencephalon is known as the **pons** (bridge). In addition to nerve fibers, the pons contains the **pontine nuclei**, which originate in the alar plates of the metencephalon and myelencephalon (Fig. 18.19, *arrows*).

### *Cerebellum*

The dorsolateral parts of the alar plates bend medially and form the **rhombic lips** (Fig. 18.18). In the caudal portion of the metencephalon, the rhombic lips are widely separated, but immediately below the mesencephalon, they approach each other in the midline (Fig. 18.20). As a result of a further deepening of the pontine flexure, the rhombic lips compress cephalocaudally and form the **cerebellar plate** (Fig. 18.20). In a 12-week embryo, this plate shows a small midline portion, the **vermis**, and two lateral portions, the **hemispheres**. A transverse fissure soon separates the **nodule** from the vermis and the lateral **flocculus** from the hemispheres (Fig. 18.20*B*). This **flocculonodular** lobe is phylogenetically the most primitive part of the cerebellum.

Initially, the **cerebellar plate** consists of neuroepithelial, mantle, and marginal layers (Fig. 18.21*A*). During further development, a number of cells formed by the neuroepithelial layer migrate to the surface of the cerebellum to form the **external granular layer**. Cells of this layer retain their ability to divide and form a proliferative zone on the surface of the cerebellum (Fig. 18.21*B*,*C*).

In the sixth month of development, the external granular layer gives rise to various cell types. Some of these cells migrate toward the differentiating Purkinje cells, which themselves are migrating in the opposite direction as they move toward the surface (Fig. 18.22), and give rise to the **inner layer of granule cells**, later called the **granule cell layer** in the fully differentiated cerebellum. **Basket** and **stellate**

**Table 18.2 Nuclei Derived from Basal and Alar Lamina in Metencephalon**

| | | | | |
|---|---|---|---|---|
| **Basal Lamina** | | | | |
| Medial ↓ | Somatic efferent | | Abducent nucleus | Supplies lateral rectus muscle in the eyeball |
| Lateral | Special visceral efferent | | Nuclei of the trigeminal and facial nerves | Innervates the musculature of the first and second pharyngeal arches |
| | General visceral efferent | | Superior salivatory nucleus (facial nerve) and inferior salivatory nucleus (glossopharyngeal nerve) | Secretomotor to submandibular and sublingual glands (facial nerve) Secretomotor to parotid gland (glossopharyngeal nerve) |
| **Alar Lamina** | | | | |
| Medial ↓ | Special visceral afferent | | Facial nerve | Conveys taste sensation from the anterior two-third of the tongue |
| | Somatic afferent | General somatic afferent | Chief and spinal sensory nuclei of the trigeminal nerve | Conveys proprioception, touch, pain, and temperature from head and neck |
| | | Special somatic afferent | Vestibular and cochlear nuclei (VIII nerve) | Conveys sensation of hearing and balance |
| Lateral | | | | |

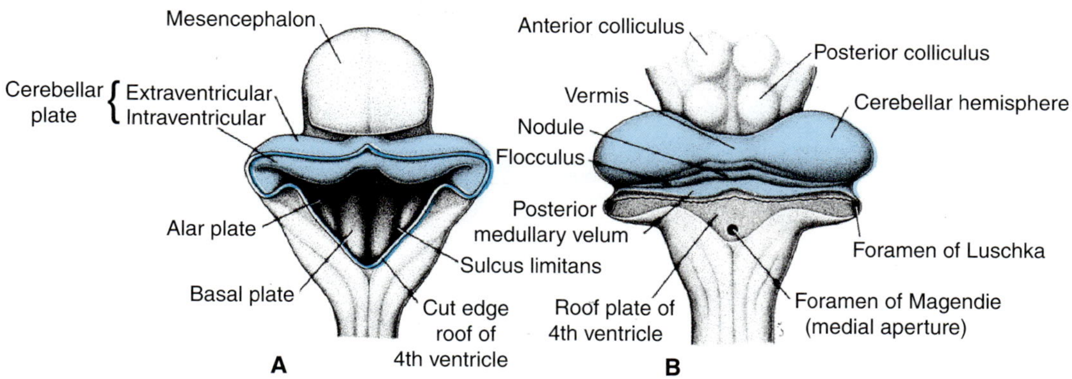


**FIGURE 18.20** **A.** Dorsal view of the mesencephalon and rhombencephalon in an 8-week embryo. The roof of the fourth ventricle has been removed, allowing a view of its floor. **B.** Similar view in a 4-month embryo. Note the choroidal fissure and the lateral and medial apertures in the roof of the fourth ventricle.

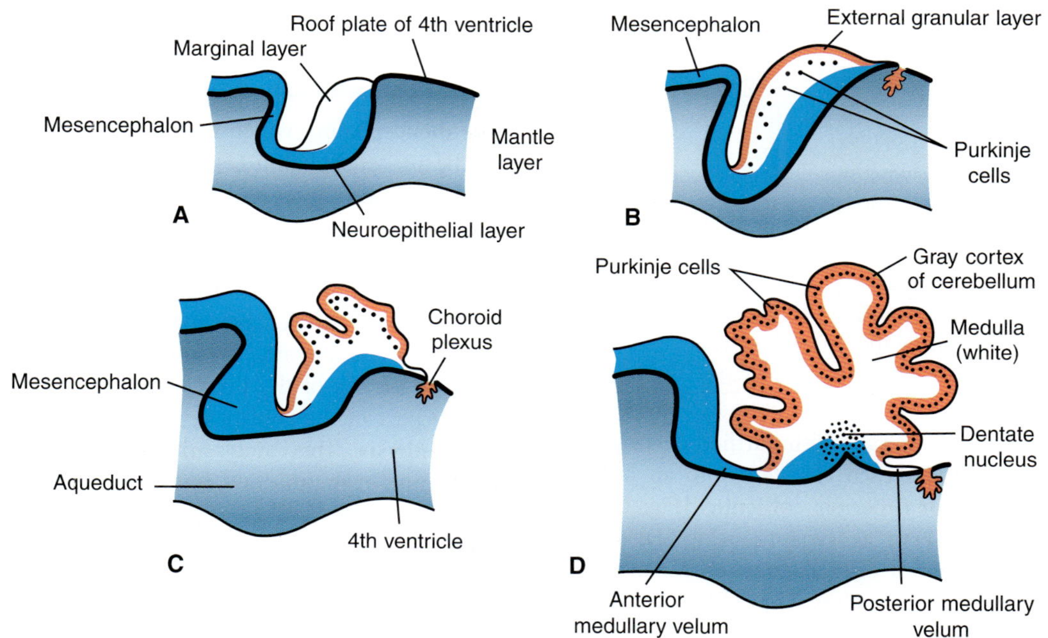


**FIGURE 18.21** Sagittal sections through the roof of the metencephalon showing development of the cerebellum. **A.** 8 weeks (~30 mm). **B.** 12 weeks (70 mm). **C.** 13 weeks. **D.** 15 weeks. Note formation of the external granular layer on the surface of the cerebellar plate **(B,C)**. During later stages, cells of the external granular layer migrate inward to mingle with Purkinje cells and form the definitive cortex of the cerebellum. The dentate nucleus is one of the deep cerebellar nuclei. Note the anterior and posterior velum.

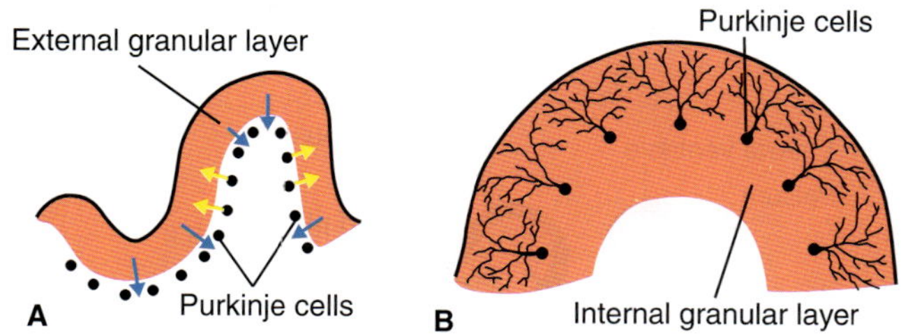


**FIGURE 18.22** Stages in development of the cerebellar cortex. **A.** The external granular layer on the surface of the cerebellum forms a proliferative layer from which some cells migrate inward (*arrows*) to form an internal layer of granule cells that is later called the granule cell layer in the fully differentiated cerebellum. Basket and stellate cells are derived from proliferating cells in the cerebellar white matter. **B.** Postnatal cerebellar cortex showing differentiated Purkinje cells, the molecular layer on the surface, and the internal granular layer beneath the Purkinje cells.

**cells** are produced by proliferating cells in the cerebellar white matter. The cortex of the cerebellum, consisting of Purkinje cells, Golgi II neurons, and neurons produced by the external granular layer, reaches its definitive size after birth (Fig. 18.22*B*). The deep cerebellar nuclei, such as the **dentate nucleus**, reach their final position before birth (Fig. 18.21*D*).

## Mesencephalon: Midbrain

In the mesencephalon (Fig. 18.23), each basal plate contains two groups of motor nuclei (Table 18.3).

The marginal layer of each basal plate enlarges and forms the **crus cerebri**. These crura serve as pathways for nerve fibers descending from the cerebral cortex to lower centers in the pons and spinal cord. Initially, the alar plates of the mesencephalon appear as two longitudinal elevations separated by a shallow

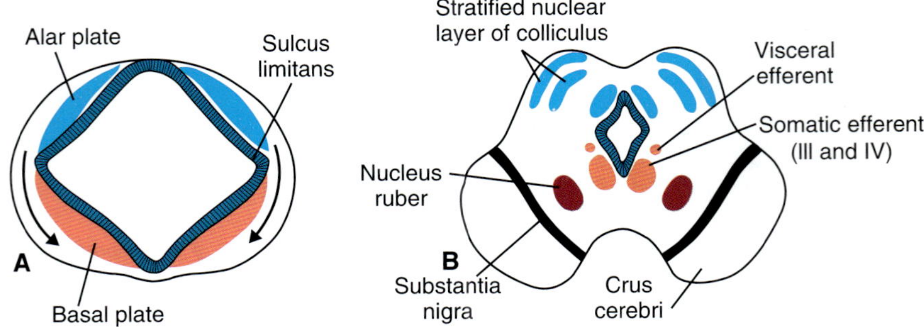


**FIGURE 18.23 A,B.** Position and differentiation of the basal and alar plates in the mesencephalon at various stages of development. *Arrows* in **(A)** indicate the path followed by cells of the alar plate to form the nucleus ruber and substantia nigra. Note the various motor nuclei in the basal plate.

**Table 18.3 Nuclei Derived from Basal and Alar Lamina in Mesencephalon**

| | | | |
|---|---|---|---|
| **Basal Lamina** | | | |
| Medial ↓ | Somatic efferent | Motor nucleus of oculomotor and trochlear nerves | Supply extraocular muscles |
| Lateral | General visceral efferent | Edinger–Westphal nucleus of the oculomotor nerve | Supplies ciliaris and sphincter pupillae muscles in the eyeball |
| **Alar Lamina** | | | |
| | General sensory afferent | Mesencephalic nucleus of the trigeminal nerve | Sensations from head and neck |

midline depression (Fig. 18.23). With further development, a transverse groove divides each elevation into an **anterior** (superior) and a **posterior** (inferior) **colliculus** (Fig. 18.23*B*). The posterior colliculi serve as synaptic relay stations for auditory reflexes; the anterior colliculi function as correlation and reflex centers for visual impulses. The colliculi are formed by waves of neuroblasts migrating into the overlying marginal zone. Here they are arranged in layers (Fig. 18.23*B*).

## Prosencephalon: Forebrain

The **prosencephalon** consists of the **telencephalon**, which forms the cerebral hemispheres, and the **diencephalon**, which forms the optic cup and stalk, pituitary, thalamus, hypothalamus, and epiphysis.

### *Diencephalon*

#### Roof Plate and Epiphysis

The diencephalon, which develops from the median portion of the prosencephalon (Figs. 18.5 and 18.17), is thought to consist of a roof plate and two alar plates but to lack floor and basal plates (interestingly, *SHH*, a ventral midline marker, is expressed in the floor of the diencephalon, suggesting that a floor plate does exist). The roof plate of the diencephalon consists of a single layer of ependymal cells covered by vascular mesenchyme. Together, these layers give rise to the **choroid plexus** of the third ventricle (Fig. 18.30). The most caudal part of the roof plate develops into the **pineal body**, or **epiphysis**. This body initially appears as an epithelial thickening in the midline, but by the seventh week, it begins to evaginate (Figs. 18.24 and 18.25). Eventually, it becomes a solid organ on the roof of the mesencephalon (Fig. 18.30) that serves as a channel through which light and darkness affect endocrine and behavioral rhythms. In the adult, calcium is frequently deposited in the epiphysis and then serves as a landmark on radiographs of the skull.

#### Alar Plate, Thalamus, and Hypothalamus

The alar plates form the lateral walls of the diencephalon. A groove, the **hypothalamic sulcus**, divides the plate into a

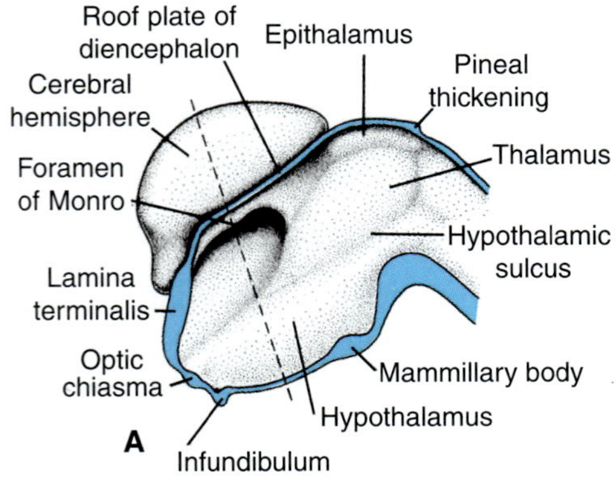


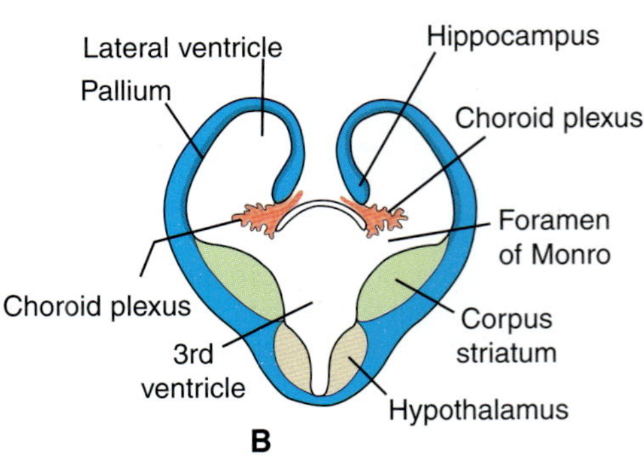


**FIGURE 18.24 A.** Medial surface of the right half of the prosencephalon in a 7-week embryo. **B.** Transverse section through the prosencephalon at the level of the *broken line* in **(A)**. The corpus striatum bulges out in the floor of the lateral ventricle and the foramen of Monro.

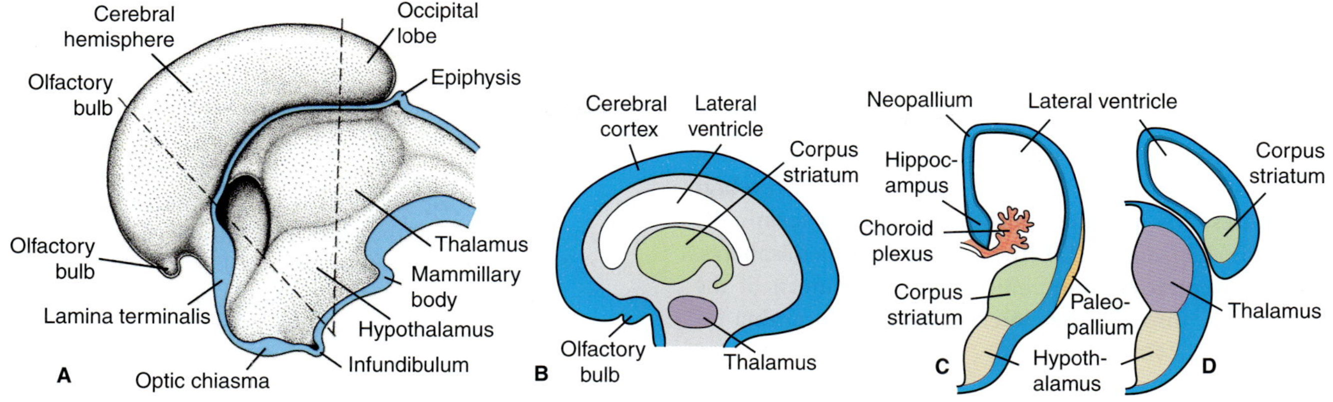


**FIGURE 18.25** **A.** Medial surface of the right half of the telencephalon and diencephalon in an 8-week embryo. **B.** Schematic showing the relationship of the lateral ventricle, corpus striatum, and thalamus. **C,D.** Transverse sections through the right half of the telencephalon and diencephalon at the level of the *broken lines* in **(A)**.

dorsal and a ventral region, the **thalamus** and **hypothalamus**, respectively (Figs. 18.24 and 18.25).

As a result of proliferative activity, the thalamus gradually projects into the lumen of the diencephalon. Frequently, this expansion is so great that thalamic regions from the right and left sides fuse in the midline, forming the **massa intermedia**, or **interthalamic connexus**.

The hypothalamus, forming the lower portion of the alar plate, differentiates into a number of nuclear areas that regulate the visceral functions, including sleep, digestion, body temperature, and emotional behavior. One of these groups, the **mammillary body**, forms a distinct protuberance on the ventral surface of the hypothalamus on each side of the midline (Figs. 18.24*A* and 18.25*A*).

## Hypophysis or Pituitary Gland

The hypophysis, or pituitary gland, develops from two completely different parts: (1) an ectodermal outpocketing of the **stomodeum** (primitive oral cavity) immediately in front of the oropharyngeal membrane, known as **Rathke pouch**, and (2) a downward extension of the diencephalon, the **infundibulum** (Fig. 18.26).

When the embryo is approximately 3 weeks old, Rathke pouch appears as an evagination of the oral cavity and subsequently grows dorsally toward the infundibulum. By the end of the second month, it loses its connection with the oral cavity and is then in close contact with the infundibulum.

During further development, cells in the anterior wall of Rathke pouch increase rapidly in number and form the **anterior lobe of the hypophysis**, or **adenohypophysis** (Fig. 18.26*B*). A small extension of this lobe, the **pars tuberalis**, grows along the stalk of the infundibulum and eventually surrounds it (Fig. 18.26*C*). The posterior wall of Rathke pouch develops into the **pars intermedia**, which in humans seems to have little significance.

The infundibulum gives rise to the **stalk** and the **pars nervosa**, or **posterior lobe of the hypophysis** (neurohypophysis) (Fig. 18.26*C*). It is composed of neuroglial cells.

*Clinical Correlates*

### Hypophyseal Defects

Occasionally, a small portion of Rathke pouch persists in the roof of the pharynx as a **pharyngeal hypophysis**. **Craniopharyngiomas** arise from remnants of Rathke pouch. They may form within the sella turcica or along the stalk of the pituitary but usually lie above the sella. They may cause hydrocephalus and pituitary dysfunction (e.g., diabetes insipidus, growth failure).



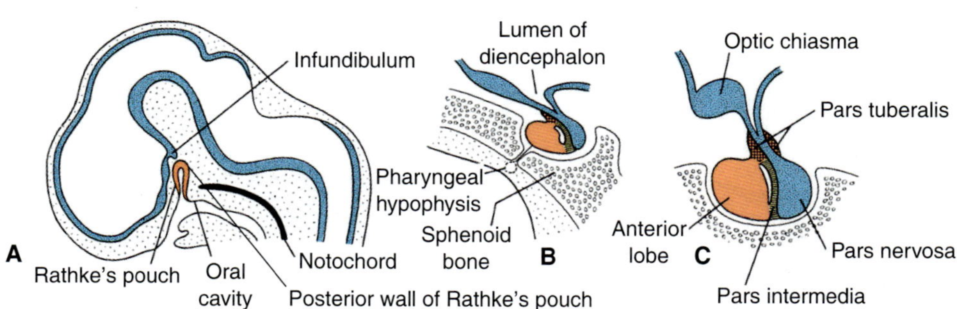


**FIGURE 18.26** **A.** Sagittal section through the cephalic part of a 6-week embryo showing Rathke pouch as a dorsal outpocketing of the oral cavity and the infundibulum as a thickening in the floor of the diencephalon. **B,C.** Sagittal sections through the developing hypophysis in the 11th and 16th weeks of development, respectively. Note formation of the pars tuberalis encircling the stalk of the pars nervosa.

In addition, it contains a number of nerve fibers from the hypothalamic area.

### Telencephalon

The telencephalon, the most rostral of the brain vesicles, consists of two lateral outpocketings, the **cerebral hemispheres**, and a median portion, the **lamina terminalis** (Figs. 18.5, 18.24, and 18.25). The cavities of the hemispheres, the **lateral ventricles**, communicate with the lumen of the diencephalon through the **interventricular foramina of Monro** (Fig. 18.24).

#### Cerebral Hemispheres

The cerebral hemispheres arise at the beginning of the fifth week of development as bilateral evaginations of the lateral wall of the prosencephalon (Fig. 18.24). By the middle of the second month, the basal part of the hemispheres (i.e., the part that initially formed the forward extension of the thalamus) (Fig. 18.24*A*) begins to grow and bulges into the lumen of the lateral ventricle and into the floor of the foramen of Monro (Figs. 18.24*B* and 18.25*A,B*). In transverse sections, the rapidly growing region has a striated appearance and is therefore known as the **corpus striatum** (Fig. 18.25*B*).

In the region where the wall of the hemisphere is attached to the roof of the diencephalon, the wall fails to develop neuroblasts and remains very thin (Fig. 18.24*B*). Here, the hemisphere wall consists of a single layer of ependymal cells covered by vascular mesenchyme, and together, they form the **choroid plexuses in each of the lateral ventricles**. The choroid plexuses should have formed in the roof of each hemisphere, but as a result of the disproportionate growth of the various parts of the hemispheres, each plexus protrudes into the lateral ventricle along the **choroidal fissure** (Figs. 18.25 and 18.27). Immediately above the choroidal fissure, the wall of the hemisphere thickens, forming the **hippocampus** (Figs. 18.24*B* and 18.25*B*). This structure's primary function is olfaction, and it bulges into the lateral ventricle.

With further expansion, the hemispheres cover the lateral aspect of the diencephalon, mesencephalon, and cephalic portion of the metencephalon (Figs. 18.27 and 18.28). The corpus striatum (Fig. 18.24*B*), being a part of the wall of the hemisphere, likewise expands posteriorly and is divided into two parts: (1) a dorsomedial portion, the **caudate nucleus**, and (2) a ventrolateral portion, the **lentiform nucleus**, which is made up of the **putamen** and **globus pallidus** (Fig. 18.27*B*). This division is accomplished by axons passing to and from the cortex of the hemisphere and breaking through the nuclear mass of the corpus striatum. The fiber bundle thus formed is known as the **internal capsule** (Fig. 18.27*B*). The caudate and lentiform nuclei (putamen and globus pallidus) are part of a collection of nuclei called the

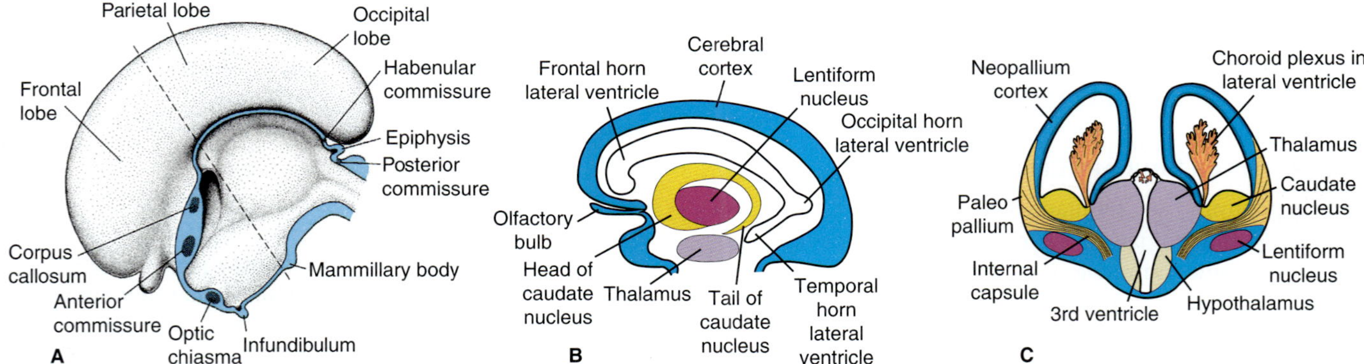


**FIGURE 18.27 A.** Medial surface of the right half of the telencephalon and diencephalon in a 10-week embryo. **B.** Schematic to indicate the relationship between the horns of the lateral ventricle, caudate and lentiform nuclei, and the thalamus. **C.** Transverse section through the hemisphere and diencephalon at the level of the *broken line* in **(A)**.

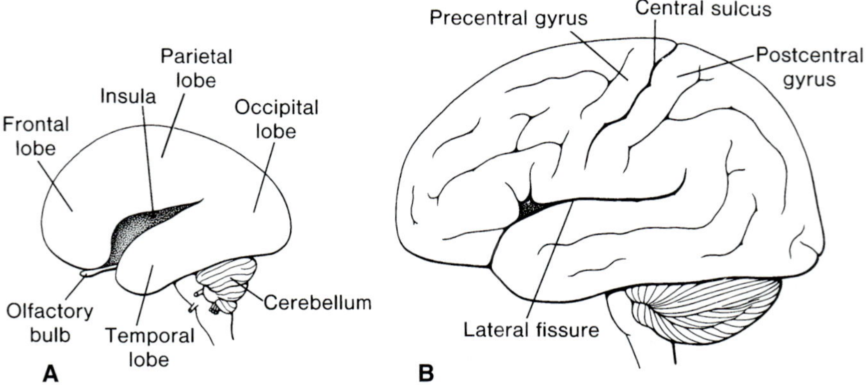


**FIGURE 18.28** Development of gyri and sulci on the lateral surface of the cerebral hemisphere. **A.** 7 months. **B.** 9 months.

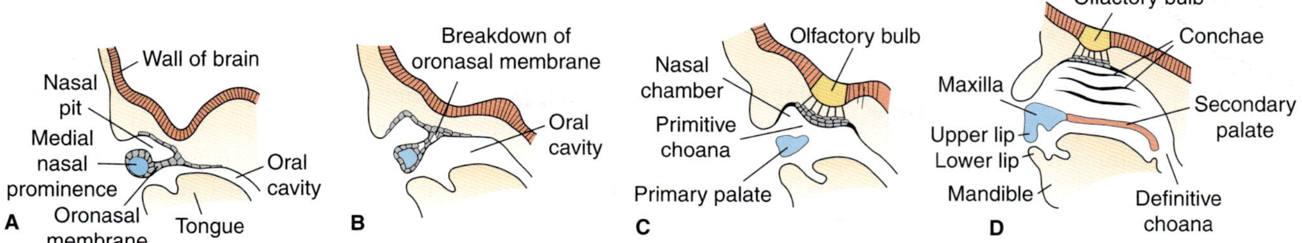


**FIGURE 18.29** **A.** Sagittal section through the nasal pit and lower rim of the medial nasal prominence of a 6-week embryo. The primitive nasal cavity is separated from the oral cavity by the oronasal membrane. **B.** Similar section as in **(A)** toward the end of the sixth week, showing breakdown of the oronasal membrane. **C.** At 7 weeks, neurons in the nasal epithelium have extended processes that contact the floor of the telencephalon in the region of the developing olfactory bulbs. **D.** By 9 weeks, definitive oronasal structures have formed, neurons in the nasal epithelium are well differentiated, and secondary neurons from the olfactory bulbs to the brain begin to lengthen. Together, the olfactory bulbs and tracts of the secondary neurons constitute the olfactory nerve (Fig. 18.30).

**basal ganglia**. These ganglia are extensively connected with the cerebral cortex, thalamus, and brainstem and play a major role in controlling voluntary movements, routine behavior, cognition, emotion, procedural learning, and eye movements.

Continuous growth of the cerebral hemispheres in anterior, dorsal, and inferior directions results in the formation of frontal, temporal, and occipital lobes, respectively. As growth in the region overlying the corpus striatum slows, however, the area between the frontal and temporal lobes becomes depressed and is known as the **insula** (Fig. 18.28*A*). This region is later overgrown by the adjacent lobes and at the time of birth is almost completely covered. During the final part of fetal life, the surface of the cerebral hemispheres grows so rapidly that a great many convolutions (**gyri**), separated by fissures and sulci, appear on its surface (Fig. 18.28*B*).

## Cortex Development

The cerebral cortex develops from the pallium (Fig. 18.24*B*), which has three regions: (1) the paleocortex (**paleopallium**), (2) the archicortex (**archipallium**), and (3) the neocortex (**neopallium**) (Figs. 18.25*C* and 18.27*C*). Phylogenetically, the archipallium is associated with the olfactory cortex and forms the hippocampus and paleopallium, which are the oldest parts of the cortex. The neopallium is the newest part of the cortex phylogenetically and comprises 90% of the cortical structure.

In the neopallium, waves of neuroblasts migrate to a subpial position and then differentiate into fully mature neurons. When the next wave of neuroblasts arrives, they migrate through the earlier formed layers of cells until they reach the subpial position. Hence, the early formed neuroblasts obtain a deep position in the cortex, whereas those formed later obtain a more superficial position.

At birth, the cortex has a stratified appearance due to differentiation of the cells in layers. The motor cortex contains a large number of **pyramidal cells**, and the sensory areas are characterized by **granular cells**.

Differentiation of the olfactory system is dependent on epithelial–mesenchymal interactions. These occur between neural crest cells and ectoderm of the frontonasal prominence to form the **olfactory placodes** (see Chapter 17, p. 245) and between these same crest cells and the palleopalial region of the telencephalon to form the **olfactory bulbs** (Fig. 18.29). Cells in the nasal placodes differentiate into primary sensory neurons of the nasal epithelium, which has axons that grow and make contact with secondary neurons in the developing olfactory bulbs (Fig. 18.29). By the seventh week, these contacts are well established. As growth of the brain continues, the olfactory bulbs and the olfactory tracts of the secondary neurons lengthen, and together they constitute the olfactory nerve (Fig. 18.30).

## Commissures

At first, each cerebral hemisphere grows as a separate structure. However, by the end of the third month, collections of nerve fibers grow across, connecting one hemisphere to the other. These fibers form in bundles, called **commissures**, and many make use of the **lamina terminalis** that forms in the cranial region of the forebrain vesicle (Figs. 18.24*A* and 18.25*A*). The lamina terminalis extends from the roof plate of the diencephalon to the optic chiasm and provides an initial connection between the hemispheres. The first of the crossing bundles to appear in the lamina terminalis is the **anterior**

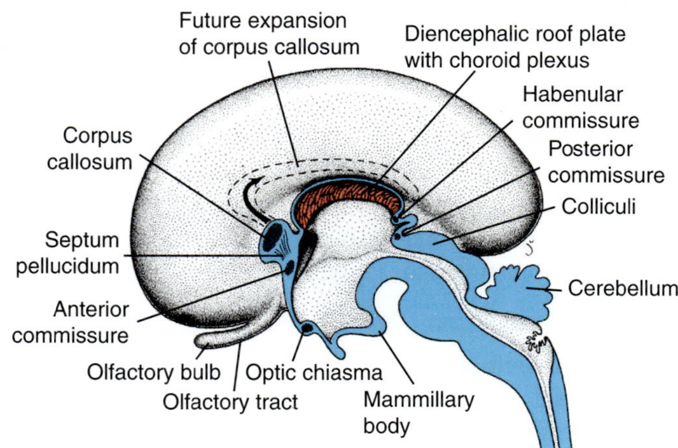


**FIGURE 18.30** Medial surface of the right half of the brain in a 4-month embryo showing the various commissures. *Broken line*, future site of the corpus callosum. The hippocampal commissure is not indicated.

Part 2

**commissure**. It consists of fibers connecting the olfactory bulb and related brain areas of one hemisphere to those of the opposite side (Figs. 18.27*A* and 18.30).

The second commissure to appear is the **hippocampal commissure (fornix)**. Its fibers arise in the hippocampus and converge on the lamina terminalis close to the roof plate of the diencephalon. From here, the fibers continue, forming an arching system immediately outside the choroid fissure, to the mammillary body and the hypothalamus.

Another important commissure is the **corpus callosum**. It appears by the 10th week of development and connects the nonolfactory areas of the right and the left cerebral cortices. Initially, it forms a small bundle in the lamina terminalis (Fig. 18.27*A*). As a result of continuous expansion of the neopallium, however, it extends first anteriorly and then posteriorly, arching over the thin roof of the diencephalon (Fig. 18.30).

In addition to the three commissures developing in the lamina terminalis, three more appear outside of this region. Two of these, the **posterior** and **habenular commissures**, are just below and rostral to the stalk of the pineal gland. The third, the **optic chiasma**, which appears in the rostral wall of the diencephalon, contains fibers from the medial halves of the retinae (Fig. 18.30).

### Meninges

The **meninges** are the three membranous layers that cover the brain and spinal cord. These membranes are derived from a combination of mesoderm and neural crest cells and begin to form in the fourth to fifth weeks. During the early fetal period, the external layer thickens to form the tough **dura mater**, whereas the inner layer forms the **pia-arachnoid mater**. The pia-arachnoid layers comprise the **leptomeninges**. Eventually, the pia mater adheres closely to the surface of the brain and spinal cord and a space forms, the **subarachnoid space**, when the pia and arachnoid separate. Cerebrospinal fluid circulates in this space between the pia mater and arachnoid mater. The space itself is traversed by arachnoid trabeculae.

The dura mater is a tough fibrous sac that encloses the arachnoid mater. In the brain, the dura mater lines the **venous sinuses**. **Arachnoid granulations**, which transfer cerebrospinal fluid back into the venous system, project into these sinuses. The dura mater also supports the brain through formation of several **septa**. One of these is the **falx cerebri** that separates the two cerebral hemispheres. Another septum, the **tentorium cerebelli**, forms a roof over the cerebellum, whereas the **falx cerebelli** extends ventrally from the tentorium cerebelli between the two cerebellar hemispheres.

### Cerebrospinal Fluid

**Cerebrospinal fluid (CSF)** is secreted by the choroid plexuses in the brain ventricles. These plexuses are modifications of the ependymal layer and produce approximately 400 to 500 mL of CSF per day. The fluid circulates through the brain ventricles leaving the lateral ventricles, for example, through the interventricular foramina, entering the third ventricle, and then passing through the **cerebral aqueduct** into the fourth ventricle (Fig. 18.30). Some CSF enters the spinal canal, and some exits the fourth ventricle through its median and lateral apertures to enter the subarachnoid space that surrounds the CNS. CSF is absorbed into the venous system from the subarachnoid space through arachnoid granulations, especially those that project into the superior sagittal sinus. CSF "floats" the brain and, thus, provides a cushion for the brain and gives it buoyancy so that its weight does not compress cranial nerves (CNs) against the inside of the skull.

## MOLECULAR REGULATION OF BRAIN DEVELOPMENT

Anteroposterior (craniocaudal) patterning of the CNS begins early in development, during gastrulation and neural induction (see Chapters 5 and 6). Once the neural plate is established, signals for segregation of the brain into forebrain, midbrain, and hindbrain regions are derived from **homeobox** genes expressed in the notochord, prechordal plate, and neural plate. The hindbrain has eight segments, the **rhombomeres**, that have variable expression patterns of the *Antennapedia* class of homeobox genes, the ***HOX*** genes (see Chapter 6, p. 75). These genes are expressed in overlapping (nested) patterns, with genes at the most 3′ end of a cluster having more anterior boundaries and paralogous genes having identical expression domains (Fig. 18.31). Genes at the 3′ end are also expressed earlier than those at the 5′ end, so that a temporal relation to the expression pattern is established. These genes, then, confer positional value along the anteroposterior axis of the hindbrain, determine the identity of the rhombomeres, and specify their derivatives. How this regulation occurs is not clear, although **retinoids (retinoic acid)** play a critical role in regulating *HOX* expression. For example, excess retinoic acid shifts *HOX* gene expression anteriorly and causes more cranial rhombomeres to differentiate into more caudal types. Retinoic acid deficiency results in a small

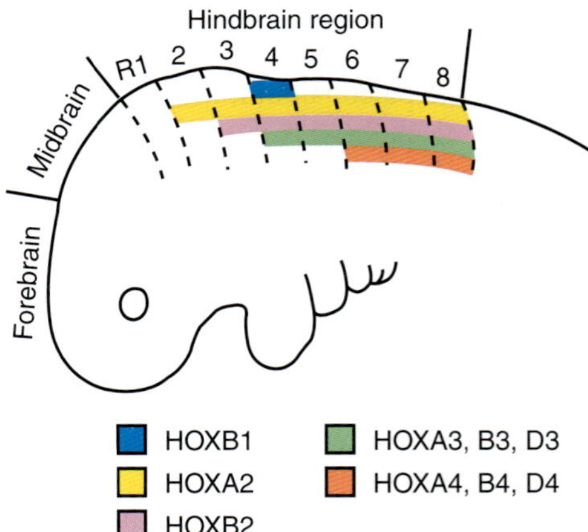


**FIGURE 18.31** Patterns of *HOX* gene expression in the hindbrain. *HOX* genes are expressed in overlapping patterns ending at specific rhombomere boundaries. Genes at the 3′ end of a cluster have the most anterior boundaries, and paralogous genes have identical expression domains. These genes confer positional value along the anterior-posterior axis of the hindbrain, determine the identity of the rhombomeres, and specify their derivatives.

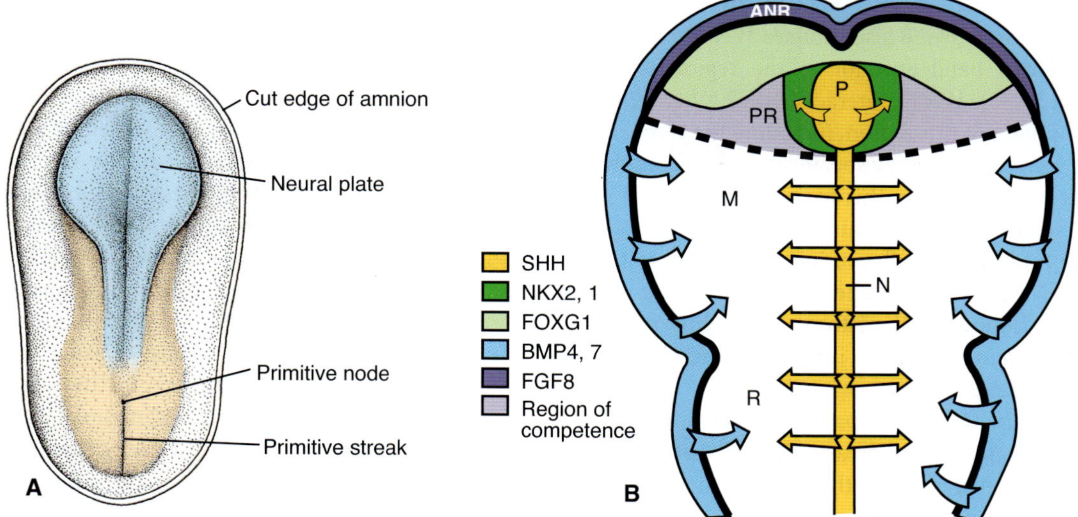


**FIGURE 18.32 A.** Dorsal view of a late presomite stage embryo at approximately 18 days showing development of the neural plate in the cranial region (*blue* area). **B.** Diagram of the cranial neural plate region shown in **(A)** (*blue* area) illustrating the organizing center known as the *anterior neural ridge* (*ANR*). This area lies in the most anterior region of the neural plate and secretes fibroblast growth factor 8 (FGF8), which induces expression of *FOXG1* in adjacent neuroectoderm. *FOXG1* regulates development of the telencephalon (cerebral hemispheres) and regional specification within the prosencephalon (*PR*). Sonic hedgehog (SHH), secreted by the prechordal plate (*P*) and notochord (*N*), ventralizes the brain and induces expression of *NKX2.1*, which regulates development of the hypothalamus. Bone morphogenetic protein 4 and 7 (BMP4 and 7), secreted by the adjacent nonneural ectoderm, control dorsal patterning of the brain. *M*, mesencephalon; *R*, rhombencephalon.

hindbrain. There is also a differential response to retinoic acid by the *HOX* genes; those at the 3′end of the cluster are more sensitive than those at the 5′ end.

Specification of the forebrain and midbrain areas is also regulated by genes containing a homeodomain. However, these genes are not of the *Antennapedia* class, whose most anterior boundary of expression stops at rhombomere 3. Thus, new genes have assumed the patterning role for these regions of the brain, which evolutionarily constitute the "new head." At the neural plate stage, ***LIM1***, expressed in the prechordal plate, and ***OTX2***, expressed in the neural plate, are important for designating the forebrain and midbrain areas, with *LIM1* supporting *OTX2* expression. (These genes are also expressed at the earliest stages of gastrulation, and they assist in specifying the entire cranial region of the epiblast.) Once the neural folds and pharyngeal arches appear, additional **homeobox** genes, including *OTX1*, *EMX1*, and *EMX2*, are expressed in specific and in overlapping (nested) patterns in the mid- and forebrain regions and specify the identity of these areas. Once these boundaries are established, two additional organizing centers appear: the **anterior neural ridge (ANR)** at the junction of the cranial border of the neural plate and nonneural ectoderm (Fig. 18.32) and the **isthmus** (Fig. 18.33) between the hindbrain and midbrain. In both locations, **fibroblast growth factor 8 (FGF8)** is the key signaling molecule, inducing subsequent gene expression that regulates differentiation. In the ANR at the four-somite stage, FGF8 induces expression of ***FOXG1***, a transcription factor (Fig. 18.32). *FOXG1* then regulates development of the telencephalon (cerebral hemispheres) and regional specification within the forebrain, including the basal telencephalon

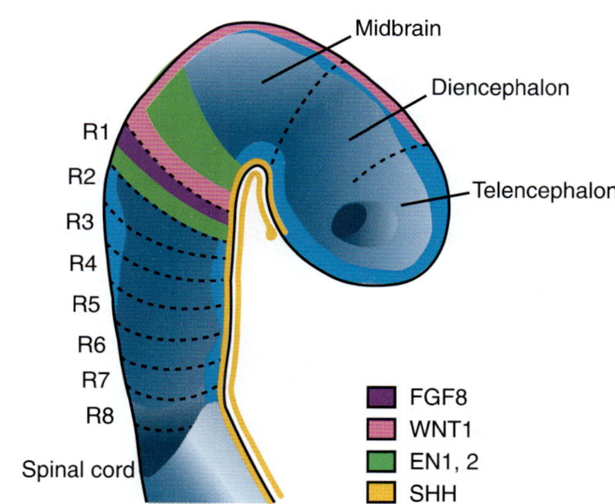


**FIGURE 18.33** Organizing center in the rhombencephalic isthmus at the boundaries between the midbrain and hindbrain. This region secretes fibroblast growth factor 8 (FGF8) in a circumferential ring that induces expression of ENGRAILED 1 and 2 (*EN1* and *EN2*) in gradients anteriorly and posteriorly from this area. *EN1* regulates development of the dorsal midbrain, and both genes participate in formation of the cerebellum. *WNT1*, another gene induced by FGF8, also assists in development of the cerebellum.

and the retina. In the isthmus, at the junction between the midbrain and hindbrain territories, *FGF8* is expressed in a ring around the circumference of this location (Fig. 18.33). FGF8 induces expression of ***ENGRAILED 1*** and ***2*** (***EN1*** and ***EN2***), two homeobox-containing genes, expressed in gradients radiating anteriorly and posteriorly from the isthmus. *EN1* regulates development throughout its expression domain, including the dorsal midbrain (tectum) and anterior

Part 2

hindbrain (cerebellum), whereas *EN2* is involved only in cerebellar development. FGF8 also induces ***WNT1*** expression in a circumferential band anterior to the region of *FGF8* expression (Fig. 18.33). *WNT1* interacts with *EN1* and *EN2* to regulate development of this region, including the cerebellum. In fact, *WNT1* may assist in early specification of the midbrain area because it is expressed in this region at the neural plate stage. *FGF8* is also expressed at this early time in mesoderm underlying the midbrain–hindbrain junction and may therefore regulate *WNT1* expression and initial patterning of this region. The constriction for the isthmus is slightly posterior to the actual midbrain–hindbrain junction, which lies at the caudal limit of *OTX2* expression.

Dorsoventral (mediolateral) patterning also occurs in the forebrain and midbrain areas. Ventral patterning is controlled by **SHH** just as it is throughout the remainder of the CNS. SHH, secreted by the prechordal plate, induces expression of ***NKX2.1***, a homeodomain-containing gene that regulates development of the hypothalamus. Importantly, SHH signaling requires cleavage of the protein, and the carboxy-terminal portion executes this process. Following cleavage of the SHH protein, cholesterol is covalently linked to the carboxy-terminus of the amino-terminal product. The amino-terminal portion retains all of the signaling properties of SHH, and its association with cholesterol assists in its distribution.

Dorsal (lateral) patterning of the neural tube is controlled by **BMP4** and **BMP7** expressed in the nonneural ectoderm adjacent to the neural plate. These proteins induce expression of *MSX1* in the midline and repress expression of *FOXG1* (Fig. 18.32). Once the neural tube is closed, BMP2 and 4 are expressed in the roof plate, and these proteins regulate expression of the transcription factor *LHX2* in the cortex. This expression then initiates a cascade of genes to pattern this region.

Expression patterns of genes regulating anterior–posterior (craniocaudal) and dorsoventral (mediolateral) patterning of the brain overlap and interact at the borders of these regions. Furthermore, various brain regions are competent to respond to specific signals and not to others. For example, only the cranial part of the neural plate expresses *NKX2.1* in response to SHH. Likewise, only the anterior neural plate expresses *FOXG1* in response to FGF8; midbrain levels express *EN2* in response to the same FGF8 signal. Thus, a **competence to respond** also assists in specifying regional differences.



## *Clinical Correlates*

### Cranial Defects

**Holoprosencephaly (HPE)** refers to a spectrum of abnormalities in which a loss of midline structures results in malformations of the brain and face. In severe cases, the lateral ventricles merge into a single **telencephalic vesicle (alobar HPE)**, the eyes are fused, and there is a single nasal chamber along with other midline facial defects (Fig. 18.34). In less severe cases, some division of the prosencephalon into two cerebral hemispheres occurs, but there is incomplete development of midline structures. Usually, the olfactory bulbs and tracts and the corpus callosum are hypoplastic or absent. In very mild cases, sometimes the only indication that some degree of HPE has occurred is the presence of a single central incisor. HPE occurs in 1/15,000 live births but is present in 1/250 pregnancies that end in early miscarriage. Mutations in ***SHH***, the gene that regulates establishment of the ventral midline in the CNS, result in some forms of HPE. Another cause is defective **cholesterol biosynthesis** leading to **Smith-Lemli-Opitz syndrome**. These children have craniofacial and limb defects, and 5% have HPE. Smith-Lemli-Opitz syndrome is an autosomal recessive condition due to abnormalities in **7-dehydrocholesterol reductase**, which metabolizes 7-dehydrocholesterol to cholesterol. Many of the defects, including those of the limbs and brain, may be due to abnormal *SHH* signaling, as cholesterol is necessary for this gene to exert its effects. Other genetic causes include mutations in the transcription factors ***SINE OCULIS HOMEOBOX 3 (SIX3)***, ***TG-INTERACTING FACTOR (TGIF)***, and the ***ZINC FINGER PROTEIN (ZIC2)***.

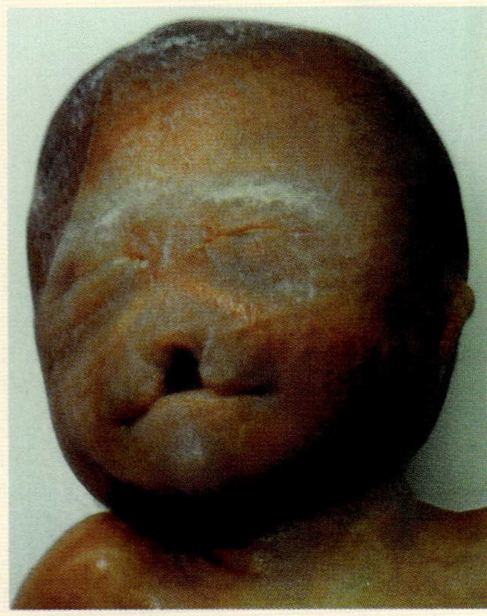

**FIGURE 18.34** Child with HPE. Note that a loss of midline tissue has resulted in a midline cleft lip, lack of nasal tissue, and eyes that are too close together (hypotelorism). In the brain, the loss of midline tissue causes the lateral ventricles to merge into a single chamber. Mutations in the gene *SHH*, which specifies the midline of the CNS at neural plate stages, are one cause for this spectrum of abnormalities.

**Schizencephaly** is a rare disorder in which large clefts occur in the cerebral hemispheres, sometimes causing a loss of brain tissue. Mutations in the homeobox gene *EMX2* appear to account for some of these cases.

Ossification defects in bones of the skull can result in **meningoceles**, **meningoencephaloceles**, and **meningohydroencephaloceles**. The most frequently affected bone is the squamous part of the occipital bone, which may be partially or totally lacking. If the opening of the occipital bone is small, only meninges bulge through it (**meningocele**), but if the defect is large, part of the brain and even part of the ventricle may penetrate through the opening into the meningeal sac (Figs. 18.35 and 18.36). The latter two malformations are known

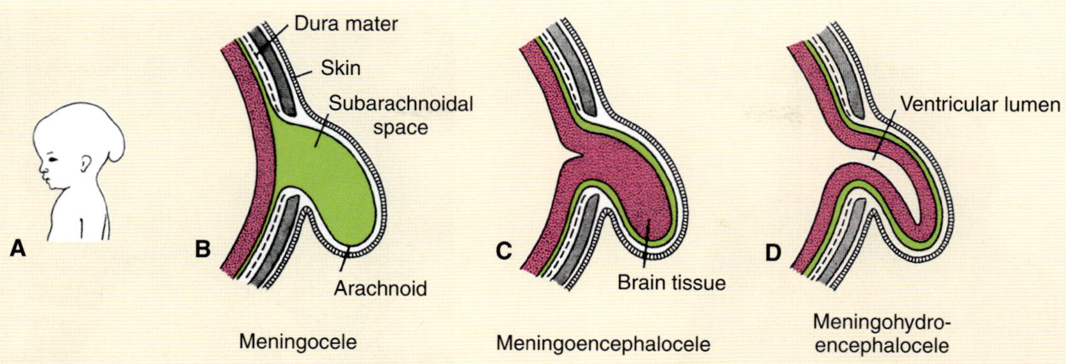


**FIGURE 18.35 A.** Profile of a child with a skull defect in the occipital region with protruding meninges and/or neural tissue. **B–D.** Drawings illustrating various types of skull defects in which meninges (meningocele **[B]**) or meninges with neural tissue (meningoencephalocele **[C]** and meningohydroencephalocele **[D]**) protrude through a bony defect. The defects usually occur in the occipital region but may involve other areas of the skull, such as the frontonasal region. In most cases, the origin of these defects is due to abnormal neural tube closure, and many can be prevented by maternal use of folic acid (400 μg daily) prior to and during pregnancy.

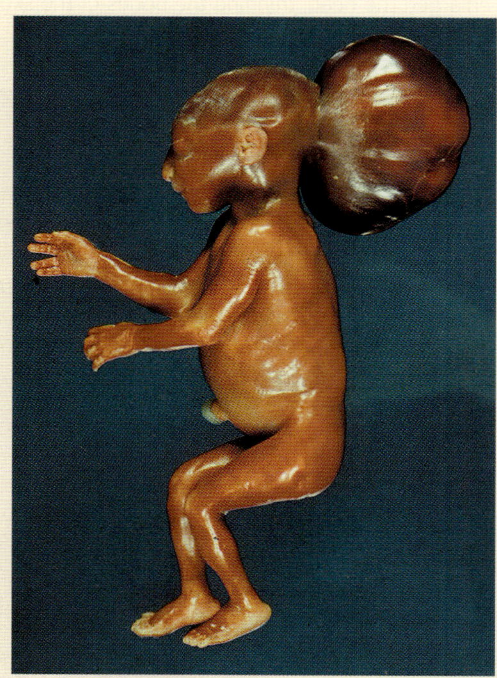

**FIGURE 18.36** Fetus with a large occipital meningoencephalocele. Some infants with smaller defects can survive with surgery, and their degree of neurological deficits depends on the amount of neural tissue that is abnormal or lost.

as **meningoencephalocele** and **meningohydroencephalocele**, respectively. These defects occur in 1/12,000 births.

**Exencephaly** is characterized by failure of the cephalic part of the neural tube to close. As a result, the vault of the skull does not form, leaving the malformed brain exposed. Later, this tissue degenerates, leaving a mass of necrotic tissue. This defect is called **anencephaly**, although the brainstem remains intact (Fig. 18.37*A*). In some cases, the closure defect of the neural tube extends caudally into the spinal cord, and the abnormality is called **craniorachischisis** (Fig. 18.37*B*). Again, there is anencephaly but with a large defect involving the spine. Because anencephalic fetuses lack a swallowing reflex, the last 2 months of pregnancy are characterized by **polyhydramnios**. The abnormality can be recognized on ultrasound, as the vault of the skull is absent. Anencephaly occurs in 1 per 5,000 births and is more common in females than in males. Like spina bifida, many of these cases can be prevented by having women take 400 μg of folic acid per day before and during early pregnancy.

**Hydrocephalus** is characterized by an abnormal accumulation of **CSF** within the ventricular system. In most cases, hydrocephalus in the newborn is due to an obstruction of the **aqueduct of Sylvius (aqueductal stenosis)**. This prevents the CSF of the lateral and third ventricles from passing into the fourth ventricle and from there into the subarachnoid space, where it would be resorbed. As a result, fluid accumulates in the lateral ventricles and presses on the brain and bones of the skull. Because the cranial sutures have not yet fused, spaces between them widen as the head expands. In extreme cases, brain tissue and bones become thin and the head may be very large (Fig. 18.38).

**Microcephaly** describes a cranial vault that is smaller than normal (Fig. 18.39). Because the size of the cranium depends on growth of the brain, the underlying defect is in brain development. Causation of the abnormality is varied; it may be genetic (autosomal recessive) or caused by prenatal insults, such as infection or exposure to drugs or other teratogens. Intellectual disability occurs in more than half the cases.

Fetal infection by toxoplasmosis may result in cerebral calcification, intellectual disability, hydrocephalus, or microcephaly. Likewise, exposure to radiation during the early stages of development may produce microcephaly. Hyperthermia (fever) produced by maternal infection or by sauna baths and hot tubs may cause spina bifida and anencephaly.

The aforementioned abnormalities are the most serious ones, and they may be incompatible with life. A great many other defects of the CNS may occur without much external manifestation. For example, the **corpus callosum** may be partially or completely absent without much functional disturbance. Likewise, partial or complete absence of the cerebellum may result in only a slight disturbance of coordination. On the other hand, cases of severe **intellectual disability** may not be associated with morphologically detectable brain abnormalities. Intellectual disability may result from genetic abnormalities (e.g., Down syndrome) or from exposures to teratogens, including infectious agents (rubella, cytomegalovirus, toxoplasmosis). The leading cause of intellectual disability is, however, **maternal alcohol abuse**.

(*Continued*)

Part 2

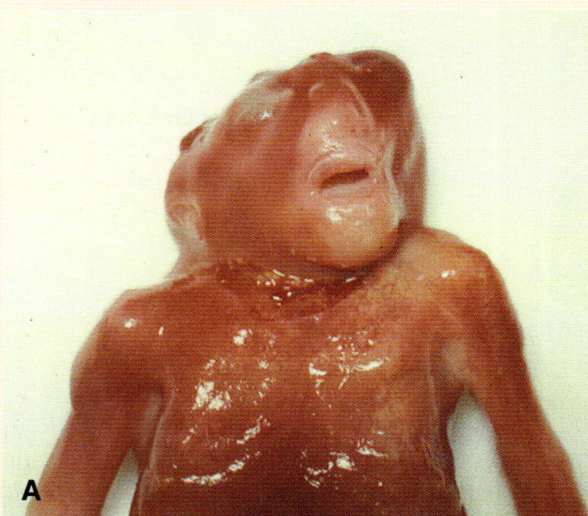


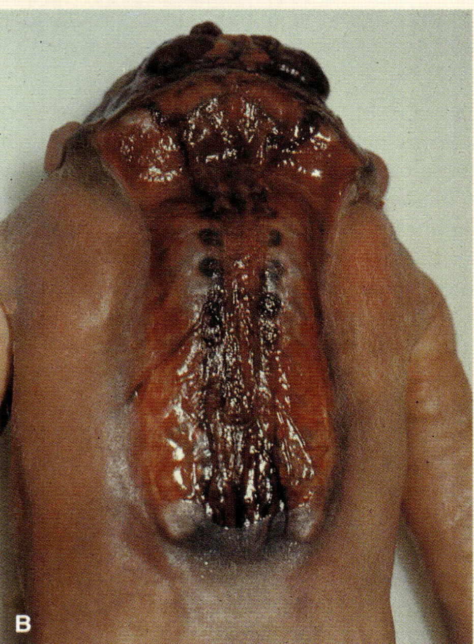


**FIGURE 18.37 A.** Fetus with anencephaly (absent brain) due to a lack of closure of the cranial neural folds. Once the folds fail to close, neural tissue is disorganized and is exposed to amniotic fluid, which causes necrosis and loss of tissue. This defect is always fatal, and most pregnancies with such cases are terminated. **B.** Fetus with anencephaly and craniorachischisis. The neural tube has failed to close in cranial and upper spinal cord regions resulting in massive necrosis of neural tissue. The defects illustrated in **(A)** and **(B)** can be prevented by maternal use of folic acid (400 μg daily) prior to and during pregnancy.

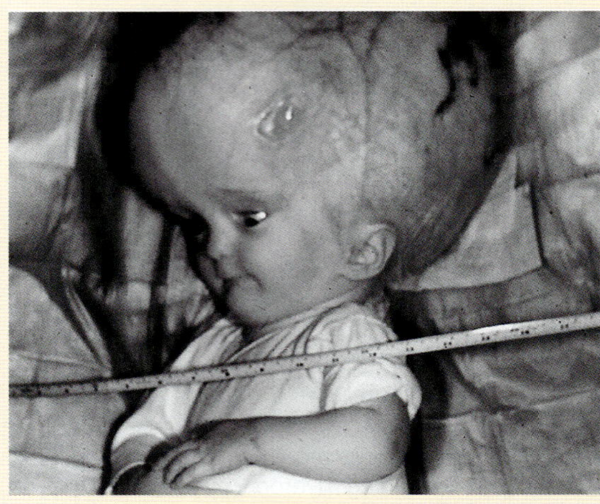

**FIGURE 18.38** Child with severe hydrocephalus. Because the cranial sutures had not closed, pressure from the accumulated CSF enlarged the head, thinning the bones of the skull and cerebral cortex.

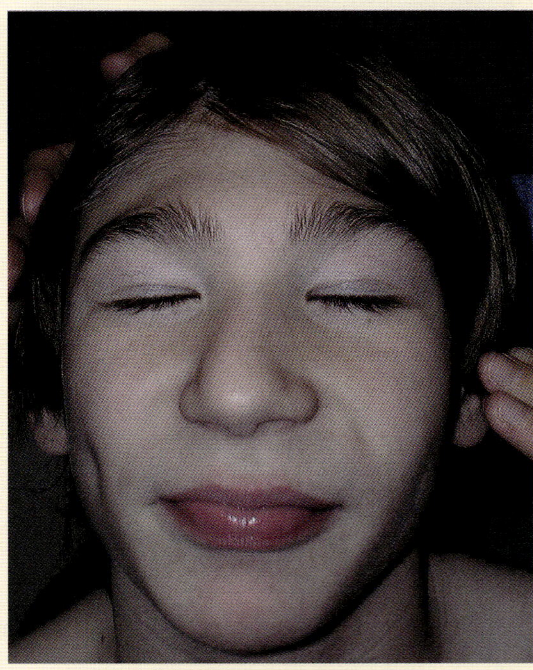

**FIGURE 18.39** Child with microcephaly. This abnormality, due to poor growth of the brain, is frequently associated with intellectual disability.



## ■ CRANIAL NERVES

By the fourth week of development, nuclei for all 12 CNs are present. All except the olfactory (I) and optic (II) nerves arise from the brainstem, and of these, only the oculomotor (III) arises outside the region of the hindbrain. In the hindbrain, proliferation centers in the neuroepithelium establish eight distinct segments, the rhombomeres. These rhombomeres give rise to motor nuclei of CNs IV, V, VI, VII, IX, X, XI, and XII (Figs. 18.17 and 18.40). Establishment of this segmental pattern appears to be directed by mesoderm collected into somitomeres beneath the overlying neuroepithelium.

Motor neurons for cranial nuclei are within the brainstem, whereas sensory ganglia are outside of the brain. Thus, the organization of CNs is homologous to that of spinal nerves, although not all CNs contain both motor and sensory fibers (Table 18.4).

Cranial nerve sensory ganglia originate from a series of **ectodermal placodes** and **neural crest cells**. Ectodermal placodes include the **nasal**, **otic**, and four **epipharyngeal**

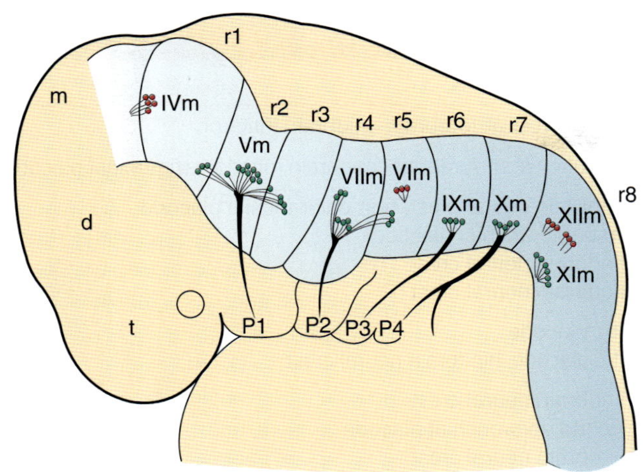


**FIGURE 18.40** Segmentation patterns in the brain and mesoderm that appear by the *25th day of development*. The *hindbrain* (coarse stipple) is divided into eight rhombomeres (*r1–r8*), and these structures give rise to the cranial motor nerves (*m*). *P1–P4*, pharyngeal (branchial) arches; *t*, telencephalon; *d*, diencephalon; *m*, mesencephalon.

**placodes** represented by ectodermal thickenings dorsal to the pharyngeal (branchial) arches (Table 18.5; see also Fig. 17.2). Epipharyngeal placodes contribute to ganglia for nerves of the pharyngeal arches (V, VII, IX, and X). Parasympathetic (visceral efferent) ganglia are derived from neural crest cells, and their fibers are carried by CNs III, VII, IX, and X (Table 18.4).

## ■ AUTONOMIC NERVOUS SYSTEM

The ANS is composed of motor (efferent) fibers that innervate smooth and cardiac muscle and secretory glands, and therefore, it is sometimes called the visceral motor system. The system is divided into two parts: a **sympathetic** portion and a **parasympathetic** portion, and both parts rely on two neurons to provide innervation, a **preganglionic** and a **postganglionic neuron**. Preganglionic neurons have their cell bodies in the gray matter of the CNS; postganglionic neurons have their cell bodies located outside of the CNS in **autonomic ganglia** and their fibers terminate on target

**Table 18.4 Origins of Cranial Nerves and Their Composition**

| Cranial Nerve | Brain Region | Type | Innervation |
|---|---|---|---|
| Olfactory (I) | Telencephalon | SA | Nasal epithelium (smell) |
| Optic (II) | Diencephalon | SA | Retina (vision) |
| Oculomotor (III) | Mesencephalon | SE<br>GVE | Sup., inf., med. Rectus, inf. Oblique, levator palpebrae sup. m.<br>(ciliary ganglion) Sphincter pupillae, ciliary m. |
| Trochlear (IV) | Metencephalon | GSE | Sup. oblique m. |
| Trigeminal (V) | Metencephalon | GSA (trigeminal ganglion)<br>SVE (branchiomotor) | Skin, mouth, facial m., teeth, ant. two-thirds of tongue<br>proprioception: skin, muscles, joints<br>M. of mastication, mylohyoid, ant. belly of digastric, tensor veli palatini, tensor tympani |
| Abducens (VI) | Metencephalon | SE | Lateral rectus m. |
| Facial (VII) | Metencephalon | SA (geniculate ganglion)<br>GSA (geniculate ganglion)<br>SVE (branchiomotor)<br>GVE | Taste ant. two-thirds of tongue<br>Skin ext. auditory meatus ant. two-thirds of tongue<br>M. of facial expression, stapedius, stylohyoid, post, belly of digastric<br>Submandibular, sublingual, and lacrimal glands |
| Vestibulocochlear (VIII) | Metencephalon | SA (vestibular and spiral ganglia) | Semicircular canals, utricle, saccule (balance), spiral organ of Corti (hearing) |
| Glossopharyngeal (IX) | Myelencephalon | SA (inferior ganglion)<br>GVA (superior ganglion)<br>GSA (inferior ganglion)<br>SVE (branchiomotor)<br>GVE (otic ganglion) | Post. one-third of tongue (taste)<br>Parotid gland, carotid body and sinus, middle ear<br>External ear<br>Stylopharyngeus<br>Parotid gland |
| Vagus (X) | Myelencephalon | SA (inferior ganglion)<br>GVA (superior ganglion)<br>GSA (superior ganglion)<br>SVE (branchiomotor)<br>GVE (ganglia at or near viscera) | Palate and epiglottis (taste)<br>Pharynx, larynx, trachea, heart, esophagus, stomach, intestines<br>Base of tongue, external auditory meatus<br>Constrictor m. pharynx, intrinsic m. larynx, sup. two-thirds esophagus<br>Trachea, bronchi, digestive tract, heart |
| Spinal accessory (XI) | Myelencephalon | SVE (branchiomotor)<br>SE | Sternocleidomastoid, trapezius m.<br>Soft palate, pharynx (with X) |
| Hypoglossal (XII) | Myelencephalon | SE | M. of tongue (except palatoglossus) |

*SA*, special afferent; *SE*, general somatic efferent; *sup.*, superior; *inf.*, inferior; *med.*, medial; *m.*, muscle; *GVE*, general visceral efferent; *GSE*, general somatic efferent; *GSA*, general somatic afferent; *ant.*, anterior; *SVE*, special visceral efferent (supplying striated muscles derived from the pharyngeal (branchial) arches); *ext.*, external; *post.*, posterior; *GVA*, general visceral afferent.

**Table 18.5 Contributions of Neural Crest Cells and Placodes to Ganglia of the Cranial Nerves**

| Nerve | Ganglion | Origin |
|---|---|---|
| Oculomotor (III) | Ciliary (visceral efferent) | Neural crest at forebrain–midbrain junction |
| Trigeminal (V) | Trigeminal (general afferent) | Neural crest at forebrain–midbrain junction, trigeminal placode |
| Facial (VII) | Superior (general and special afferent)<br>Inferior (geniculate) (general and special afferent)<br>Sphenopalatine (visceral efferent)<br>Submandibular (visceral efferent) | Hindbrain neural crest, first epibranchial placode<br>First epibranchial placode<br>Hindbrain neural crest<br>Hindbrain neural crest |
| Vestibulocochlear (VIII) | Acoustic (cochlear) (special afferent)<br>Vestibular (special afferent) | Otic placode<br>Otic placode, hindbrain neural crest |
| Glossopharyngeal (IX) | Superior (general and special afferent)<br>Inferior (petrosal) (general and special afferent)<br>Otic (visceral efferent) | Hindbrain neural crest<br>Second epibranchial placode<br>Hindbrain neural crest |
| Vagus (X) | Superior (general afferent)<br>Inferior (nodose) (general and special afferent)<br>Vagal parasympathetic (visceral efferent) | Hindbrain neural crest<br>Hindbrain neural crest; third, fourth epibranchial placodes<br>Hindbrain neural crest |

organs. In general, **norepinephrine** is the neurotransmitter employed by the sympathetic system, whereas **acetylcholine** is employed by the parasympathetic system.

## Sympathetic Nervous System

Cell bodies of preganglionic neurons of the sympathetic nervous system are located in the **intermediolateral cell columns (horns) of the spinal cord at the levels of T1–L2** (Fig. 18.42). Cell bodies for postganglionic neurons are located in **paravertebral ganglia** on each side of the vertebral column and in **prevertebral (preaortic) ganglia** located around major vessels branching from the aorta (celiac, superior mesenteric, and inferior mesenteric arteries; Fig. 18.42). Paravertebral ganglia are linked by fibers and form the right and left **sympathetic trunks (chain ganglia)**. All of these ganglia originate from neural crest cells of the thoracic region that migrate during the fifth week of development (Fig. 18.41). Crest cells forming the sympathetic trunk ganglia also migrate cranially and caudally to extend these trunks into cervical and pelvic regions. Migration and positioning of these crest cells is regulated by BMPs secreted by the dorsal aorta that act as chemoattractants for the migrating cells.

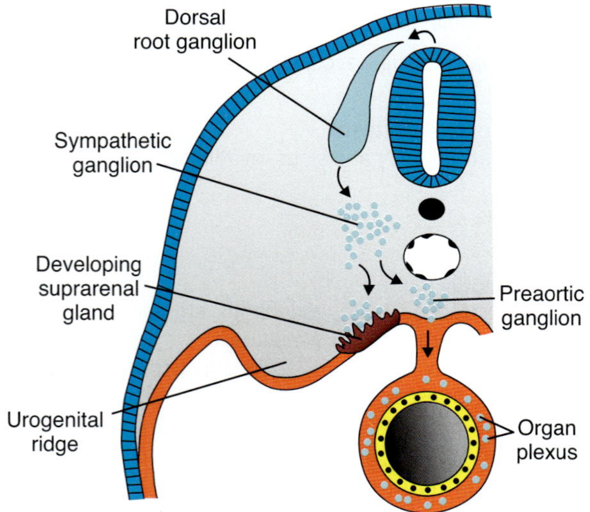


**FIGURE 18.41** Formation of the sympathetic ganglia. Neural crest cells (light blue) migrate from the neural tube and form the dorsal root ganglia, all of the sympathetic ganglia, and the adrenal medulla.

Preganglionic sympathetic fibers originating from cell bodies in the spinal cord from T1 to L2 exit via ventral roots (because they are motor fibers), enter a spinal nerve, then a ventral primary ramus, and, almost immediately, enter a white ramus communicans to reach the sympathetic trunk (Fig. 18.42). Once in the trunk, they can synapse at the segment they entered, ascend or descend to synapse on cranial or caudal neurons, or they can pass through the trunks without synapsing and travel to prevertebral ganglia to synapse. Preganglionic fibers traveling to prevertebral ganglia are collected into groups called abdominopelvic splanchnic nerves: These include the greater (T5–T9), lesser (T10–T11), least (T12), and lumbar splanchnic nerves (Fig. 18.42). Postganglionic fibers from the sympathetic trunk ganglia to blood vessels, arrector pili muscles (goose bumps), and sweat glands in the head and neck, body wall, and limbs travel from the sympathetic trunk through **gray rami communicantes** to ventral rami of all 31 spinal nerves and travel on blood vessels to reach their destinations (Fig. 18.42). Postganglionic fibers from lower cervical and upper thoracic trunk ganglia exit the trunks as collections of fibers called the cardiopulmonary splanchnic nerves on their way to innervate the heart and lungs (Fig. 18.42). Postganglionic fibers from prevertebral (preaortic) ganglia travel via blood vessels to innervate the abdominal organs and genitalia. Note that because cell bodies of preganglionic neurons are located in spinal cord segments T1–L2, these segments will be the only ones to have **white rami communicantes**. However, because each spinal nerve receives fibers from postganglionic neurons, every ventral primary rami of every spinal nerve will be connected to a gray rami communicantes.

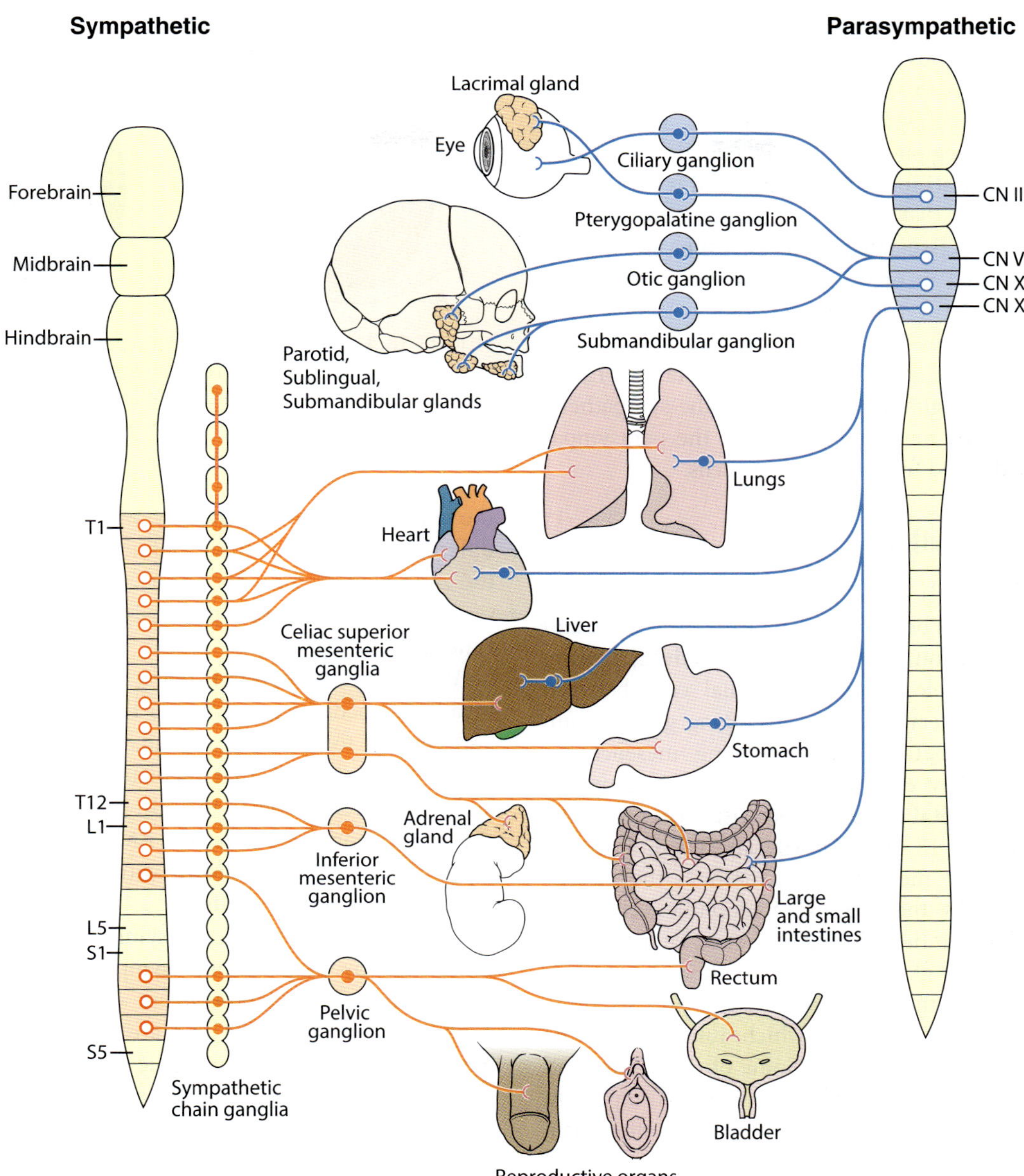


**FIGURE 18.42** Diagram of the sympathetic and parasympathetic divisions of the autonomic nervous system. Preganglionic sympathetic neurons arise from two sources in the intermediolateral cell columns of the spinal cord: thoracolumbar outflow from T1 to L2, 3 and sacral outflow from S2 to S4. From thoracolumbar segments, fibers travel to the sympathetic chain ganglia (trunks) via ventral roots of spinal nerves and then white rami communicans. In the trunks, they may synapse at the level they entered, ascend or descend to synapse at other levels, or pass through without synapsing. Postganglionic fibers traveling from the trunks to blood vessels, arrector pili muscles, and sweat glands travel by gray rami communicans to all 31 spinal nerves. Preganglionic fibers that do not synapse form abdominopelvic splanchnic nerves on their way to prevertebral ganglia. Preganglionic parasympathetic cell bodies lie in the brainstem in cranial nerve nuclei CN III (oculomotor), CN VII (facial), CN IX (glossopharyngeal), and CN X (vagus). Postganglionic neuron cell bodies serving structures in the head and neck region lie in the ciliary (CN III), pterygopalatine and submandibular (CN VII), and otic (CN XI) ganglia. Postganglionic neurons associated with the vagus nerve (CN X) serving thoracic and abdominal structures are usually located on or in the organs that are being innervated.

Part 2

## Parasympathetic Nervous System

Preganglionic parasympathetic neuron cell bodies are located in the brainstem and the sacral region (S2–S4) of the spinal cord and consequently are sometimes called the craniosacral portion of the ANS (Fig. 18.42). **Preganglionic parasympathetic fibers** from nuclei in the brainstem travel via the **oculomotor (CN III), facial (CN VII), glossopharyngeal (CN IX),** and **vagus (CN X) nerves** to structures in the head and neck. The vagus nerve also supplies parasympathetic innervation to most of the visceral organs down to the region of the proximal third of the transverse colon (Fig. 18.42). Preganglionic fibers from the sacral component of the system exit the spinal cord via the ventral roots of spinal nerves from S2 to S4 and then leave the ventral primary rami of these nerves as the pelvic splanchnic nerves to provide innervation to the remaining portion of the gastrointestinal tract from the distal two-thirds of the transverse colon to the rectum (Fig. 18.42). Some of these fibers also travel to the bladder and erectile tissue of the genitalia. Postganglionic parasympathetic neuron cell bodies in the cranial region reside in four ganglia: the **ciliary (CN III)**, **pterygopalatine** and **submandibular (CN VII)**, and **otic (CN IX**; Fig. 18.42). Postganglionic neurons in the thorax and abdomen associated with the **vagus nerve (CN X)** are usually located in or on the organ innervated. This arrangement is also true for postganglionic cell bodies of pelvic splanchnic nerves in the pelvic region, which exist individually or as smaller ganglia in the walls of target organs, such as the enteric ganglia of the gut. As in the sympathetic system, postganglionic neurons throughout the parasympathetic system are derived from neural crest cells.

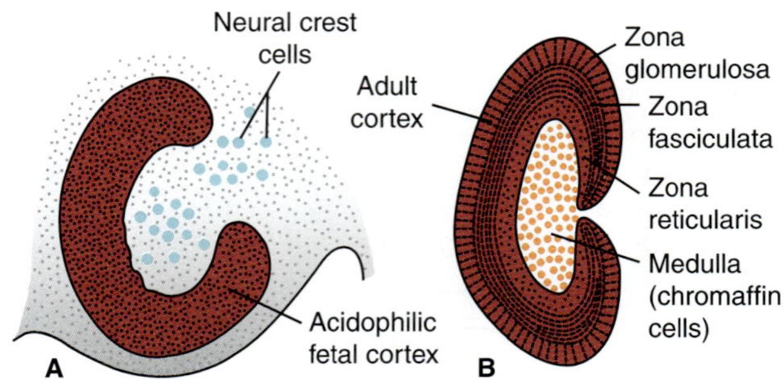


**FIGURE 18.43 A.** Neural crest cells penetrating the fetal cortex of the suprarenal gland. **B.** Neural crest cells form the medulla of the adrenal gland and differentiate into chromaffin cells. Later in development, the definitive cortex almost completely surrounds the medulla.

## Suprarenal (Adrenal) Gland

The suprarenal (adrenal) gland develops from two components: (1) a mesodermal portion, which forms the **cortex**, and (2) an ectodermal portion, which forms the **medulla**. During the fifth week of development, mesothelial cells between the root of the mesentery and the developing gonad begin to proliferate and penetrate the underlying mesenchyme (Fig. 18.41). Here, they differentiate into large acidophilic cells, which form the **fetal cortex**, or **primitive cortex**, of the suprarenal gland (Fig. 18.43*A*). Shortly afterward, a second wave of cells from the mesothelium penetrates the mesenchyme and surrounds the original acidophilic cell mass. These cells, smaller than those of the first wave, later form the **definitive cortex** of the gland (Fig. 18.43). These are steroid-producing cells and in the second trimester begin secreting dehydroepiandrosterone (DHEA), which functions in the synthesis of androgen and estrogen. Some of this compound is converted to estrogen by the placenta, which is important for maintaining the placenta and pregnancy. Soon after birth, the fetal cortex regresses rapidly, whereas the remaining cells differentiate into the three definitive layers of the cortex: the zona glomerulosa, zona fasciculata, and zona reticularis (Fig. 18.43*B*). The cortex primarily secretes cortisol, aldosterone, and androgens.

While the fetal cortex is being formed, **neural crest cells** invade its medial aspect, where they are arranged in cords and clusters to form the medulla of the gland (Figs. 18.41 and 18.43*A*). Signals that regulate migration of these cells and their specification to the adrenal medulla emanate from the dorsal aorta and include BMPs. When differentiated, these cells stain yellow-brown with chrome salts and hence are called **chromaffin cells** (Fig. 18.43*B*). These cells represent modified postganglionic sympathetic neurons that are innervated by preganglionic sympathetic fibers and when stimulated produce epinephrine (adrenaline) and norepinephrine (noradrenaline) that are released directly into the bloodstream. During embryonic life, chromaffin cells are scattered widely throughout the embryo, but in the adult, the only persisting group is in the medulla of the adrenal glands.

### *Clinical Correlates*

#### Pheochromocytomas

**Pheochromocytomas** are rare tumors involving chromaffin cells that result in excessive production and release of epinephrine and norepinephrine causing paroxysmal episodes of hypertension, increased heart rate, headaches, and other associated symptoms. Most occur in the adrenal medulla, but approximately 10% occur in other sites, usually the abdomen. Twenty-five percent are familial and have been associated with mutations in the *RET* gene that plays a role in neural crest cell migration.

#### Congenital Megacolon (Hirschsprung Disease)

**Congenital megacolon (Hirschsprung disease)** results from a failure of parasympathetic ganglia to form in the wall of a part or all of the colon and rectum because the neural crest cells fail to migrate. Most familial cases of Hirschsprung disease are caused by mutations in the ***RET* gene**, which codes for a cell membrane **tyrosine kinase receptor**. This gene on chromosome 10q11 is essential for neural crest cell migration. The ligand for the receptor is **GLIAL CELL–DERIVED NEUROTROPHIC GROWTH FACTOR** secreted by mesenchyme cells through which crest cells migrate. Receptor ligand interactions then regulate crest cell migration. Consequently, if there are abnormalities in the receptor, migration is inhibited, and no parasympathetic ganglia form in affected areas. The rectum is involved in nearly all cases, and the rectum and sigmoid are involved in 80% of affected infants. The transverse and ascending portions of the colon are involved in only 10% to 20%. The colon is dilated above the affected region, which has a small diameter because of tonic contraction of noninnervated musculature.

Part 2

## SUMMARY

- The central nervous system (CNS) **originates in the ectoderm** and appears as the **neural plate** at the middle of the third week (Fig. 18.1).
- After the edges of the plate fold, the **neural folds** approach each other in the midline to fuse into the **neural tube** (Figs. 18.2 and 18.3).
- The cranial end closes at approximately day 25, and the caudal end closes at day 28.
- The CNS then forms a tubular structure with a broad cephalic portion, the **brain**, and a long caudal portion, the **spinal cord**.
- Failure of the neural tube to close results in defects such as **spina bifida** (Figs. 18.15 and 18.16) and **anencephaly** (Fig. 18.37); these defects can be prevented by **folic acid.**
- The **spinal cord**, which forms the caudal end of the CNS, is characterized by the **basal plate** containing the **motor neurons**, the **alar plate** for the **sensory neurons**, and a **floor plate** and a **roof plate** as connecting pathways between the two sides (Fig. 18.8).
- **Spinal nerves** form from each segment of the spinal cord. These nerves have their motor nuclei in the basal plate (inside the cord) and their sensory cell bodies in spinal ganglia derived from neural crest cells (outside the cord).
- **SHH** ventralizes the neural tube in the spinal cord region and induces the floor and basal plates. **BMP4 and BMP7**, expressed in nonneural ectoderm, maintain and upregulate expression of *PAX3* and *PAX7* in the alar and roof plates.
- The **brain** can be divided into the **brainstem**, which is a continuation of the spinal cord and resembles that structure in its organization of basal and alar plates, and the **higher centers**, the cerebellum and cerebral hemispheres, which accentuate the alar plates.
- After closure of the neural tube, the brain consists of three vesicles: **the rhombencephalon (hindbrain), mesencephalon (midbrain),** and **prosencephalon (forebrain)**.
- Later, these primary vesicles subdivide into five different regions (Fig. 18.5). The **rhombencephalon** is divided into (1) the **myelencephalon**, which forms the **medulla oblongata** (this region has a basal plate for somatic and visceral efferent neurons and an alar plate for somatic and visceral afferent neurons) (Fig. 18.18), and (2) the **metencephalon**, with its typical basal (efferent) and alar (afferent) plates (Fig. 18.19).
- This brain vesicle is also characterized by formation of the **cerebellum** (Fig. 18.20), a coordination center for posture and movement, and the **pons**, the pathway for nerve fibers between the spinal cord and the cerebral and the cerebellar cortices (Fig. 18.19).
- The **mesencephalon**, or **midbrain**, does not subdivide and resembles the spinal cord with its basal efferent and alar afferent plates. The mesencephalon's alar plates form the anterior and posterior colliculi as relay stations for visual and auditory reflex centers, respectively (Fig. 18.23).
- The prosencephalon also subdivides into the diencephalon posteriorly and the telencephalon anteriorly.
- The diencephalon consists of a thin roof plate and a thick alar plate in which the **thalamus** and **hypothalamus** develop (Figs. 18.24 and 18.25). It participates in formation of the pituitary gland, which also develops from Rathke pouch (Fig. 18.26). Rathke pouch forms the **adenohypophysis**, the **intermediate lobe**, and **pars tuberalis**, and the diencephalon forms the **posterior lobe**, the **neurohypophysis**, which contains neuroglia and receives nerve fibers from the hypothalamus.
- The telencephalon consists of two lateral outpocketings, the **cerebral hemispheres**, and a median portion, the **lamina terminalis** (Fig. 18.27).
- The lamina terminalis is used by the commissures as a connection pathway for fiber bundles between the right and left hemispheres (Fig. 18.30).
- The cerebral hemispheres, originally two small outpocketings (Figs. 18.24 and 18.25), expand and cover the lateral aspect of the diencephalon, mesencephalon, and metencephalon (Figs. 18.26, 18.27, and 18.28).
- Eventually, nuclear regions of the telencephalon come in close contact with those of the diencephalon (Fig. 18.27).
- The **ventricular system**, containing **cerebrospinal fluid (CSF)**, extends from the lumen in the spinal cord to the fourth ventricle in the rhombencephalon through the narrow aqueduct in the mesencephalon (**aqueduct of Sylvius**) and to the third ventricle in the diencephalon. By way of the **foramina of Monro**, the ventricular system extends from the third ventricle into the lateral ventricles of the cerebral hemispheres. CSF is produced in the **choroid plexuses** of the third, fourth, and lateral ventricles. Blockage of CSF in the ventricular system or subarachnoid space results in **hydrocephalus.**
- The brain is patterned along the anteroposterior (craniocaudal) and dorsoventral (mediolateral) axes.
- ***HOX* genes** pattern the anteroposterior axis in the hindbrain and specify rhombomere identity. Other transcription factors containing a homeodomain pattern the anteroposterior axis in the forebrain and midbrain regions, including ***LIM1*** and ***OTX2***.
- Two other organizing centers, the **anterior neural ridge (ANR)** and the **rhombencephalic isthmus**, secrete **FGF8**, which serves as the inducing signal for these areas. In response to this growth factor, the cranial end of the forebrain expresses ***FOXG1***, which regulates development of the telencephalon, and the isthmus expresses ***ENGRAILED* genes** that regulate differentiation of the cerebellum and the roof of the midbrain.
- As it does throughout the CNS, **SHH**, secreted by the prechordal plate and notochord, ventralizes the forebrain and midbrain areas. **BMP4 and BMP7**, secreted by nonneural ectoderm, induce and maintain expression of dorsalizing genes.
- There are **12 cranial nerves**, and most of these originate from the hindbrain. Motor neurons for each of the nerves are located within the brain, whereas sensory neurons

(*Continued*)

originate outside of the brain from ectodermal placodes and neural crest cells (Tables 18.4 and 18.5). In this regard, organization of the sensory and motor cell bodies for these nerves is similar to that for spinal nerves.

- The **autonomic nervous system (ANS)** consists of **sympathetic** and **parasympathetic** components. This is a two-neuron system with **preganglionic** and **postganglionic** fibers. Preganglionic neurons for the sympathetic system lie in the intermediate (lateral) horns of the spinal cord from T1 to L2; its postganglionic neurons lie in the **sympathetic trunks and paravertebral (preaortic) ganglia** along the aorta.
- Parasympathetic preganglionic neurons have their nuclei in the brainstem (associated with **CNs III, VII, IX, and X**) and in the **sacral region** of the spinal cord (S2–S4); postganglionic nuclei reside in ganglia that usually lie close to the organs they innervate. Neural crest cells form all of the ganglia for the ANS.
- The **suprarenal (adrenal) gland** is derived from two sources: (1) mesoderm from the posterior body wall that proliferates to form the **fetal cortex** that is replaced by a second proliferation of these cells that form the **definitive cortex**. This part of the gland produces steroids and plays a role in maintaining pregnancy by secreting DHEA that is converted by the placenta to estrogen; (2) **neural crest cells** that migrate from the neural folds and form the **medulla** of the gland. These cells differentiate into **chromaffin cells** and represent modified postganglionic sympathetic neurons. When stimulated by preganglionic neurons, they secrete **epinephrine (adrenalin)** and **norepinephrine (noradrenaline)** directly into the bloodstream.

Part 2

## Self-Assessment

### Comprehensive Questions

1. Write a short note on cranial nerves of the general visceral afferent column.
2. Write a short note on the embryological basis of spina bifida.
3. How are cranial nerves and spinal nerves similar? How are they different?
4. What components come together to form a spinal nerve? What is the difference between a dorsal root, ventral root, dorsal primary ramus, and ventral primary ramus?
5. What are the two parts of the ANS? Where are their respective preganglionic neurons located? What cells give rise embryologically to their postganglionic neurons?
6. Write a note on the embryological basis of holoprosencephaly.

### Problem Solving Questions

1. At what level is a spinal tap performed? From an embryological standpoint, why is this possible?
2. A 23-year-old primigravida presented to an obstetrics clinic with 19 weeks of pregnancy. Her antenatal scan showed absence of calvarium with only the basilar parts of the occipital bone being seen. Rudimentary malformed nervous tissue was observed through the cranial defect. There was no abnormality detected in the spine and the spinal cord. The lab investigations showed high levels of maternal serum alpha-fetoprotein (MSAFP). Her general built was poor and she had poor nutritional status. She was not taking any vitamin supplements as well. She was immediately advised for medical termination of pregnancy. What is the probable diagnosis and the embryological basis for this anomaly? At what age can it be detected on USG? What measures can be taken by the lady to prevent such an anomaly in future pregnancies?
3. A multigravida female $G_2P_1L_1$ presented in an obstetrics clinic with 18 weeks of pregnancy. Her antenatal ultrasound scans showed absence of cerebellum in the posterior cranial fossa. The cerebellar tonsils were observed herniating down from the posterior cranial fossa through the foramen magnum. Dilation of bilateral lateral ventricles were also observed. The spine showed a large vertebral arch defect in the thoracolumbar region. What is the probable diagnosis?
4. Prenatal ultrasound reveals an infant with an enlarged head and expansion of both lateral ventricles. What is this condition called, and what might have caused it?

### Multiple Choice Questions

1. The spinal cord develops from which of the following?
   (a) Neural tube
   (b) Notochord
   (c) Primitive streak
   (d) Rhombencephalon
2. What is the adult representation of the location of anterior neuropore?
   (a) Septum transversum
   (b) Terminal ventricle
   (c) Lamina terminalis
   (d) Foramen of Monro
3. A 1-year-old baby with loss of pharyngeal reflex was diagnosed to have infantile progressive bulbar palsy. Which of the following gives rise to the affected structure?
   (a) Prosencephalon
   (b) Mesencephalon
   (c) Rhombencephalon
   (d) Diencephalon
4. Which of the following neural tube defects is characterized by gapes in vertebral arches?
   (a) Encephalocele
   (b) Spina bifida
   (c) Hydrocephaly
   (d) Syringomyelia
5. Which of the following brainstem nuclei is not derived from the alar plate?
   (a) Inferior olivary
   (b) Substantia nigra
   (c) Dentate
   (d) Hypoglossal
6. Adrenal medulla develops from
   (a) Basal plate of neural tube
   (b) Alar plate of neural tube

(c) Yolk sac
(d) Neural crest

7. Transcription factor responsible for ventralization of neural tube is
   (a) PAX
   (b) BMP4
   (c) SHH
   (d) TGF-b
8. Anencephaly occurs due to failure in closure of
   (a) Spinous process
   (b) Anterior neuropore
   (c) Posterior neuropore
   (d) Entire neural tube
9. Anterior lobe of the pituitary gland develops from
   (a) Diencephalon
   (b) Rathke's pouch
   (c) Nasopharynx
   (d) Oropharynx
10. The neural tube finally develops into how many dilatations called vesicles?
   (a) 2
   (b) 3
   (c) 4
   (d) 5

**Answers**

1. (a) 2. (c) 3. (c) 4. (b) 5. (d) 6. (d) 7. (c) 8. (b) 9. (b) 10. (d)

CHAPTER

# 19 Ear

**Specific Learning Objectives**

- Development of
  - Internal ear
  - Middle ear
  - External ear
- Hearing
- Clinical correlates

**Competency Covered**

AN43.4 Describe the development of the face and branchial apparatus.

Part 2

In the adult, the ear forms one anatomic unit serving both hearing and equilibrium. In the embryo, however, it develops from three distinctly different parts: (1) the **external ear**, the sound-collecting organ; (2) the **middle ear**, a sound conductor from the external to the internal ear; and (3) the **internal ear**, which converts sound waves into nerve impulses and registers changes in equilibrium.

## INTERNAL EAR

The first indication of the developing ear can be found in embryos of approximately 22 days as a thickening of the surface ectoderm on each side of the rhombencephalon (Fig. 19.1). These thickenings, the **otic placodes**, invaginate rapidly and form the **otic** or **auditory vesicles (otocysts)** (Fig. 19.2). Cells from the otocyst differentiate and form ganglion cells for the statoacoustic (vestibulocochlear) ganglia (Fig. 19.2*C*). During later development, each vesicle divides into (1) a ventral component that gives rise to the **saccule** and **cochlear duct** and (2) a dorsal component that forms the **utricle**, **semicircular canals**, and **endolymphatic duct** (Figs. 19.3, 19.4, 19.5, and 19.6). Together, these epithelial structures form the **membranous labyrinth**.

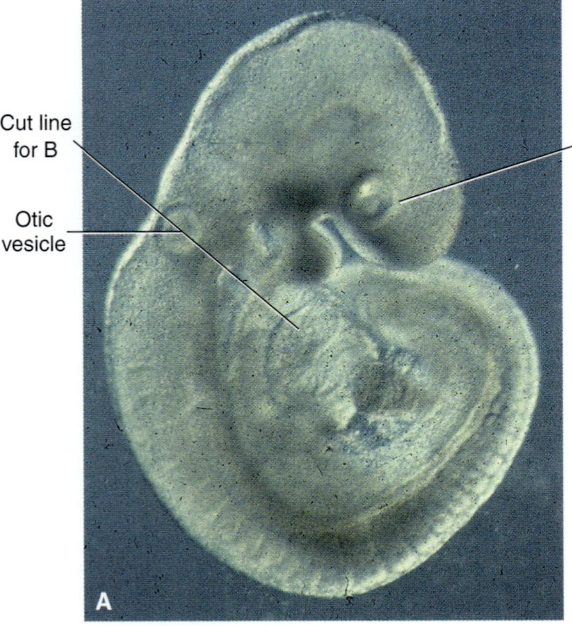


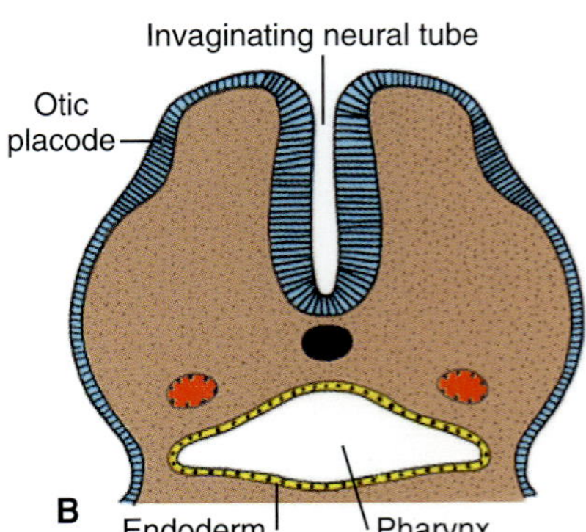


**FIGURE 19.1** **A.** An embryo at the end of the fourth week of development showing the otic and optic vesicles. **B.** Region of the rhombencephalon showing the otic placodes in a 22-day embryo.

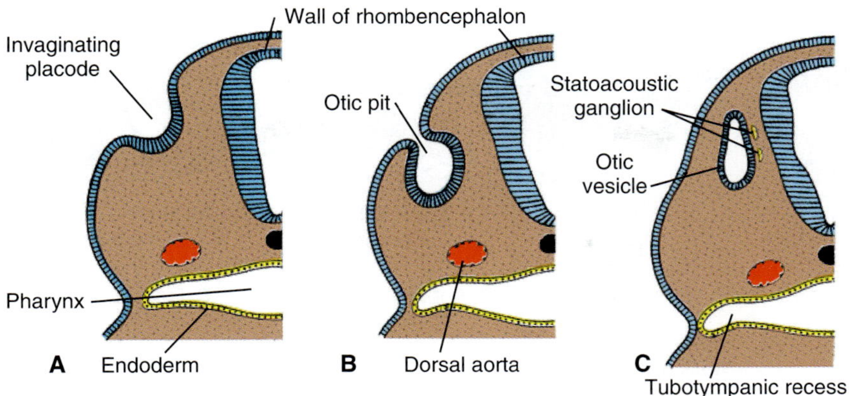


**FIGURE 19.2** Transverse sections through the region of the rhombencephalon showing formation of the otic vesicles. **A.** 24 days. **B.** 27 days. **C.** 4.5 weeks. Neurons derived from the otic vesicle (otocyst) form the statoacoustic (vestibulocochlear) ganglia.

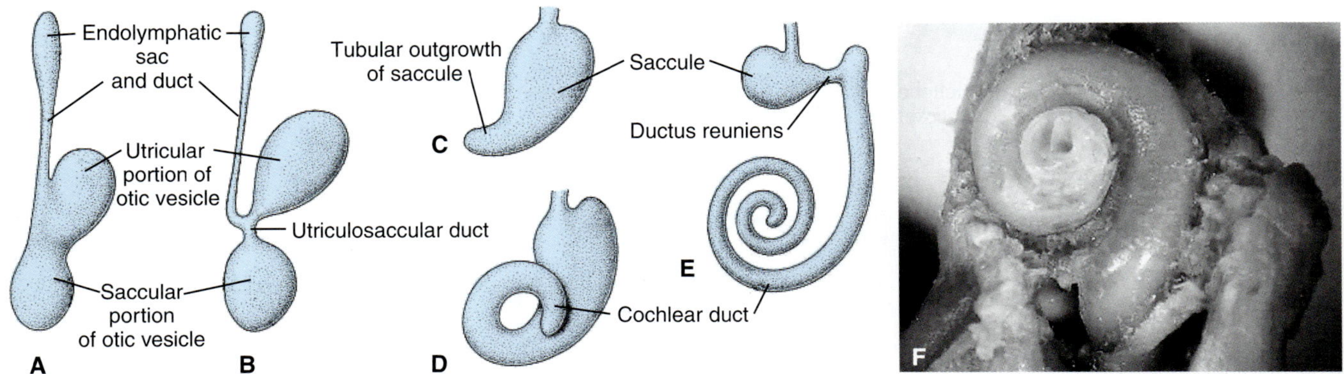


**FIGURE 19.3 A,B.** Development of the otocyst showing a dorsal utricular portion with the endolymphatic duct and a ventral saccular portion. **C–E.** Cochlear duct at 6, 7, and 8 weeks, respectively. **F.** A human cochlea showing two and half turns at 30 weeks of gestation. Note formation of the ducts of the ductus reuniens and utriculosaccular duct in the schematic diagrams.

Part 2

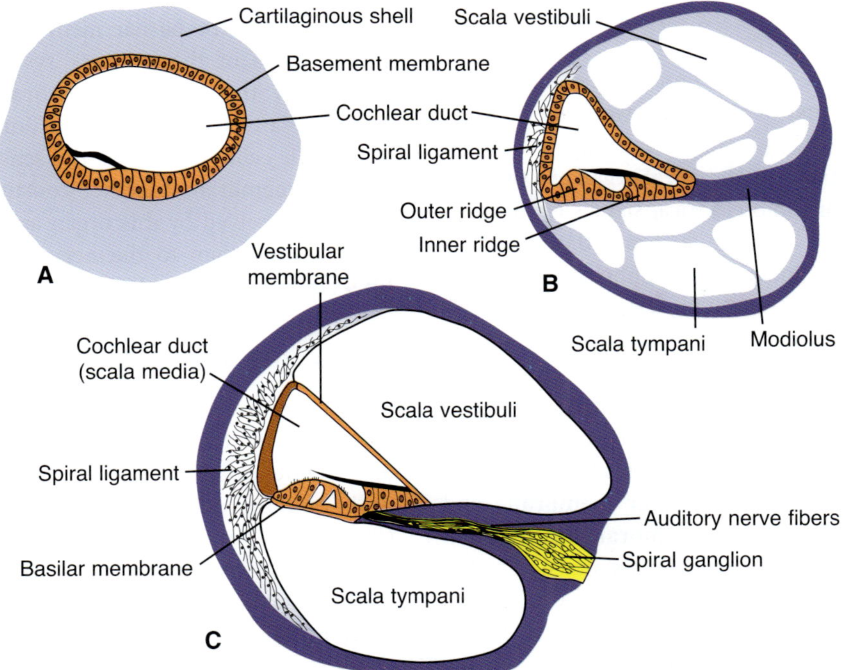


**FIGURE 19.4** Development of the scala tympani and scala vestibuli. **A.** The cochlear duct is surrounded by a cartilaginous shell. **B.** During the 10th week, large vacuoles appear in the cartilaginous shell. **C.** The cochlear duct (scala media) is separated from the scala tympani and the scala vestibuli by the basilar and vestibular membranes, respectively. Ganglion cells from the vestibulocochlear nerve (cranial nerve VIII) form the spiral ganglion and extend processes to innervate the hair cells.

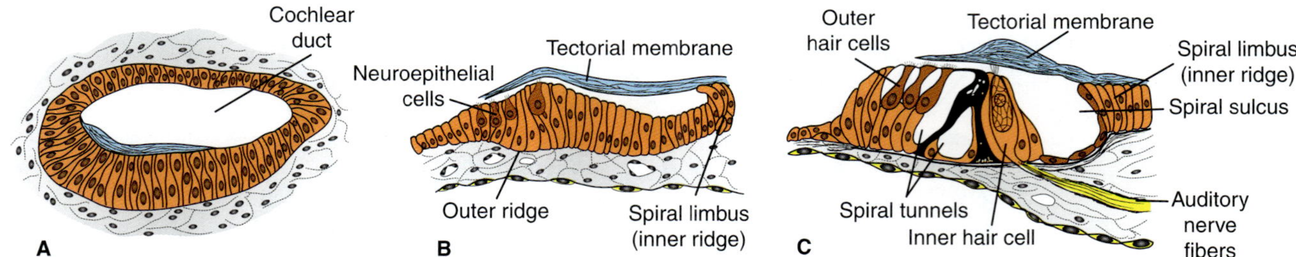


**FIGURE 19.5** Development of the organ of Corti. **A.** 10 weeks. **B.** Approximately 5 months. **C.** Full-term infant.

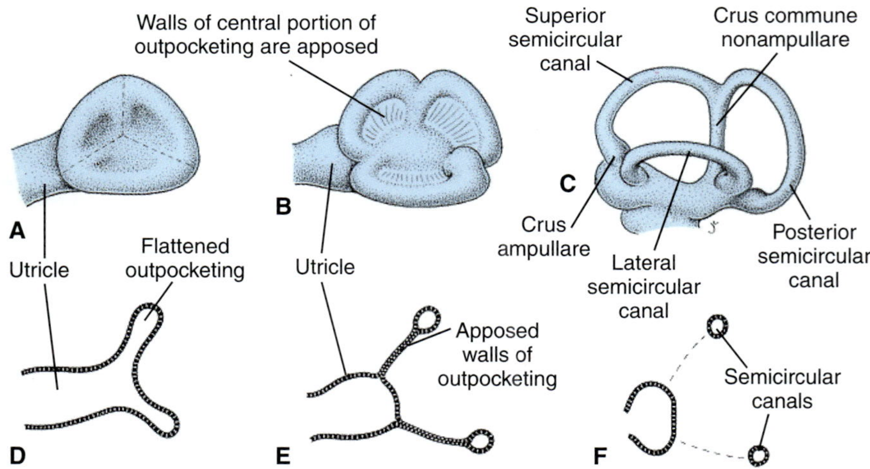


**FIGURE 19.6** Development of the semicircular canals. **A.** 5 weeks. **B.** 6 weeks. **C.** 8 weeks. **D–F.** Apposition, fusion, and disappearance, respectively, of the central portions of the walls of the semicircular outpocketings. Ampullae in the semicircular canals contain sensory cells arranged in a crest, the crista ampullaris, for maintaining.

## Saccule, Cochlea, and Organ of Corti

In the sixth week of development, the saccule forms a tubular outpocketing at its lower pole (Fig. 19.3*C–E*). This outgrowth, the **cochlear duct**, penetrates the surrounding mesenchyme in a spiral fashion until the end of the eighth week, when it has completed 2.5 turns (Fig. 19.3*D–F*). In the seventh week, cells of the cochlear duct differentiate into the **spiral organ of Corti** that transduces sound vibrations into electrical signals for hearing. A connection between the cochlear duct and the remaining portion of the saccule is maintained but confined to a narrow pathway, the **ductus reuniens** (Fig. 19.3*E*; see also Fig. 19.8).

Mesenchyme surrounding the cochlear duct soon differentiates into cartilage (Fig. 19.4*A*). In the 10th week, this cartilaginous shell undergoes vacuolization, and two perilymphatic spaces, the **scala vestibuli** and **scala tympani**, are formed (Fig. 19.4*B,C*). The cochlear duct is then separated from the scala vestibuli by the **vestibular membrane** and from the scala tympani by the **basilar membrane** (Fig. 19.4*C*). The lateral wall of the cochlear duct remains attached to the surrounding cartilage by the **spiral ligament**, whereas its median angle is connected to and partly supported by a long cartilaginous process, the **modiolus**, the future axis of the bony cochlea (Fig. 19.4*B*).

Initially, epithelial cells of the cochlear duct are alike (Fig. 19.4*A*). With further development, however, they form two ridges: the **inner ridge**, the future **spiral limbus**, and the **outer ridge** (Fig. 19.4*B*). The outer ridge forms **one row of inner** and **three or four rows of outer hair cells**, lying on the basilar membrane. The hair cells are the sensory cells of the auditory system (Fig. 19.5). They are covered by the **tectorial membrane**, a fibrillar gelatinous substance attached to the spiral limbus that rests on the tip of the hair cells (Fig. 19.5). The sensory cells (hair cells) and tectorial membrane together constitute the **organ of Corti**. Impulses received by this organ are transmitted to the spiral ganglion and then to the nervous system by the **auditory fibers of cranial nerve VIII** (Figs. 19.4 and 19.5).

## Utricle and Semicircular Canals

During the sixth week of development, **semicircular canals** appear as flattened outpocketings of the utricular part of the otic vesicle (Fig. 19.6*A,B*). Central portions of the walls of these outpocketings eventually appose each other (Fig. 19.6*B,C*) and disappear, giving rise to three semicircular canals (Fig. 19.6; see also Fig. 19.8). Whereas, one end of each canal dilates to form the **crus ampullare**, the other, the **crus nonampullare**, does not widen (Fig. 19.6). Because two of the latter type fuse, however, only five crura enter the utricle, three with an ampulla and two without.

Cells in the ampullae form a crest, the **crista ampullaris**, containing sensory cells for maintenance of equilibrium. Similar sensory areas, the **maculae acusticae**, develop in the walls of the utricle and saccule. Impulses generated in sensory cells of the cristae and maculae as a result of a change in position of the body are carried to the brain by **vestibular fibers of cranial nerve VIII**.

During formation of the otic vesicle, a small group of cells breaks away from its wall and forms the **statoacoustic ganglion** (Fig. 19.2*C*). Other cells of this ganglion are derived from the neural crest. The ganglion subsequently splits into **cochlear** and **vestibular** portions, which supply sensory cells of the organ of Corti and those of the saccule, utricle, and semicircular canals, respectively.

## MIDDLE EAR

### Tympanic Cavity and Auditory Tube

The **tympanic cavity**, which originates in the endoderm, is derived from the **first pharyngeal pouch** (Figs. 19.2 and 19.7). This pouch expands in a lateral direction and the distal part of the pouch, the **tubotympanic recess**, widens and gives rise to the primitive tympanic cavity. The proximal part remains narrow and forms the **auditory tube (eustachian tube)** (Figs. 19.7*B* and 19.8), through which the tympanic cavity communicates with the nasopharynx.

### Ossicles

The **malleus** and **incus** are derived from cartilage of the **first pharyngeal arch**, and the **stapes** is derived from that of the **second arch** (Fig. 19.9*A*). Although the ossicles appear during the first half of fetal life, they remain embedded in mesenchyme until the eighth month (Fig. 19.9*B*), when the surrounding tissue dissolves (Figs. 19.7, 19.8, and 19.9*B*). The endodermal epithelial lining of the primitive tympanic cavity then extends along the wall of the newly developing space. The tympanic cavity is now at least twice as large as before. When the ossicles are entirely free of surrounding mesenchyme, the endodermal epithelium connects them in a mesentery-like fashion to the wall of the cavity (Fig. 19.9*B*). The supporting ligaments of the ossicles develop later within these mesenteries.

Because the malleus is derived from the first pharyngeal arch, its muscle, the **tensor tympani**, is innervated by the **mandibular branch of the trigeminal nerve**. The **stapedius**

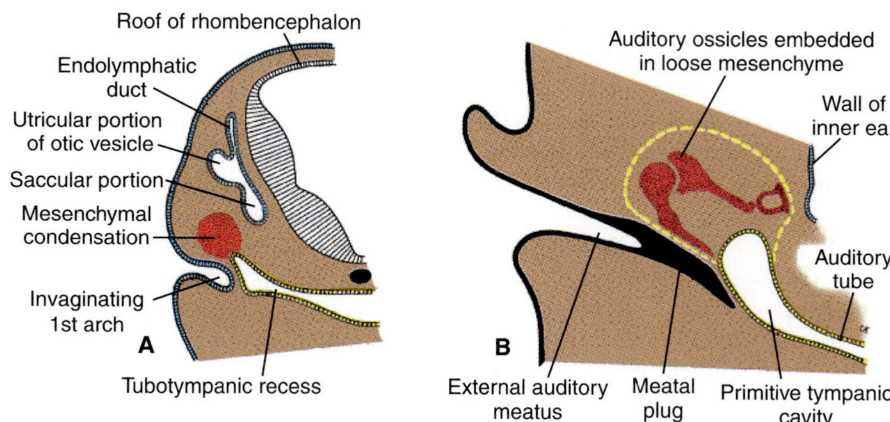


**FIGURE 19.7 A.** Transverse section of a 7-week embryo in the region of the rhombencephalon, showing the tubotympanic recess, the Invaginating 1st arch, and mesenchymal condensation, foreshadowing development of the ossicles. **B.** Middle ear showing the cartilaginous precursors of the auditory ossicles. *Thin yellow line* in mesenchyme indicates future expansion of the primitive tympanic cavity.

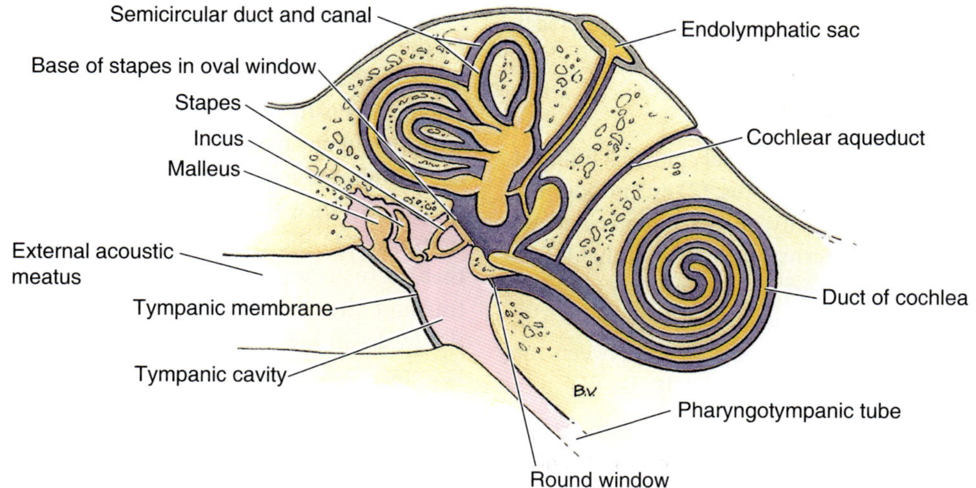


**FIGURE 19.8** Ear showing the external auditory meatus, the middle ear with its ossicles, and the inner ear.

Part 2

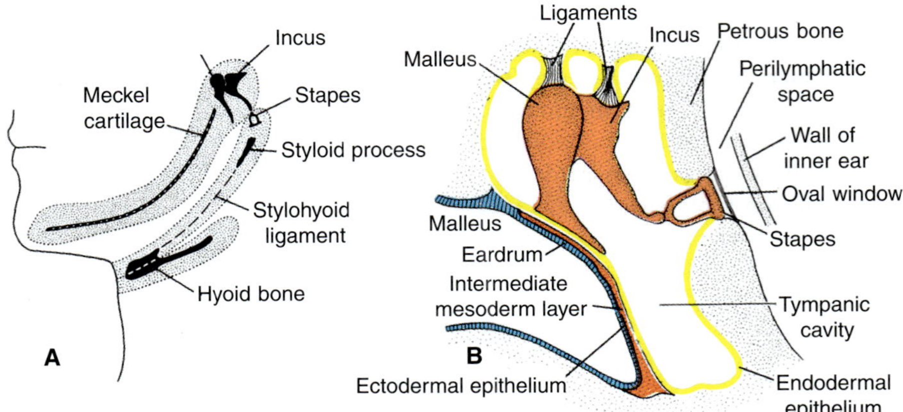


**FIGURE 19.9 A.** Derivatives of the first three pharyngeal arches. The malleus and incus form at the dorsal tip of the first arch and the stapes at that of the second arch. **B.** Middle ear showing the handle of the malleus in contact with the eardrum. The stapes will establish contact with the membrane in the oval window. The wall of the tympanic cavity is lined with endodermal epithelium.

**muscle**, which is attached to the stapes, is innervated by the **facial nerve**, the nerve to the second pharyngeal arch.

During late fetal life, the tympanic cavity expands dorsally by vacuolization of surrounding tissue to form the **tympanic antrum**. After birth, the epithelium of the tympanic cavity invades the bone of the developing **mastoid process**, and epithelium-lined air sacs are formed (**pneumatization**). Later, most of the mastoid air sacs come in contact with the antrum and tympanic cavity. Expansion of inflammations of the middle ear into the antrum and mastoid air cells is a common complication of middle ear infections.

## EXTERNAL EAR

### External Auditory Meatus

The **external auditory meatus** develops as an invagination of first arch tissue and not from the first pharyngeal cleft as previously believed (Fig. 19.7*A*). At the beginning of the third month, epithelial cells at the bottom of the meatus proliferate, forming a solid epithelial plate, the meatal plug (Fig. 19.7*B*). In the seventh month, this plug dissolves, and the epithelial lining of the floor of the meatus participates in formation of the definitive eardrum. Occasionally, the meatal plug persists until birth, resulting in congenital deafness.

### Eardrum or Tympanic Membrane

The eardrum is made up of (1) an ectodermal epithelial lining at the bottom of the external auditory meatus, (2) an endodermal epithelial lining of the tympanic cavity, and (3) an intermediate layer of connective tissue (mesodermal) (Fig. 19.9*B*) that forms the fibrous stratum. The major part of the eardrum is firmly attached to the handle of the malleus (Figs. 19.8 and 19.9*B*), and the remaining portion forms the separation between the external auditory meatus and the tympanic cavity.

### Auricle

The **auricle**, or external ear, develops from proliferation of tissues derived from the neural crest at the dorsal ends of the **first** and **second pharyngeal arches**, on either side of the first pharyngeal cleft (Fig. 19.10). Proliferation of tissue from the second arch forms nearly all of the external ear, whereas the first arch contributes the tragus and the external auditory meatus (Fig. 19.10). The process involves molecular pathways regulating *HOXA2* expression: First arch tissues are *HOXA2*$^-$; whereas second arch tissues are *HOXA2*$^+$. Mutations in genes involved in these pathways cause many external ear malformations, including duplications, tags, and pits (see Clinical Correlates, p. 289). Such malformations are common because of the complexity of external ear morphology. Furthermore, because neural crest cells give rise to the external ear, as well as several other organs and tissues, external ear defects often occur in combination with abnormalities in those structures, such as the face, skull, and heart. Initially, the external ears are in the lower neck region (Fig. 19.10*A*,*B*), but growth of the body and ramus of the mandible posteriorly and cranially moves the external ears to the side of the head at the level of the eyes.

## HEARING

Hearing is dependent on sound waves that cause vibrations in the tympanic membrane, which is held tightly like the surface of a drum by the tensor tympani muscle. If too loud a sound, causing potentially damaging vibrations, occurs, the tensor tympani together with the stapedius muscle stretches the membrane even tighter to prevent it from vibrating too forcefully. Once the tympanic membrane vibrates, it causes movement of the ear ossicles, the malleus, incus, and stapes that serve to amplify the force of the sound wave and to transmit the pressure of the wave to the cochlea through the oval window (Fig. 19.8). Amplification results from two factors: (1) The large size difference between the tympanic membrane (55 mm$^2$) and the oval window (3.2 mm$^2$), where the stapes attaches, results in greater energy produced by the membrane to be transferred and amplified at the oval window; (2) because of its shape, the malleus acts like a lever to increase the force received by the stapes (Figs. 19.8 and 19.9*B*).

Part 2

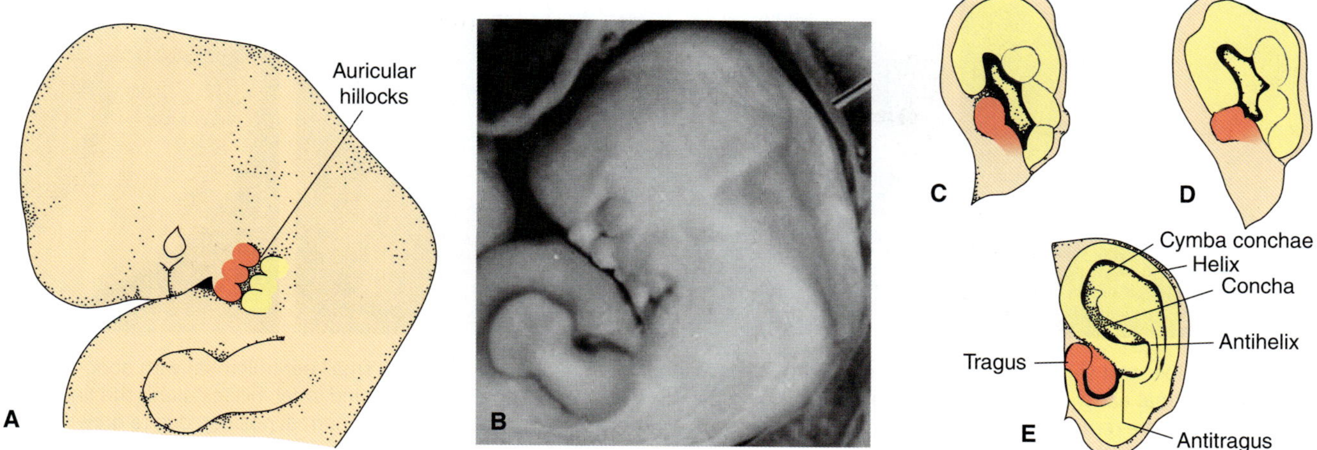


**FIGURE 19.10 A.** Drawing of a 6-week-old embryo showing a lateral view of the head and six auricular hillocks surrounding the dorsal end of the first pharyngeal cleft. **B.** Six-week-old human embryo showing a stage of external ear development similar to that depicted in **(A)**. **C–E.** Growth of tissues from the second arch (*yellow*) forms most of the external ear. Tissue from the first arch (*red*) forms the tragus and invaginates to form the external auditory meatus. The first pharyngeal cleft is overgrown by second arch tissue and disappears. Note that the ear is part of the mandibular portion of the first pharyngeal arch and that the ear lies horizontally at the side of the neck. At this stage, the mandible is small. As the mandible grows anteriorly and posteriorly, the ears, which are located immediately posterior to the mandible, will be repositioned into their characteristic location at the side of the head.

Pressure produced by movement of the stapes at the oval window creates a fluid wave in the cochlea that is balanced by movement of the round window (Fig. 19.8). The fluid wave moves small regions of the basilar membrane (Fig. 19.4) and the location of these regions is determined in part by the amplitude (loudness) and frequency (pitch) of the wave. Near the oval window, the basilar membrane is attached by shorter, stiffer fibers to the side of the cochlea; farther along the cochlea, the fibers are longer and more flexible. Based on these fiber characteristics and the frequency of the wave, the wave reaches a point where it resonates with the fibers and moves the basilar membrane. This movement is sensed by adjacent hair cells that send impulses back through nerve fibers of the acoustic segment of the statoacoustic nerve (Figs. 19.4*C* and 19.5*C*). High frequencies (high pitch) are heard near the oval window where fibers connecting the basilar membrane are shorter and stiffer; lower frequencies are heard farther up the cochlea where the fibers are longer and more flexible. Note that the human fetus is able to perceive sound stimulus by 20–24 weeks of development.

Part 2

## *Clinical Correlates*

### Hearing Loss and External Ear Abnormalities

**Congenital hearing loss** may be due to abnormalities of the hair cells or auditory nerve ganglia (**sensorineural loss**) or to structural defects in the external ear canal, eardrum, or ear ossicles (**conductive hearing loss**). Fifty percent of cases are genetic and may involve autosomal dominant or recessive or X-linked genes. In Treacher Collins syndrome, malformations in the external ear and ear canal and the ear ossicles can all be involved in causing varying degrees of conductive hearing loss. In Down syndrome, hearing loss may be caused by sensorineural and/or conductive abnormalities. Most cases caused by other factors are characterized by sensorineural defects. These factors include **prenatal infections** (rubella, cytomegalovirus, herpes simplex), **prematurity**, and **maternal diabetes**. **Accutane (retinoids)** can cause both types of deafness.

The most common ear ossicle to be involved in conductive hearing loss is the **stapes**, and this fact may be due to its unique origin because its footplate is derived from neural crest cells and paraxial mesoderm. Neural crest cells direct formation of the footplate and of the oval window. Without directive signals from the neural crest, neither the footplate nor the oval window develops properly. Stapes fixation (ankylosis) is the most common abnormality and usually involves both ears.

**External ear defects** are common; they include minor and severe abnormalities (Fig. 19.11). They are significant from the standpoint of the psychological and emotional trauma they may cause and for the fact that they are often associated with other malformations. This association is due in part to the fact that external ears are derived from neural crest cells and this cell type contributes to development of many other structures, including the face, skull, and heart. Thus, external ear defects serve as clues to examine infants carefully for other abnormalities. **All of the frequently occurring chromosomal syndromes and most of the less common ones have ear anomalies as one of their characteristics.**

**Preauricular appendages and pits** (Fig. 19.11*C,D*) are skin tags and shallow depressions, respectively, anterior to the ear. Pits arise when invagination of first arch tissues to form the external auditory meatus fails to occur properly. Appendages can occur when misexpression of genes regulating development of the external ears results in duplications of tissue growth and differentiation. Like other external ear defects, both are often associated with other malformations.

(*Continued*)

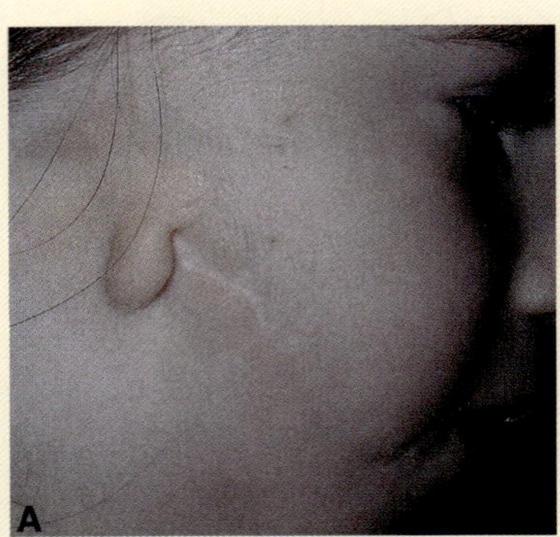

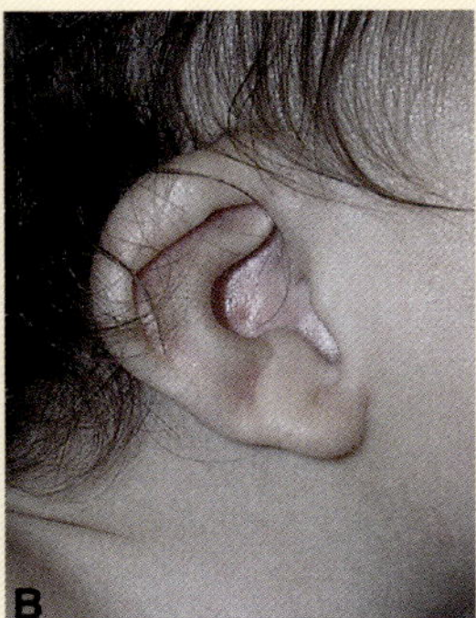

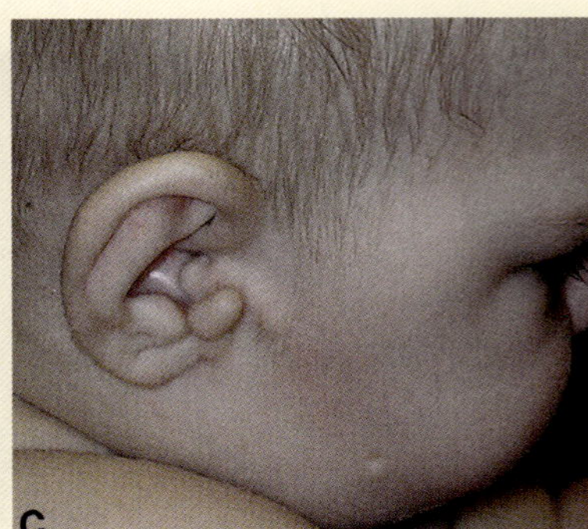

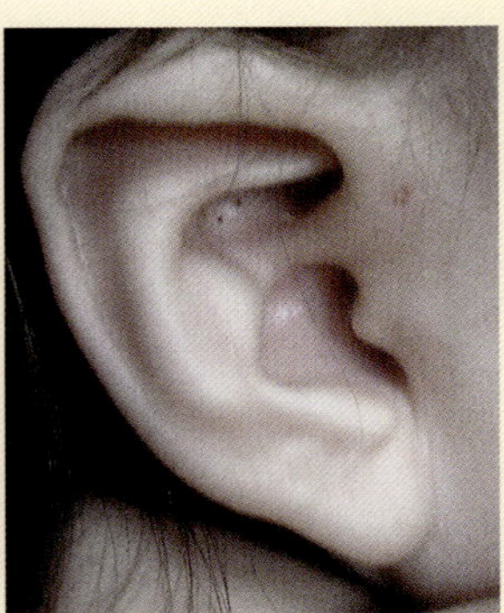

**FIGURE 19.11** External ear defects. **A.** Almost complete absence (anotia) of the external ear. **B.** A small ear (microtia) with abnormal features. **C.** Abnormal ear with preauricular appendages (skin tags). Note also the slight depression and small hillock along the line of the mandible. These are remnants of ear development and indicate the path of the ear as it moved to its normal position due to growth of the mandible. **D.** Preauricular pit.

## SUMMARY

- The ear consists of three parts that have different origins but that function as one unit.
- The **internal ear** originates from the otic placode close to the rhombencephalon.
- The otic placode invaginates to form the **otic vesicle**.
- The otic vesicle in the fourth week of development detaches from surface ectoderm.
- This vesicle divides into a ventral component, which gives rise to the **saccule** and **cochlear duct** and a dorsal component, which gives rise to the **utricle**, **semicircular canals**, and **endolymphatic duct** (Figs. 19.3, 19.6, and 19.8).
- The epithelial structures thus formed are known collectively as the **membranous labyrinth**. Except for the **cochlear duct**, which forms the **organ of Corti**, all structures derived from the membranous labyrinth are involved with equilibrium.
- The **middle ear**, consisting of the **tympanic cavity** and **auditory tube**, is lined with epithelium of endodermal origin and is derived from the first pharyngeal pouch.
- The auditory tube extends between the tympanic cavity and the nasopharynx.
- The **ossicles**, which transfer sound from the tympanic membrane to the oval window, are derived from the first (**malleus** and **incus**) and second (**stapes**) pharyngeal arches (Fig. 19.9).
- The **external auditory meatus** develops from the first pharyngeal arch as an invagination of the ectoderm and is separated from the tympanic cavity by the tympanic membrane (eardrum).
- The eardrum consists of (1) an ectodermal epithelial lining, (2) an intermediate layer of mesenchyme, and (3) an endodermal lining from the first pharyngeal pouch.
- The **auricle** develops from six mesenchymal hillocks (Fig. 19.10) along the first and second pharyngeal arches. Defects in the auricle are often associated with other congenital malformations.

## Self-Assessment

### Comprehensive Questions

1. Write a note on the development of the organ of Corti.
2. Discuss the role of tensor tympani at very-high-frequency sound waves.

### Problem Solving Questions

1. The otic placode plays a major role in formation of the internal (inner ear). What is a placode, and where does the otic placode form? What structures does it contribute to the inner ear?
2. What is the embryologic origin of the tympanic (middle ear) cavity, auditory tube, and tympanic membrane (eardrum)?
3. A newborn has bilateral microtia. Should you be concerned about other malformations? What cell population might be involved in the embryologic origin of the defect?

### Multiple Choice Questions

1. Tympanic membrane is formed by all of the following except
   (a) Ectodermal epithelial lining
   (b) Endodermal epithelial lining
   (c) Intermediate layer of mesoderm
   (d) Neural crest cells
2. External auditory meatus develops from
   (a) Invagination of first arch tissue
   (b) First pharyngeal cleft
   (c) First pharyngeal pouch
   (d) Meatal plug
3. Malleus and stapes are derived from
   (a) Malleus from the first pharyngeal arch and stapes from the second pharyngeal arch

(b) Both from the second pharyngeal arch
(c) Both from the first pharyngeal arch
(d) Stapes from the first pharyngeal arch and malleus from the second pharyngeal arch

4. Tympanic cavity develops from
(a) First pharyngeal pouch
(b) Second pharyngeal pouch
(c) First pharyngeal arch
(d) Second pharyngeal arch

5. Otic placode develops from ectodermal thickening close to
(a) Telencephalon
(b) Diencephalon
(c) Mesencephalon
(d) Rhombencephalon

6. Sensorineural hearing loss is due to abnormalities in all of the following except
(a) Hair cells
(b) Cochlear nerve
(c) External auditory canal
(d) Cochlear ganglion

7. Tensor tympani is supplied by
(a) Mandibular nerve
(b) Facial nerve
(c) Vestibular nerve
(d) Cochlear nerve

**Answers**

1. (d) 2. (a) 3. (a) 4. (b) 5. (d) 6. (c) 7. (a)

CHAPTER

# 20 Eye



### Specific Learning Objectives

- Formation of optic cup, optic vesicle, and lens vesicle
- Development of iris, ciliary body, and retina
- Development of lens, sclera, choroid, and cornea
- Formation of optic nerve
- Molecular regulation of eye development
- Clinical correlates

### Competency Covered

AN43.4 Describe the development and developmental basis of congenital anomalies of the eye.

## OPTIC CUP AND LENS VESICLE

The developing eye appears in the 22-day embryo as a pair of shallow grooves on the sides of the forebrain (Fig. 20.1). With closure of the neural tube, these grooves form outpocketings of the forebrain, the optic vesicles. These vesicles subsequently come in contact with the surface ectoderm and induce changes in the ectoderm necessary for lens formation (Fig. 20.1). Shortly thereafter, the optic vesicle begins to invaginate and forms the double-walled optic cup (Figs. 20.1 and 20.2*A*). The inner and outer layers of this cup are initially separated by a lumen, the intraretinal space (Fig. 20.2*B*), but soon this lumen disappears, and the two layers appose each other (Fig. 20.2*D*,*E*). Invagination is not only restricted to the central portion of the cup but also involves a part of the inferior surface (Fig. 20.2*A*) that forms the choroid fissure. Formation of this fissure allows the hyaloid artery to reach the inner chamber of the eye (Fig. 20.3; see also Fig. 20.7). During the seventh week, the lips of the choroid fissure fuse, and the mouth of the optic cup becomes a round opening, the future pupil.

During these events, cells of the surface ectoderm, initially in contact with the optic vesicle, begin to elongate and form the lens placode (Fig. 20.1). This placode subsequently invaginates and develops into the lens vesicle. During the fifth week, the lens vesicle loses contact with the surface ectoderm and lies in the mouth of the optic cup (Figs. 20.2C to E, 20.3, and 20.4).

During these events, cells of the surface ectoderm, initially in contact with the optic vesicle, begin to elongate and form the lens placode (Fig. 20.1). This placode subsequently invaginates and develops into the lens vesicle. During the fifth week, the lens vesicle loses contact with the surface ectoderm and lies in the mouth of the optic cup (Figs. 20.2*C*–*E* and 20.3).

## RETINA, IRIS, AND CILIARY BODY

The outer layer of the optic cup, which is characterized by small pigment granules, is known as the **pigmented layer** of

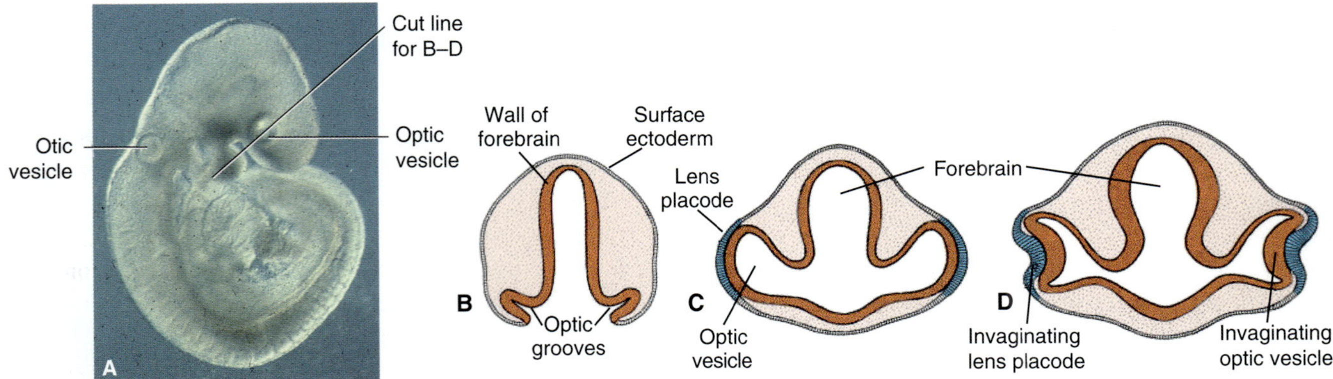


**FIGURE 20.1 A.** Embryo at the end of 4 weeks of development showing the otic and optic vesicles. **B.** Transverse section through the forebrain of a 22-day embryo (~14 somites) showing the optic grooves. **C.** Transverse section through the forebrain of a 4-week embryo showing the optic vesicles in contact with the surface ectoderm. Note the slight thickening of the ectoderm (lens placode). **D.** Transverse section through the forebrain of a 5-mm embryo showing invagination of the optic vesicle and the lens placode.

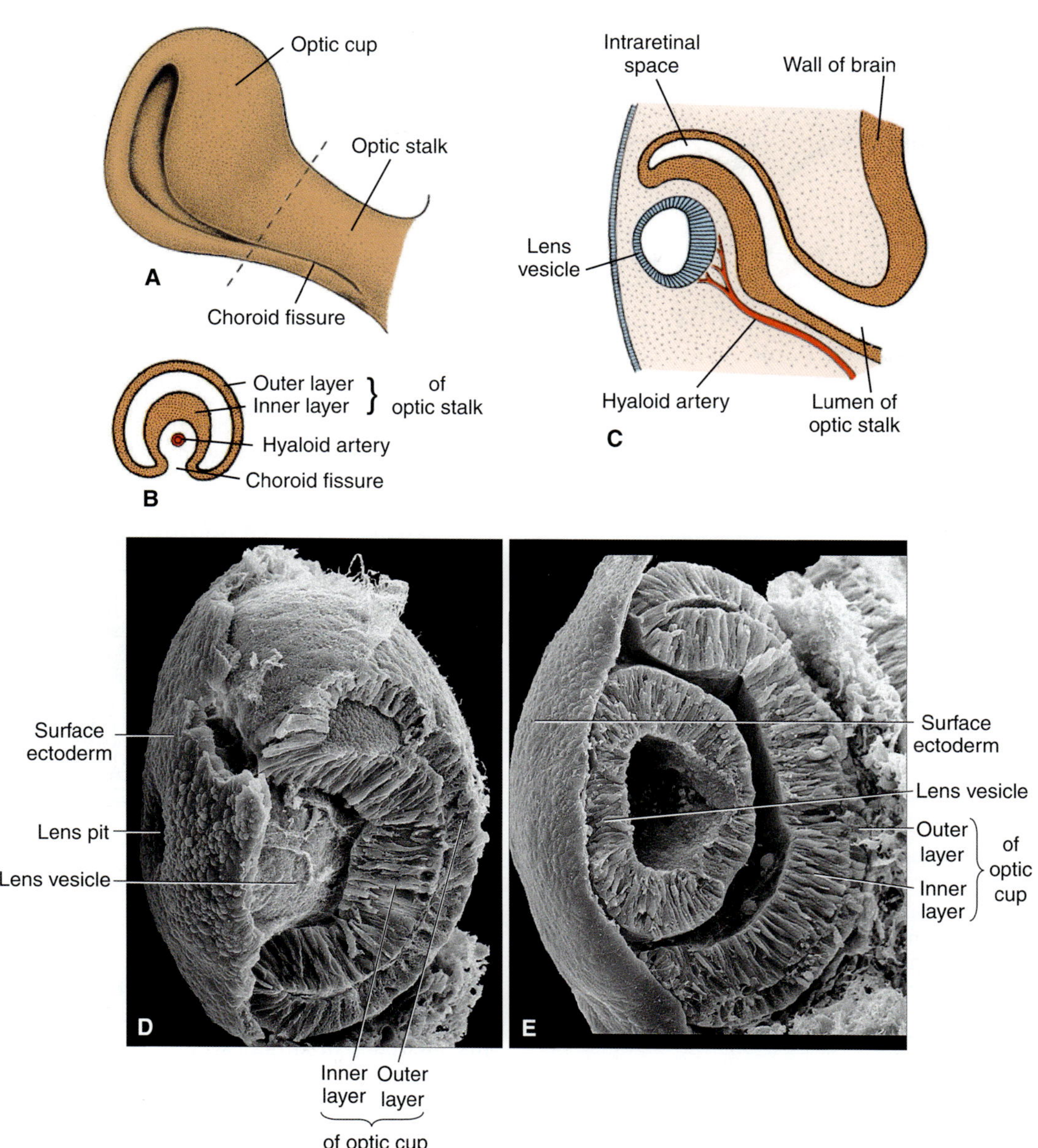


**FIGURE 20.2** **A.** Ventrolateral view of the optic cup and optic stalk of a 6-week embryo. The choroid fissure on the undersurface of the optic stalk gradually tapers off. **B.** Transverse section through the optic stalk as indicated in **(A)**, showing the hyaloid artery in the choroid fissure. **C.** Section through the lens vesicle, the optic cup, and optic stalk at the plane of the choroid fissure. **D.** Scanning electron micrograph through the eye at 6 weeks of development. The lens vesicle has not quite finished detaching from the surface ectoderm, and the two layers of the optic cup have formed. **E.** Scanning electron micrograph through the eye at 6.5 weeks of development. The lens is completely detached from the surface ectoderm and will soon start to form lens fibers.

the retina (Fig. 20.2*D,E*; see also Fig. 20.7). Development of the inner **(neural) layer** of the optic cup is more complicated. The posterior four-fifths, the **pars optica retinae**, contains cells bordering the intraretinal space (Fig. 20.3) that differentiate into the photoreceptive **rods** and **cones** (Fig. 20.5). Rods are more numerous (120 million) and more sensitive than cones (6 to 7 million) but do not detect color like the cones. Adjacent to this photoreceptive layer is the mantle layer, which, as in the brain, gives rise to neurons and supporting cells, including the **outer nuclear layer**, **inner nuclear layer**, and **ganglion cell layer** (Fig. 20.5). On the surface is a fibrous layer that contains axons of nerve cells of the deeper layers. Nerve fibers in this zone converge toward the optic stalk, which develops into the optic nerve (Fig. 20.3). Hence, light impulses pass through most layers of the retina before they reach the rods and cones.

The anterior fifth of the inner layer, the **pars ceca retinae**, remains one cell layer thick. It later divides into the **pars iridica retinae**, which forms the inner layer of the iris, and the **pars ciliaris retinae**, which participates in formation of the **ciliary body** (Figs. 20.6 and 20.7).

Meanwhile, the region between the optic cup and the overlying surface epithelium is filled with loose mesenchyme (Figs. 20.2*C* and 20.7). The **sphincter** and **dilator pupillae** muscles form in this tissue (Fig. 20.6). These muscles develop from the underlying ectoderm of the optic cup. In the adult, the iris is formed by the pigment-containing external layer,

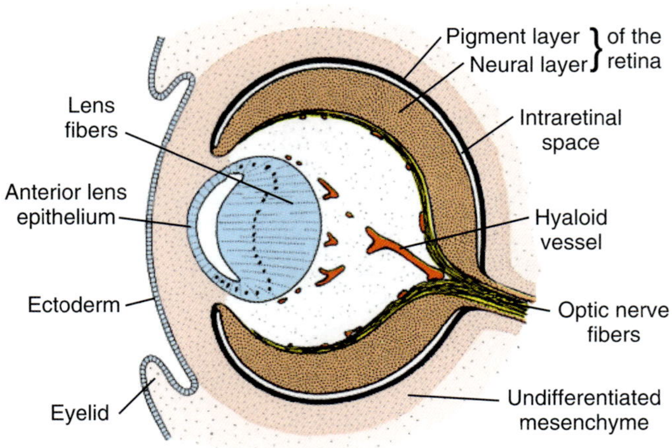


**FIGURE 20.3** Section through the eye of a 7-week embryo. The eye primordium is completely embedded in mesenchyme. Fibers of the neural retina converge toward the optic nerve.

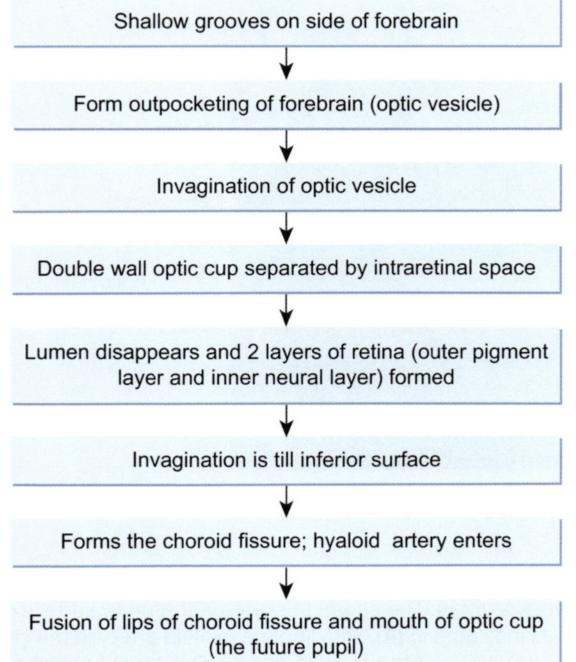


**FIGURE 20.4** Formation of eyeball.

the unpigmented internal layer of the optic cup, and a layer of richly vascularized connective tissue that contains the pupillary muscles (Fig. 20.6).

The **pars ciliaris retinae** is easily recognized by its marked folding (Figs. 20.6*B* and 20.7). Externally, it is covered by a layer of mesenchyme that forms the **ciliary muscle**; on the inside, it is connected to the lens by a network of elastic fibers, the **suspensory ligament** or zonula (Fig. 20.7). Contraction of the ciliary muscle changes tension in the ligament and controls curvature of the lens.

## LENS

Shortly after formation of the lens vesicle (Fig. 20.2*C*), cells of the posterior wall begin to elongate anteriorly and form long

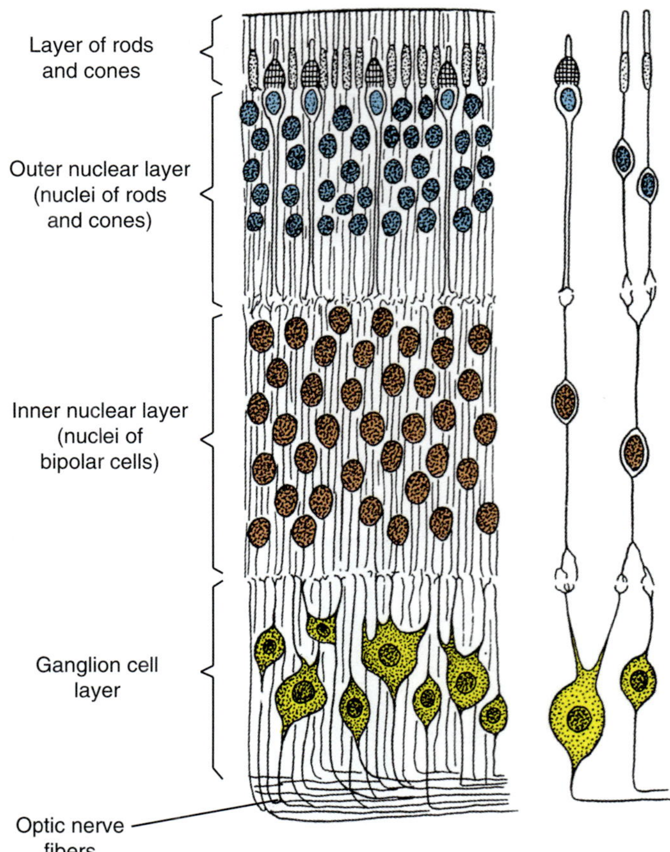


**FIGURE 20.5** Various layers of the pars optica retinae in a fetus of approximately 25 weeks.

fibers that gradually fill the lumen of the vesicle (Fig. 20.3). By the end of the seventh week, these **primary lens fibers** reach the anterior wall of the lens vesicle. Growth of the lens is not finished at this stage, however, because new (secondary) lens fibers are continuously added to the central core.

## CHOROID, SCLERA, AND CORNEA

At the end of the fifth week, the eye primordium is completely surrounded by loose mesenchyme (Fig. 20.3). This tissue soon differentiates into an inner layer comparable with the pia mater of the brain and an outer layer comparable with the dura mater. The inner layer later forms a highly vascularized pigmented layer known as the **choroid**; the outer layer develops into the sclera and is continuous with the dura mater around the optic nerve (Fig. 20.7).

Differentiation of mesenchymal layers overlying the anterior aspect of the eye is different. The **anterior chamber** forms through vacuolization and splits the mesenchyme into an inner layer in front of the lens and iris, the **iridopupillary membrane**, and an outer layer continuous with the sclera, the **substantia propria** of the **cornea** (Fig. 20.7). The anterior chamber itself is lined by flattened mesenchymal cells. Hence, the cornea is formed by (1) an epithelial layer derived from the surface ectoderm; (2) the **substantia propria** or **stroma**, which is continuous with the sclera; and (3) an epithelial layer, which

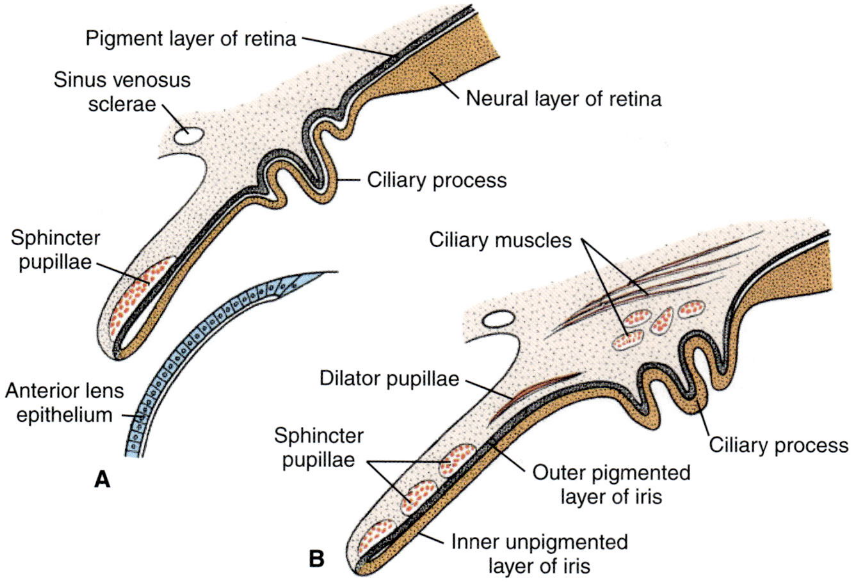


**FIGURE 20.6** Development of the iris and ciliary body. The rim of the optic cup is covered by mesenchyme, in which the sphincter and dilator pupillae develop from the underlying ectoderm.

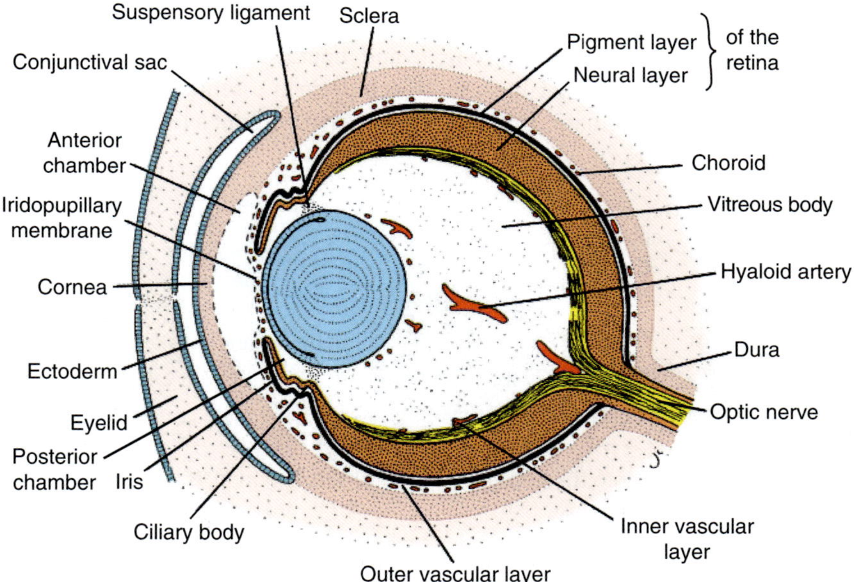


**FIGURE 20.7** Section through the eye of a 15-week fetus showing the anterior chamber, iridopupillary membrane, inner and outer vascular layers, choroid, and sclera.



borders the anterior chamber. The iridopupillary membrane in front of the lens disappears completely. The **posterior chamber** is the space between the iris anteriorly and the lens and ciliary body posteriorly. The anterior and posterior chambers communicate with each other through the pupil and are filled with fluid called the **aqueous humor** produced by the ciliary process of the ciliary body. The clear aqueous humor circulates from the posterior chamber into the anterior chamber providing nutrients for the avascular cornea and lens. From the anterior chamber, the fluid passes through the **scleral venous sinus** (canal of Schlemm) at the iridocorneal angle where it is resorbed into the bloodstream. Blockage of the flow of fluid at the canal of Schlemm is one cause of **glaucoma**.

## ■ VITREOUS BODY

Mesenchyme not only surrounds the eye primordium from the outside but also invades the inside of the optic cup by way of the choroid fissure. Here, it forms the hyaloid vessels, which during intrauterine life supply the lens and form the vascular layer on the inner surface of the retina (Fig. 20.7). In addition, it forms a delicate network of fibers between the lens and retina. The interstitial spaces of this network later fill with a transparent gelatinous substance, forming the **vitreous body** (Fig. 20.7). The hyaloid vessels in this region are obliterated and disappear during fetal life, leaving behind the hyaloid canal.

## OPTIC NERVE

The optic cup is connected to the brain by the optic stalk, which has a groove, the **choroid fissure**, on its ventral surface (Figs. 20.2 and 20.3). In this groove are the hyaloid vessels. The nerve fibers of the retina returning to the brain lie among cells of the inner wall of the stalk (Fig. 20.8). During the seventh week, the choroid fissure closes, and a narrow tunnel forms inside the optic stalk (Fig. 20.8*B*). As a result of the continuously increasing number of nerve fibers, the inner wall of the stalk grows, and the inside and outside walls of the stalk fuse (Fig. 20.8*C*). Cells of the inner layer provide a network of neuroglia that supports the optic nerve fibers.

The optic stalk is thus transformed into the **optic nerve**. Its center contains a portion of the hyaloid artery, later called the **central artery of the retina**. On the outside, a continuation of the choroid and sclera, the **pia arachnoid** and **dura** layer of the nerve, respectively, surround the optic nerve.

## MOLECULAR REGULATION OF EYE DEVELOPMENT

***PAX6*** is the key regulatory gene for eye development. It is a member of the ***PAX*** (paired box) family of transcription factors and contains two DNA-binding motifs that include a paired domain and a paired-type homeodomain. Initially, this transcription factor is expressed in a band in the anterior neural ridge of the neural plate before neurulation begins (Fig. 20.9*A,B*; see also Fig. 18.32). At this stage, there is a single eye field that later separates into two optic primordia (Fig. 20.9*B*). The signal for separation of this field is **SONIC HEDGEHOG (SHH)** expressed in the prechordal plate. *SHH* expression upregulates ***PAX2*** in the center of the eye field and downregulates ***PAX6*** (Fig. 20.9*C*). Later, this pattern is maintained so that *PAX2* is expressed in the optic stalks and *PAX6* is expressed in the optic cup and overlying surface ectoderm that forms the lens. As development proceeds, it appears that *PAX6* is not essential for optic cup formation. Instead, this process is regulated by interactive signals between the optic vesicle and surrounding mesenchyme and the overlying surface ectoderm in the lens-forming region (Fig. 20.10). Thus, fibroblast growth factors (FGFs) from the surface ectoderm promote differentiation of the neural (inner layer) retina, whereas transforming growth factor β (TGF-β), secreted by surrounding mesenchyme, directs formation of the pigmented (outer) retinal layer. Downstream from these gene products, the transcription factors *MITF* and *CHX10* are expressed and direct differentiation of the pigmented and neural layer, respectively (Fig. 20.10). Thus, the lens ectoderm is essential for proper formation of the optic cup, such that without a lens placode, no cup invagination occurs.

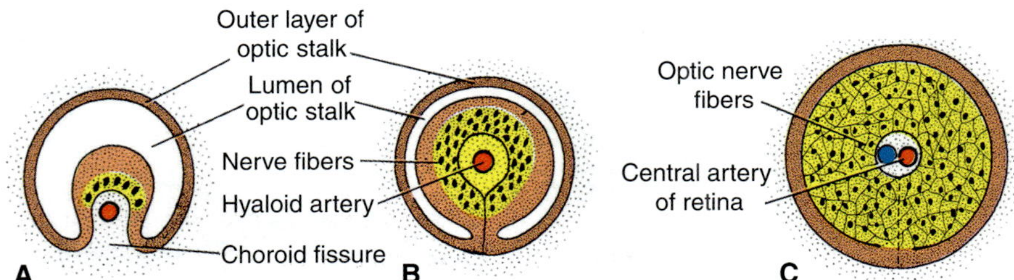


**FIGURE 20.8** Transformation of the optic stalk into the optic nerve. **A.** Sixth week (9 mm). **B.** Seventh week (15 mm). **C.** Ninth week. Note the central artery of the retina in the optic nerve.

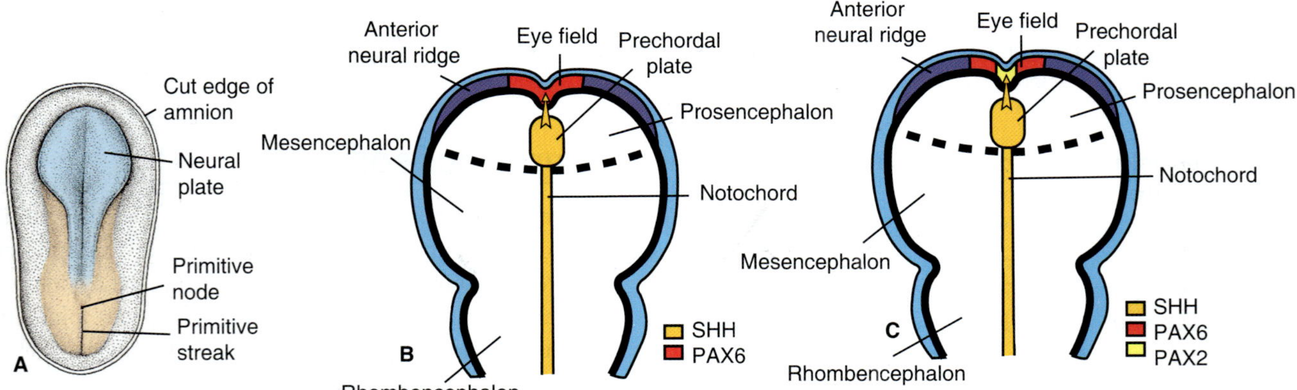


**FIGURE 20.9 A.** Dorsal view of the cranial neural plate region (*blue* area) in a presomite stage embryo at 3 weeks' gestation. **B,C.** Drawings of the cranial neural plate region depicted in **(A)** showing the initial stages of eye development. The transcription factor *PAX6* is the master gene for eye development, and it is initially expressed in a band in the center of the anterior neural ridge **(B)**. Sonic hedgehog (SHH), secreted by the prechordal plate, inhibits the expression of *PAX6* in the midline and upregulates expression of *PAX2* in this same location **(C)**. *PAX2* then regulates optic stalk differentiation, whereas *PAX6* continues to regulate differentiation of the eyes.

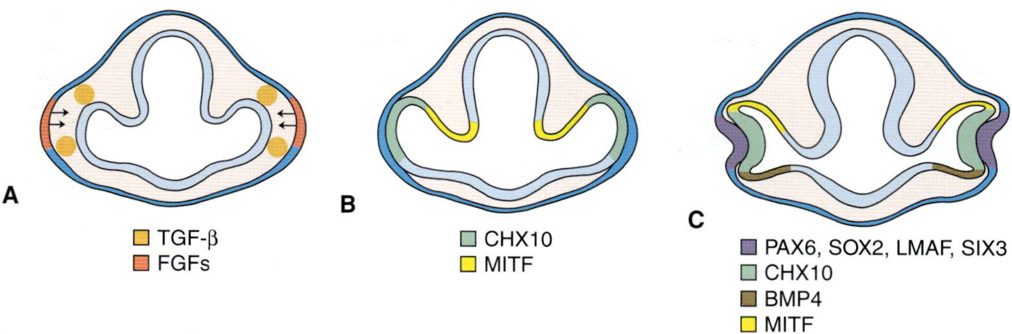


**FIGURE 20.10** Drawing showing molecular regulation of epithelial–mesenchymal interactions responsible for patterning eye development. **A.** Once *PAX6* establishes the eye field, fibroblast growth factors (FGFs), secreted by surface ectoderm in the prospective lens-forming region overlying the optic vesicle, promote differentiation of the neural retinal layer, whereas members of the transforming growth factor β (TGF-β) family, secreted by surrounding mesenchyme, promote differentiation of the pigmented retinal layer. These external signals cause regionalization of the inner and outer layers of the optic cup and upregulate downstream genes, including *CHX10* and *MITF*, that regulate continued differentiation of these structures. **B,C.** In addition to its role in determining the eye fields, *PAX6* regulates lens development. Thus, *PAX6* upregulates *SOX2* expression in the prospective lens, whereas BMP4 secreted by the outer vesicle upregulates the transcription factor *LMAF*. Once this gene is activated, *PAX6* induces expression of the homeodomain-containing genes *SIX3* and *PROX1*. The combined expression of *PAX6*, *SOX2*, *LMAF*, and *PROX1* leads to crystallin formation. *SIX3* assists in regulating this process by inhibiting the crystallin gene.

Differentiation of the lens depends on *PAX6*, although the gene is not responsible for inductive activity by the optic vesicle. Instead, *PAX6* acts in the surface ectoderm to regulate lens development (Fig. 20.10*C*). This expression upregulates the transcription factor *SOX2* and also maintains *PAX6* expression in the prospective lens ectoderm. In turn, the optic vesicle secretes BMP4, which also upregulates and maintains *SOX2* expression as well as expression of *LMAF*, another transcription factor (Fig. 20.10*C*). Next, the expression of two homeobox genes, *SIX3* and *PROX1*, is regulated by *PAX6*. The combined expression of *PAX6*, *SOX2*, and *LMAF* initiates expression of genes responsible for lens crystallin formation, including *PROX1*. *SIX3* also acts as a regulator of crystallin production by inhibiting the crystallin gene. Finally, *PAX6*, acting through *FOX3*, regulates cell proliferation in the lens.



## Clinical Correlates

### Eye Abnormalities

**Coloboma** may occur if the choroid fissure fails to close. Normally, this fissure closes during the seventh week of development (Fig. 20.8). When it does not, a cleft persists. Although such a cleft is usually in the iris only–**coloboma iridis** (Fig. 20.11*A*)–it may extend into the ciliary body, the retina, the choroid, and the optic nerve. Coloboma is a common eye abnormality frequently associated with other eye defects. Colobomas (clefts) of the eyelids may also occur. Mutations in the ***PAX2*** gene have been linked with optic nerve colobomas and may play a role in the other types as well. Renal defects also occur with mutations in *PAX2* as part of the **renal coloboma syndrome** (see Chapter 16).

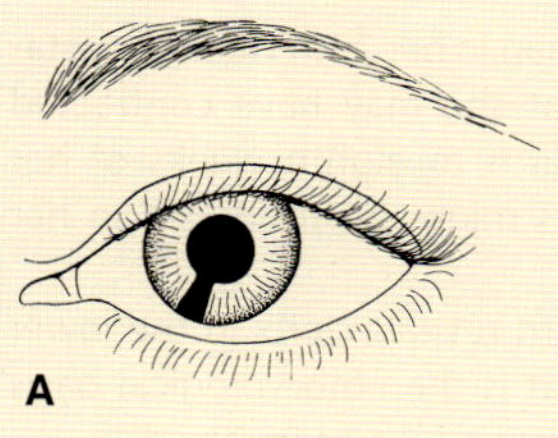


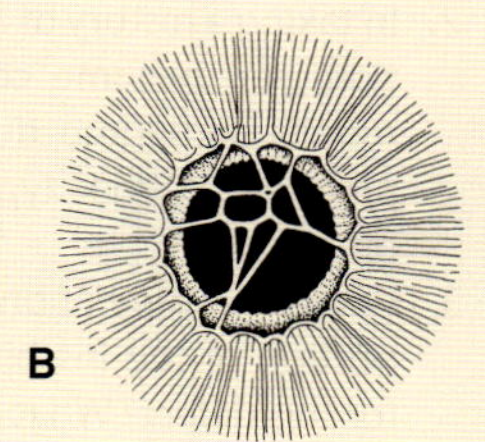


**FIGURE 20.11** **A.** Coloboma iris. **B.** Persistence of the iridopupillary membrane.

The **iridopupillary membrane** (Fig. 20.11*B*) may persist instead of being resorbed during formation of the anterior chamber.

**Congenital cataracts** cause the lens to become opaque during intrauterine life. Although this anomaly is usually genetically determined, many children born to mothers who had rubella (German measles) between the fourth and seventh weeks of pregnancy had cataracts. If the mother is infected after the seventh week of pregnancy, the lens escapes damage, but the child may have hearing loss as a result of cochlear abnormalities. Because of the MMR (measles, mumps, and rubella) vaccine, congenital rubella syndrome has been nearly eradicated in the United States.

The **hyaloid artery** may persist to form a cord or cyst. Normally, the distal portion of this vessel degenerates, leaving the proximal part to form the central artery of the retina.

In **microphthalmia**, the eye is too small; the eyeball may be only two-thirds of its normal volume. Usually associated with other ocular abnormalities, microphthalmia can result from intrauterine infections, such as cytomegalovirus and toxoplasmosis.

**Anophthalmia** is absence of the eye. In some cases, histological analysis reveals some ocular tissue. The defect is usually accompanied by severe cranial abnormalities.

**Congenital aphakia** (absence of the lens) and **aniridia** (absence of the iris; Fig. 20.12) are rare anomalies that result

(*Continued*)

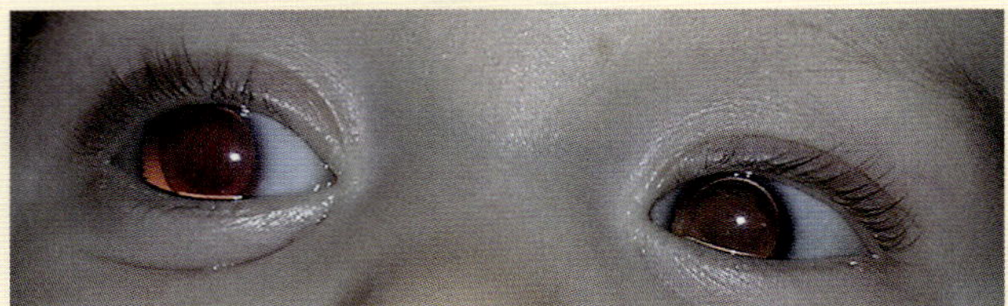

**FIGURE 20.12** Patient with aniridia (absence of the iris), which can be due to mutations in *PAX6*.

from disturbances in induction and development of tissues responsible for formation of these structures. Mutations in **PAX6** result in aniridia and may also contribute to anophthalmia and microphthalmia.

**Cyclopia** (single eye) and **synophthalmia** (fusion of the eyes) comprise a spectrum of defects in which the eyes are partially or completely fused (Fig. 20.13). The defects are caused by a loss of midline tissue that may occur as early as days 19 to 21 of gestation or at later stages when facial development is initiated. This loss results in underdevelopment of the forebrain and frontonasal prominence. These defects are invariably associated with a brain defect called **holoprosencephaly**, in which the cerebral hemispheres are partially or completely merged into a single telencephalic vesicle. Factors associated with holoprosencephaly include alcohol, maternal diabetes, mutations in *SHH*, and abnormalities in cholesterol metabolism that may disrupt SHH signaling (see Chapter 18).

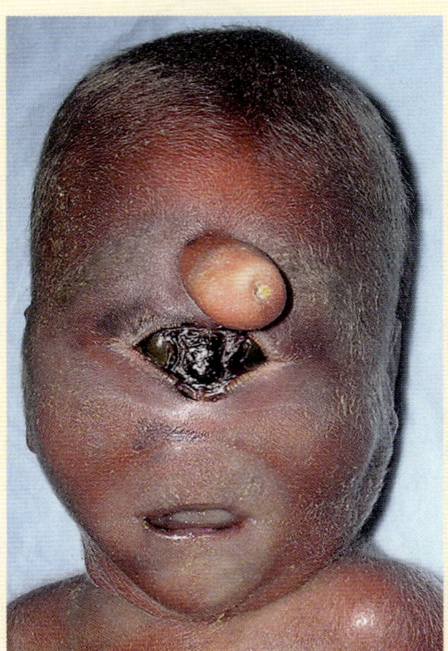

**FIGURE 20.13** Synophthalmia. The eyes are fused because loss of midline structures prevented the eye fields from separating. Such babies also have severe cranial defects, including holoprosencephaly (see Chapter 18).

Part 2

## SUMMARY

- The eyes begin to develop as a pair of outpocketings that will become the **optic vesicles** on each side of the forebrain at the end of the fourth week of development (Fig. 20.1).
- The optic vesicles contact the surface ectoderm and induce **lens** formation. When the optic vesicle begins to invaginate to form the pigment and neural layers of the retina, the lens placode invaginates to form the lens vesicle.
- Through a groove at the inferior aspect of the optic vesicle, the **choroid fissure**, the **hyaloid artery (later the central artery of the retina)** enters the eye (Fig. 20.3).
- Nerve fibers of the eye also occupy this groove to reach the optic areas of the brain.
- The cornea is formed by (1) a layer of surface ectoderm; (2) the stroma, which is continuous with the sclera; and (3) an epithelial layer bordering the anterior chamber (Fig. 20.7).
- ***PAX6***, the master gene for eye development, is expressed in the single eye field at the neural plate stage. The eye field is separated into two optic primordia by SHH, which upregulates ***PAX2*** expression in the optic stalks while downregulating *PAX6*, restricting this gene's expression to the optic cup and lens.
- Epithelial–mesenchymal interactions between prospective lens ectoderm, optic vesicle, and surrounding mesenchyme then regulate lens and optic cup differentiation (Figs. 20.9 and 20.10).

## Self-Assessment

### Comprehensive Questions

1. Describe the formation of lens.
2. Describe the formation of retina.

### Problem Solving Questions

1. A newborn has unilateral aphakia (absent lens). What is the embryological origin of this defect?
2. In taking a history of a young woman in her 10th week of gestation, you become concerned that she may have contracted rubella sometime during the fourth to eighth weeks of her pregnancy. What types of defects might be produced in her offspring?
3. Physical examination of a newborn reveals clefts in the lower portion of the iris bilaterally. What is the embryological basis for this defect? What other structures might be involved?

## Multiple Choice Questions

1. Optic vesicle develops from the side of
   (a) Prosencephalon
   (b) Diencephalon
   (c) Metencephalon
   (d) Mesencephalon
2. Hyaloid artery forms
   (a) Ophthalmic artery
   (b) Stapedial artery
   (c) Central artery of retina
   (d) Ciliary artery
3. A baby is born with cataract. The mother was possibly infected with
   (a) Toxoplasmosis
   (b) Cytomegalovirus
   (c) Rubella
   (d) HIV
4. Lens vesicle develops due to induction of
   (a) Surface ectoderm with forebrain
   (b) Optic vesicle with surface ectoderm
   (c) Optic stalk with optic vesicle
   (d) Thickening of surface ectoderm
5. Optic nerve is derived from
   (a) Optic stalk
   (b) Diencephalon
   (c) Neural layer of optic vesicle
   (d) Pituitary stalk
6. Outer layer of optic cup forms
   (a) Neural layer
   (b) Pigment layer
   (c) Optic nerve
   (d) Choroid

### Answers

1. (b) 2. (c) 3. (c) 4. (b) 5. (a) 6. (b)

CHAPTER

# 21 Integumentary System

## Specific Learning Objectives

- Development of epidermis
- Dermis
- Pigment disorders
- Dermatoglyphics
- Hair, nails, sweat glands
- Mammary glands and abnormalities

## Competency Covered

AN9.3 Describe the development of the breast.

Part 2

## SKIN

The skin is the largest organ in the body and has a dual origin: (1) A superficial layer, the **epidermis**, develops from the surface ectoderm. (2) A deep layer, the **dermis**, develops from the underlying mesenchyme.

### Epidermis

Initially, the embryo is covered by a single layer of ectodermal cells (Fig. 21.1*A*). In the beginning of the second month, this epithelium divides, and a layer of flattened cells, the **periderm**, or **epitrichium**, is laid down on the surface (Fig. 21.1*B*). With further proliferation of cells in the basal layer, a third, intermediate zone is formed (Fig. 21.1*C*). Finally, at the end of the fourth month, the epidermis acquires its definitive arrangement, and four layers can be distinguished (Fig. 21.1*D*):

The **basal layer**, or **germinative layer**, is responsible for production of new cells. This layer later forms ridges and hollows, which are reflected on the surface of the skin in the fingerprint.

A thick **spinous layer** consists of large polyhedral cells containing fine tonofibrils.

The **granular layer** contains small keratohyalin granules in its cells.

The **horny layer**, forming the tough scale-like surface of the epidermis, is made up of closely packed dead cells containing keratin.

Cells of the **periderm** are usually cast off during the second part of intrauterine life and can be found in the amniotic fluid. During the first 3 months of development, the epidermis is invaded by cells arising from the **neural crest**. These cells synthesize melanin pigment in melanosomes. As melanosomes accumulate, they are transported down dendritic processes of melanocytes and are transferred intercellularly to keratinocytes of the skin and hair bulb. In this manner, pigmentation of the skin and hair is acquired.

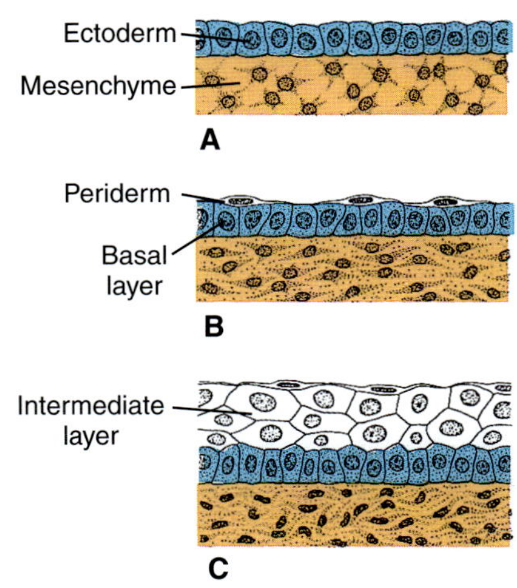


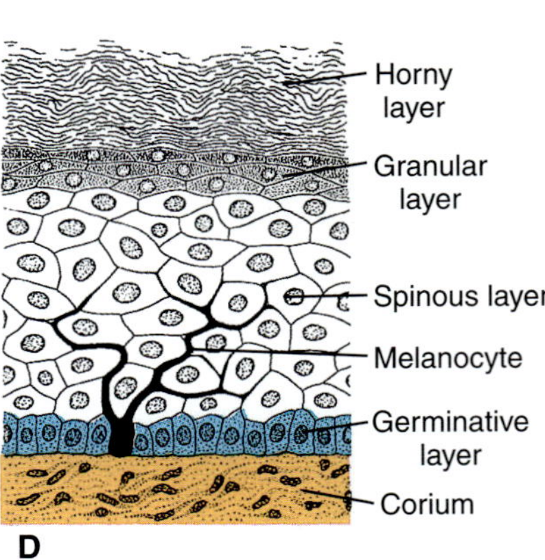


**FIGURE 21.1** Formation of the skin at various stages of development. **A.** 5 weeks. **B.** 7 weeks. **C.** 4 months. **D.** Birth.

## Clinical Correlates

### Pigmentary Disorders

A large number of pigmentary disorders occur, and these can be classified as diseases of melanocyte development, function, and survival. Examples of abnormalities of melanocyte function include **piebaldism** (patchy absence of hair and skin pigment) and **Waardenburg syndrome (WS)**, which feature patches of white skin and hair. There are several types of WS, but they share some common characteristics, including patches of white hair (usually a forelock), heterochromia iris (eyes of different colors), white patches of skin, and deafness. The defects arise because of faulty migration or proliferation of neural crest cells (absence of melanocytes derived from these cells in the stria vascularis in the cochlea accounts for deafness in these diseases). Some types of WS result from mutations in ***PAX3***, including WS1 and WS3.

Diseases of melanocyte function include the various forms of **albinism** characterized by globally reduced or absent pigmentation in the skin, hair, and eyes. These cases are classified as different types of **oculocutaneous albinism (OCA)**. In most cases, abnormalities of melanin synthesis or processing produce the abnormalities.

**Vitiligo** results from a loss of melanocytes due to an autoimmune disorder. There is patchy loss of pigment from affected areas, including the skin and overlying hair and the oral mucosa. Vitiligo is also associated with other autoimmune diseases, particularly of the thyroid.

### Fingerprints

The epidermal ridges that produce typical patterns on the surface of the fingertips, palms of the hand, and soles of the feet are genetically determined. They form the basis for many studies in medical genetics and criminal investigations (**dermatoglyphics**). In children with chromosomal abnormalities, the epidermal pattern on the hand and fingers is sometimes used as a diagnostic tool.

## Clinical Correlates

### Keratinization of the Skin

**Ichthyosis**, excessive keratinization of the skin, is characteristic of a group of hereditary disorders that are usually inherited as an autosomal recessive trait but may also be X-linked. In severe cases, ichthyosis may result in a grotesque appearance, as in the case of a **harlequin fetus** (Fig. 21.2).

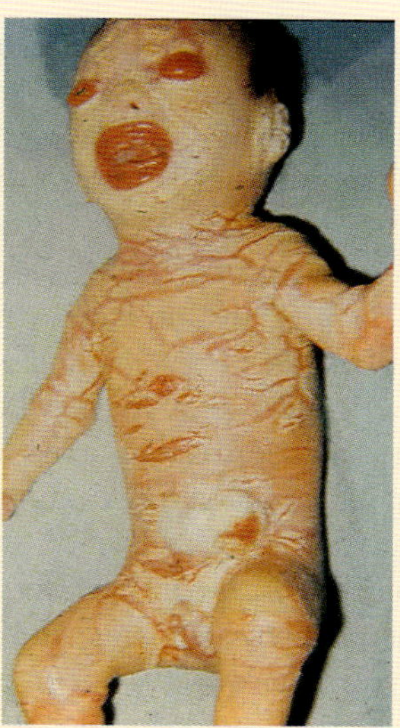

**FIGURE 21.2** Ichthyosis in a harlequin fetus with massive thickening of the keratin layer, which cracks to form fissures between thickened plaques.

### Dermis

**Dermis** is derived from mesenchyme that has three sources: (1) lateral plate mesoderm supplying cells for dermis in the limbs and body wall, (2) paraxial mesoderm supplying cells for dermis in the back, and (3) neural crest cells supplying cells for dermis in the face and neck. During the third and fourth months, this tissue, the **corium** (Fig. 21.1*D*), forms many irregular papillary structures, the **dermal papillae**, which project upward into the epidermis. Most of these papillae contain a small capillary or a sensory nerve end organ. The deeper layer of the dermis, the **subcorium**, contains large amounts of fatty tissue.

At birth, the skin is covered by a whitish paste, the **vernix caseosa**, formed by secretions from sebaceous glands and degenerated epidermal cells and hairs. It protects the skin against the macerating action of amniotic fluid.

## ■ HAIR

Hairs begin development as solid epidermal proliferations from the germinative layer that penetrates the underlying dermis (Fig. 21.3*A*). At their terminal ends, hair buds invaginate. The invaginations, the **hair papillae**, are rapidly filled with mesoderm in which vessels and nerve endings develop (Fig. 21.3*B*,*C*). Soon, cells in the center of the hair buds become spindle-shaped and keratinized, forming the **hair shaft**, whereas peripheral cells become cuboidal, giving rise to the **epithelial hair sheath** (Fig. 21.3*B*,*C*).

The **dermal root sheath** is formed by the surrounding mesenchyme. A small smooth muscle, also derived from mesenchyme, is usually attached to the dermal root sheath. The muscle is the **arrector pili muscle**. Continuous proliferation of epithelial cells at the base of the shaft pushes the hair upward, and by the end of the third month, the first hairs appear on the surface in the region of the eyebrow and upper lip. The first hair that appears, **lanugo hair**, is shed at about the time of birth and is later replaced by coarser hairs arising from new hair follicles.

The epithelial wall of the hair follicle usually shows a small bud penetrating the surrounding mesoderm (Fig. 21.3*C*). Cells from these buds form the **sebaceous glands**. Cells from the central region of the gland degenerate, forming a fat-like substance (**sebum**) secreted into the hair follicle, and from there, they reach the skin.

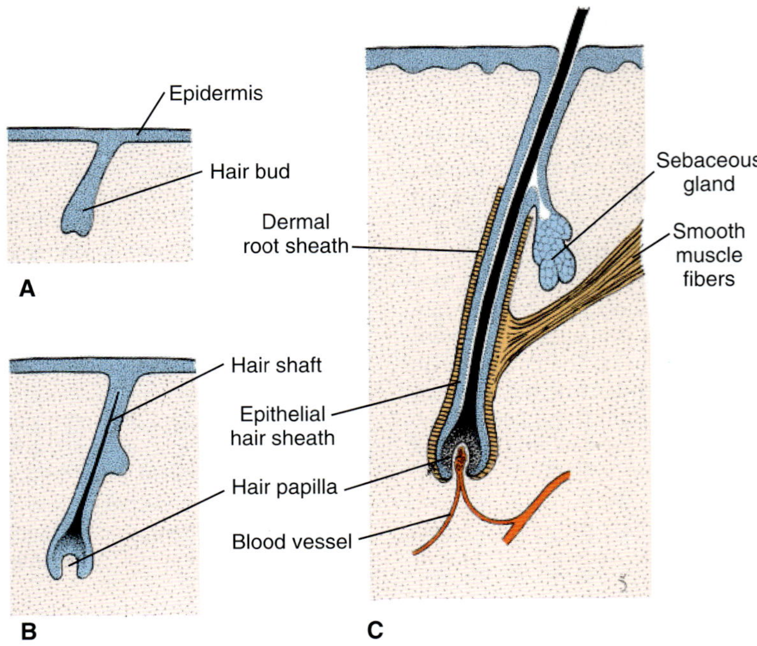


**FIGURE 21.3** Development of a hair and a sebaceous gland. **A.** 4 months. **B.** 6 months. **C.** Newborn.

Part 2

### Clinical Correlates

#### Abnormalities of Hair Distribution

**Hypertrichosis** (excessive hairiness) is caused by an unusual abundance of hair follicles. It may be localized to certain areas of the body, especially the lower lumbar region covering a spina bifida occulta defect or may cover the entire body (Fig. 21.4).

**Atrichia**, the congenital absence of hair, is usually associated with abnormalities of other ectodermal derivatives, such as teeth and nails.

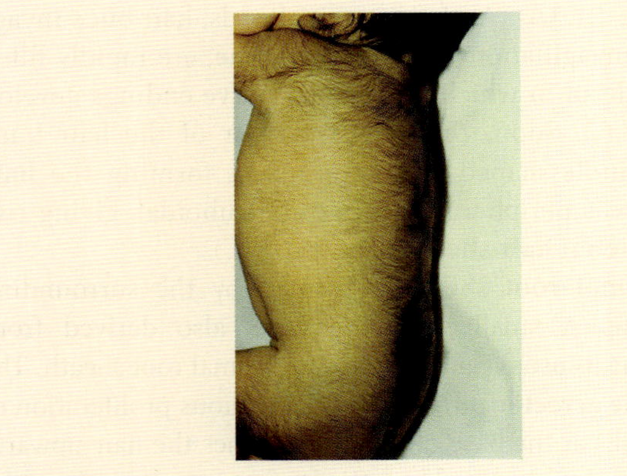

**FIGURE 21.4** Child with hypertrichosis.

## FINGERNAILS AND TOENAILS

By the end of the third month, thickenings in the epidermis appear at the tips of the digits to form the **nail fields**. From this location, these fields migrate to the dorsal side of each digit and grow proximally, forming the **nail root**, whereas proliferation of tissue surrounding each nail field creates a shallow depression for each nail. From the nail root, epidermis differentiates into fingernails and toenails that do not reach the tips of the digits until the ninth month of development.

## SWEAT GLANDS

There are two types of sweat glands: **eccrine** and **apocrine**. Eccrine sweat glands form in the skin over most parts of the body beginning as buds from the germinative layer of the epidermis. These buds grow into the dermis, and their end coils to form the secretory parts of the glands. Smooth muscle cells associated with the glands also develop from the epidermal buds. These glands function by merocrine mechanisms (exocytosis) and are involved in temperature control.

Apocrine sweat glands develop anywhere there is body hair, including the face, axillae, and pubic region. They begin to develop during puberty and arise from the same epidermal buds that produce hair follicles. Hence, these sweat glands open onto hair follicles instead of skin. The sweat produced by these glands contains lipids, proteins, and pheromones, and odor originating from this sweat is due to bacteria that break down these products. It should be noted that these glands classified as apocrine because a portion of the secretory cells is shed and incorporated into the secretion.

## MAMMARY GLANDS

Mammary glands are modified sweat glands and first appear as bilateral bands of thickened epidermis called the **mammary lines** or **mammary ridges**. In a 7-week embryo, these lines extend on each side of the body from the base of the forelimb to the region of the hind limb (Fig. 21.5C). Although the major

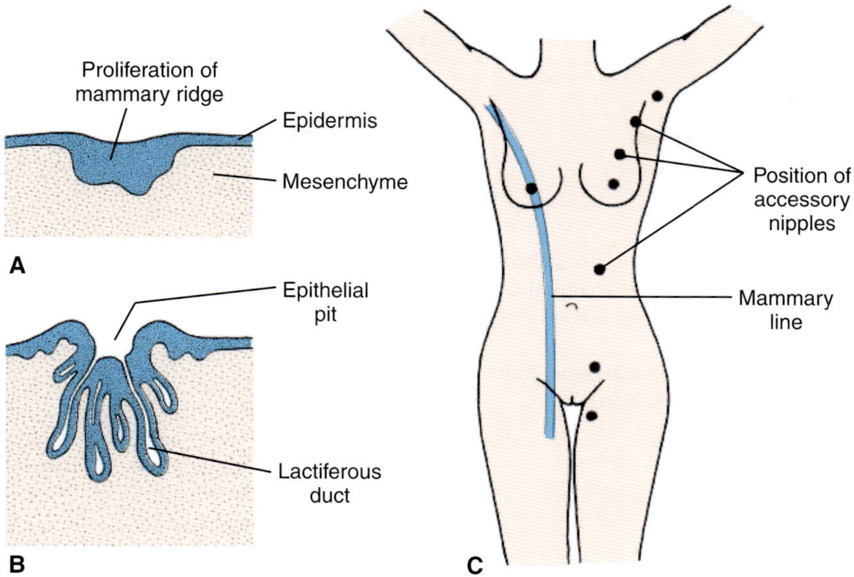


**FIGURE 21.5** **A,B.** Sections through the developing mammary gland at the third and eighth months, respectively. **C.** Positions of accessory nipples (*blue line*, mammary line).

part of each mammary line disappears shortly after it forms, a small portion in the thoracic region persists and penetrates the underlying mesenchyme (see Fig. 21.5*A*). Here it forms 16 to 24 sprouts, which in turn give rise to small, solid buds. By the end of prenatal life, the epithelial sprouts are canalized and form the **lactiferous ducts**. Initially, the **lactiferous ducts** open into a small epithelial pit (Fig. 21.5*B*). Shortly after birth, this pit is transformed into the **nipple** by proliferation of the underlying mesenchyme. At birth, lactiferous ducts have no alveoli and therefore no secretory apparatus. At puberty, however, increased concentrations of estrogen and progesterone stimulate branching from the ducts to form alveoli and secretory cells.

Part 2

## Clinical Correlates

### Mammary Gland Abnormalities

**Polythelia** is a condition in which accessory nipples have formed resulting from the persistence of fragments of the mammary line (Fig. 21.5*C*). Accessory nipples may develop anywhere along the original mammary line (Fig. 21.6) but usually appear in the axillary region.

**Polymastia** occurs when a remnant of the mammary line develops into a complete breast.

**Inverted nipple** is a condition in which the lactiferous ducts open into the original epithelial pit that has failed to evert.

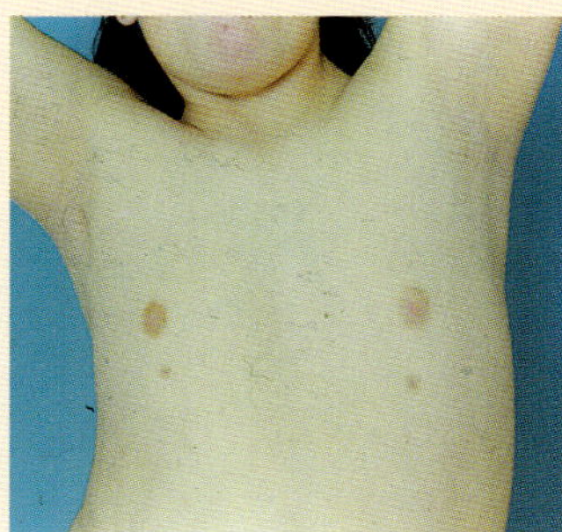

**FIGURE 21.6** Child with bilateral polythelia (supernumerary nipples).


## SUMMARY

- The skin and its associated structures, hair, nails, and glands, are derived from surface ectoderm.
- **Melanocytes**, which give the skin its color, are derived from **neural crest cells**, which migrate into the epidermis.
- The production of new cells occurs in the **germinative** layer. After moving to the surface, cells are sloughed off in the horny layer (Fig. 21.1).
- The **dermis**, the deep layer of the skin, is derived from lateral plate mesoderm (limbs and body wall), from dermatomes that form from somites in paraxial mesoderm (back), and from neural crest cells (face and neck).
- **Hairs** develop from downgrowth of epidermal cells into the underlying dermis. By about 20 weeks, the fetus is covered by downy hair, **lanugo hair**, which is shed at the time of birth.
- **Sebaceous glands**, **sweat glands**, and **mammary glands** all develop from epidermal proliferations.
- Supernumerary nipples (**polythelia**) and breasts (**polymastia**) are relatively common (Figs. 21.5 and 21.6).

## Self-Assessment

### Comprehensive Questions

1. Write briefly on melanocytes.
2. Write briefly on milk ridge.

### Problem Solving Questions

1. A woman appears to have accessory nipples in her axilla and on her abdomen bilaterally. What is the embryological basis for these additional nipples, and why do they occur in these locations?
2. At birth, a new born baby is covered by a whitish paste. What is it called and how is it formed? What is its function?

### Multiple Choice Questions

1. Melanocytes are derived from
   (a) Neural crest
   (b) Ectoderm
   (c) Paraxial mesoderm
   (d) Epidermal ridges
2. Lanugo hair present in newborn sheds at
   (a) One month after birth
   (b) One week after birth
   (c) At birth
   (d) Before birth
3. Mammary glands are modified
   (a) Sebaceous glands
   (b) Sweat glands
   (c) Serous and mucous acinar glands
   (d) Holocrine glands
4. Dermis is a derivative of
   (a) Ectoderm
   (b) Mesoderm
   (c) Endoderm
   (d) Neural crest
5. Vitiligo results due to absence/thinning of
   (a) Stratum corneum
   (b) Stratum spinosum
   (c) Dendritic layer
   (d) Melanocytes

### Answers

1. (a) 2. (c) 3. (b) 4. (b) 5. (d)

# Part 3

# Molecular Regulation and Signaling Pathways

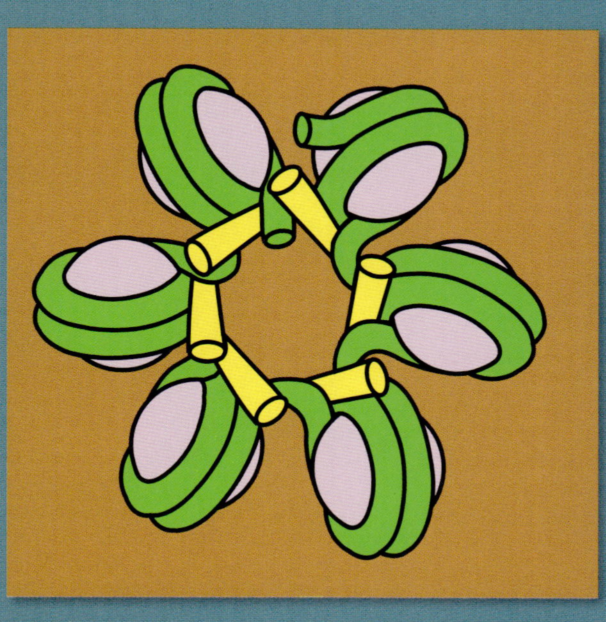

CHAPTER

# 22 Introduction to Molecular Regulation and Signaling

## Specific Learning Objectives

- Gene transcription
- Regulations of gene transcription
- Induction and organ formation
- Cell signaling and signal transduction pathways
  - Paracrine
  - Juxtacrine
- Paracrine signaling factors
  - Fibroblast growth factors
  - Hedgehog proteins
  - WNT proteins
  - TGFβ superfamily
- Important signaling pathways during development
  - Sonic hedgehog (SHH)
  - Planar cell polarity
  - Notch pathway

## Competencies Covered

BI7.1 Describe the structure and functions of DNA and RNA and outline the cell cycle.

BI7.2 Describe the processes involved in replication and repair of DNA and the transcription and translation mechanisms.

BI7.3 Describe gene mutations and the basic mechanism of regulation of gene expression.

Molecular biology has opened the doors to new ways to study embryology and to enhance our understanding of normal and abnormal development. Sequencing the human genome, together with creating techniques to investigate gene regulation at many levels of complexity, has taken embryology to the next level. Thus, from the anatomical to the biochemical to the molecular level, the story of embryology has progressed, and each chapter has enhanced our knowledge.

Embryonic development is directed by **genomes** that contain all of the information required to make an individual. The information is encoded in **DNA** in sequences called **genes** that code for proteins. In turn, proteins regulate expression of other genes and act as signal molecules to orchestrate development. Although initially it was believed that genes are the blueprint for life and they determine our phenotype (genetic determinism), however, the recent concept of epigenetics highlights that our external and internal environment modulate the expression of our genes independent of any change in the nucleotide sequence.

There are approximately 23,000 genes in the human genome, which represents only one-fifth of the number (100,000) predicted prior to completion of the Human Genome Project. Because of various levels of regulation, however, the number of proteins derived from these genes is closer to the original predicted number of genes. What has been disproved is the one gene–one protein hypothesis. Thus, through a variety of mechanisms, a single gene may give rise to many proteins.

Gene expression is a highly regulated process and is regulated at several levels: (1) Different genes may be transcribed, (2) DNA transcribed from a gene may be selectively processed to regulate which RNAs reach the cytoplasm to become messenger RNAs (mRNAs), (3) mRNAs may be selectively translated, (4) proteins made from the mRNAs may be differentially modified , and (5) there are a huge number of noncoding RNA which regulate the expression of genes.

## GENE TRANSCRIPTION

Genes are contained in a complex of DNA and proteins (mostly histones) called **chromatin**, and its basic unit of structure is the **nucleosome** (Fig. 22.1). Each nucleosome is composed of an octamer of **histone proteins** and approximately 140 base pairs of DNA. Nucleosomes themselves are joined into clusters by binding of DNA existing between nucleosomes (**linker DNA**) with other histone proteins (H1 histones; Fig. 22.1). DNA can be tightly coiled. In this inactive state, chromatin appears as beads of nucleosomes on a string of DNA and is referred to as **heterochromatin**. For transcription to occur, this DNA must be uncoiled from the beads. In this uncoiled state, chromatin is referred to as **euchromatin**.

Genes reside within the DNA strand and contain regions called **exons**, which can be translated into proteins, and **introns**, which are interspersed between exons and which are not transcribed into proteins (Fig. 22.2). In addition to exons and introns, a typical gene includes the following: a **promoter**

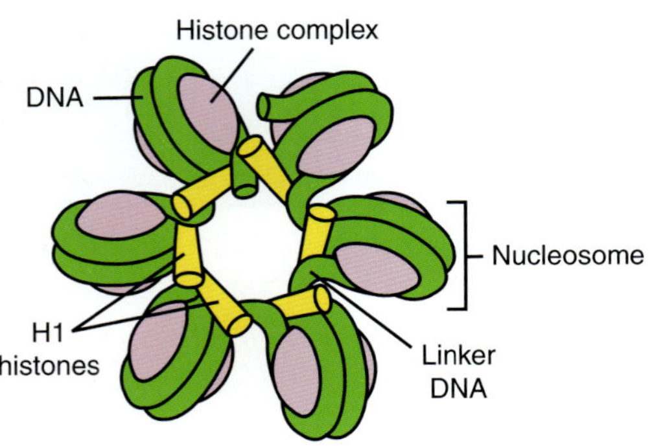


**FIGURE 22.1** Drawing showing nucleosomes that form the basic unit of chromatin. Each nucleosome consists of an octamer of histone proteins and approximately 140 base pairs of DNA. Nucleosomes are joined into clusters by linker DNA and other histone proteins.

**region** that binds **RNA polymerase** for the initiation of **transcription**; a **transcription initiation site**; a **translation initiation site** to designate the first amino acid in the protein; a **translation termination codon**; and a **3′** untranslated region that includes a sequence (the poly A addition site) that assists with stabilizing the mRNA, allows it to exit the nucleus, and permits it to be translated into protein (Fig. 22.2). By convention, the 5′ and the 3′ regions of a gene are specified in relation to the RNA transcribed from the gene. Thus, DNA is transcribed from the 5′ to the 3′ end, and the promoter region is upstream from the transcription initiation site (Fig. 22.2). The promoter region, where the RNA polymerase binds, usually contains the sequence TATA, and this site is called the **TATA box** (Fig. 22.2). In order to bind to this site, however, the polymerase requires additional proteins called **transcription factors** (Fig. 22.3). Transcription factors also have a specific **DNA-binding domain** plus a **transactivating domain** that activates or inhibits transcription of the gene whose promoter or enhancer it has bound. In combination with other proteins, transcription factors activate gene expression by causing the DNA nucleosome complex to unwind, by releasing the polymerase so that it can transcribe the DNA template At least four *cis*-acting DNA elements regulate the initiation of transcription by RNA polymerase II (RNPII). The first of these elements is the core promoter; it determines where RNPII binds to DNA and where it begins copying DNA into RNA. The other three types of regulatory DNA sequences called proximal promoter elements, enhancers, and silencers influence the efficiency or rate of transcription initiation by RNPII from the core promoter element.

**Enhancers** are regulatory elements of DNA that activate utilization of promoters to control their efficiency and the rate of transcription from the promoter. Enhancers can reside anywhere along the DNA strand and do not have to reside close to a promoter. Like promoters, enhancers bind transcription factors (through the transcription factor's transactivating domain) and are used to regulate the timing of a gene's expression and its cell-specific location. For example, separate enhancers in a gene can be used to direct the same gene to be expressed in different tissues. The *PAX6* transcription factor, which participates in pancreas, eye, and neural tube development, contains three separate enhancers, each of which regulates the gene's expression in the appropriate tissue. Enhancers act by altering chromatin to expose the promoter or by facilitating binding of the RNA polymerase.

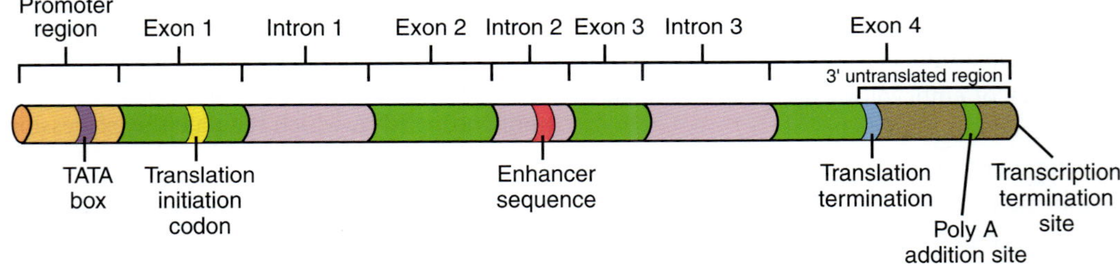


**FIGURE 22.2** Drawing of a "typical" gene showing the promoter region containing the TATA box; exons that contain DNA sequences that are translated into proteins; introns; the transcription initiation site; the translation initiation site that designates the code for the first amino acid in a protein; and the 3′ untranslated region that includes the poly A addition site that participates in stabilizing the mRNA, allows it to exit the nucleus, and permits its translation into a protein.

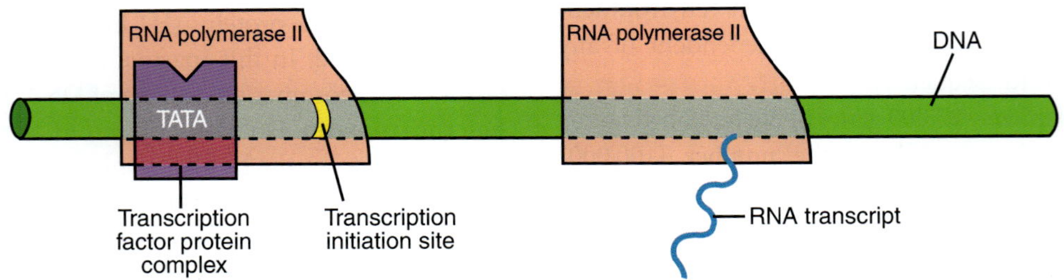


**FIGURE 22.3** Drawing showing binding of RNA polymerase II to the TATA box site of the promoter region of a gene. This binding requires a complex of proteins plus an additional protein called a *transcription factor*. Transcription factors have their own specific DNA-binding domain and function to regulate gene expression.

Sometimes, enhancers can inhibit transcription and are called **silencers**. This phenomenon allows a transcription factor to activate one gene while silencing another by binding to different enhancers. Thus, transcription factors themselves have a DNA-binding domain specific to a region of DNA plus a transactivating domain that binds to a promoter or an enhancer and activates or inhibits the gene regulated by these elements. Complementing the *cis*-acting regulatory sequences are various *trans*-acting factors that facilitate RNPII binding and therefore the initiation of transcription. These proteins are referred to as transcription factors. There are two broad categories of transcription factors, the general transcription factors that are absolutely required for RNPII-mediated transcription and the transcriptional activators and repressors that influence the efficiency or rate of RNPII transcription initiation. These transcription factors (activators and repressors) bind to enhancers and silencer elements and regulate transcription initiation by aiding or preventing the assembly of preinitiation complexes.

### DNA Methylation Represses Transcription

Methylation of cytosine bases in the promoter regions of genes represses transcription of those genes. Thus, some genes are silenced by this mechanism. For example, one of the X chromosomes in each cell of a female is inactivated (**X chromosome inactivation**) by this methylation mechanism. Similarly, genes in different types of cells are repressed by methylation, such that muscle cells make muscle proteins (their promoter DNA is mostly unmethylated) but not blood proteins (their DNA is highly methylated). In this manner, each cell can maintain its characteristic differentiated state. Genomic imprinting responsible for the monoallelic expression of the genes depending on the sex of inheritance is also a mechanism whereby silencing occurs by methylation of cytosine bases clustered at CpG islands at the promoter of genes. Approximately 40 to 60 human genes are imprinted, and their methylation patterns are established during spermatogenesis and oogenesis. Methylation silences DNA by inhibiting binding of transcription factors and is further stabilized by post-translational modification of amino terminal ends of histone proteins forming nucleosomes.

## ■ OTHER REGULATORS OF GENE EXPRESSION

The initial transcript of a gene is called **nuclear RNA (nRNA)** or sometimes **premessenger RNA**. nRNA is longer than mRNA because it contains introns that are removed (**spliced out**) as the nRNA moves from the nucleus to the cytoplasm. In fact, this splicing process provides a means for cells to produce different proteins from a single gene. For example, by removing different introns, exons are "spliced" in different patterns, a process called **alternative splicing** (Fig. 22.4). The process is carried out by **spliceosomes**, which are complexes of **small nuclear RNAs (snRNAs)** and proteins that recognize specific splice sites at the 5′ or the 3′ ends of the nRNA. Proteins derived from the same gene are called **splicing isoforms** (also called **splice variants** or **alternative splice forms**), and these afford the opportunity for different cells to use the same gene to make proteins specific for that cell type. For example, isoforms of the *WT1* gene have different functions in gonadal versus kidney development.

Even after a protein is made (translated), there may be **posttranslational modifications** that affect its function. For example, some proteins have to be cleaved to become active, or they might have to be phosphorylated. Others need to combine with other proteins or be released from sequestered sites or be targeted to specific cell regions. Thus, there are many regulatory levels for synthesizing and activating proteins, such that although only 23,000 genes exist, the potential number of proteins that can be synthesized is probably closer to five times the number of genes.

## ■ INDUCTION AND ORGAN FORMATION

Organs are formed by interactions between cells and tissues. Most often, one group of cells or tissues causes another set of cells or tissues to change their fate, a process called **induction**. In each such interaction, one cell type or tissue is the **inducer** that produces a signal, and one is the **responder** to

Part 3

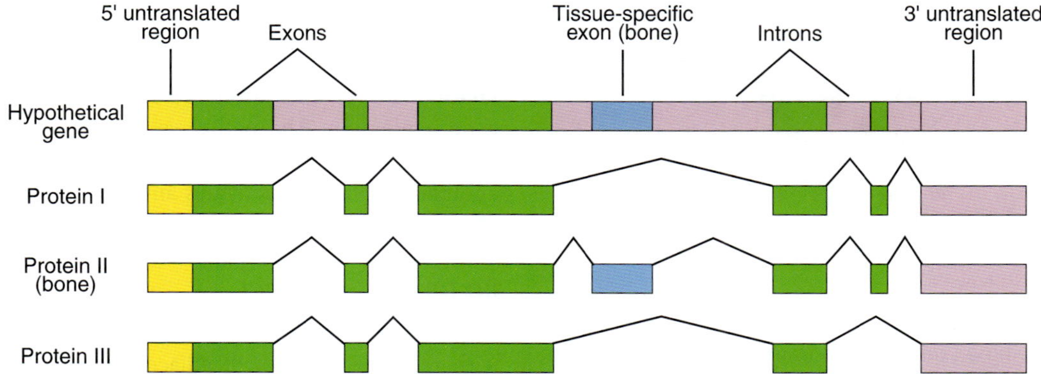


**FIGURE 22.4** Drawing of a hypothetical gene illustrating the process of alternative splicing to form different proteins from the same gene. Spliceosomes recognize specific sites on the initial transcript of nRNA from a gene. Based on these sites, different introns are "spliced out" to create more than one protein from a single gene. Proteins derived from the same gene are called *splicing isoforms*.

that signal. The capacity to respond to such a signal is called **competence**, and competence requires activation of the responding tissue by a **competence factor**. Many inductive interactions occur between epithelial and mesenchymal cells and are called **epithelial–mesenchymal interactions** (Fig. 22.5). Epithelial cells are joined together in tubes or sheets, whereas mesenchymal cells are fibroblastic in appearance and dispersed in extracellular matrices (Fig. 22.5). Examples of epithelial–mesenchymal interactions include the following: gut endoderm and surrounding mesenchyme to produce gut-derived organs, including the liver and pancreas; limb mesenchyme with overlying ectoderm (epithelium) to produce limb outgrowth and differentiation; and endoderm of the ureteric bud and mesenchyme from the metanephric blastema to produce nephrons in the kidney. Inductive interactions can also occur between two epithelial tissues, such as induction of the lens by epithelium of the optic cup. Although an initial signal by the inducer to the responder initiates the inductive event, **crosstalk** between the two tissues or cell types is essential for differentiation to continue (Fig. 22.5, *arrows*). Another feature is the reciprocal nature of several inductive interactions. Once the lens is formed, it can then induce other tissues. One of the responding tissues is the optic vesicle itself. Thus, the inducer becomes the induced. Under the influence of factors secreted by the lens, the optic vesicle becomes the optic cup and the wall of the optic cup further differentiates into neural and pigmented retina. This is known as reciprocal inductions. The ectoderm above it is also being induced to form the cornea. In reciprocal inductions, a structure does not need to be fully differentiated in order to have a function.

**Concept of undifferentiated cells forming a differentiated tissue/organ**

Undifferentiated cells (responder) are induced by another group of cells (inducer) to get differentiated. The process is **induction**.

(Inducer) ⟶ (Responder)

The process of responding by responder and induction by inducer is competence (depends on competency factor).

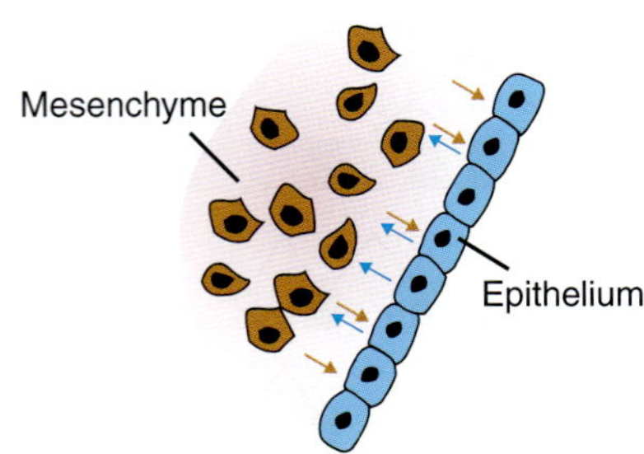


**FIGURE 22.5** Drawing illustrating an epithelial–mesenchymal interaction. Following an initial signal from one tissue, a second tissue is induced to differentiate into a specific structure. The first tissue constitutes the inducer, and the second is the responder. Once the induction process is initiated, signals (*arrows*) are transmitted in both directions to complete the differentiation process.

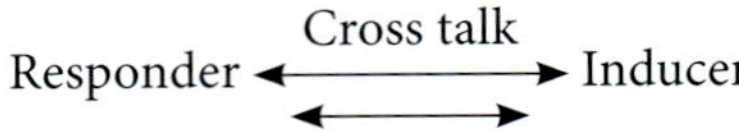


Once induced, there is cross talk (bilateral interaction) between the group of inducer cells and responder cells to form the differentiated organ/tissue.

## CELL SIGNALING

Cell-to-cell signaling is essential for induction, for conference of competency to respond, and for crosstalk between inducing and responding cells. These lines of communication are established by **paracrine interactions**, whereby proteins synthesized by one cell diffuse over short distances to interact with other cells, or by **juxtacrine interactions**, which do not involve diffusable proteins. The diffusable proteins responsible for paracrine signaling are called **paracrine factors** or **growth and differentiation factors (GDFs)**.

### Signal Transduction Pathways

#### *Paracrine Signaling*

When proteins synthesized by one cell can diffuse over small distances to induce changes in the neighboring cells, the event is called paracrine interaction. The diffusible proteins are called paracrine factors or growth and differentiating factors. Paracrine factors act by receptor binding and then initiate a series of enzymatic reactions which regulate transcription factors. Paracrine factors act by **signal transduction pathways** either by activating a pathway directly or by blocking the activity of an inhibitor of a pathway (inhibiting an inhibitor, as is the case with hedgehog signaling). Signal transduction pathways include a **signaling molecule** (the **ligand**) and a **receptor** (Fig. 22.6). The receptor spans the cell membrane and has an **extracellular domain** (the **ligand-binding region**), a **transmembrane domain**, and a **cytoplasmic domain**. When a ligand binds its receptor, it induces a conformational change in the receptor that activates its cytoplasmic domain. Usually, the result of this activation is to confer enzymatic activity to the receptor, and most often, this activity is a **kinase** that can **phosphorylate** other proteins using ATP as a substrate. In turn, phosphorylation activates these proteins to phosphorylate additional proteins, and thus, a cascade of protein interactions is established that ultimately activates a **transcription factor**. This transcription factor then activates or inhibits gene expression. The pathways are numerous and complex and in some cases are characterized by one protein inhibiting another that in turn activates another protein (much like the situation with hedgehog signaling).

#### *Juxtacrine Signaling*

In juxtacrine signaling, proteins from inducing cells interact with receptor proteins of adjacent responding cells without diffusing from the cell producing it. Thus, the inducing proteins remain bound to the inducing cell surface. **Juxtacrine signaling** is mediated through signal transduction pathways

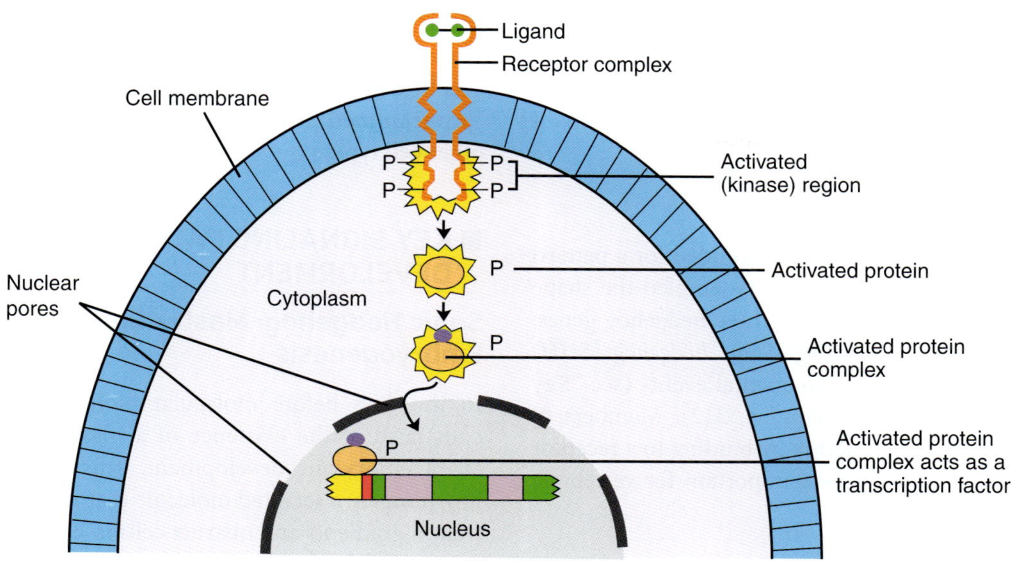


**FIGURE 22.6** Drawing of a typical signal transduction pathway involving a ligand and its receptor. Activation of the receptor is conferred by binding to the ligand. Typically, the activation is enzymatic involving a tyrosine kinase, although other enzymes may be employed. Ultimately, kinase activity results in a phosphorylation cascade of several proteins that activates a transcription factor for regulating gene expression.

as well but does not involve diffusable factors. Instead, there are three ways juxtacrine signaling occurs: (1) A protein on one cell surface interacts with a receptor on an adjacent cell in a process analogous to paracrine signaling (Fig. 22.6). The **Notch pathway** represents an example of this type of signaling (see "Key Signaling Pathways for Development," p. 312). (2) Ligands in the extracellular matrix secreted by one cell interact with their receptors on neighboring cells. The extracellular matrix is the milieu in which cells reside. This milieu consists of large molecules secreted by cells including **collagen**, **proteoglycans** (**chondroitin sulfates**, **hyaluronic acid**, etc.), and **glycoproteins**, such as **fibronectin** and **laminin**. These molecules provide a substrate for cells on which they can anchor or migrate. For example, laminin and type IV collagen are components of the **basal lamina** for epithelial cell attachment, and fibronectin molecules form scaffolds for cell migration. Receptors that link extracellular molecules such as fibronectin and laminin to cells are called **integrins**. These receptors "integrate" matrix molecules with a cell's **cytoskeletal machinery** (e.g., **actin microfilaments**), thereby creating the ability to migrate along matrix scaffolding by using contractile proteins, such as **actin**. Also, integrins can induce gene expression and regulate differentiation as in the case of chondrocytes that must be linked to the matrix to form cartilage. (3) There is direct transmission of signals from one cell to another by **gap junctions**. These junctions occur as channels between cells through which small molecules and ions can pass. Such communication is important in tightly connected cells like epithelia of the gut and neural tube because they allow these cells to act in concert. The junctions themselves are made of **connexin proteins** that form a channel, and these channels are "connected" between adjacent cells.

It is important to note that there is a great amount of redundancy built into the process of signal transduction. For example, paracrine signaling molecules often have many family members such that other genes in the family may compensate for the loss of one of their counterparts. Thus, the loss of function of a signaling protein through a gene mutation does not necessarily result in abnormal development or death. In addition, there is crosstalk between pathways, such that they are intimately interconnected. These connections provide numerous additional sites to regulate signaling.

## Paracrine Signaling Factors

There is a large number of **paracrine signaling factors** acting as ligands, which are also called **GDFs**. Most are grouped into four families, and members of these same families are used repeatedly to regulate development and differentiation of organ systems. Furthermore, the same GDFs regulate organ development throughout the animal kingdom from *Drosophila* to humans. The four groups of GDFs include the **fibroblast growth factor (FGF)**, **WNT**, **hedgehog**, and **transforming growth factor-β (TGF-β)** families. Each family of GDFs interacts with its own family of receptors, and these receptors are as important as the signal molecules themselves in determining the outcome of a signal.

### *Fibroblast Growth Factors*

Originally named because they stimulate the growth of fibroblasts in culture, there are now approximately two dozen **FGF** genes that have been identified, and they can produce hundreds of protein isoforms by altering their RNA splicing or their initiation codons. FGF proteins produced by these genes activate a collection of **tyrosine receptor kinases** called **fibroblast growth factor receptors (FGFRs)**. In turn, these receptors activate various signaling pathways. FGFs are particularly important for angiogenesis, axon growth, and mesoderm differentiation.

Although there is redundancy in the family, such that FGFs can sometimes substitute for one another, individual FGFs may be responsible for specific developmental events. For example, FGF8 is important for development of the limbs and parts of the brain.

### Hedgehog Proteins

The ***hedgehog*** gene was named because it coded for a pattern of bristles on the leg of *Drosophila* that resembled the shape of a hedgehog. In mammals, there are three hedgehog genes: ***desert***, ***Indian***, and ***sonic hedgehog***. *Sonic hedgehog* (*SHH*) is involved in a multitude of developmental events (see "Key Signaling Pathways for Development," p. 312). Members of the hedgehog protein family function by binding to a receptor called Patched. This pathway is very important for vertebrate limb and neural differentiation.

### WNT Proteins

There are at least 15 different **WNT** genes that are related to the segment polarity gene, *wingless* in *Drosophila*. Their receptors are members of the **frizzled family** of proteins. WNT proteins are involved in regulating proliferation of stem cells, regulating limb patterning, midbrain development, and some aspects of somite and urogenital differentiation among other actions. WNT proteins have a lipid molecule covalently bound to them and these hydrophobic molecules are critical for the functioning of WNT proteins and increase their concentration in the cell membrane.

### The TGF-β Superfamily

The **TGF-β** superfamily has more than 30 members and includes the **TGF-βs**, the **bone morphogenetic proteins (BMPs)**, the **activin family**, VgI family, glial-derived neurotrophic factor (GDNF), the **müllerian inhibiting factor (MIF, anti-müllerian hormone)**, and others. The first member of the family, TGF-β1, was isolated from virally transformed cells. TGF-β members are important for extracellular matrix formation, epithelial branching that occurs in lung, kidney, and salivary gland development, and enteric neuron differentiation. The BMP family induces bone formation and is involved in regulating cell division, cell death (apoptosis), and cell migration among other functions.

### Other Paracrine Signaling Molecules

Another group of paracrine signaling molecules important during development are neurotransmitters, including **serotonin, γ-amino butyric acid (GABA), epinephrine**, and **norepinephrine**, that act as ligands and bind to receptors just as proteins do. These molecules are not just transmitters for neurons; they also provide important signals for embryological development. For example, serotonin (5-HT) acts as a ligand for a large number of receptors, most of which are G protein–coupled receptors. Acting through these receptors, 5-HT regulates a variety of cellular functions, including cell proliferation and migration, and is important for establishing laterality, gastrulation, heart development, and other processes during early stages of differentiation. Norepinephrine also acts through receptors and appears to play a role in **apoptosis (programmed cell death)** in the interdigital spaces and in other cell types.

## KEY SIGNALING PATHWAYS FOR DEVELOPMENT

### Sonic Hedgehog: Master Gene for Embryogenesis

In the days before molecular biology, embryologists were convinced of the existence of a master signal that directed all of embryonic development. This signal would act as a **morphogen**, a secreted molecule that would establish concentration gradients and instruct cells in how to become different tissues and organs. Although we now know that there are a multitude of signaling molecules that coordinately regulate development, the protein **SHH** comes closest to being the master morphogen of them all. This protein is involved in development of the vasculature, left–right axis formation, midline, cerebellum, neural patterning, limbs, smooth muscle patterning, heart, gut, pharynx, lungs, pancreas, kidneys, bladder, hair follicles, teeth, thymocytes, inner ear, eyes, and taste buds: a veritable plethora of developmental events. Sonic signaling is via the pathway shown in Figure 22.7. The protein binds to its receptor **Patched (Ptc)**, a protein that normally inhibits the receptor-like protein **Smoothened (Smo)**. Upon binding of SHH to Ptc, Ptc activity is eliminated, the inhibition of Smo is removed, and Smo is activated to, ultimately, upregulate activity of the ***GLI*** family (1 to 3) of transcription factors that control expression of target genes. The specificity of *SHH* expression in different cell types is regulated by multiple enhancer elements acting independently to control *SHH* transcription in different cells and tissues.

The SHH protein has some unique characteristics, including the fact that after translation, it is cleaved and **cholesterol** is added to the C-terminus of its N-terminal domain. It is the addition of cholesterol that links SHH to the plasma membrane. Then, a palmitic acid moiety is added to the N-terminus and SHH becomes fully functional. Its release from the plasma membrane is produced by the transmembrane protein **Dispatched**, and at this point, SHH can establish the concentration gradients characteristic of its action as a morphogen.

### The Planar Cell Polarity: Convergent Extension Pathway

The **planar cell polarity (PCP) pathway** regulates the process of **convergent extension** whereby a tissue becomes longer and narrower (Fig. 22.8*A*). For example, during neural tube formation (neurulation), the neural plate narrows and elongates to form the neural groove between the neural folds. Similarly, during gastrulation, cells move medially and the embryonic axis elongates. Other examples of convergent extension include elongation of the cardiac outflow tract and movement

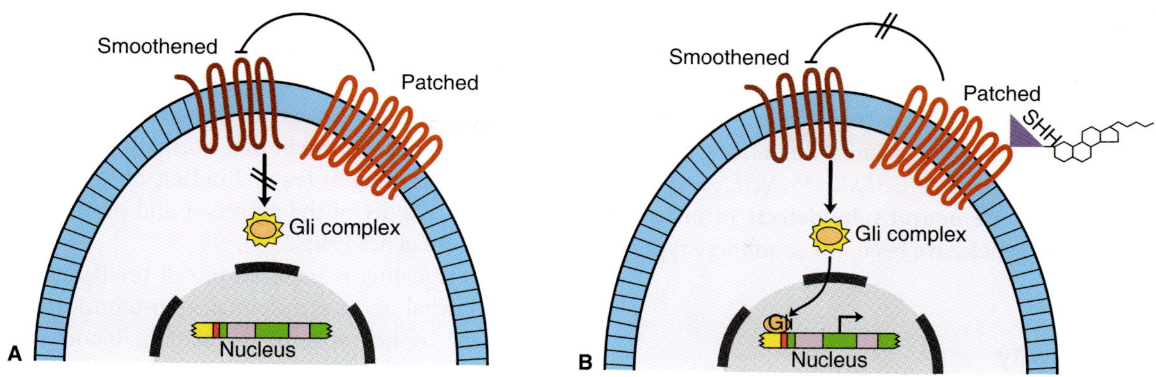


**FIGURE 22.7** Drawings illustrating the sonic hedgehog (SHH) signaling pathway. **A.** Drawing of a cell showing Patched inhibition of Smoothened that blocks activation of the GLI proteins that normally transduce the SHH signal. **B.** Drawing showing SHH binding to its receptor Patched, that removes Patched's inhibition of Smoothened. Activation of Smoothened then upregulates the GLI transcription factors that bind to DNA and control downstream effector genes in the SHH pathway.

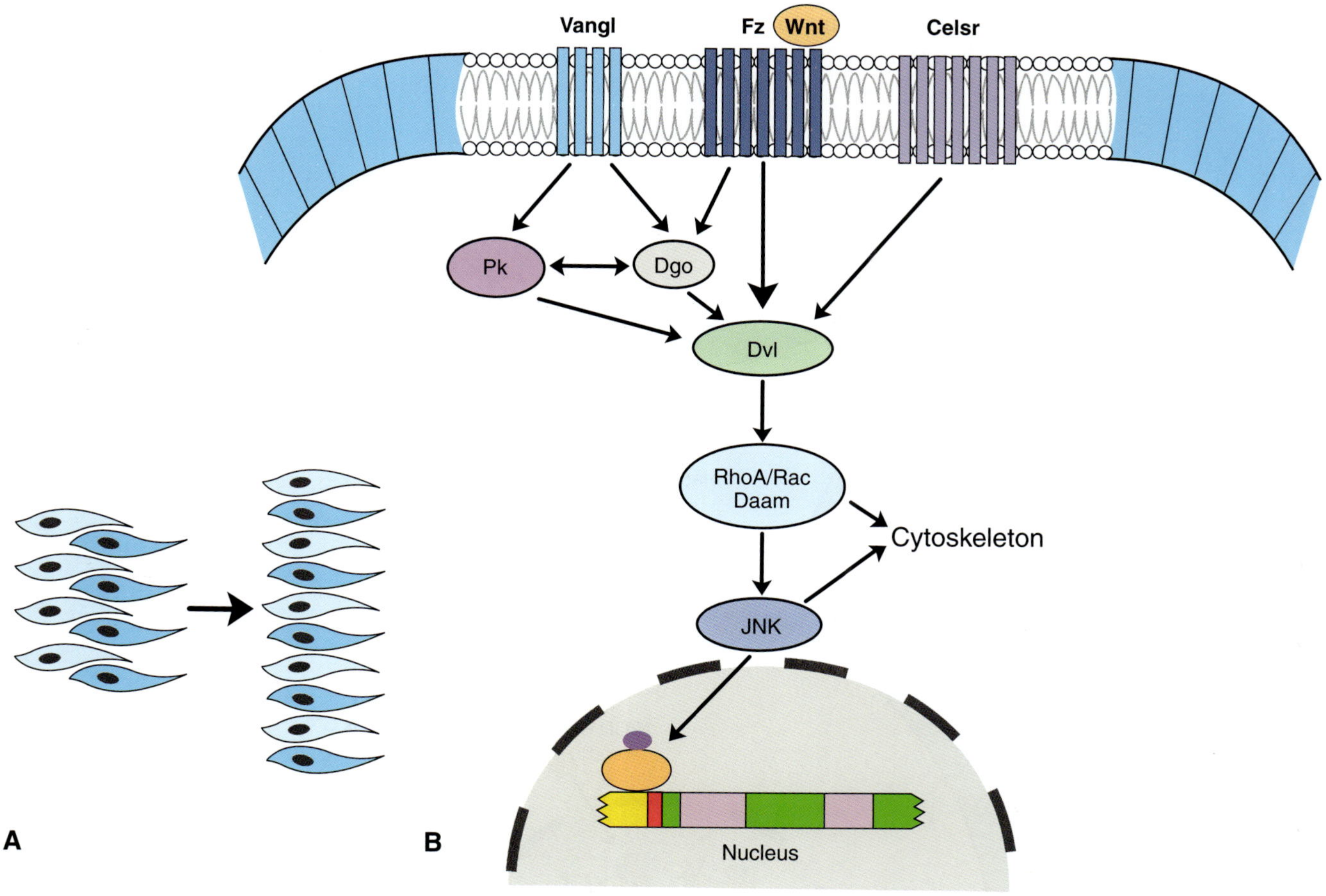

**FIGURE 22.8** **A.** Drawing illustrating the process of convergent extension whereby cells intercalate with their neighbors to increase the long axis of a tissue, such as occurs during lengthening of the neural tube during neurulation. Convergent extension is dependent on the PCP pathway (the reorganization of cells and cell sheets in the plane of a tissue) that is regulated by the noncanonical *WNT* signaling pathway **(B)**. Wnt binds to its receptor Frizzled, which, together with two other transmembrane proteins *Celsr* and *Vangl*, activate *DISHEVELLED*. Dishevelled then acts through *Rho* and *Rac* kinases to upregulate c-Jun N-terminal kinases (*JNK*) that control cytoskeletal changes and downstream effectors, including transcription factors.

of the lateral body wall folds toward the midline. Convergent extension requires changes in cell shape together with cell movement and intercalation with other cells (Fig. 22.8*A*).

PCP refers to the reorganization of cells and cell sheets in the plane of a tissue, such as occurs during convergent extension. The principal PCP signaling pathway is the noncanonical **WNT** pathway, which includes the Wnt receptor **Frizzled (Fz)** and two other transmembrane proteins called **Celsr** and **Vangl** (Fig. 22.8*B*). These transmembrane proteins primarily target activation of *DISHEVELLED (DVL)*, either

Part 3

directly or through downstream effectors, such as Prickle (Pk) and Diego (Dgo). In turn, Dvl regulates signaling via the Rho and Rac kinases to upregulate c-Jun N-terminal kinases (JNK) that control cytoskeletal changes and other downstream effectors including transcription factors. Mutations in many of these genes, including *FZ, CELSR, VANGL,* and *DVL* have been shown to cause **neural tube defects** in mice and mutations in *VANGL* genes have been linked to these types of defects in humans.

## The *Notch* Pathway

**Notch** transmembrane receptors bind to transmembrane ligands of the **DSL (Delta/Serrate/LAG-2)** family, which requires cell-to-cell contact (juxtacrine signaling) for signaling to occur. In mammals, there are four Notch family members and five transmembrane ligands (Jagged 1 and 2 and Delta 1 to 3). Binding of one of these proteins to a Notch receptor causes a conformational change in the Notch protein such that part of it on the cytoplasmic side of the membrane is cleaved. The pathway is very straightforward in that there are no second messengers involved. Thus, the cleaved portion of the protein enters the nucleus directly and binds to a DNA-binding protein that normally represses transcription of Notch target genes. Binding of Notch removes the inhibitory activity of the repressor and permits activation of downstream genes (Fig. 22.9).

*Notch* signaling is involved in cell proliferation, apoptosis, and epithelial to mesenchymal transitions. It is especially important in neuronal differentiation, blood vessel formation and specification (angiogenesis), somite segmentation, pancreatic β-cell development, B- and T-cell differentiation in the immune system, development of inner ear hair cells, and septation of the outflow tract of the heart. Mutations in *JAG1* or *NOTCH2* cause **Alagille syndrome** characterized by cardiac outflow tract defects as well as skeletal, ocular, renal, and hepatic abnormalities. *JAG1* mutations have also been linked to cases of tetralogy of Fallot (a cardiac outflow tract defect).

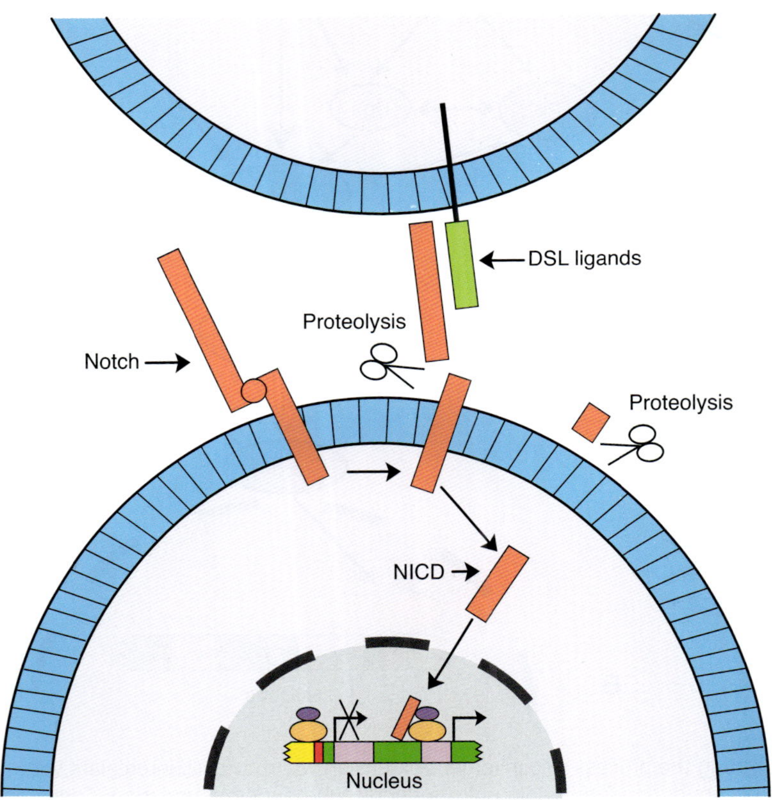


**FIGURE 22.9** Drawing illustrating signaling via the *Notch* pathway. Notch receptors located on one cell bind a ligand from the *DSL* family (Jagged or Serrate) that are located on an adjacent cell (juxtacrine signaling), and this receptor–ligand interaction activates a proteolytic enzyme that cleaves the Notch protein to produce the activated membrane anchored Notch extracellular truncation (NEXT). NEXT is then cleaved by an intracellular secretase enzyme that results in the release of Notch intracellular domain (NICD) that represents the active signaling portion of the original Notch receptor. NICD translocates directly to the nucleus where it binds to transcription repressors and removes their inhibitory activity on downstream target genes of the Notch pathway.

## SUMMARY

- During the past century, embryology has progressed from an observational science to one involving sophisticated technological and molecular advances.
- Observations and modern techniques provide a clearer understanding of the origins of normal and abnormal development and, in turn, suggest ways to prevent and treat birth defects. In this regard, knowledge of gene function has created entire new approaches to the subject.
- There are approximately 23,000 genes in the human **genome**, but these genes code for approximately 100,000 proteins.
- Genes are contained in a complex of DNA and proteins called **chromatin**, and its basic unit of structure is the nucleosome.
- Chromatin appears tightly coiled as beads of nucleosomes on a string and is called **heterochromatin**. For transcription to occur, DNA must be uncoiled from the beads as **euchromatin**.
- Genes reside within strands of DNA and contain regions that can be translated into proteins, called **exons**, and untranslatable regions, called **introns**.
- A typical gene also contains a **promoter region** that binds **RNA polymerase** for the initiation of transcription; a **transcription initiation site**, to designate the first amino acid in the protein; a **translation termination codon**; and a **3′** untranslated region that includes a sequence (the poly A addition site) that assists with stabilization of the mRNA.
- The RNA polymerase binds to the promoter region that usually contains the sequence TATA, the **TATA box**. Binding requires additional proteins called **transcription factors**.
- Methylation of cytosine bases in the promoter region silences genes and reduces gene expression. This process along with histone tail modifications is responsible for **X chromosome inactivation** whereby the expression of genes on one of the X chromosomes in females is silenced and is also the underlying mechanism for genomic **imprinting** in which either a paternal or a maternal gene expression is repressed and there is monoallelic expression of the genes.
- Different proteins can be produced from a single gene by the process of **alternative splicing** that removes different introns using **spliceosomes**. Proteins derived in this manner are called **splicing isoforms** or **splice variants**. Also, proteins may be altered by **posttranslational modifications**, such as phosphorylation or cleavage.
- **Induction** is the process whereby one group of cells or tissues (the **inducer**) causes another group (the **responder**) to change their fate. The capacity to respond is called **competence** and must be conferred by a **competence factor**. Many inductive phenomena involve **epithelial–mesenchymal interactions**.
- **Signal transduction pathways** include a signaling molecule (the **ligand**) and a **receptor**. The receptor usually spans the cell membrane and is activated by binding with its specific ligand. Activation usually involves the capacity to phosphorylate other proteins, most often as a **kinase**. This activation establishes a cascade of enzyme activity among proteins that ultimately activates a transcription factor for initiation of gene expression.
- Cell-to-cell signaling may be **paracrine**, involving **diffusable factors**, or **juxtacrine**, involving a variety of **nondiffusable factors**. Proteins responsible for paracrine signaling are called **paracrine factors** or **GDFs**.
- There are four major families of GDFs: **FGFs**, **WNTs**, **hedgehogs**, and **TGF-βs**.
- In addition to proteins, **neurotransmitters**, such as **serotonin (5-HT)** and **norepinephrine**, also act through paracrine signaling, serving as ligands and binding to receptors to produce specific cellular responses. Juxtacrine factors may include products of the extracellular matrix, ligands bound to a cell's surface, and direct cell-to-cell communications.
- There are many cell signaling pathways important for development, but two key pathways involve the protein **SHH** and the **noncanonical *WNT* pathway**, better known as the **PCP pathway** that regulates **convergent extension**.
  - ***SHH*** is almost a **master gene**, and when this gene's protein product binds to its receptor **patched**, it removes patched's inhibition of **smoothened**. Once activated, smoothened causes upregulation of the ***GLI*** family of transcription factors that control downstream signaling by SHH. SHH is a diffusible factor with a cholesterol molecule bound to it, and it serves as a **morphogen** by establishing concentration gradients that regulate cell responses. SHH signaling is involved in many developmental events, including establishing the midline and left–right asymmetry and in patterning many different organs.
  - The **PCP** regulates movements of cells and sheets of cells in the plane of a tissue, such that the cells intercalate with other cells in such a way that the tissue elongates, a process called **convergent extension**. These types of cell movements are responsible for lengthening the embryo and the neural tube during gastrulation and neurulation, respectively.
- Several genes are involved in regulating this process, including **WNT** and its receptor **FRIZZLED**, ***CELSR***, and ***VANGL*** that code for transmembrane proteins, and ***DISHEVELLED*** that codes for a protein that acts through Rho and Rac kinases to affect the cytoskeleton and other genes regulating cell movements. Mutations in these genes cause neural tube defects in mice, and those involving VANGL have been linked to these defects in humans.
- These pathways have numerous connections and do not function independent of each other. These pathways reinforce each other. Each cell has several receptors and thus each cell receives many signals simultaneously. In addition, a single receptor can activate several different pathways.

## Self-Assessment

### Comprehensive Questions

1. What is meant by "competence to respond" as part of the process of induction? What tissues are most often involved in induction? Give two examples.
2. What is reciprocal induction?
3. Under normal conditions, FGFs and their receptors (FGFRs) are responsible for growth of the skull and development of the cranial sutures. How might these signaling pathways be disrupted? Do these pathways involve paracrine or juxtacrine signaling? Can you think of a way that loss of expression of one FGF might be circumvented?
4. What is genomic imprinting?
5. What is an epithelial–mesenchymal interaction?

### Multiple Choice Questions

1. The number of genes in the human genome is
   (a) 3000
   (b) 13,000
   (c) 23,000
   (d) 33,000
2. In a rapidly dividing cell, the chromatin in nucleus is
   (a) Euchromatic
   (b) Heterochromatic
   (c) Few cells are euchromatic while few are heterochromatic
   (d) No change is seen in the state of chromatin
3. Paracrine signal transduction involves
   (a) Diffusible factors in cell-to-cell signaling
   (b) Nondiffusible factors
   (c) Impermeable factors
   (d) No ligand or receptor is required
4. Planar cell polarity is seen in tissue extension involving
   (a) Lateral folding
   (b) Notochord formation
   (c) Neural tube formation
   (d) Elongation of gut tube
5. Different proteins can be obtained from a gene by a process called
   (a) Induction
   (b) Mutations
   (c) Alternate splicing
   (d) RNA polymerase

### Answers

1. (b) 2. (a) 3. (a) 4. (c) 5. (c)

# Appendix

# Answers to Problem Solving Questions

## Chapter 2

1. Down syndrome is caused by Trisomy 21 in 95% of the cases. This trisomy is caused by nondisjunction of chromosomes during meiosis. 4% of the cases are attributed to unbalanced translocations between chromosome 21 and chromosome 13, 14, 15, or 21. The risk of these chromosomal abnormalities increases in the oocytes of the mother as her age advances thereby resulting in Down syndrome.
2. The parents need to consult the doctor who will investigate for hormones and normal morphology of the female reproductive tract. Genetic analysis for any chromosomal anomaly for any abnormalities like Turner syndrome may need to be performed.
3. Linked genes are the genes that are located on one chromosome, cannot segregate, and are inherited together. Example in humans is the gene for hair and eye color.
4. Prader-Willi syndrome is an example of genomic imprinting where the characteristics depend on whether the genetic material is inherited from mother or the father. Prader-Willi syndrome is a result of microdeletion in the paternal genome on the long arm of chromosome 15: 15q11- 15q13. Hence, it is a structural chromosomal abnormality. All the genes present in this segment undergo deletion. Such sites on the chromosome are called contiguous gene complexes. These can be identified by fluorescence in situ hybridization. The affected individual will show hypotonia, obesity, intellectual disability, hypogonadism, and undescended testis.

## Chapter 3

1. Pelvic inflammatory diseases, such as gonorrhea, are a major cause of occluded oviducts (uterine tubes). Although the patient may be cured, scarring closes the lumen of the tubes and prevents the passage of sperm to the oocyte and of the oocyte to the uterine cavity. IVF can overcome the difficulty by fertilizing the woman's oocytes in culture and transferring them to her uterus for implantation.
2. The couple has no physical or functional problems. For pregnancy, it is essential that the couple has unprotected physical contact during or around the time of ovulation. Ovulation usually occurs during the middle of the menstrual cycle and is usually accompanied by rise in the basal body temperature of the female. Charting the body temperature and noting this rise can be helpful.
3. Emergency contraceptive pills, which are high dose of progestin or in combination with estrogen, have to be taken by the female within 120 hours of unprotected intercourse to prevent pregnancy. Examples: Mifepristone (RU-486) and ulipristal acetate.

## Chapter 4

1. It is not clear why the conceptus is not rejected by the maternal system. Recent evidence suggests that secretion of immunosuppressive molecules, such as cytokines and proteins, and expression of unrecognizable antigens of the major histocompatibility complex protect the conceptus from rejection. In some cases, maternal immunological responses do adversely affect pregnancy, as in some cases of autoimmune disease. Thus, patients with systemic lupus erythematosus have poor reproductive outcomes and histories of multiple spontaneous abortions. It has not been conclusively shown that maternal antibodies can cause birth defects.
2. In some cases, trophoblastic tissue is the only tissue in the uterus, and embryo-derived cells are either absent or present in small numbers. This condition is termed as *hydatidiform mole*, which, because of its trophoblastic origin, secretes human chorionic gonadotropin and mimics the initial stages of pregnancy. Most moles are aborted early in pregnancy, but those containing remnants of an embryo may remain into the second trimester. If pieces of trophoblast are left behind following spontaneous abortion or surgical removal of a mole, cells may continue to proliferate and form tumors known as *invasive moles*, or *choriocarcinoma*. Because early trophoblast development is controlled by paternal genes, it is thought that the origin of moles may be from fertilization of an ovum without a nucleus.
3. The most likely diagnosis is an ectopic pregnancy in the uterine tube, which can be confirmed by ultrasound. Implantation in a uterine tube results from poor transport of the zygote and may be a result of scarring. As with Down syndrome, the frequency of ectopic pregnancy increases with maternal age over 35 years.
4. The earliest method to detect pregnancy is a urine pregnancy test. The syncytiotrophoblast of the placenta starts to secrete human chorionic gonadotrophin in the second week of intrauterine life. By the end of second week, the levels are sufficient enough to be detected in the urine by radioimmunoassay. This is the basis for pregnancy testing.

## Chapter 5

1. Unfortunately, consuming large quantities of alcohol at any stage during pregnancy may adversely affect embryonic development. In this case, the woman has exposed the embryo during the third week of gestation (assuming that fertilization occurred at the midpoint of the menstrual cycle), at the time of gastrulation. This stage is particularly vulnerable to insult by alcohol and may result in fetal alcohol syndrome (intellectual disability, abnormal facies) (see Chapter 9). Although fetal alcohol syndrome is most

common in offspring of alcoholic mothers, no *safe* levels of blood alcohol concentration have been established for embryogenesis. Therefore, because alcohol causes birth defects and is the leading cause of intellectual disability, it is recommended that women who are planning a pregnancy or who are already pregnant refrain from use of any alcohol.

2. Such a mass is probably a sacrococcygeal teratoma. These tumors arise as remnants of the primitive streak, usually in the sacral region. The term *teratoma* refers to the fact that the tumor contains different types of tissues. Because it is derived from the streak, which contains cells for all three germ layers, it may contain tissues of ectoderm, mesoderm, or endoderm origin. Such tumors are three times as common in female fetuses as in male fetuses.
3. The baby has a severe form of caudal dysgenesis called *sirenomelia* (mermaid-like). Sirenomelia, which occurs in varying degrees, is probably caused by abnormalities in gastrulation in caudal segments. It was initially termed *caudal regression*, but it is clear that structures do not regress; they simply do not form. Also known as *caudal agenesis* and *sacral agenesis*, sirenomelia is characterized by varying degrees of flexion, inversion, lateral rotation, and occasional fusion of the lower limbs; defects in lumbar and sacral vertebrae; renal *agenesis*; imperforate anus; and agenesis of internal genital structures except the testes and ovaries. Its cause is unknown. It occurs sporadically but is most frequently observed among infants of diabetic mothers.
4. This patient has left-sided laterality sequence and should be evaluated for additional defects. Sidedness is established at the time of primitive streak formation (gastrulation) and is regulated by genes, such as *NODAL*, and *PITX2* which become restricted in their expression. Partial reversal of left–right asymmetry is more often associated with other defects than complete asymmetry (situs inversus).
5. As you listen to your patient's request to take one of the selective serotonin reuptake inhibitors (SSRIs) medications, you remember the thalidomide tragedy and its lesson that women who are planning to get pregnant or who already are should beware of taking any substance that could be harmful to their unborn baby. Also, you are aware of scientific studies showing that serotonin is an important signaling molecule during embryonic development, especially for establishing the left–right (laterality) axis, and you have read the epidemiological literature that establishes an association between the SSRIs and birth defects. Therefore, you advise your patient not to take the drugs. Instead, you try to get her involved in an exercise program and other social activities that have a similar efficacy as the SSRIs for preventing most levels of depression. Only in severe cases of anxiety and depression might an alternative strategy, including medication be advisable.

## Chapter 6

1. This is a spina bifida type of neural tube defect. This results from the failure of closure of neural tube in the 3rd and 4th week of development. It may be a meningocele (herniation of meninges alone) or a meningomyelocele (herniation of neural tissue along with overlying meninges). Since neural tissue is seen herniating in this case, it is a meningomyelocele. Most commonly involved segments are lumbosacral segments. Consumption of folic acid 400 µg/day routinely and then 4000 µg/day 1 month prior to next conception and continued till first trimester should be recommended in this case to reduce the risk of recurrence in subsequent pregnancies.
2. The probable cause could be intrauterine growth retardation or constitutionally small baby. In the beginning of the third month, the size of the head is maximum in proportion to the body.
3. The cloaca is the endoderm lined terminal part of the hindgut. Its ventral aspect comes in direct contact with the surface ectoderm without any intervening mesoderm. This forms the cloacal membrane. In the 7th week, the urorectal septum descends down to fuse with cloacal membrane and divides it into an anal membrane and a urogenital membrane. The cloacal membrane ruptures in the 7th week creating the anal opening for the hindgut and a ventral opening for the urogenital sinus. Imperforate anus occurs when the anal membrane fails to break down.

## Chapter 7

1. There are two mechanisms explaining the origin of this type of diaphragmatic hernia. First, the esophageal region of the foregut may have failed to lengthen. This growth is necessary to position the stomach in the abdomen. Otherwise, the stomach fails to move into the abdominal region and remains in the thoracic cavity. Second, muscle cells may have failed to migrate into the area of the left pleuroperitoneal membrane, resulting in a weakened area and a subsequent herniation of the stomach back into the pleural cavity. This second mechanism is more common than failure of the esophageal region to grow. The degree of hypoplasia of the lungs resulting from compression by abdominal viscera determines the fate of the infant. Treatment requires surgical repair of the defect and attempts to correct the malformation in utero have been made.
2. The defect is gastroschisis. It occurs because of a weakness in the body wall caused by abnormal closure of the ventral body wall. Because the bowel is not covered by the amnion, it may become necrotic because of exposure to the amniotic fluid. It is also possible for the bowel loops to twist around themselves (volvulus), cutting off their blood supply and producing an infarction. Gastroschisis is not associated with genetic abnormalities and only 15% have other malformations. Therefore, if damage to the bowel is not too extensive, survival rates are good.
3. During the fourth week, the septum transversum, which forms the central tendon of the diaphragm, lies opposite cervical segments three to five (C3–C5). As the embryo grows and the head fold curves ventrally, the position of the septum transversum (diaphragm) shifts caudally into the thoracic cavity. Musculature for the diaphragm is derived from the original cervical segments located at its site of

origin, however. Therefore, because muscle cells always carry the nerve from their site of origin to wherever they migrate, it is the phrenic nerve from C3, C4, and C5 that innervates the diaphragm (C3, C4, and C5 keep the diaphragm alive).

## Chapter 8

1. The expected date of delivery is calculated by adding 40 weeks or 280 days to the first day of the last menstrual period. Therefore, the EDD in this case comes out to be 27th October 2023.
2. An excess of amniotic fluid is called *hydramnios* or *polyhydramnios*, and many times (35%) the cause is unknown (idiopathic). A high incidence (25%) is also associated with maternal diabetes and with birth defects that interfere with fetal swallowing, such as esophageal atresia and anencephaly.
3. No. She is not correct. The placenta does not act as a complete barrier, and many compounds cross freely, especially lipophilic substances, such as toluene and alcohol. Furthermore, early in pregnancy, the placenta is not completely developed, and the embryo is particularly vulnerable. These early weeks are also very sensitive to insult by compounds such as toluene, which causes toluene embryopathy.
4. **Preeclampsia** is the condition in this case, which is characterized by maternal hypertension and proteinuria due to reduced organ perfusion and occurs in approximately 5% of pregnancies. The condition may progress to eclampsia, which is characterized by seizures, In India, toxemia due to eclampsia is responsible for 10% of maternal mortality. Preeclampsia begins suddenly anytime from approximately 20 weeks' gestation to term and may result in fetal growth retardation, fetal death, or death of the mother. In fact, preeclampsia is a leading cause of maternal mortality.
5. An extremely long umbilical cord may encircle the neck of the fetus, usually without increased risk, but sometimes it can cause strangulation and cause fetal death.
6. This is a case of twinning where one twin is lost during the course of pregnancy. The incidence of twinning may be much higher than the number observed at birth because twins are conceived more often than they are born. This case is referred to as **vanishing twin**. This disappearance, which occurs in the first trimester or the early second trimester, may result from resorption or formation of a fetus papyraceus.

## Chapter 9

1. Neural tube defects, such as spina bifida and anencephaly, produce elevated α-fetoprotein (AFP) levels, as do abdominal defects, such as gastroschisis and omphalocele. Maternal serum AFP levels are also elevated, so that they may be used as a screen to be confirmed by amniocentesis. Ultrasonography is used to confirm the diagnosis.
2. Because Down syndrome is a chromosomal abnormality resulting most commonly from trisomy 21 (see Chapter 2), cells or fetal DNA can be collected for genetic analysis. Noninvasive Prenatal Screening (NIPS) procedures include collecting cells and/or cell-free DNA (cfDNA) from maternal blood. A positive result is then confirmed by invasive procedures such as amniocentesis or chorionic villus biopsy. Chorionic villus sampling (CVS) has the advantage that sufficient cells can be obtained immediately to do the analysis, whereas cells collected by amniocentesis, which is not usually done prior to 14 weeks' gestation, must be cultured for approximately 2 weeks to obtain sufficient numbers. The risk of fetal loss following CVS is 1%, which is about twice as high as that of amniocentesis.
3. Status of the fetus is critical for managing pregnancy, delivery, and postnatal care. Size, age, and position are important for determining the time and mode of delivery. Knowing whether birth defects are present is important for planning postnatal care. Tests for determining fetal status are dictated by maternal history and factors that increase risk, such as exposure to teratogens, chromosome abnormalities in either parent, advanced maternal age, or the birth of a previous infant with a birth defect.
4. Factors that influence the action of a teratogen are (1) genotype of the mother and conceptus, (2) dose and duration of exposure to the agent, and (3) stage of embryogenesis when exposure occurs. Most major malformations are produced during the embryonic period (teratogenic period), the third to eighth weeks of gestation. Stages prior to this time, however, including the preimplantation period and after the eighth week (fetal period) remain susceptible. The brain, for example, remains sensitive to insult throughout the fetal period. No stage of pregnancy is free of risk from teratogenic insult.
5. The woman is correct that drugs may be teratogenic. Severe hyperthermia such as this, however, is known to cause neural tube defects (spina bifida and anencephaly) at this stage of gestation. Therefore, one must weigh the risk of teratogenicity of an antipyretic agent with a low teratogenic potential, such as low-dose aspirin, against the risk of hyperthermia. Interestingly, malformations have been associated with sauna-induced hyperthermia. No information about exercise-induced hyperthermia and birth defects is available, but strenuous physical activity (running marathons) raises body temperature significantly and probably should be avoided during pregnancy.
6. Because more than 50% of pregnancies are unplanned, all women of childbearing age should consume 400 μg of folic acid daily as a supplement to prevent neural tube defects. If a woman has not been taking folate and is planning a pregnancy, she should begin the supplement 3 months prior to conception and continue throughout gestation. Folic acid is nontoxic even at high doses, can prevent up to 70% of neural tube defects, and may prevent conotruncal heart defects and facial clefts.
7. The woman's concerns are valid, as infants of insulin-dependent diabetic mothers have an increased incidence of birth defects, including a broad spectrum of minor and major anomalies. Placing the mother under strict metabolic control using multiple insulin injections prior to conception and throughout pregnancy, significantly

reduces the incidence of abnormalities and affords the greatest opportunity for a normal pregnancy. A similar scenario occurs with women who have phenylketonuria. Strict management of these patients' disease prior to conception and during pregnancy virtually eliminates the risk of congenital defects in the offspring. Both situations stress the need for planning pregnancies and for avoiding potential teratogenic exposures, especially during the first 8 weeks of gestation, when most defects are produced.

8. **Valproic acid** increases the risk for several defects, including atrial septal defects (ASD), cleft palate, hypospadias, polydactyly, and craniosynostosis, but the highest risk is for the neural tube defect, spina bifida. An antenatal scan should be done to see the effects before advising to continue or terminate the pregnancy.
9. Hydrops fetalis is a condition in the fetus characterized by an accumulation of excessive fluid or edema of subcutaneous spaces and effusions into body cavities such as pleural and pericardial cavities. It results from fetal anemia caused by maternal antibody response against fetal blood cells. The fetal anemia can have either an immune or a non-immune cause. In this condition, the heart has to pump greater volume of blood to deliver the same amount of oxygen leading to fetal hydrops in most severe cases. Rh negativity is the cause of immune-mediated hydrops fetalis in this case.

## Chapter 10

1. Cranial sutures are fibrous regions between flat bones of the skull. Membranous regions where more than two bones meet are known as *fontanelles*, the largest of which is the anterior fontanelle (soft spot). These sutures and fontanelles permit (1) molding of the head as it passes through the birth canal and (2) growth of the brain. Growth of the skull, which continues after birth as the brain enlarges, is greatest during the first 2 years of life. Premature closure of one or more sutures (craniosynostosis) results in deformities in the shape of the head, depending on which sutures are involved. Craniosynostosis is often associated with other skeletal defects, and evidence suggests that genetic factors are important in the causation (see Table 10.1). Defects of the long bones and digits are often associated with other malformations and should prompt a thorough examination of all systems. Clusters of defects that occur simultaneously with a common cause are called *syndromes*, and limb anomalies, especially of the radius and digits, are common components of such clusters. Diagnosis of syndromes is important in determining recurrence risks and thus in counseling parents about subsequent pregnancies.
2. Formation of the vertebrae is a complex process involving growth and fusion of the caudal portion of one sclerotome with the cranial portion of an adjacent one. Not surprisingly, mistakes occur, and they result in fusions and increases and decreases in the number of vertebrae (Klippel-Feil sequence). In some cases, only half a vertebra forms (hemivertebra), resulting in asymmetry and lateral curvature of the spine (scoliosis). *HOX* (homeobox) genes that pattern the vertebra may have mutations that cause part of one not to form properly. Scoliosis may also be caused by weakness of back muscles.
3. This is a case of achondroplasia which is a type of skeletal dysplasia. The gene affected is *FGFR3*. This disorder has an autosomal dominant inheritance, and 90% cases appear sporadically due to new mutations.
4. The anomaly in this case is cleidocranial dysostosis. In this anomaly, there is late closure of fontanelles and decreased mineralization of cranial sutures. This leads to bossing of frontal, parietal, and occipital bones. The clavicles are often underdeveloped or missing in this condition.
5. This condition is known as scoliosis (lateral bending of vertebral column). The vertebrae develop from the resegmentation of sclerotome portion of somites. In this process, the caudal half of each sclerotome fuses with the cranial part of subsequent sclerotome to form the vertebrae. This patterning is regulated by HOX genes. Sometimes abnormal fusion of sclerotomes may lead to asymmetrical vertebra or half of a vertebra may be missing. Such defects lead to scoliosis.
6. Spina bifida results from the failure of closure of neural tube anywhere from the cervical region to the caudal region during the 3rd and 4th week of development. Most commonly involved segments are lumbosacral segments. It may be of two types: spina bifida occulta or cystica. In spina bifida occulta, spinal cord is intact with unfused vertebral arches but covered with skin whereas in spina bifida cystica, meninges alone or with neural tissue may protrude through the vertebral defect. The herniation of meninges alone is called meningocele and herniation of meninges with neural tissue is called meningomyelocele. Rachischisis is a severe type of neural tube defect where there the neural folds remain as a flattened mass of primitive neural tissue. It can be diagnosed antenatally by ultrasound and by detection of alpha-feto protein levels in maternal serum and amniotic fluid. To reduce the occurrence of these defects, all women are advised to consume 400 μg of folic acid per day starting from one month prior to conception and to continue throughout pregnancy. A woman with a history of neural tube defect must take 400 μg folic acid/day routinely and then 4000 μg/day 1 month prior to next conception and continued till first trimester.

## Chapter 11

1. There is absence of the pectoralis minor and partial or complete absence of the pectoralis major muscle. The defect known as *Poland anomaly* is the most likely diagnosis. Poland anomaly is often associated with shortness of the middle digits (brachydactyly) and digital fusion (syndactyly). Loss of the pectoralis major muscle produces little or no loss of function because other muscles compensate. The defect's disfiguring characteristics can be quite concerning, however, especially in females.
2. Innervation for muscles is derived from the vertebral level from which the muscle cells originate, and this relation is

maintained regardless of where the muscle cells migrate. Thus, myoblasts forming the diaphragm originate from cervical segments 3, 4, and 5, migrate to the thoracic region, and carry their nerves with them.

3. This is a case of muscular dystrophy. Since all the male children are affected but the female offspring is healthy, this is Duchenne muscular dystrophy which is an X-linked recessive disease. There is progressive muscular wasting and weakness due to mutation in the gene for dystrophin, a muscle protein. The family has to be counseled to go for a genetic testing to confirm the diagnosis followed by physical rehabilitation of the affected children.

## Chapter 12

1. Defects of the long bones and digits are often associated with other malformations and should prompt a thorough examination of all systems. Clusters of defects that occur simultaneously with a common cause are called *syndromes*, and limb anomalies, especially of the radius and digits, are common components of such clusters. Diagnosis of syndromes is important in determining recurrence risks and thus in counseling parents about subsequent pregnancies.
2. **Marfan syndrome** is caused by mutations in the ***FIBRILLIN* (*FBN1*)** gene located on chromosome 15q21.1. Affected individuals are usually tall and slender with long thin limbs and a long thin face. Other characteristics include sternal defects (pectus excavatum or carinatum), joint hyperflexibility, dilatation and/or dissection of the ascending aorta, and dislocation of the lens of the eye.

## Chapter 13

1. A four-chambered view is sought in ultrasound scans of the heart. The chambers are divided by the atrial septum superiorly, the ventricular septum inferiorly, and the endocardial cushions surrounding the atrioventricular canals laterally. Together, these structures form a cross with integrity readily visualized by ultrasound. In this case, however, the fetus probably has a ventricular septal defect, the most commonly occurring heart malformation, in the membranous portion of the septum. The integrity of the great vessels should also be checked carefully because the conotruncal septum dividing the aortic and pulmonary channels must come into contact with the membranous portion of the interventricular septum for this structure to develop normally.
2. Because neural crest cells contribute to much of the development of the face and to the conotruncal septum, these cells have probably been disrupted. Crest cells may have failed to migrate to these regions, failed to proliferate, or may have been killed. Retinoic acid (vitamin A) is a potent teratogen that targets neural crest cells among other cell populations. Because retinoids are effective in treating acne, which is common in young women of childbearing age, great care should be employed before prescribing the drug to this cohort.
3. Endocardial cushion tissue is essential for proper development of these structures. In the common atrioventricular canal, the superior, the inferior, and two lateral endocardial cushions divide the opening and contribute to the mitral and tricuspid valves in the left and right atrioventricular canals. In addition, the superior and inferior cushions are essential for complete septation of the atria by fusion with the septum primum and of the ventricles by forming the membranous part of the interventricular septum. Cushion tissue in the conus and truncus forms the conotruncal septum, which spirals down to separate the aorta and pulmonary channels and to fuse with the inferior endocardial cushion to complete the interventricular septum. Therefore, any abnormality of cushion tissue may result in a number of cardiac defects, including atrial and ventricular septal defects, transposition of the great vessels, and other abnormalities of the outflow tract.
4. In the development of the vascular system for the head and neck, a series of arterial arches forms around the pharynx. Most of these arches undergo alterations, including regression, as the original patterns are modified. Two such alterations that produce difficulty swallowing are (1) double aortic arch, in which a portion of the right dorsal aorta (that normally regresses) persists between the seventh intersegmental artery and its junction with the left dorsal aorta, creating a vascular ring around the esophagus, and (2) right aortic arch, in which the ascending aorta and the arch form on the right. If in such cases the ligamentum arteriosum remains on the left, it passes behind the esophagus and may constrict it.
5. **Tetralogy of Fallot** is the most frequently occurring abnormality of the **conotruncal** region due to an unequal division of the conus resulting from anterior displacement of the conotruncal septum. Displacement of the septum produces four cardiovascular alterations: (1) a narrow right ventricular outflow region, **pulmonary infundibular stenosis**; (2) a large defect of the interventricular septum; (3) an overriding aorta that arises directly above the septal defect; and (4) hypertrophy of the right ventricular wall because of higher pressure on the right side.

## Chapter 14

1. This infant most likely has some type of tracheoesophageal atresia with or without a tracheoesophageal fistula. The baby cannot swallow, and this condition results in polyhydramnios. The defect is caused by abnormal partitioning of the trachea and esophagus by the tracheoesophageal septum. These defects are often associated with other malformations, including a constellation of vertebral anomalies, anal atresia, cardiac defects, renal anomalies, and limb defects known as the *VACTERL association*.
2. There is insufficient production of surfactant in neonates born prematurely. Surfactant is necessary for reducing surface tension between air–blood surfaces in the alveoli permitting normal lung function. Alveoli collapse due to deficiency of surfactant in preterm neonates resulting in

respiratory distress syndrome. Administration of steroids during pregnancy and use of artificial surfactants can improve the prognosis for these infants.

3. This is a case of congenital diaphragmatic hernia due to defect in the development of the diaphragm. The diaphragm develops from the following sources: Septum transversum (central tendon), pleuroperitoneal membranes, somites of 3rd to 5th cervical segments (muscular part), and dorsal mesentery of the esophagus (crura of diaphragm). Failure of pleuroperitoneal membranes to close the pericardioperitoneal canals results in diaphragmatic hernia. The pleural and peritoneal cavities are communicating with each other allowing abdominal viscera, mostly coils of small intestine to herniate into the thorax. If the defect is huge, part of liver, stomach, or spleen can also herniate. This results in reduced space for the lungs to develop and they become hypoplastic.

   Most common is the Bochdalek's hernia (90% cases) where there is a defect in the posterolateral part usually on the left side. As a result, the heart is also shifted to the right side. Musculoskeletal deformities such as scoliosis may also be seen due to mechanical effects.

## Chapter 15

1. The baby most likely has some type of esophageal atresia and/or tracheoesophageal fistula. In 90% of these cases, the proximal part of the esophagus ends in a blind pouch, and a fistula connects the distal part with the trachea. Polyhydramnios results because the baby cannot swallow amniotic fluid. Aspiration of fluids at birth may cause pneumonia. The defect is caused by an abnormal partitioning of the respiratory diverticulum from the foregut by the tracheoesophageal septum.
2. The most likely diagnosis is an omphalocele resulting from a failure of herniated bowel to return to the abdominal cavity at 10 to 12 weeks of gestation. Because the bowel normally herniates into the umbilical cord, it is covered by amnion. This situation is in contrast to gastroschisis, in which loops of bowel herniate through an abdominal wall defect and are not covered by amnion. The prognosis is not good because 25% of infants with omphalocele die before birth, 40% to 88% have associated anomalies, and approximately 15% show chromosomal abnormalities. If no other complicating defects are present, surgical repair is possible, and in experienced hands, survival is 100%.
3. This infant has an imperforate anus with a rectovaginal fistula, part of an anorectal atresia complex. She appears to have a high anorectal atresia because the fistula connects the rectum to the vagina, accounting for meconium (intestinal contents) in this structure. The defect was probably caused by a cloaca that was too small, so that the cloacal membrane was shortened posteriorly. This condition causes the opening of the hindgut to shift anteriorly. The smaller the cloaca is posteriorly, the farther anteriorly the hindgut opening shifts, resulting in a higher defect.

## Chapter 16

1. The three systems to form are the pronephros, mesonephros, and metanephros—all derivatives of the intermediate mesoderm. They form in succession in a cranial-to-caudal sequence. Thus, the pronephros forms in cervical segments at the end of the third week but is rudimentary and rapidly regresses. The mesonephros, which begins early in the fourth week, extends from thoracic to upper lumbar regions. It is segmented in only its upper portion and contains excretory tubules that connect to the mesonephric (Wolffian) duct. This kidney also regresses but may function for a short time. It is more important because the tubules and collecting ducts contribute to the genital ducts in the male. Collecting ducts near the testes form the efferent ductules, whereas the mesonephric duct forms the epididymis, ductus deferens, and ejaculatory duct. In the female, these tubules and ducts degenerate because maintaining them depends on testosterone production. The metanephros lies in the pelvic region as a mass of unsegmented mesoderm (metanephric blastema) that forms the definitive kidneys. Ureteric buds grow from the mesonephric ducts and, on contact with the metanephric blastema, induce it to differentiate. The ureteric buds form collecting ducts and ureters, whereas the metanephric blastema forms nephrons (excretory units), each of which consists of a glomerulus (capillaries) and renal tubules.
2. Both the ovaries and testes develop in the abdominal cavity from intermediate mesoderm along the urogenital ridge. Both also descend by similar mechanisms from their original position, but the uterus prevents migration of the ovary out of the abdominal cavity. In the male, however, a mesenchymal condensation, the gubernaculum (which also forms in females but attaches to the uterus), attaches the caudal pole of the testis, first to the inguinal region and then to the scrotal swellings. Growth and retraction of the gubernaculum, together with increasing intra-abdominal pressure, cause the testis to descend. Failure of these processes causes undescended testes, known as *cryptorchidism*. Approximately 2% to 3% of term male infants have an undescended testicle, and in 25% of these, the condition is bilateral. In many cases, the undescended testis descends by age 1 year. If it does not, testosterone administration (because this hormone is thought to play a role in descent) or surgery may be necessary. Fertility may be affected if the condition is bilateral.
3. Male and female external genitalia pass through an indifferent stage during which it is impossible to differentiate between the two sexes. Under the influence of testosterone, these structures assume a masculine appearance, but the derivatives are homologous between males and females. These homologies include (1) the clitoris and penis, derived from the genital tubercle; (2) the labia majora and scrotum, derived from the genital swellings that fuse in the male; and (3) the labia minora and penile urethra, derived from the urethral folds that fuse in the male. During early stages, the

genital tubercle is larger in the female than in the male, and this has led to misidentification of sex by ultrasound.

4. The uterus is formed by fusion of the lower portions of the paramesonephric (Müllerian) ducts. Numerous abnormalities have been described; the most common consists of two uterine horns (bicornuate uterus). Complications of this defect include difficulties in becoming pregnant, high incidence of spontaneous abortion, and abnormal fetal presentations. In some cases, a part of the uterus has a blind end (rudimentary horn), causing problems with menstruation and abdominal pain.

## Chapter 17

1. Neural crest cells are important for craniofacial development because they contribute to so many structures in this region. They form all of the bones of the face and the anterior part of the cranial vault and the connective tissue that provides patterning of the facial muscles. They also contribute to cranial nerve ganglia, meninges, dermis, odontoblasts, and stroma for glands derived from pharyngeal pouches. In addition, crest cells from the hindbrain region of the neural folds migrate ventrally to participate in septation of the conotruncal region of the heart into aortic and pulmonary vessels. Unfortunately, crest cells appear to be vulnerable to a number of compounds, including alcohol and retinoids, perhaps because they lack catalase and superoxide dismutase enzymes that scavenge toxic-free radicals. Many craniofacial defects result from insults on neural crest cells and may be associated with cardiac abnormalities because of the contribution of these cells to heart morphogenesis.
2. The child may have DiGeorge anomaly, which is characterized by these types of craniofacial defects and partial or complete absence of thymic tissue. Loss of thymic tissue compromises the immune system, resulting in numerous infections. Damage to neural crest cells is the most likely cause of the sequence because these cells contribute to development of all of these structures, including the stroma of the thymus. Teratogens, such as alcohol, have been shown to cause these defects experimentally.
3. Children with midline clefts of the lip often have intellectual disabilities. Median clefts are associated with loss of other midline structures, including those in the brain. In its extreme form, the entire cranial midline is lost, and the lateral ventricles of the cerebral hemispheres are fused into a single ventricle, a condition called *holoprosencephaly*. Midline clefts, induced as the cranial neural folds begin to form (approximately days 19 to 21), result from the loss of midline tissue in the prechordal plate region.
4. The child most likely has a thyroglossal cyst that results from incomplete regression of the thyroglossal duct. These cysts may form anywhere along the line of descent of the thyroid gland as it migrates from the region of the foramen cecum of the tongue to its position in the neck. A cyst must be differentiated from ectopic glandular tissue, which may also remain along this pathway.
5. This condition is an oblique facial cleft formed due to the failure of maxillary prominence along the line of the nasolacrimal groove. As a result the nasolacrimal groove is exposed and can lead to purulent discharge.

## Chapter 18

1. A spinal tap is performed between vertebra L4 and vertebra L5 because the spinal cord ends at the L2–L3 level. Thus, it is possible to obtain cerebrospinal fluid at this level without damaging the cord. The space is created because after the third month, the cord, which initially extended the entire length of the vertebral column, does not lengthen as rapidly as the dura and vertebral column do, so that in the adult, the spinal cord ends at the L2–L3 level.
2. Anencephaly is the result of failure of closure in the cephalic part of neural tube. This condition leads to nonformation of cranial vault of skull leaving the malformed brain exposed to the exterior which later degenerates into necrotic mass. Anencephaly is incompatible with life. There is a risk of recurrence of a neural tube defect in future pregnancies as well. Antenatal folic acid therapy is a great preventive measure leading to reduced risk of anencephaly in all pregnancies and especially in cases with history of neural tube defects. Diagnosis of anencephaly can be made on USG as early as 10 weeks. In case of this female, since she has already had a baby with NTD, she should consume 400 µg folic acid daily. Later, when she plans a pregnancy, she should increase it to 4000 µg per day beginning at least 1 month before conception and continuing through the first trimester.
3. Arnold-Chiari malformation is the caudal displacement and herniation of cerebellum through foramen magnum, which obstructs the flow of cerebrospinal fluid and causes the hydrocephalus. Herniation of the cerebellum occurs because the spinal cord is tethered to the vertebral column due to its abnormal development. As the vertebral column lengthens, tethering of the cord pulls the cerebellum into the foramen magnum, cutting off the flow of cerebrospinal fluid.
4. This condition, hydrocephalus, results from a blockage in the flow of cerebrospinal fluid from the lateral ventricles through the foramina of Monro and the cerebral aqueduct into the fourth ventricle and out into the subarachnoid space, where it would be resorbed. In most cases, blockage occurs in the cerebral aqueduct in the midbrain. It may result from genetic causes (X-linked recessive) or viral infection (toxoplasmosis, cytomegalovirus).
5. The autonomic nervous system is composed of the sympathetic and parasympathetic systems. The sympathetic portion has its preganglionic neurons located in the intermediate horn of the spinal cord from T1–L2. The parasympathetic portion has a craniosacral origin with its preganglionic neurons in the brain and spinal cord (S2–S4). The cranial outflow is carried by cranial nerves III, VII, IX, and X. Postganglionic cell bodies for both systems are derived from neural crest cells.
6. It refers to a spectrum of anomalies where there is incomplete development of midline structures involving brain

and face. The lateral ventricles are fused, the eyes are close together, or fused. There is a single nasal chamber. The olfactory bulbs, tracts, and corpus callosum may be absent. There may be a single central incisor. There are several genetic causes for holoprosencephaly. Most common include: mutation in Sonic Hedgehog gene, defective cholesterol synthesis (Smith–Lemli–Opitz syndrome), mutation in SIX3, TGIF, and zinc finger protein ZIC2.

## Chapter 19

1. A placode is a region of cuboidal ectoderm that thickens by assuming a columnar shape. The otic placodes form on both sides of the hindbrain and then invaginate to form otic vesicles. Placodes give rise to sensory organs, and the otic placodes are no exception. Thus, from the otic vesicle, tubular outpocketings form and differentiate into the saccule, utricle, semicircular canals, and the endolymphatic and cochlear ducts. Together, these structures constitute the membranous labyrinth of the internal ear.
2. The tympanic (middle ear) cavity is derived from the first pharyngeal pouch and therefore is lined by endoderm. The pouch expands laterally to incorporate the ear ossicles and create the middle ear cavity, whereas the medial portion lengthens to form the auditory tube that maintains an open connection to the pharynx. The tympanic membrane (eardrum) forms when ectoderm cells on the surface of the first pharyngeal arch invaginate to form the external auditory meatus and canal. As the ectoderm invaginates toward the middle ear cavity, mesenchyme between the invaginating cells and endoderm lining the cavity becomes very thin. Thus, the tympanic membrane is formed between the external auditory meatus and the underlying middle ear cavity and it is comprised of three layers: (1) ectoderm and (2) mesenchyme from the first pharyngeal arch and (3) endoderm from the first pharyngeal pouch when this structure forms the middle ear cavity.
3. Microtia involves defects of the external ear that range from small but well-formed ears to absence of the ear (anotia). Other defects occur in 20% to 40% of children with microtia or anotia, including the oculoauriculovertebral spectrum (hemifacial microsomia), in which case the craniofacial defects may be asymmetrical. Because the external ear is derived from hillocks on the first two pharyngeal arches, which are largely formed by neural crest cells, this cell population plays a role in most external ear malformations.

## Chapter 20

1. The lens forms from a thickening of ectoderm (lens placode) adjacent to the optic cup. Lens induction may begin very early, but contact with the optic cup plays a role in this process as well as in maintenance and differentiation of the lens. Therefore, if the optic cup fails to contact the ectoderm or if the molecular and cellular signals essential for lens development are disrupted, a lens will not form.
2. Rubella is known to cause cataracts, microphthalmia, congenital deafness, and cardiac malformations. Exposure during the fourth to eighth week places the offspring at risk for one or more of these birth defects.
3. As the optic cup reaches the surface ectoderm, it invaginates, and along its ventral surface, it forms a fissure that extends along the optic stalk. It is through this fissure that the hyaloid artery reaches the inner chamber of the eye. Normally, the distal portion of the hyaloid artery degenerates, and the choroid fissure closes by fusion of its ridges. If this fusion does not occur, colobomas occur. These defects (clefts) may occur anywhere along the length of the fissure. If they occur distally, they form colobomas of the iris; if they occur more proximally, they form colobomas of the retina, choroid, and optic nerve, depending on their extent. Mutations in *PAX2* can cause optic nerve colobomas and may be responsible for other types as well. Also, mutations in this gene have been linked to renal defects and renal coloboma syndrome.

## Chapter 21

1. Mammary gland formation begins as budding of epidermis into the underlying mesenchyme. These buds normally form in the pectoral region along a thickened ridge of ectoderm, the mammary or milk line. This line or ridge extends from the axilla into the thigh on both sides of the body. Occasionally, accessory sites of epidermal growth occur, so that extra nipples (polythelia) and extra breasts (polymastia) appear. These accessory structures always occur along the milk line and usually in the axillary region. Similar conditions also occur in males.
2. At birth, the skin is covered by a whitish paste, the **vernix caseosa**, formed by secretions from sebaceous glands and degenerated epidermal cells and hairs. It protects the skin against the macerating action of amniotic fluid.

# Assessing Learning Outcomes

*Essential questions which address the learning outcomes of a competent medical undergraduate are presented below:*

## Write short notes on the following topics:

1. Differences between embryonic and adult stem cells
2. Steps and results of fertilization
3. Capacitation
4. Ectopic pregnancy
5. Anatomical basis of contraception
6. Hormonal control during phases of the menstrual cycle
7. Amniotic cavity
8. Primitive streak
9. Notochord
10. Gastrulation
11. Neural tube formation/Neurulation
12. Placental barrier structure and function
13. Types of placenta
14. Placental circulation
15. Chorionic villi and their functions
16. Umbilical cord
17. Twinning
18. Formation and derivatives of somites
19. Development of body cavities
20. Development of diaphragm
21. Development of atrial and ventricular septum
22. Fetal circulation
23. Circulatory changes at birth
24. Development of diaphragm
25. Development of tongue and its innervation
26. Pharyngeal arches
27. Development of thyroid
28. Cloaca
29. Rotation of midgut
30. Development of IVC
31. Portal vein
32. Optic placode
33. Otic placode
34. Development of pituitary
35. Development of adrenal

## Enumerate the following:

1. Derivatives of notochord
2. Derivatives of yolk sac
3. Derivatives of alar plate
4. Derivatives of endocardial cushion
5. Abnormal implantation sites
6. Derivatives of neural crest
7. Derivatives of ectoderm, endoderm, and mesosderm
8. Derivatives of foregut, mid gut, and hind gut
9. Skeletal/muscular derivatives of pharyngeal arches
10. Derivatives of pharyngeal pouch/clefts
11. Adult derivatives of ventral mesogastrium
12. Adult derivatives of mesonephric duct in males and females
13. Derivatives of paramesonephric duct in females and males

## Write embryological basis of the following anomalies and mention their causes:

1. Chromosomal abnormalities: Down's, Klinefelter's, Turner's, Trisomy 13 and 18
2. Meningocele
3. Meningomyelocele
4. Spine bifida
5. Anencephaly
6. Hydrocephalus
7. Diaphragmatic hernia
8. Atrial septal defects
9. Fallot's tetralogy
10. Patent ductus arteriosus
11. Retroesophageal subclavian artery
12. Tracheoesophageal fistula
13. Respiratory distress syndrome
14. Annular pancreas
15. Meckel's diverticulum/vitellointestinal duct
16. Malrotation of gut
17. Subhepatic cecum
18. Omphalocele
19. Polycystic kidney
20. Horse shoe kidney
21. Double ureter
22. Retrocaval ureter
23. Hypospadias and epispadias
24. Bicornuate uterus
25. Undescended testis
26. Branchial cyst
27. Cervical sinus
28. Lingual thyroid
29. Thyroglossal cyst
30. Cleft palate and lip
31. Oblique facial cleft
32. De George's syndrome

# Glossary of Key Terms

## A

**Abaxial domain** Mesodermal domain composed of the parietal layer of lateral plate mesoderm and somite cells from the myotome and sclerotome regions that migrate across the lateral somitic frontier.

**Acrosome reaction** Release of enzymes from the acrosome on the head of sperm that assists in sperm penetration of the zona pellucida. Zona proteins induce the reaction following sperm binding.

**Adenohypophysis** Anterior portion of the pituitary derived from Rathke pouch.

**Alar plates** Sensory area in the dorsal region of the spinal cord and brain.

**Allantois** Vestigial structure that serves as a respiratory and waste storage organ for avian embryos. It extends from the ventral region of the urogenital sinus to the umbilicus. Later, its distal portion, called the *urachus*, becomes a fibrous cord and forms the median umbilical ligament. If it remains patent, then it may form a urachal fistula or cyst in this region.

**Alternative splicing** Process of removing ("splicing out") introns to create different proteins from the same gene.

**Alveolar cells** Cells lining the alveoli. Type I cells are involved in gas exchange. Type II cells produce surfactant.

**Amelia** Complete absence of a limb.

**Amniocentesis** Procedure used to withdraw amniotic fluid for analysis of factors, such as $\alpha$-fetoprotein (AFP) and cells (chromosomes), which provide information about the status of the fetus.

**Amniochorionic membrane** Membrane formed when expansion of the amniotic cavity obliterates the chorionic cavity causing the amnion to contact the chorion and the two to fuse. The amniochorionic membrane serves as a hydrostatic wedge during the initiation of labor.

**Amnion** Membrane derived from the epiblast that surrounds the fluid-filled amniotic cavity around the embryo and fetus. The fluid cushions the fetus and forms a hydrostatic wedge to assist with dilation of the cervix during labor. The fluid itself can be used for analysis of fetal well-being.

**Amniotic bands** Pieces of amnion that tear loose and can wrap themselves around digits and limbs causing constrictions and amputations or can be swallowed by the fetus causing disruptions in facial development. The origin of bands is unknown.

**Anencephaly** Neural tube defect in which the cranial neural folds fail to close, leading to tissue degeneration and little or no formation of higher brain centers, cerebral cortex, etc. The abnormality is lethal, but 70% of these defects can be prevented by daily maternal use of 400 μg of folic acid beginning 2 to 3 months prior to conception and continuing throughout pregnancy.

**Angiogenesis** Formation of blood vessels by sprouting from existing vessels.

**Annulus fibrosis** Outer ring of fibrous tissue in an intervertebral disc.

**Anterior visceral endoderm (AVE)** Collection of endoderm cells at the cranial end of the bilaminar disc responsible for inducing the head region through secretion of transcription factors, including *OTX2*, *LIM1*, and *HESX1*.

**Anti-Müllerian hormone (AMH)** Another term for Müllerian-inhibiting substance produced by Sertoli cells that causes regression of the Müllerian (paramesonephric) ducts in males.

**Aortic arch** Branch from the aortic sac to the dorsal aorta traveling in the center of each pharyngeal arch. Initially, there are five pairs, but these undergo considerable remodeling to form definitive vascular patterns for the head and neck, aorta, and pulmonary circulation.

**Apical ectodermal ridge (AER)** Layer of thickened ectoderm at the distal tip of the limb that controls outgrowth of the limb by maintaining a rapidly proliferating population of adjacent mesoderm cells, called the progress zone.

**Apoptosis** Programmed cell death, for example, between the digits.

**Arachnoid mater** The middle layer of the meninges covering the brain and spinal cord. It attaches to the dura and cerebrospinal fluid flows in the subarachnoid space between the arachnoid mater and pia mater.

**Arthrogryposis** Severe joint contractures in the limbs. May be caused by neurological defects, muscular abnormalities, or anomalies of joint formation.

**Atresia** Congenital absence of an opening or lumen, for example, gut atresia.

**Autonomic nervous system (ANS)** Composed of the sympathetic and parasympathetic nervous systems that control smooth muscle and glands.

## B

**Basal plates** Motor area in the ventral portion of the spinal cord and brain.

**Bladder exstrophy** Ventral body wall defect caused by lack of closure of the lateral body wall folds in the pelvic region resulting in protrusion of the bladder through the defect.

**Blastocyst** Stage of embryogenesis at the time of implantation where outer trophoblast cells form a fluid-filled sphere with a small group of embryoblast cells, the inner cell mass, at one pole.

**Bone morphogenetic proteins (BMPs)** Members of the transforming growth factor β family that serve as signal molecules for a number of morphogenetic events, including dorsalizing the central nervous system, participating in bone formation, etc.

**Bowman capsule** Cup-shaped structure at the end of each proximal convoluted tubule that partially surrounds a glomerulus.

**Brachycephaly** Type of craniosynostosis in which the coronal sutures close prematurely resulting in a tall, short head shape.

**Brachydactyly** Short digits.

**Brain vesicles** Once the neural tube closes, expanded spaces in the brain fill with fluid to form three primary brain vesicles: the prosencephalon (forebrain), mesencephalon (midbrain), and rhombencephalon (hindbrain). These three primary vesicles form five definitive vesicles: The prosencephalon divides into the telencephalon and diencephalon, the mesencephalon does not divide, and the rhombencephalon forms the metencephalon and myelencephalon.

**Brainstem** "Lower" centers of the brain, including the myelencephalon, pons of the metencephalon, and the mesencephalon.

## C

**Capacitation** A period of sperm conditioning in the female reproductive tract lasting about 7 hours that is required for sperm to be able to fertilize an egg.

**Cardiac looping** Bending of the heart tube positions the heart in the left thoracic region and creates the "typical" heart shape with the atria posterior to the ventricles.

**Cardinal veins** System of anterior, posterior, and common cardinal veins that drain the head and body of the embryo in the late third and early fourth weeks.

**Caudal dysgenesis** Also called sirenomelia or mermaid syndrome, it is caused by insufficient production of mesoderm by the primitive streak. Consequently, there are not enough cells to form the lower part of the body so that the legs are fused. Renal agenesis is usually the cause of death. The defects are most often observed in infants from insulin-dependent diabetics.

**Cerebral aqueduct (of Sylvius)** Lumen of the mesencephalon that connects the third and fourth ventricles. It is often the site for abnormalities that impede the flow of cerebrospinal fluid and cause hydrocephalus.

**Chiari malformation** A congenital defect in which the cerebellum herniates through the foramen magnum, as for example happens with a tethered spinal cord in cases of spina bifida. The defect is usually associated with hydrocephalus due to compression that affects the flow of cerebrospinal fluid.

**Chondrocranium** Part of the neurocranium that forms the base of the skull and arises by first establishing cartilage models for the bones (endochondral ossification).

**Chorion** Multilayered structure consisting of the somatic layer of extraembryonic mesoderm, cytotrophoblast, and syncytiotrophoblast. It contributes the fetal portion of the placenta, including the villi and villus lakes.

**Chorion frondosum (leafy chorion)** Embryonic side of the chorion, where villi form.

**Chorion laeve (smooth chorion)** Abembryonic side of the chorion, where villi regress, leaving a smooth surface.

**Chorionic cavity** Space formed between the extraembryonic mesoderm lining the cytotrophoblast (somatic extraembryonic mesoderm) and that surrounding the yolk sac and embryo (splanchnic extraembryonic mesoderm). The chorionic cavity will eventually be obliterated by expansion of the amniotic cavity and fusion of the amnion with the chorion.

**Choroid plexuses** Vascularized structures formed in the lateral, third, and fourth ventricles that produce cerebrospinal fluid.

**Cloaca** Common chamber for the hindgut and urinary systems. Its anterior portion forms the urogenital sinus, and its posterior portion forms the anus.

**Cloacal membrane (plate)** Membrane formed at the caudal end of the embryo from adhesion between epiblast and hypoblast cells. Later, it covers the cloaca and eventually breaks down to form openings into the urogenital sinus and anus.

**Coloboma** Defect in the eye due to incomplete closure of the optic fissure. Usually, these defects are restricted to the iris.

**Compaction** Process whereby cells of the morula stage form tight junctions to seal themselves in preparation for forming and pumping fluid into the blastocyst cavity.

**Congenital malformation** Synonymous with the term *birth defect*, it refers to any structural, behavioral, functional, or metabolic disorder present at birth.

**Connecting stalk** Mesodermal connection that connects the embryo to the placenta. It contains the allantois and umbilical vessels and will be incorporated into the umbilical cord with the yolk sac (vitelline) stalk (duct).

**Conus cordis** Another term for the conus arteriosus referring to the proximal portion of the outflow tract of the heart.

**Cotyledons** Compartments (15 to 20) in the placenta formed when decidual septa grow into the intervillous spaces. These septa never reach the chorionic plate so that there is communication between cotyledons.

**Cranial nerves (CNs)** Twelve pairs of nerves associated with the brain, with all but two (the olfactory and optic) originating from the brainstem.

**Craniosynostosis** Premature closure of one or more cranial sutures, leading to an abnormally shaped skull. A major cause is mutations in fibroblast growth factor receptors (FGFRs).

**Crista terminalis** Ridge of tissue in the right atrium between the original trabeculated part of the right atrium and the smooth-walled part derived from the sinus venosus.

**Cryptorchidism** Failure of one or both testes to descend to the scrotum.

**Cytotrophoblast** Proliferative inner layer of the trophoblast.

## D

**Deformations** Altered development of structures caused by mechanical forces, for example, clubfeet resulting from too little room in the amniotic cavity.

**Dermatome** Dorsal portion of each somite that forms the dermis of the skin of the back. Dermatomes are segmented and supplied by spinal nerves from the segments at which they originated. This segmental pattern is maintained as they migrate over the body. Thus, each region that they occupy on the skin is also called a dermatome and is innervated by the same spinal nerve that originally supplied the dermatome region of the somite.

**Diaphysis** Shaft of the long bones.

**Diencephalon** Derived from the caudal portion of the prosencephalon (forebrain) and forms the thalamus, hypothalamus, posterior lobe of the pituitary, optic stalks (nerves), and other structures.

**Dihydrotestosterone** Converted from testosterone and responsible for the differentiation of the mesonephric duct and external genitalia.

**Diploid** The normal chromosome complement present in somatic cells. In these cells, chromosomes appear as 23 homologous pairs to form the diploid number of 46.

**Disruptions** Term used to describe birth defects resulting from destructive processes that alter a structure after it had formed normally, for example, vascular accidents that cause bowel atresias and amniotic bands that cause limb or digit amputations.

**Dizygotic twins** Twins formed from two eggs, the most common form of twinning (66%).

**Dorsal mesentery** Double layer of peritoneum suspending the gut tube from the dorsal body wall from the lower end of the esophagus to the rectum. Later, as the gut grows and rotates, some parts of the dorsal mesentery are lost as portions of the gut fuse to the posterior body wall, that is, parts of the duodenum and colon.

**Dorsal primary ramus** Branch of a spinal nerve that innervates intrinsic back muscles, derived from primaxial muscle cells, and skin over the back.

**Dorsal root** Sensory fibers passing from a dorsal root ganglion to the spinal cord.

**Dura mater** Tough outer covering of the meninges over the brain and spinal cord. In the brain, it forms septa for support and dural sinuses for return of venous blood and cerebrospinal fluid to the circulation.

**Dysmorphology** Study of the causes, prognoses, treatment, and prevention of birth defects. Usually, a dysmorphologist is a clinical geneticist in a genetics department.

## E

**Ectoderm** One of the three basic germ layers that forms skin, the central nervous system, hair, and many other structures.

**Ectopia cordis** Ventral body wall defect resulting from lack of closure of the lateral body wall folds in the thoracic region causing the heart to lie outside the thoracic cavity.

**Ectopic** Something that is not in its normal position, for example, an embryo's implantation site.

**Ectrodactyly** Missing digits.

**Efferent ductules** Tubules that connect the rete testis to the mesonephric duct for the passage of sperm from the seminiferous tubules to the epididymis. The tubules are derived from nephric tubules of the mesonephric kidney.

**Embryogenesis** Another term for organogenesis, meaning the period of organ formation from approximately the third to eighth weeks after fertilization.

**Endocardial cushions** Structures consisting of loose connective tissue covered by endothelium that are responsible for most septation processes occurring in the heart.

**Endochondral ossification** Mechanism for forming bone by first establishing a cartilaginous model followed by ossification. This type of bone formation is characteristic of the bones of the limbs and base of the skull.

**Endoderm** One of the three basic germ layers that form the gut and its derivatives.

**Enhancers** Regulatory elements of DNA that activate utilization of promoters, control promoter efficiency, and regulate the rate of transcription.

**Epiblast** Dorsal (top) layer of cells comprising the bilaminar germ disc during the second week of development. The hypoblast forms the ventral layer. All tissues of the embryo are derived from the epiblast.

**Epibranchial placodes** Four thickened regions of ectoderm lying dorsal to the pharyngeal arches that form sensory ganglia for cranial nerves V, VII, IX, and X.

**Epididymis** Highly convoluted region derived from the mesonephric duct and used for sperm storage.

**Epiphyseal plate** Cartilaginous region between the diaphysis and epiphysis of the long bones that continues to produce bone growth by endochondral ossification until the bones have acquired their full length. Then these plates disappear (close).

**Epiphysis** End of the long bones.

**Epiploic foramen (of Winslow)** Opening between the lesser and greater sacs in the abdominal cavity located at the free margin of the lesser omentum between the duodenum and the liver. In its ventral border lie the common bile duct, hepatic artery, and portal vein (the portal triad).

**Epithelial–mesenchymal interactions** Process whereby virtually every organ is formed. Examples include limb ectoderm and underlying mesenchyme, gut endoderm and surrounding mesenchyme, ureter epithelium and metanephric mesenchyme, etc. Signals pass back and forth between these cell types to regulate organ differentiation.

**Exon** Region of a gene that can be transcribed into a protein.

## F

**Falciform ligament** Part of the ventral mesentery that attaches the liver to the ventral body wall.

**Fibroblast growth factors (FGFs)** Signal proteins in a large family having over 15 members. They are involved in a number of embryological events, including formation of the sutures and bones of the skull. Mutations in their receptors (FGFRs) cause a variety of craniofacial abnormalities, including many forms of craniosynostosis.

**Fistula** An abnormal passageway.

**Folic acid** A "B" vitamin that can prevent approximately 70% of neural tube defects if taken as a 400-µg supplement by mothers beginning 2 to 3 months prior to conception and continuing throughout pregnancy.

**Fontanelle** Wide spaces in the skull created where more than two bones meet. The largest is the anterior fontanelle, sometimes called the "soft spot," located where the two parietal and two frontal bones meet.

**Foramen cecum** Pit at the junction of the anterior two-thirds and posterior one-third of the tongue representing the site of origin of the thyroid gland.

**Foramen ovale** Opening in the interatrial septum that permits shunting of blood from right to left during fetal development.

**Foregut** Part of the gut tube beginning caudal to the pharynx just proximal to the lung bud and extending to a point just distal to the liver bud. It forms the esophagus, stomach, and part of the duodenum, in addition to the lungs, liver, gallbladder, and pancreas, which all form from diverticula (buds) off the gut tube.

**Fossa ovalis** Depression on the right side of the interatrial septum formed when the septum primum and septum secundum are pressed against each other and the foramen ovale is closed at birth.

## G

**Gastroschisis** Ventral body wall defect resulting from a lack of closure of the lateral body wall folds in the abdominal region resulting in protrusion of intestines and sometimes other organs through the defect.

**Gastrulation** Process of forming the three primary germ layers from the epiblast involving movement of cells through the primitive streak to form endoderm and mesoderm.

**Germ layers** Three basic cell layers of ectoderm, mesoderm, and endoderm derived from the process of gastrulation. These layers form all of the structures in the embryo.

**Glomerulus** Tuft of capillaries formed in the Bowman capsule at the end of each proximal convoluted tubule.

**Gray rami communicantes** Connections carrying postganglionic sympathetic fibers from ganglia in the sympathetic trunks to spinal nerves. Gray rami exist at all levels of the spinal cord.

**Greater omentum** Double layer of peritoneum formed from dorsal mesentery and extending down over the intestines from the greater curvature of the stomach. It serves as a storage site for fat and can wall off pockets of infection (the police officer of the abdomen).

**Greater sac** Most of the abdominal cavity with exception of the lesser sac lying dorsal to the lesser omentum. The two sacs are connected via the epiploic foramen (of Winslow).

**Growth factors** Proteins that act as signal molecules that are usually secreted and have their signals transduced by receptors on target cells.

**Gubernaculum** Condensation of mesenchyme extending from the testis to the floor of the scrotum that assists in descent of the testis from the posterior abdominal wall to the scrotum.

## H

**Haploid** Term used to denote the number of chromosomes in the gametes (23), which is half the number present in somatic (diploid) cells.

**Hindgut** Part of the gut tube extending from the distal one-third of the transverse colon to the upper portion of the anal canal. It forms part of the transverse colon, the descending colon, the sigmoid colon, the rectum, and the upper part of the anal canal.

**Holoprosencephaly** Defect where so much midline tissue for the face and brain has been lost that the two lateral ventricles fuse together and appear as one.

**Homeobox genes** Transcription factors that contain a homeobox, a specific DNA-binding motif (sequence) within a region called the homeodomain. These genes are important for patterning the embryonic axis, establishing different regions of the brain, determining the origin and type of gut derivatives, patterning the limbs, and other similar phenomena.

**Hydatidiform mole** Trophoblast forms placental tissue, but with no embryo. Moles express only paternal genes and probably arise from fertilization of an enucleated egg followed by duplication of the paternal chromosomes to restore a diploid number. Moles secrete high concentrations of human chorionic gonadotropin and may become invasive (malignant).

**Hydrocephalus** Increased amounts of cerebrospinal fluid in the brain leading to increased intracranial pressure; usually due to a block in the circulatory pattern of the fluid, which most often occurs in the cerebral aqueduct of Sylvius in the mesencephalon. If the cranial sutures have not fused, the child's head enlarges, sometimes to great proportions if the pressure is not relieved.

**Hyperplasia** An increase in cell number.

**Hypertrophy** An increase in size of a part or organ.

**Hypoblast** Ventral layer of the bilaminar germ disc. Contributes to formation of the yolk sac and extraembryonic mesoderm but not to tissues of the embryo.

**Hypospadias** An opening of the urethra along the ventral aspect of the penis or scrotum.

## I

**Induction** Process whereby one population of cells or a tissue causes another set of cells or tissues to change their fate. Thus, one cell type is the inducer, and one is the responder.

**Inguinal canal** Oblique passageway from the lower abdomen to the scrotum for the testes. Forms in female fetuses as well.

**Inner cell mass** Cluster of cells segregated to one pole of the blastocyst and from which the entire embryo develops.

**Intermaxillary segment** Formed from the medial nasal processes; it includes the philtrum region of the upper lip, the upper jaw component housing the four incisor teeth, and the primary palate.

**Intermediate column** Origin of the sympathetic cell bodies (lateral horn cells) in the spinal cord from T1–L2.

**Intermediate mesoderm** Mesoderm-derived layer lying between the paraxial and lateral plate layers and responsible for forming much of the urogenital system.

**Intervertebral disc** Cushioning disc formed between each vertebra consisting of a central gelatinous portion, the nucleus pulposus, and an outer ring of fibrous tissue called the annulus fibrosus.

**Intramembranous (membranous) ossification** Formation of bone directly from mesenchyme cells, such as in the flat bones of the skull.

**Intron** Region of a gene that cannot be transcribed into a protein.

## J

**Juxtacrine signaling** Type of cell-to-cell signaling that does not use diffusable proteins. There are three types: (1) a protein (ligand) on one cell surface reacts with its receptor on another cell surface, (2) ligands in the extracellular matrix secreted by one cell interact with another, and (3) direct transmission of signals via gap junctions.

## K

**Karyotype** Chromosomal makeup of an individual.

## L

**Lateral horn** Origin of neurons (intermediate columns) for the sympathetic nervous system lying in the lateral region of the spinal cord from T1 to L1–L2.

**Lateral plate mesoderm** Mesoderm-derived tissue that splits into splanchnopleure (visceral) and somatopleure (parietal) layers surrounding the organs and body cavity.

**Lateral somitic frontier** Border between each somite and the parietal layer of lateral plate mesoderm. Some cells from the myotome and sclerotome regions of each somite migrate across the frontier to enter the lateral plate mesoderm and with it forms the abaxial domain.

**Laterality sequences (heterotaxy)** Right and left sides are established during gastrulation in the third week of development. Patients with defects in sidedness, such that they are primarily bilaterally right or left sided, have laterality sequences.

**Lesser omentum** Double layer of ventral mesentery extending from the liver to the proximal end of the duodenum and lesser curvature of the stomach.

**Lesser sac** Space behind the lesser omentum that communicates with the rest of the abdominal cavity (greater sac) via the epiploic foramen (of Winslow).

**Ligand** A signal molecule.

## M

**Mantle layer** Inner layer of the neural tube containing neurons (gray matter).

**Marginal layer** Peripheral layer of the neural tube containing nerve fibers (white matter).

**Meiosis** Cell divisions that take place in the germ cells to generate male and female gametes. Meiosis requires two cell divisions to reduce the number of chromosomes from 46 to the haploid number of 23.

**Membranous ossification** Process of forming bone directly from mesenchyme. This process is characteristic of the flat bones of the cranial vault.

**Meninges** The three membranous layers, pia mater, arachnoid mater, and dura mater, that cover the brain and spinal cord.

**Meningocele** Neural tube defect in which a sac of fluid-filled meninges protrudes through an opening in the skull or vertebrae.

**Meningoencephalocele** Herniation of meninges and brain tissue through a defect in the skull, usually in the occipital region.

**Meromelia** Partial absence of a limb.

**Mesencephalon** One of the three primary brain vesicles that does not subdivide.

**Mesenchyme** Any loosely organized tissue composed of fibroblast-like cells and extracellular matrix regardless of the origin of the cells.

**Mesentery** A collection of connective tissues that maintains the gut tube and its derivatives in their normal anatomical positions. In the abdomen, dorsal mesentery extends from the lower portion of the esophagus to the rectum as a continuous sheet of tissue attached to the posterior body wall and providing a pathway for blood vessels, lymphatics, and nerves to the gut tube and its derivatives. Dorsal mesentery is continuous with ventral mesentery and forms the lesser omentum and falciform ligament.

**Mesoderm** One of three basic germ layers that form blood vessels, bone, connective tissue, and other structures.

**Mesonephric ducts (Wolffian ducts)** Collecting ducts for the mesonephric kidney that regress in female fetuses but form the epididymis, ductus deferens, seminal vesicle, and ejaculatory ducts in male fetuses.

**Mesonephros** Primitive kidney that forms tubules and ducts in the thoracic and lumbar regions. Most of these structures degenerate, but the main duct (mesonephric duct) and some of the tubules contribute to the male reproductive system.

**Metanephros** Definitive kidney formed from metanephric mesoderm (metanephric blastema) in the pelvic region.

**Metencephalon** Derived from the cranial portion of the rhombencephalon (hindbrain) and forms the cerebellum and pons.

**Microphthalmia** A smaller than normal eye, usually associated with other ocular abnormalities. May be caused by intrauterine infections, such as cytomegalovirus.

**Midgut** Part of the gut tube extending from immediately distal to the liver bud to the proximal two-thirds of the transverse colon. It forms part of the duodenum, jejunum, ileum, cecum, appendix, ascending colon, and part of the transverse colon. Early in development, it forms the primary intestinal loop with the superior mesenteric artery as its axis. This loop is involved in gut rotation and physiological umbilical herniation and is connected to the yolk sac by the vitelline duct.

**Mitosis** The process whereby one cell divides giving rise to two daughter cells each with 46 chromosomes.

**Monozygotic twins** Twins formed from a single oocyte. Splitting may occur at the two-cell stage or after formation of the germ disc but usually takes place at the time of inner cell mass formation.

**Morphogen** Molecule secreted at a distance that can induce cells to differentiate. The same morphogen can induce more than one cell type by establishing a concentration gradient.

**Mosaicism** The presence of two or more genetically different cell lines in the same individual. The mosaicism may be germ line, in which case the individual shows no traits of the genetic abnormality but can pass it on to their offspring; or it may occur in somatic cells, in which case the individual may exhibit varying characteristics of the genetic abnormality, such as in Down syndrome.

**Müllerian inhibiting substance (MIS)** Another term for anti-Müllerian hormone. Produced by Sertoli cells and causes regression of the Müllerian (paramesonephric) ducts in male fetuses.

**Myelencephalon** Derived from the caudal portion of the rhombencephalon (hindbrain) and forms the medulla oblongata.

**Myelomeningocele** Protrusion of meninges and spinal cord tissue through a defect in the vertebral arch called spina bifida.

**Myotome** Muscle-forming region of a somite formed by myocytes derived from the ventrolateral and dorsomedial regions that coalesce beneath the dermatome. These cells remain in the primaxial domain and form the intrinsic back muscles, intercostal and cervical muscles, and some muscles of the upper limb girdle.

## N

**Nephron** Functional unit of the kidney consisting of the proximal and distal convoluted tubules, loop of Henle, Bowman capsule, and a glomerulus.

**Neural crest cells** Cells of the neuroepithelium that form at the tips ("crest") of the neural folds and then migrate to other regions to form many structures, including spinal ganglia, bones and connective tissue of the face, septa for the outflow tract of the heart, some cranial nerve ganglia, ganglia for the gut tube (enteric ganglia), melanocytes, etc. These cells are vulnerable to teratogenic insult and provide a rationale for why many children with facial clefts also have cardiac defects.

**Neurocranium** Part of the skull that forms a protective case around the brain (the other part of the skull is the viscerocranium or face). It consists of two parts, the membranous neurocranium or flat bones of the skull, and the cartilaginous neurocranium or chondrocranium, forming the base of the skull.

**Neuromeres** Brain segments associated with somitomeres. They are especially prominent in the hindbrain where they are called rhombomeres.

**Neuropores** Cranial and caudal openings in the neural tube that exist from the time that closure of the neural folds is initiated until it is complete, that is, unclosed portions of the closing neural tube.

**Neurulation** Process of transforming the neural plate into the neural tube. Neurulation begins in the third week and ends at 28 days. Failure of the neural folds to close the tube results in neural tube defects, including anencephaly and spina bifida.

**Notochord** An extended column of midline cells lying immediately ventral to the floor plate of the central nervous system and extending from the hypophysis to the end of the spinal cord. It is important for inducing the neural plate, the ventral (motor) region of the brain and spinal cord, and the sclerotome portion of the somites to form vertebrae. The major signal molecule for these phenomena is sonic hedgehog (SHH).

**Nucleosome** Basic unit of structure of chromatin, containing a complex of histone proteins and approximately 140 base pairs of DNA.

**Nucleus pulposus** Central gelatinous portion of an intervertebral disc derived from proliferation of notochord cells.

## O

**Omental bursa (lesser peritoneal sac)** Space created posterior to the stomach by gut rotation. This space connects to the rest of the peritoneal cavity (greater peritoneal sac) through the epiploic foramen (of Winslow).

**Omentum** Fold of mesentery passing from the stomach to the liver (lesser omentum) or from the stomach to the transverse colon and beyond (greater omentum).

**Omphalocele** Ventral body wall defect caused by failure of physiologically herniated loops of bowel to return to the body cavity in the 10th week.

**Organogenesis** Period of development when the organ primordia are established, usually considered to be from the beginning of the third week to the end of the eighth week of gestation. This is the time when organs are most sensitive to insult, and induction of most birth defects occurs.

**Oropharyngeal membrane** Membrane formed at the cranial end of the germ disc by adhesion between epiblast and hypoblast cells. Later, it covers the opening of the oral cavity and breaks down as the pharynx develops. (The old term was *buccopharyngeal membrane*.)

**Outer cell mass** Cells that surround the blastocyst cavity and cover the inner cell mass and that will form the trophoblast.

## P

**Palpebral fissures** The opening between the eyelids.

**Paracrine signaling** Type of signaling from one cell to another where proteins synthesized by one cell diffuse short distances to interact with other cells.

**Paramesonephric ducts (Müllerian ducts)** Ducts that parallel the mesonephric duct and extend from the abdominal cavity to the posterior wall of the urogenital sinus. These ducts regress in the male fetus but form the uterus, uterine (fallopian) tubes, and upper part of the vagina in female fetuses.

**Paraxial mesoderm** Mesoderm-derived tissue along the axis of the embryo responsible for forming somites and somitomeres.

**Parenchyma** The specific cells of a gland or organ held together by connective tissue called the stroma.

**Parietal** Pertaining to the wall of any cavity.

**Parturition** Birth.

**Pericardioperitoneal canal** Openings from the abdomen to the thorax posterior to the septum transversum that are closed by the pleuroperitoneal membranes during formation of the diaphragm.

**Peritoneal ligaments** Thickenings of peritoneum that join organs together. For example, the spleen and kidney by the lienorenal ligament and the liver to the duodenum by the hepatoduodenal ligament.

**Pharyngeal arches** Bars of mesenchyme derived from mesoderm and neural crest cells that form in five pairs around the pharynx, somewhat like the gills (branchia) of a fish. They are covered by ectoderm externally and endoderm internally. Clefts are present externally between pairs of arches, whereas pouches are present between arches internally. However, there is no communication between clefts and pouches.

**Pharyngeal cleft** Ectoderm-lined indentation between pharyngeal arches on their external surfaces.

**Pharyngeal pouch** Endoderm-lined indentation between pharyngeal arches on their internal surfaces.

**Phenotype** Physical characteristics of an individual.

**Philtrum** The depression in the midline of the upper lip formed by the medial nasal prominences.

**Phocomelia** Partial absence of a limb (a type of meromelia) in which the long bones are missing or very short resulting in the hand or foot attached to the side of the body.

**Pia mater** Thin membranous inner layer of the meninges that is applied to the surface of the brain and spinal cord.

**Placode** A thickened region of ectoderm that forms sensory organs and ganglia. Examples include the nasal, otic, lens, and epibranchial placodes.

**Pleuropericardial folds** Extensions of mesoderm from the lateral body wall that meet in the midline to separate the pleural and pericardial cavities. The folds carry the phrenic nerve with them, contribute to the parietal pericardium, and form the fibrous pericardium.

**Pleuroperitoneal folds** Extensions of mesoderm that extend from the body wall to meet the septum transversum and mesentery of the esophagus, thereby closing the pericardioperitoneal canals during formation of the diaphragm.

**Polydactyly** Extra digits.

**Prechordal plate** Collection of mesoderm cells lying between the oropharyngeal membrane and the cranial end of the notochord. These cells represent some of the first to pass through the primitive streak and are important for forebrain induction using sonic hedgehog as a signal molecule.

**Primary heart field (PHF)** Cardiac progenitor cells that have migrated through the primitive streak and positioned themselves in the splanchnic (visceral) layer of lateral plate mesoderm in a horseshoe shape cranial to the cranial region of the neural plate. These cells will coalesce to form the heart tube and will contribute to the formation of the atria, left ventricle, and right ventricle.

**Primary intestinal loop** Loop formed around the superior mesenteric artery by the midgut. It rotates and lengthens as it herniates into the umbilicus in the sixth week. It then continues its growth and rotation as it reenters the abdominal cavity beginning in the 10th week.

**Primary palate** Formed by the medial nasal prominences as part of the intermaxillary segment. It fuses with the secondary palate.

**Primaxial domain** Region of mesoderm around the neural tube that contains only somite-derived (paraxial mesoderm) cells.

**Primitive body cavity** Created by ventral body wall closure, this space extends from the cervical region to the pelvis. It will be divided by the diaphragm into thoracic and peritoneal cavities and by the pleuropericardial folds into the pleural and pericardial cavities.

**Primitive node** Elevated region around the cranial end of the primitive streak that is known as the "organizer" because it regulates important processes such as laterality and formation of the notochord.

**Primitive pit** Depression in the primitive node.

**Primitive streak** Groove formed in the epiblast at the caudal end of the bilaminar germ disc stage embryo through which epiblast cells migrate to form endoderm and mesoderm during gastrulation.

**Primordial germ cells** Cells responsible for differentiating into eggs and sperm. They migrate from the wall of the yolk sac to the genital ridges.

**Processus vaginalis** Outpocketing of peritoneum that precedes the testis through the inguinal canal. Once it reaches the scrotum, it pinches off from the abdominal cavity and forms the tunica vaginalis of the testis. If it fails to pinch off, then it can serve as a path for herniation of bowel through the canal into the scrotum, forming an inguinal (indirect) hernia.

**Proctodeum** Ectodermally lined pit that invaginates to form the lower third of the anal canal. Initially, this region is separated from the remainder of the anal canal by the anal membrane (once the posterior portion of the cloacal membrane), which breaks down to permit continuity between the two parts of the canal.

**Progress zone** Proliferating population of mesenchyme cells immediately beneath the apical ectodermal ridge (AER). By signaling through FGFs, the AER maintains the progress zone and promotes proximodistal growth of the limb.

**Promoter region** Site in a typical gene that binds RNA polymerase for the initiation of transcription.

**Pronephros** Primitive kidney that forms a few nonfunctional vestigial tubules in the cervical region.

**Prosencephalon** One of three primary brain vesicles that form the telencephalon and diencephalon.

## R

**Rathke pouch** Outpocketing of ectoderm from the roof of the oral cavity that forms the anterior portion (adenohypophysis) of the pituitary.

**Rectouterine pouch (Douglas pouch)** Depression between the vagina and rectum. This site is the most common place for an ectopic pregnancy within the peritoneal cavity (the most common site of all is in the ampullary region of the uterine tube).

**Renal corpuscle** Combination of Bowman capsule and a glomerulus.

**Retroperitoneal** Posterior to the parietal peritoneum covering the body wall.

**Rhombencephalon** One of three primary brain vesicles that form the metencephalon and myelencephalon.

**Rhombomere** One of eight segments that forms in the rhombencephalon that contributes to development of cranial nerve nuclei and gives rise to neural crest cells that migrate to the pharyngeal arches.

**Round ligament of the liver (ligamentum teres hepatis)** Formed by the obliterated umbilical vein that runs in the free margin of the falciform ligament.

## S

**Scaphocephaly** Type of craniosynostosis in which the sagittal suture closes prematurely resulting in a long, narrow head shape.

**Sclerotome** Ventromedial part of each somite that forms the vertebrae.

**Secondary heart field (SHF)** Group of cells in the visceral (splanchnic) layer of lateral plate mesoderm lying beneath the floor of the posterior part of the pharynx. Regulated by neural crest cells migrating in the region, SHF cells contribute to formation of the right ventricle and outflow tract (conus cordis and truncus arteriosus) of the heart.

**Secondary palate** Derived from the maxillary processes of the first arch and includes the soft and hard palates. Fuses with the primary palate anteriorly.

**Septum primum** First septum to grow down from the roof of the common atrium and contributes to the interatrial septum. Prior to contact with the atrioventricular endocardial cushions, programmed cell death creates a new opening in this septum to maintain communication between the atrial chambers. This septum will form the valve of the foramen ovale.

**Septum secundum** Second septum to grow down from the roof of the common atrium toward the atrioventricular endocardial cushions. It never makes contact with the cushions, such that an oblique opening, the foramen ovale, is created between the septum secundum and septum primum that allows shunting of blood from the right atrium to the left during fetal development. At birth, this opening is closed when the septum primum is pressed against the septum secundum and the adult pattern of blood flow is established.

**Septum transversum** Mesoderm tissue originally lying cranial to the heart but repositioned between the heart and connecting stalk by cranial folding of the embryo. It gives rise to the central tendon of the diaphragm, connective tissue for the liver, and ventral mesentery.

**Situs inversus** Complete reversal of left- and right-sidedness of the organs in the thorax and abdomen.

**Somatic (parietal) mesoderm** That layer of lateral plate mesoderm associated with ectoderm. It forms the parietal pleura, parietal peritoneum, etc.

**Somatopleure** Combination of the parietal (somatic) layer of the lateral plate mesoderm and the adjacent layer of ectoderm.

**Somites** Epithelial balls of cells formed in segmental pairs along the neural tube from paraxial mesoderm. Somites differentiate into vertebrae, muscles of the back and body wall, and dermis of the skin.

**Somitomeres** Loosely organized segmented collections of paraxial mesoderm in the cranial region. Somitomeres form muscles and bones of the face and skull.

**Sonic hedgehog** Secreted protein that acts as a morphogen in several embryonic sites, including the limbs, somites, gut formation, and establishment of the midline in the central nervous system.

**Spina bifida** Neural tube defect that involves incomplete development of the vertebral arches with or without defects of the underlying neural tube. If only the vertebrae are involved, the defect is called spina bifida occulta because it is usually skin-covered and not visible from the surface. If the underlying neural tube is affected, then the defect is called spina bifida cystica. Seventy percent of these defects can be prevented by daily maternal use of 400 μg of folic acid beginning 2 to 3 months prior to conception and continuing throughout pregnancy.

**Spinal ganglion (dorsal root ganglion)** Ganglion derived from neural crest cells that lie outside the spinal cord and houses the sensory cell bodies for a spinal nerve.

**Spinal nerve** Nerve formed by the junction of dorsal and ventral roots at each intervertebral foramen.

**Splanchnic nerves** Preganglionic sympathetic and parasympathetic fibers in the thorax (greater [T5–T9], lesser [T10 and T11], and least [T12] splanchnic nerves; sympathetic), lumbar region (lumbar splanchnic nerves [L1 and L2]; sympathetic), and pelvic region (pelvic splanchnic nerves S2–S4; parasympathetic).

**Splanchnopleure** Combination of the visceral (splanchnic) layer of lateral plate mesoderm with the adjacent layer of endoderm.

**Stenosis** A narrowing of a canal or orifice.

**Stomodeum** The ectodermally lined primitive oral cavity, separated from the pharynx by the oropharyngeal membrane, that later breaks down.

**Stroma** Connective tissue of glands.

**Surfactant** Phospholipid made by alveolar type II cells that reduces surface tension in alveoli, which is essential for respiration. Production does not begin until the end of the sixth month, making it difficult for premature infants born before this time to survive.

**Suture** Narrow seams of connective tissue that separate the flat bones of the skull allowing molding of the skull through the birth canal and growth and expansion as the brain grows.

**Sympathetic trunks (chain ganglia)** Paired collections of sympathetic ganglia lying on the posterior body wall lateral to the vertebral bodies. Sometimes called sympathetic chain ganglia.

**Syncytiotrophoblast** Outer multinucleated layer of the trophoblast that serves to invade the endometrium of the uterus.

**Syndactyly** Fusion of one or more digits.

**Syndrome** A group of abnormalities occurring together that have a known cause, for example, Down syndrome and fetal alcohol syndrome (FAS).

## T

**Telencephalon** Derived from the most cranial portion of the prosencephalon (forebrain) and forms the cerebral hemispheres.

**Teratogen** A factor that causes a birth defect, such as a drug or environmental toxicant.

**Teratology** Science that studies the origin, causes, and prevention of birth defects.

**Teratoma** Tumor-containing derivatives from all three germ layers. They may arise from remnants of the primitive streak or from germ cells that do not migrate successfully to the gonadal ridges. The most common ones are caudal teratomas arising in the buttocks region.

**Thyroglossal duct** Duct formed along the path of thyroid migration extending in the midline from the foramen cecum in the tongue to the neck.

**Tracheoesophageal septum** Septum that separates the trachea from the gut tube.

**Transcription factors** Proteins that have DNA-binding sites that regulate the expression of downstream genes.

**Trophoblast** Outer cell layer surrounding the blastocyst from which placental tissues are derived.

**Truncus arteriosus** Distal portion of the outflow tract of the primitive heart tube that connects to the aortic sac and that becomes septated to form the ascending aorta and pulmonary artery.

## U

**Urachus** Vestigial remnant of the allantois from the ventral surface of the urogenital sinus to the umbilicus that normally regresses to a fibrous cord, forming the median umbilical ligament. Sometimes it may remain patent to form a urachal fistula or cyst.

**Urogenital ridge** Bilateral epithelial-covered elevation of intermediate mesoderm that lies in the lower thoracic and lumbar regions and that forms the mesonephric kidneys and the gonads.

**Urorectal septum** Wedge of mesoderm that grows down between the hindgut and primitive urogenital sinus, partially separating these two structures. The caudal end of the septum forms the perineal body.

**Uterovesical pouch** Depression between the vagina and the bladder.

## V

**Vasculogenesis** Formation of blood vessels from blood islands in situ.

**Ventral mesentery** Double layer of peritoneum derived from the septum transversum and extending from the liver to the ventral body wall (the falciform ligament) and from the liver to the stomach and duodenum (lesser omentum).

**Ventral primary ramus** Ventral branch of a spinal nerve that innervates limb and trunk muscles except the intrinsic ("true") back muscles, which are innervated by dorsal primary rami.

**Ventral root** Motor fibers passing from ventral horn cells in the spinal cord to a spinal nerve.

**Visceral** Relating to the organs of the body.

**Visceral (splanchnic) layer** That part of the lateral plate mesoderm that is associated with endoderm and forms the visceral pleura, visceral peritoneum, etc.

**Viscerocranium** Part of the skull that comprises the bones of the face (the other part of the skull is the neurocranium).

**Vitelline duct** Connection between the yolk sac and the primary intestinal loop of the midgut through the connecting stalk. Failure of this duct to degenerate results in fistulas and diverticula (Meckel diverticulum) from the small intestine to the umbilicus.

## W

**White rami communicantes** Connections carrying preganglionic sympathetic fibers from spinal nerves to the sympathetic trunks. White rami exist only at levels T1–L2.

## Y

**Yolk sac** Structure located ventral to the bilaminar germ disc derived from the hypoblast. It is the site of origin of the first blood cells and remains attached to the midgut via the vitelline (yolk sac) duct until late in development.

## Z

**Zone of polarizing activity (ZPA)** Population of mesoderm cells at the posterior border of the limb next to the apical ectodermal ridge that regulates anterior–posterior patterning of the limb.

# Index

**Note**: Page numbers followed by *t* and *f* indicate table and figure respectively.

## N



## O



## P

## R



## S